D1047666

NOV 0 9 2007

THE WASHINGTON MANUAL OF ONCOLOGY
Second Edition

THE WASHINGTON MANUAL OF ONCOLOGY
Second Edition

Editor

Ramaswamy Govindan, MD

Associate Professor
Division of Oncology
Alvin J. Siteman Cancer Center at
Washington University School of Medicine
St. Louis, Missouri

Wolters Kluwer
Health
Philadelphia · Baltimore · New York · London
Buenos Aires · Hong Kong · Sydney · Tokyo

Lippincott
Williams & Wilkins

Senior Executive Editor: Jonathan W. Pine
Senior Managing Editor: Anne E. Jacobs
Project Manager: Alicia Jackson
Senior Manufacturing Manager: Benjamin Rivera
Director of Marketing: Sharon Zinner
Design Coordinator: Terry Mallon
Cover Designer: Larry Didona
Production Services: Laserwords Private Limited, Chennai, India

530 Walnut Street
Philadelphia, PA 19106 USA
LWW.com

Library of Congress Cataloging-in-Publication Data
The Washington manual of oncology / [edited by] Ramaswamy Govindan. —2nd ed.
    p. ; cm.
  Includes bibliographical references and index.
  ISBN 978-0-7817-8402-3 (alk. paper)
  1. Cancer—Handbooks, manuals, etc. 2. Oncology—Handbooks, manuals. etc. I. Govindan, Ramaswamy. II. Washington University (Saint Louis, Mo.). School of Medicine. III. Title: Manual of oncology.
  [DNLM: 1. Neoplasms—physiopathology—Handbooks. 2. Neoplasms—therapy—Handbooks. QZ 39 W319 2008]
  RC262.5.W375 2008
  616.99′4—dc22
                                                                        2007031801

Care has been taken to confirm the accuracy of the information presented and to describe generally accepted practices. However, the authors, editors, and publisher are not responsible for errors or omissions or for any consequences from application of the information in this book and make no warranty, expressed or implied, with respect to the currency, completeness, or accuracy of the contents of the publication. Application of the information in a particular situation remains the professional responsibility of the practitioner.

The authors, editors, and publisher have exerted every effort to ensure that drug selection and dosage set forth in this text are in accordance with current recommendations and practice at the time of publication. However, in view of ongoing research, changes in government regulations, and the constant flow of information relating to drug therapy and drug reactions, the reader is urged to check the package insert for each drug for any change in indications and dosage and for added warnings and precautions. This is particularly important when the recommended agent is a new or infrequently employed drug.

Some drugs and medical devices presented in the publication have Food and Drug Administration (FDA) clearance for limited use in restricted research settings. It is the responsibility of the health care provider to ascertain the FDA status of each drug or device planned for use in their clinical practice.

To purchase additional copies of this book, call our customer service department at (800) 638-3030 or fax orders to (301) 223-2320. International customers should call (301) 223-2300.

Visit Lippincott Williams & Wilkins on the Internet: at LWW.com. Lippincott Williams & Wilkins customer service representatives are available from 8:30 am to 6 pm, EST.

10 9 8 7 6 5 4 3 2 1

Dedicated to the memory of Matthew A. Arquette, MD, my dear friend, former colleague, and the Associate Editor of the first edition of The Washington Manual of Oncology

$\mathcal{T}$he past four years since the first edition of *The Washington Manual of Oncology* have witnessed a steady progress in the treatment of a wide variety of malignancies. In keeping with these changes, we have made extensive revisions to the new edition of the manual. Almost all of the chapters have been extensively revised and rewritten. The new slate of contributing authors, with their perspectives and valuable insight, has contributed significantly to the freshness of this edition. We have made changes even while correcting final page proofs to incorporate some of the new information from the recently concluded meeting of the American Society of Clinical Oncology. As before, this manual is written keeping the trainees in mind while also providing a quick update for the practitioners of oncology. It is our hope that you, the reader, find this manual practical, useful, and stimulating.

Ramaswamy Govindan, MD

PREFACE TO THE FIRST EDITION

These are exciting times in oncology. The novel imaging techniques, improved supportive care, and the availability of several new agents that have novel mechanisms of action hold considerable promise in improving the outcomes of cancer patients. In this era of information overload, it is critically important to have a practical manual that is helpful to physicians taking care of patients with cancer.

The chapters are arranged in a logical order beginning with evaluation of symptoms and proceeding in an orderly fashion through the work-up, staging, and stage-directed therapy, and finally ending with discussion on epidemiology and current focus of research. We have embarked on this first edition of *The Washington Manual of Oncology* to provide a very practical manual that is helpful to medical residents, fellows in training, nurse practitioners, and other practitioners of clinical oncology. Our plan is to publish this book in a timely fashion every two years to keep the information current and up-to-date.

Ramaswamy Govindan, MD

I want to thank the individual contributors, who are all my dear and well-respected colleagues, for their efforts. As I have found over the years, a number of individuals also work behind the scenes to produce a book. At Lippincott Williams & Wilkins, Jonathan Pine, Senior Executive Editor, was truly a pleasure to work with and has provided great leadership, and Anne Jacobs, Senior Managing Editor, was instrumental in keeping the project moving and persistent with follow-up, even when I was delinquent repeatedly in keeping up the deadlines. At Laserwords, Gopika Sasidharan was remarkable in delivering the page proofs on time and very skillful and was very patient while working with me. I am grateful to my nursing and secretarial staff for their help while I was busy working on this project. I would like to specifically thank my remarkable secretary, Starlene Drennen, for her assistance. My work was made not only easy but also pleasurable by the great working environment at Washington University School of Medicine in St. Louis. I owe a particular debt of gratitude to the leadership provided by three individuals in the Department of Medicine—Mathew J Ellis, M.D., John F. DiPersio, M.D., Ph.D., and Kenneth S. Polonsky, M.D. Finally, my two adorable children, Ashwin and Akshay, and my lovely wife, Prabha, make everything worthwhile.

CONTENTS

PRINCIPLES AND PRACTICE OF SURGERY IN CANCER THERAPY

Elbert Y. Kuo, Steven E. Finkelstein, and Rebecca L. Aft

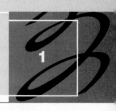

I. **THE CHANGING ROLE OF THE SURGICAL ONCOLOGIST IN THE 21ST CENTURY.** Early cancer therapy centered on surgical excision as the primary treatment modality for solid tumors. It was theorized that cancer spread occurred sequentially from the primary site to the regional lymph nodes and then on to distant sites. Therefore, it was hypothesized that complete local excision of all cancerous cells would lead to effective disease control. In patients with untreated cancer, median survival was frequently measured in months. Early *en bloc* resection of tumors with contiguous normal surrounding tissue and lymph nodes led to improved overall survival. As a consequence, increasingly aggressive and extensive resections of malignant tumors were performed. As the initial improvement in survival began to plateau, it became apparent that successively larger resections to obtain locoregional control of larger tumors did not necessarily translate into further survival benefit. This led to the testing and development of screening strategies and adjuvant therapies. The current role for the surgeon in the management of patients with cancers involves a broad spectrum of surgical procedures for diagnosis, local control, cure, and palliation.

II. **DIAGNOSTIC PROCEDURES: ACQUISITION OF MATERIAL FOR DIAGNOSIS.** Once a lesion has been identified, one role of the surgical oncologist is to provide adequate material for definitive diagnosis. The method of biopsy requires consideration of the differential diagnosis, amount of tissue needed for definitive diagnosis, location of the lesion, and potential forms of treatment. It is preferable to perform biopsies of lesions at the periphery where viable tumor is located, because the cores of solid tumors may be necrotic. This also allows the pathologist to evaluate the invasion into normal tissue since some tumors (thyroid) have low mitotic rates and bland cytologic features, which are insufficient for determining malignancy. General principles for biopsy include sampling representative tissue, obtaining adequate tissue for diagnosis, procuring viable tissue, minimizing contamination of adjacent uninvolved tissues, orienting the tissue for margin analysis, and providing tissue to the pathologist in the appropriate conditions (fresh or fixed).

A. **Fine needle aspiration cytology.** Fine needle aspiration (FNA) yields a smear of single cells and aggregates for cytologic analysis. The biopsy is performed using a 22- to 25-gauge needle, which can be percutaneously guided to most anatomic sites. Although the track of the needle is theoretically contaminated with malignant cells, in practice, FNA-track metastases are rarely a clinical problem. Cells are collected in the hub of the needle and subsequently expelled onto slides. The slides are air dried or sprayed with a cytofixative for staining. The most common stains used for analysis are Papanicolaou for nuclear morphology and Diff-Quick for cytoplasmic features. Diagnosis is based on the cytologic features of the cells including cohesiveness, nuclear and cytoplasmic morphology, and number. An advantage of FNA is that a wide area of the tumor can be sampled. The limitations of FNA include (a) small sample size; (b) lack of information on histologic architecture that cannot distinguish between *in situ* and invasive tumors (breast, thyroid); (c) inability to obtain grade of tumors; and (d) interpretation of certain immunohistochemical stains. FNA can be useful for diagnosing recurrent lymphoma; however, for a primary diagnosis of lymphoma, more tissue may be required.

B. **Core needle biopsy.** Core needle biopsies yield fragments of tissue, which allow the evaluation of tumor architecture. The biopsy is performed using 14- to 16-gauge needles specifically designed for this purpose (Tru-Cut, Bioptry). Larger biopsy specimens that sample larger areas of tissue can be obtained with vacuum-assisted devices (Vicora, Mammotome). The procedure is performed by anesthetizing the skin overlying the lesion, puncturing the skin with a no. 11 blade, inserting the biopsy needle into the tumor, and deploying the biopsy device. Core needle biopsies can be combined with imaging such as mammography (stereotactic core biopsy), computed tomography (CT), or ultrasonography. A false-negative biopsy may result if the needle misses or skives (pares) the malignant tumor, which may occur with very sclerotic cancers such as in the breast. The most common complication of core needle biopsies is bleeding, and the procedure should be cautiously performed in patients with coagulopathies. In addition, masses near large vascular structures, hollow organs, or in the central nervous system (CNS) are not amenable to this procedure.

C. Cutaneous punch biopsy. Punch biopsies are used to obtain tissue from cutaneous lesions using 2- to 6-mm round surgical blades. A full-thickness skin specimen including subcutaneous fat is obtained. The procedure is performed by anesthetizing the skin and advancing the punch blade into the lesion. The core tissue is removed from the wound with a forceps, and the tissue base is divided with scissors. The wound can be closed with a single absorbable suture. The procedure is simple to perform, with few complications, and is useful for obtaining tissue for pathologic diagnosis from suggestive skin lesions (melanoma, basal cell, or squamous cell carcinoma) that may subsequently require definitive surgical resection.

D. Open biopsy

1. Incisional biopsy. Occasionally neoplasms are not amenable to percutaneous needle biopsy because of anatomic location, requirements for large amounts of tissue for diagnosis (sarcomas), or concern regarding sampling errors in diffuse lesions. An incisional biopsy is the most expedient method for obtaining tissue for definitive diagnosis. These procedures are usually performed in an outpatient surgical setting. Incisional biopsies are performed by placing an incision directly over the lesion after anesthetizing the skin. A wedge of tissue large enough for accurate diagnosis is removed from the periphery of the lesion. Excellent hemostasis must be obtained to avoid hematogenous seeding. The biopsy incision should be planned such that it can be included in the tissue to be removed by subsequent definitive surgery (longitudinal for limb sarcomas) because some tumors have a propensity for seeding the biopsy incision. A biopsy site that is far removed from the potential operative incision can severely jeopardize later attempts for surgical control of the tumor or potential limb-sparing procedures and can result in a compromised surgery.

2. Excisional biopsy. Excisional biopsies remove the entire lesion and are best suited for small lesions. This may be curative for small cancers (melanoma, breast cancer, sarcoma, basal cell carcinomas). Depending on the size of the lesion and the closure required, excisional biopsies can be performed as an office-based procedure or in the operating room. All specimens should be oriented for accurate margin assessment. This allows the surgeon to resect additional tissue for inadequate or close margins.

III. STAGING: DETERMINING THE EXTENT OF DISEASE AND RESECTABILITY. When distant disease is suspected, most cancers can be staged with CT, positron emission tomography (PET), magnetic resonance imaging (MRI), or bone radionuclide scans. However, surgical staging procedures for melanoma, breast cancer, a subset of abdominal malignancies, and thoracic malignancies are more sensitive than currently available radiographic modalities and alter patient management in a large percentage of cases.

A. Mediastinoscopy. Mediastinoscopy is used for the preoperative staging of bronchogenic carcinoma and evaluation of mediastinal adenopathy. It is the most accurate method for staging mediastinal lymph nodes. The procedure is performed under general anesthesia. A transverse surgical incision is made above the sternal notch, and a mediastinoscope is inserted along the trachea. Lymph node can be biopsied from the pretracheal, subcarinal, and paratracheal node stations and examined for metastatic disease. The procedure is highly sensitive (100%) and specific (90%) in staging of bronchogenic carcinoma and has low morbidity and mortality. Recently, techniques in endoscopic ultrasound (EUS) and endobronchial ultrasound (EBUS) have been developed to get needle biopsies of mediastinal lymph nodes. Together these techniques, (EUS, EBUS, mediastinoscopy) are important tools to help stage mediastinal lymph nodes.

B. Laparotomy. Radiographic staging and laparoscopy have largely replaced laparotomy. Laparotomy is used selectively for staging ovarian and nonseminomatous testicular cancers. The procedure is performed under general anesthesia through a midline incision. The procedure has low morbidity and short recovery. Complications include infection, bleeding, wound dehiscence, and rare events related to exploration of the intraabdominal contents and general anesthesia.

C. Laparoscopy. The role of laparoscopy for the diagnosis and treatment of patients with cancer has greatly expanded over the last decade. Laparoscopy is now considered an effective tool for diagnosis and staging of intraabdominal malignancies (liver, pancreas, stomach, and medullary thyroid carcinoma). Laparoscopy has been shown to decrease the incidence of unnecessary laparotomies for unresectable disease in up to 70% of patients with abdominal malignancies. Diagnostic laparoscopy for staging is usually performed at the time of a planned laparotomy. If distant or unresectable disease is found, then an unnecessary laparotomy is avoided. The procedure is performed under general anesthesia. A laparoscope is introduced through an infraumbilical port after the abdomen is insufflated with carbon dioxide. Placement of accessory ports aids in dissection and retraction, which allow most intraabdominal organs to be viewed. Biopsies of solid organs, lymph nodes, and suggestive lesions can be obtained. When laparoscopy is combined with intraoperative ultrasonography, lesions deep in the parenchyma of an organ can be identified, as well as tumor invasion into adjacent structures, such as major blood vessels. This is especially useful in evaluation of the liver and pancreatic malignancies and may be the most sensitive imaging technique for the detection of liver metastases. The procedure has few complications and may be performed on an outpatient basis. Port-site metastasis and intraabdominal spread by the pneumoperitoneum, although of theoretical concern, are rare (less than 1.0% of cases).

D. Lymphadenectomy. The location, type of cancer, and clinical evidence of nodal involvement are the major considerations in performing lymphadenectomy. Presence and extent of nodal involvement is the most accurate risk indicator of distant disease development for many cancers. In general, regional lymph nodes should be removed when the likelihood of metastases is high or if lymph nodes are found by clinical examination to be involved. If possible, regional lymph nodes should be removed at the time of the primary surgery. If a lymph node is found to exceed 3 cm in size, the tumor likely has extranodal extension and involves the perinodal fat. These lymph nodes should be resected with surrounding fat and, if of low morbidity, the adjacent nerves (intercostal brachial sensory nerve of the axilla). Studies are on to determine the survival benefit of lymphadenectomies in cancer resections (stomach, pancreas, breast). The major morbidity of regional lymphadenectomy is limb lymphedema and injury to adjacent nerves.

E. Sentinel lymph node biopsy. Sentinel lymph node biopsy (SLNB) is based on data demonstrating hierarchical lymphatic drainage occurring from the primary tumor to the first draining lymph node (sentinel lymph node [SLN]) and then to the remaining nodes in the regional lymphatic basin. Numerous studies have demonstrated that localized malignancies metastasize to the SLN before involving other nodes in the basin. Therefore, the presence or absence of metastatic disease in the SLN predicts the status of the entire regional lymphatic basin. SLNB is currently used for staging the axilla in breast cancer and regional nodal basins in melanoma. Two techniques are used for lymphatic mapping, which may be used independently or in combination. The first technique involves the injection of a radiolabeled colloid around the lesion, which is followed radiographically and/or intraoperatively by using the gamma probe. The second technique employs isosulfan blue, which is injected intraoperatively around the tumor and allowed to percolate through the lymphatics. In both techniques, an incision is made at the edge of the nodal basin, and the SLN is identified by tracing blue or radioactive lymphatic channels to the first blue or radioactive node. If more than one nodal basin is potentially involved, then preoperative lymphoscintigraphy may be performed to identify the draining nodal basins. In experienced hands, the procedure has very high specificity and sensitivity. The advantages of SLNB are selective lymph node dissections in those patients who would benefit most, avoiding the morbidity associated with lymph node clearance in those patients with low risk of disease, and the ability to perform immunohistochemical stains or polymerase chain reaction (PCR) to detect micrometastatic disease. Disadvantages of SLNB are related to the skill of the operator, which may result in a significant false-negative rate.

IV. SURGICAL TREATMENT. Surgical planning involves consideration of the tumor stage and location, the general health of the patient, expected morbidity and mortality of the procedure, probability of successful treatment, and the availability and effectiveness of other treatment modalities. Surgical resection of solid tumors provides excellent local control and is currently the only curative option for most solid tumors.

A. Primary resection

   1. Principles of surgical resection. The primary goal of cancer surgery is the complete extirpation of local and regional disease for local control and for decreasing the risk of local recurrence. This involves removing the primary lesion with adequate margins of normal surrounding tissue to minimize the risk of local recurrence. The stage, mechanisms of local spread, morbidity, and mortality of the procedure must be taken into consideration before any surgical procedure is undertaken. In patients with metastatic disease, long-term control may not be as important as it is in patients who have localized disease, which may be surgically curable, although in these cases surgery can be palliative. Knowledge of the most common avenues of spread for the various histologic types of cancers is essential for successful local control. Depending on the cell of origin, cancers may spread mucosally, submucosally, along fascial planes, or along nerves (Table 1.1). With advances in anesthesia, postoperative care, and reconstructive procedures, large surgical procedures can be performed safely in elderly patients and patients with multiple comorbid conditions. Intraoperatively, successful resection requires good exposure, excision of previous biopsy sites, maintaining a bloodless surgical field to visualize the extent of tumor spread, and *en bloc* resection of the tumor and surrounding normal tissue. Local recurrence or wound seeding can be theoretically minimized by minimal manipulation of the tumor, confining dissection to normal tissue, and early ligation of major feeding vessels at their origin. Complete removal of the tumors has many favorable effects including minimizing residual disease and eliminating hypoxic, poorly vascularized cells, which are drug and radiation resistant.

   2. Premalignant lesions and prophylactic surgery. Surgery is indicated for premalignant lesions and noninvasive cancers of the skin, mouth, cervix, colon, breast, and thyroid, although only a proportion of such lesions may progress to malignancy (Table 1.2). Several inherited disorders associated with increased cancer risk have been described. Surgery can significantly reduce cancer occurrence (Table 1.3).

B. Operative principles

   1. Anatomy. The anatomic location of cancers is an important consideration in surgical planning. Some tumors cannot be adequately treated by surgical resection alone because of anatomic constraints, which may result in incomplete excision (nasopharynx). Residual microscopic disease after surgical resection can sometimes be treated effectively with adjuvant radiation therapy to decrease local recurrence. Those patients whose lesions are intimately involved with major blood vessels (lung/aorta) or bilaterally involve an essential organ (liver)

TABLE 1.1 Adequate Tissue Margins for Primary Malignancy Treated with Surgery Alone

Tissue	Margin	Rationale
Melanoma		
Thin (<0.75 mm)	1 cm	Localized
Thick (>1.0 mm)	2 cm	Increased risk of local recurrence
Sarcoma	Excise entire muscle group or 1 cm	—
Breast, invasive	1 cm	Must be combined with radiation therapy because of multifocality
Colon	2–5 cm	—
Esophagus	10 cm	Potential for extensive submucosal spread
Squamous cell carcinoma of head/neck	1 cm	May be limited by adjacent structures
Lung	Excise lobe or lung	—
Pancreas	1 mm–1 cm	Margins may be limited by surrounding vessels
Liver	1 cm	—
Basal cell carcinoma	2 mm	Very localized malignant area
Stomach	6 cm	Intramural spread

or those with a limited life expectancy due to the natural history of the disease may not benefit from surgical resection.

2. **Neoadjuvant therapy before resection.** If a lesion is resectable and localized at the time of diagnosis, then surgery should be performed. Large lesions or lesions invading into surrounding structures that are not initially resectable may be amenable to volume reduction with initial (neoadjuvant) chemotherapy or radiation therapy. This strategy has allowed successful but more limited, less morbid resections or function-preserving resections of many cancers (colorectal, breast, larynx, pancreatic cancers). In addition, the response to neoadjuvant therapy is useful for monitoring response to various treatment regimens. If a pathologic complete response is possible, the surgical site should be marked with metallic clips at the time of biopsy for future identification at the time of surgery. Disadvantages of neoadjuvant therapy are the possible delays in undergoing standard curative therapy.

    Preoperative radiation therapy may be used alone or in combination with chemotherapy to reduce tumor size before resection. Advantages of preoperative radiation therapy are potentially smaller treatment fields and

TABLE 1.2 Surgery for *in situ* Disease and Atypia

Organ	Pathology	Detection method
Cervix	Atypia	Papanicolaou test
Mouth	Dysplasia	Oral examination
Gastroesophageal tract	Dysplasia (Barrett) leukoplakia	Endoscopy
Breast	*In situ*	Mammogram/physical examination

TABLE 1.3	Prophylactic Surgery	
Disorder	**Cancer risk**	**Surgery**
Familial polyposis coli	100% risk	Colectomy
Ulcerative colitis	With dysplasia, >50% risk	Colectomy
MEN II/FMTC	100% medullary thyroid cancer (genetic screening)	Thyroidectomy
BRCA1/2	>60% breast cancer	Mastectomy

FMTC, familial medullary thyroid cancer; MEN, multiple endocrine neoplasia.

reduced potential seeding of the tumor during surgery. Disadvantages of preoperative radiotherapy include the resulting fibrosis, which may obscure resection margins and increase the difficulty and morbidity of the surgery. Preoperative radiation therapy renders the wound edges functionally ischemic, which may affect the type of reconstruction performed and tissue resected or result in increased wound complications. Although neoadjuvant therapy may decrease the size of the lesion, there is generally little benefit in overall survival.

C. **Extent of resection.** Extent of resection depends on the organ involved and method of local spread. Adequate margins range from 1 mm to 5 cm for cutaneous and hollow organ tumors (Table 1.1). Resections for solid organ tumors are usually guided by the blood supply, and usually resection of a lobe (liver, lung) or the entire organ (kidney) or a partial resection (pancreas) is performed. The most efficacious method for local control and prevention of local recurrence is wide excision. This may require encompassing any biopsy incision or needle tract into the *en bloc* excision. If the malignancy is adherent to a contiguous organ, then a partial resection of the latter organ may be performed to obtain negative margins. Most solid tumors have a propensity for dissemination through local lymphatics to regional lymph nodes. If a lymph node in the draining area exceeds 3 cm in size, the tumor is likely extranodal and involves the perinodal fat. Local excision is then inadequate and *en bloc* resection of the organ, regional lymph nodes, and adjacent involved regions should be performed. To prevent seeding of tumor, the no-touch technique can be used, which includes minimal palpation of the tumor and early ligation of the blood supply to limit dislodgement of the tumor cells into the venous circulation. Although the ability of these techniques to reduce local recurrence is controversial, their theoretic value has led to widespread acceptance. If a second area of the body requires surgery at the time of tumor excision, gloves, gowns, sheets, and instruments must be changed. This further prevents transplantation of tumor to a distant site.

If margins are positive after resection, options include further surgery, adjuvant therapy, or careful follow-up. If microscopic tumor is found at the resection margin, adjuvant postoperative radiation may be given. However, this may be associated with a higher risk of tumor recurrence, poorer cosmetic results, and more radiation complications due to the higher radiation doses required (breast, sarcoma, head/neck cancers). These patients may benefit from reexcision of the tumor bed to achieve microscopically clear margins if this is technically feasible. In these cases, the potential morbidity and mortality of repeat surgery should be assessed.

D. **Laparoscopic and laparoscopy-assisted surgeries.** Laparoscopic or laparoscopy-assisted tumor resections are increasingly being performed worldwide. The most common laparoscopic cancer surgery performed is colectomy. Laparoscopy-assisted distal pancreatectomies, gastrectomies, esophagectomies and video-assisted thoracic (VAT) lobectomies are becoming more common. In general, laparoscopic procedures result in shorter hospital stay, less intraoperative blood loss, decreased requirement for analgesics, and earlier return to normal activities. Concerns have been raised regarding margin width and *en bloc* resection of draining nodal basins; however, studies examining these issues for colectomy have reported no significant difference. Indeed, data is emerging suggesting that this holds true for other laproscopic resection options.

V. METASTASES AND RECURRENT DISEASE

A. Distant metastasis. With many types of cancer, death is often the result of metastatic disease. It is often assumed that the patient with disseminated disease is not a candidate for surgical procedures. However, subsets of patients with isolated metastases are amenable to a complete surgical resection (hepatic and pulmonary) with resulting increased survival. Excisions of symptomatic metastases that cannot be treated by other means are appropriate for resection to improve quality of life (melanoma, breast, thyroid, and other endocrine cancers). This includes patients with subcutaneous metastases that present cosmetic problems and bowel metastases that cause obstruction or bleeding. Patients with multiple metastases to the lung or liver should be considered for resection if the metastases are present in only one organ system, if there is adequate normal parenchyma remaining after resection, and if the operative risk is minimal. The longer the time interval between initial diagnosis and the appearance of metastatic disease, the more likely it is that surgery will be beneficial and result in increased overall survival. Resection of a small number of pulmonary metastases from sarcoma or localized lung and liver metastases from colorectal cancers will result in increased survival for approximately 25% of patients. In breast cancer, there is emerging evidence that surgery of the breast improves overall survival in patients with metastatic disease.

B. Resection for recurrent locoregional disease. Local recurrence of cancer can result from incomplete excision at the initial surgery, the presence of residual cancer cells distant from the primary lesion, or second primary tumors that develop in residual normal tissue. Intensive follow-up is used to detect recurrent or persistent tumors before distant dissemination occurs. With some cancers, the presence of local recurrence may signal the presence of distant disease in a proportion of patients (approximately 50% for breast cancer). Similar surgical principles apply to resection of recurrent disease.

C. Palliative surgery. Significant improvement in quality of life and alleviation of symptoms can be achieved with palliative surgery, which allows patients to resume as many of their normal daily activities as possible (Table 1.4). This includes resection for obstruction, pain, bleeding, or perforation of a hollow viscus or for hormonal effects of endocrine tumors (insulinomas, gastrinomas, medullary thyroid cancers). As laparoscopic techniques become more common, these minimally invasive approaches may provide invaluable tools for allowing patients the ability to their maximize quality of life without the morbidity associated with open surgery.

TABLE 1.4　**Palliative Surgical Procedures**

Presentation	Surgical procedure
Malignant pleural effusion	Thoracostomy tube, sclerosis
Biliary obstruction	Stent or choledochojejunostomy
Bowel obstruction, large	Colostomy with mucous fistula
Bowel obstruction, small	Resection, bypass, gastrostomy tube
Bowel obstruction, duodenal	Gastrojejunostomy
Esophageal obstruction	Stent, gastrostomy tube
Locally advanced breast cancer	Salvage mastectomy

VI. RECONSTRUCTION: FUNCTIONAL AND COSMETIC. Advances in the understanding of the tissue blood supply have allowed improvements in the coverage of surgical defects after cancer resections. Rarely are disfiguring primary closures or skin grafts the only option. Two advances have led to major changes in plastic reconstructions of cancer resections. The first was the anatomic elucidation of muscular blood supply, which allowed tissue associated with a defined vascular network to be moved to a defect within reach of its pedicle. The second advance was in the field of microsurgery, which allowed muscle flaps with the overlying subcutaneous fat and skin to be detached from their original blood supply and reanastomosed to vessels in a different anatomic area. These advances meant that multiple-stage reconstructions were no longer required to bring well-vascularized tissue into a surgical defect. This decreases the risk of postoperative wound complications and avoids delays in commencing adjuvant therapy. Currently, immediate reconstruction is frequently performed during the same surgery as an oncologic resection. With these new techniques, large amounts of tissues can be reliably transplanted to fill dead spaces, pad and cover susceptible organs or structures, and provide restoration of form, function, and contour. Free and pedicled tissue transfers are used for reconstruction after surgery for the breast, mandibular area, and perineum. Commonly used donor myocutaneous flaps include the latissimus dorsi, rectus abdominis, and gracilis muscles. If bone is required, fibula-based flaps are commonly used. Flap success rate is 95%, and multiple studies have demonstrated improved quality of life with reconstruction procedures and no decrement in the ability to detect recurrence. In those patients requiring adjuvant therapy, reconstruction does not delay the time to initiation of treatment. Disadvantages of reconstruction are secondary problems at the donor site and increased operative time.

VII. NEWER TREATMENT MODALITIES

    A. Cryotherapy. Intraoperative cryoablation is regarded as an effective form of palliative therapy and may cure some patients with small tumors. Intraoperative ultrasonography is used to monitor hepatic cryosurgery for nonresectable disease. Hepatic cryotherapy involves the freezing and thawing of liver tumors by means of a cryoprobe inserted into the tumors. During freeze/thaw cycles, intracellular and extracellular ice forms, leading to tumor destruction. Tumors are then left *in situ* to be absorbed. Cryosurgery can treat multiple lesions and allows salvage of more uninvolved liver parenchyma than does surgical resection. Postoperative complications include hemorrhage, biliary fistula, myoglobinuria, and acute renal failure. Overall morbidity rates range from 6% to 50%. Mortality rates range from 0% to 8%. Hepatic cryosurgery is an option for patients with isolated liver metastases from colorectal cancer that are not surgically resectable but are limited enough to allow cryoablation of all lesions. It is unclear whether cryoablation will lead to survival equivalent to that after surgical resection.

    B. Radiofrequency ablation. This technique involves percutaneous or intraoperative insertion of a radiofrequency (RF) probe into the center of a hepatic tumor under ultrasonography or CT guidance. RF energy is then emitted from the electrode and absorbed by the surrounding tissue. This process generates heat, leading to coagulation necrosis of the treated tissue. The initial limitation of this therapy was the small (1.5 cm) diameter of necrosis achievable with a single RF probe. Newer probes allow treatment of larger volumes. The primary advantage of RF ablation over cryosurgery lies in the low incidence of complications and the ease of performance under CT or ultrasonography guidance. RF ablation can be performed percutaneously, thereby avoiding laparotomy or laparoscopy.

VIII. SURGICAL INTERVENTION FOR ONCOLOGIC EMERGENCIES. Although true oncologic emergencies are rare, surgeons are often consulted regarding the management of complications that are a result of tumor progression or cytotoxic therapy.

    A. Bowel perforation. Perforation of the gastrointestinal (GI) tract in patients with cancer carries a high morbidity and mortality. Although most perforations are from benign causes (diverticulitis, appendicitis, peptic ulcer disease), they can also occur as a result of chemotherapy or radiation therapy or as a primary presentation of a malignancy. Undiagnosed colorectal cancers can present with perforation as a result of full-thickness colonic involvement or proximal perforation from a distal obstructing mass. The latter perforations most frequently occur at the cecum. The response of some malignancies, such as GI lymphomas, is so great to chemotherapy that full-thickness necrosis of the bowel wall occurs. Patients undergoing cancer therapy are often immunosuppressed and malnourished, which masks the traditional signs of a perforation (peritonitis, leukocytosis, fever, tachycardia). Immunosuppression and poor nutrition are associated with an increase in the operative mortality and morbidity of these patients. Mortality rates as high as 80% have been reported in patients who undergo an emergency laparotomy and in those who have metastatic disease and are undergoing chemotherapy. Comfort care and nonsurgical treatments should be discussed in patients with an overall poor prognosis. In patients who undergo abdominal exploration, ostomies, gastrostomy, and feeding jejunostomy tubes should be considered.

B. Bowel obstruction. Intestinal obstruction is commonly found in cancer patients presenting with nausea, vomiting, abdominal distention, and obstipation. Benign sources of obstruction such as adhesions from previous surgery and radiation enteritis account for approximately one third of cases in these patients. Primary (ovarian, colonic, and stomach) malignancies or metastatic disease (lung, breast, and melanoma) are the cause of intestinal obstruction in two thirds of cases. In a small percentage of cancer patients, functional obstruction can also occur without a mechanical cause from electrolyte abnormalities, radiation therapy, malnutrition, narcotic analgesics, and prolonged immobility. In these patients, correction of the underlying cause and bowel decompression are the cornerstones of treatment. The approach to the diagnosis and treatment of obstruction in patients with cancer should be similar to that for patients with benign disease. All patients should be initially resuscitated with IV fluids, have electrolyte abnormalities corrected, be decompressed with a nasogastric tube, and have urine output monitored. Patients who have signs of compromised bowel viability or perforation (abdominal tenderness, leukocytosis, fever, persistent tachycardia, free intra-abdominal air) should undergo immediate exploratory laparotomy. Patients with a complete bowel obstruction rarely respond to medical management and require surgical exploration. Between 25% and 50% of patients with a partial small bowel obstruction will resolve their obstruction with conservative measures. Those patients who do not demonstrate resolution after a finite period or progress to complete obstruction should undergo laparotomy. A colonic obstruction should be excluded before surgical intervention with a water-soluble contrast enema. CT scans of the abdomen with oral and rectal contrast can be helpful for determining the presence of a transition point, bowel wall thickening, or the presence of recurrent disease. Cancer patients with benign obstructions from adhesions or internal herniation benefit from surgery. If malignant obstruction is present, resection or bypass of the obstructed segment may be performed; however, only 35% of patients will have durable relief of symptoms after surgical treatment. These patients should be strongly considered for gastrostomy tube placement at the time of surgery, which provides significant palliation by relieving emesis and obviating the need for nasogastric suction. Radiation-induced enteritis may be clinically indistinguishable from adhesive small bowel obstruction. In cases of radiation enteritis, short segments of narrowed bowel may be resected; however, long segments should be treated with bypass. Surgical intervention for a malignant bowel obstruction is associated with a significant morbidity (30%) and mortality (10%) and patients have a mean survival of approximately 6 months only following laparotomy for a malignant bowel obstruction.

C. Neutropenic enterocolitis (typhlitis). Neutropenic enterocolitis most often occurs in patients who are undergoing chemotherapy and are neutropenic for more than 7 days. Symptoms include febrile neutropenia, diarrhea, abdominal distention, and right lower quadrant pain. Initially, the presentation can be very similar to appendicitis. Radiologic findings are often nonspecific or may demonstrate thickening of the cecum. Serial abdominal examinations are critical for proper diagnosis and treatment. Most episodes will resolve with conservative management with bowel rest, IV fluid resuscitation, nasogastric decompression, and broad-spectrum antibiotics. However, if patients develop perforation, uncontrolled hemorrhage, become septic, or symptoms continue to worsen despite medical therapy, a laparotomy should be performed. A right hemicolectomy with ileostomy and mucous fistula is the surgery of choice and may be reversed after several months.

D. Biliary obstruction. In addition to pancreatic and bile duct carcinomas, lymphomas, melanomas, and breast, colon, stomach, lung, and ovarian cancers can cause biliary obstruction due to metastasis to the portal lymph nodes or hilum of the liver. The prognosis for patients with biliary obstruction from metastatic disease is poor. Two-month mortality rates approaching 70% have been reported. Treatment should be aimed at preventing cholangitis and palliating jaundice. Endoscopic retrograde cholangiopancreatography (ERCP) with stent placement or percutaneous transhepatic drainage should be the initial treatment strategy.

E. Hemorrhage. Patients with malignancies who develop GI bleeding should undergo the same workup as those without malignant disease. Resuscitation, correction of coagulopathies, and a workup to define the bleeding site should be initiated immediately. Bright blood per rectum or hematemesis can give clues to a lower or upper GI source. Malignant tumors are rarely the source of significant intra-abdominal hemorrhage. If the bleeding is not at a life-threatening rate, a tagged red blood cell scan, angiography, embolization, and endoscopic interventions can all be used to diagnose and treat the hemorrhage. The timing of surgical intervention is based on the rate and volume of blood loss, the underlying pathology, and the overall prognosis of the patient.

F. Pericardial tamponade. Metastatic disease to the pericardium leading to malignant obstruction of the pericardial lymphatics is the most common cause of pericardial tamponade in cancer patients. Lung cancer, breast cancer, lymphoma, leukemia, melanoma, and primary neoplasms of the heart are most commonly implicated in tamponade. The development of symptoms in a patient depends on the rate of accumulation of the volume of the pericardial fluid and compliance of the sac. If the accumulation is gradual, more than 2 L can be found in the pericardial sac. Patients often present with vague symptoms of chest pain, dyspnea, and anxiety. On examination, decreased heart sounds, tachycardia, pulsus paradoxus, and jugular venous distention can be found. Echocardiography is the best test to determine if there is excess pericardial fluid. Pericardiocentesis with placement of a drainage catheter can be life saving in a patient in tamponade and shock. Additional options in more stable patients include tetracycline sclerosis, radiation therapy, subxiphoid pericardiotomy, window pericardectomy, and complete pericardectomy. A subxiphoid approach avoids the need for a thoracotomy.

G. Superior vena cava syndrome. Superior vena cava syndrome (SVCS) results from an impedance to outflow from the superior vena cava (SVC) due to external compression by malignancy, fibrosis, or thrombosis. In more than 95% of patients, SVCS results from a malignancy. The SVC is a thin-walled vessel in the middle mediastinum and any enlargement of the perihilar or paratracheal lymph nodes or abnormalities of the aorta, pulmonary artery, or mainstem bronchus could lead to impingement on the SVC. The SVC is responsible for venous drainage of the head, neck, upper extremities, and upper thorax. Small cell lung cancer and other pulmonary malignancies are the most common etiology of SVCS, although lymphomas, germ cell tumors, and metastatic lesions to the supraclavicular nodal basins are also responsible. In most cases, SVCS develops gradually. The most common symptoms are dyspnea and facial fullness. Other symptoms associated with SVCS are venous engorgement of the neck and chest wall, cyanosis, and upper extremity edema. Symptoms are worse when the patient bends forward or reclines. Unless SVCS causes impedence of the airway from laryngeal edema (an emergency treated with intubation, tracheostomy, or emergent radiation therapy), a thorough workup can be conducted. Chest radiography, CT, and biopsy can be useful in determining the etiology of SVC obstruction. Treatment includes diuretics, elevation of the head, and steroids, and chemotherapy and/or radiation therapy directed at treating the underlying cause. SVCS can be secondary to indwelling central venous catheters causing thrombosis. This can often be successfully treated with thrombolytic agents followed by systemic anticoagulation. Balloon angioplasty and vascular stenting can be used if initial therapies fail. Surgical innominate vein–right atrial bypass is a last option.

H. Spinal cord compression. Spinal cord compression is an acute emergency. The severity of neurologic impairment at presentation dictates the potential reversibility of symptoms. Early recognition is essential in preventing progressive or irreversible neurologic deterioration that can lead to paralysis and loss of sphincter control. Extradural metastatic lesions of the vertebral body or neural arch are the most common cause of spinal cord compression in patients with malignancies. As tumors expand, they often impinge on the anterior aspect of the spinal cord. Metastatic lesions from lung, breast, prostate cancers, and multiple myeloma are the most common lesions responsible for spinal cord compression. Of these, 10% occur in the cervical vertebrae, 70% in the thoracic vertebrae, and 20% in the lumbosacral vertebrae. 90% of patients will present with localized back pain. The pain usually precedes the onset of neurologic deterioration by weeks to months. Patients will develop motor loss and weakness followed by sensory loss. Patients often describe an ascending tingling sensation beginning in the distal extremities. The onset of urinary retention, constipation, and/or loss of bowel or bladder control is a late and ominous manifestation. In addition to plain radiographs, MRI is the study of choice for evaluating patients with suspected spinal cord compression. Gadolinium contrast provides optimal imaging of extramedullary and intramedullary lesions. In cases of rapid compression of the spinal cord, therapeutic intervention must be performed immediately to avoid irreversible neurologic deficits. The patient should be immediately started on steroids, and treatment options include radiation therapy, surgery, chemotherapy, or a combination of all three. Laminectomy is effective in managing patients with epidural masses and in select cases surgical resection of the mass may be possible. As mentioned earlier, the functional status at the time of presentation clearly correlates with the posttreatment outcome; early diagnosis and recognition is crucial.

IX. VASCULAR ACCESS

A. Central venous catheterization. Many cancer patients require frequent venous catheterization for phlebotomy, chemotherapy, or infusions. Peripheral venous sites for catheterization can become quickly exhausted because of the venotoxic effects of the cytotoxic agents, the trauma of repeated use, and the undesirability of performing access procedures in limbs with proximal lymphadenectomies. Central venous catheters are designed for repeated venous access. Although they are generally easily placed, complications include pneumothorax, hemothorax, air embolism, cardiac arrhythmia, and arterial injury. Over the long term, these catheters can cause central vein thrombosis, embolism, infection, and scarring. Relative contraindications to placement include uncorrected thrombocytopenia or coagulopathy and earlier irradiation to the head or neck, which can result in scarring. For these latter patients, an ultrasonography before the procedure may be useful to establish the patency of their veins. Patients who are hypercoagulable from their cancers may benefit from low-dose warfarin (1 to 2 mg/day) to prevent central venous thrombosis.

1. Hickman catheters/Broviac catheters. Tunneled externalized central venous catheters of the Hickman or Broviac type are available in single- to triple-lumen varieties and have wide internal diameters, which allow blood sampling and result in higher patency rates. A Dacron cuff in the extravascular subcutaneous portion of the catheter develops fibrous ingrowth, serves as a mechanical barrier to infection, and prevents accidental dislodgement. Catheters are placed percutaneously using the Seldinger technique into the subclavian or internal jugular vein or by venous cutdown into the cephalic or external jugular veins. The catheter is inserted under fluoroscopic guidance to ensure proper placement at the SVC–atrial junction. Patency can be maintained by flushing with heparinized saline (100 U/mL) every month and after each use of the catheter. If catheter thrombosis occurs, patency can be reestablished by infusing streptokinase. The catheter exit site should be cleaned and dressed every 24 to 72 hours using sterile technique. Infection may involve the device, the catheter tunnel, or the exit site. Signs of catheter-tunnel or exit-site infection include erythema, induration, and suppuration, and may necessitate catheter removal. Sepsis from catheter infection should be documented by blood cultures drawn from both the catheter and peripheral sites. Coagulase-negative staphylococci are the most common pathogens isolated. Most catheter-caused infections can be treated effectively with a 10- to 14-day course of IV antibiotics. However, persistence of positive cultures necessitates catheter removal. If untreated, catheter infections may lead to septic thrombophlebitis of the catheterized vessel, endocarditis, or a distant focus of suppuration such as osteomyelitis, septic arthritis, or disseminated abscesses. Hickman catheter–related infections are five times more common than infections in implanted ports. Disadvantages of Hickman catheters are limitations of patient activity, frequent maintenance, and malfunction due to thrombotic occlusions. Advantages are easy access with standard needles and bedside removal.

2. **Implantable catheters: Portacath, Infusaport.** Completely implantable subcutaneous catheters comprise a reservoir with a silicone septum, which is available with single and double lumens attached to a silicone catheter. Port access is performed with a Hueber needle that punctures but does not tear the silicone septum. The integrity of the septum is maintained for 1,500 to 2,000 cannulations. The port is placed in a subcutaneous pocket, and the attached catheter is threaded into the subclavian, internal jugular, or in special circumstances, into the femoral vein using fluoroscopic guidance to ensure correct positioning. Ports should be flushed monthly with heparinized saline to maintain patency. Infections may involve the port pocket, the port reservoir, or the catheter. Port-pocket infections require removal of the catheter. The main advantages of the implantable catheters are cosmesis, few restrictions on activities such as bathing, low maintenance (monthly flushing to maintain patency), and low incidence of infection, which make it ideal for intermittent long-term therapy. The main disadvantages are access, which requires trained personnel and a Hueber needle, and higher cost as compared with peripheral access.

B. **Arterial catheters: hepatic artery infusion catheters.** Hepatic artery infusion (HAI) catheters are currently under clinical trials to treat hepatic metastases and have been so for approximately 15 years. HAI chemotherapy targets liver metastases, which derive most of their blood supply from the hepatic arterial circulation, in contrast to normal liver, which derives most of its blood supply from the portal circulation. In addition, higher levels of local therapy can be achieved without concomitant systemic toxicity due to the clearance of many chemotherapeutic agents from first pass through the liver. HAI chemotherapy is generally reserved for patients without evidence of extrahepatic disease. These catheters are placed at laparotomy. Before placement, patients undergo an angiogram to define regional arterial anatomy because of the highly variant arterial anatomy in this area. The infusion port or continuous infusion pump is placed in the abdominal subcutaneous tissues over the rectus muscle fascia, and the catheter is tunneled into the abdomen. The tip of the catheter is placed in the gastroduodenal artery at its junction with the common hepatic artery. Cholecystectomy is required to prevent chemotherapy-induced chemical cholecystitis, and complete separation of the hepatic arterial circulation from the gastroduodenal blood supply must be achieved to prevent GI toxicity. Postoperatively, radiolabeled microaggregated albumin is injected into the infusion pump, and a scintillation scan is obtained to verify hepatic infusion and exclusion of extrahepatic perfusion. Chemotherapeutic agents are injected into the port reservoir, which is designed to ensure continuous infusion of a constant amount of agent. Studies have demonstrated higher response rates with HAI than with systemic chemotherapy; however, no survival advantage has been observed. Current strategies combine liver resection, residual tumor ablation, and HAI pump placement.

X. ENTERAL FEEDING TUBES. Malnutrition is common in the cancer patient and may be related to inadequate voluntary intake, altered metabolism, or the effects of therapy. Enteral alimentation can be useful before or after surgery or during therapy. Early concerns that hyperalimentation would lead to rapid tumor growth have not been borne out by experience, and in severely malnourished patients (less than 80% standard weight for height), there is a measurable improvement in operative morbidity if nutritional supplementation is provided 7 to 10 days before surgery. Postoperatively, enteral or parenteral alimentation can support the cancer patient who is unable to eat because of a healing anastomosis or a postoperative ileus. During chemotherapy or radiation therapy, inflammation, infection, or strictures may lead to inadequate oral intake requiring enteral alimentation. The route of administration of nutritional support is selected based on length of anticipated need, intestinal tract function, degree of malnutrition, access for administration, and potential complications. In patients with adequate GI function, enteral alimentation is preferred over the parenteral route. Enteral alimentation is less expensive, leads to fewer metabolic imbalances, preserves the GI architecture, and is thought to prevent bacterial translocation. The most common morbidities associated with enteral alimentation are abdominal distention, nausea, or diarrhea, which can occur in 10% to 20% of patients. These symptoms usually abate with a decreased rate of infusion or strength of the formula.

A. Gastrostomy tubes. Gastrostomy tubes (G-tubes) may be placed percutaneous or intraoperatively. They can serve the dual functions of conduits for feeding or intestinal decompression. Other advantages of a G-tube are bolus feeding with high-osmolar formulas because of the reservoir capacity of the stomach, and the ability to replace dislodged tubes easily through the gastrocutaneous fistula. Disadvantages include risk of aspiration in patients with lower esophageal sphincter dysfunction or without an intact gag reflex. Enteral feeds can be administered by bolus (200 to 400 mL over a 5- to 10-minute period) and is the preferred feeding method in ambulatory patients because it is less confining.

B. Jejunostomy tubes. Jejunostomy tubes (J-tubes) are small-caliber feeding tubes placed distal to the ligament of Treitz by laparotomy or laparoscopy. Generally the tubes are placed through a surgical Witzel tunnel to prevent obstruction proximal to the site of insertion and to reduce the risk of leak. The advantages of J-tubes are the minimal risk of aspiration and the ability to feed distal to the obstruction or fistula. Because there is no reservoir capacity, enteral feeds are administered continuously over 12- to 24-hour periods, and there is limited tolerance to high-osmolar loads. Once dislodged, these tubes are not easily replaced. In addition, because of the small caliber, these tubes may become clogged with inspissated material and require vigorous flushing to reestablish patency.

Suggested Readings

Bremers AJA, Rutgers EJT, van deVelde CJH. Cancer surgery: the last 25 years. *Cancer Treat Rev* 1999;25:333–353.

Cromheeke M, de Jong KP, Hoekstra HJ. Current treatment for colorectal cancer metastatic to the liver. *Eur J Surg Oncol* 1999;25:451–463.

Giuliano AE, Kirgan DM, Guenther M, et al. Lymphatic mapping and sentinel lymphadenectomy for breast cancer. *Ann Surg* 1995;220:391–401.

Hammoud ZT, Anderson RC, Meyers BF, et al. The current role of mediastinoscopy in the evaluation of thoracic disease. *J Thorac Cardiovasc Surg* 1999;118:894–899.

Langstein HN, Robb GL. Reconstructive approaches in soft tissue sarcoma. *Semin Surg Oncol* 1999;17:52–65.

Pollock RE, Morton DL. Principles of surgical oncology. In: Bast RC, Gansler TS, Holland JF, et al. eds. *Cancer medicine*, 5th ed. Lewiston: Marcel Dekker Inc, 2000:448–458.

Ramshaw BJ, Esartia P, Mason EM, et al. Laparoscopy for diagnosis and staging of malignancy. *Semin Surg Oncol* 1999;16:279–283.

Rosenberg SA. Principles of cancer management: surgical oncology. In: Devita VT, Hellman S, Rosenberg SA, eds. *Principles and practice of oncology*, 6th ed. Philadelphia: Lippincott Williams & Wilkins, 2001:253–264.

Shafir M. Vascular access in cancer patients. In: Bast RC, Gansler TS, Holland JF, et al. eds. *Cancer medicine*, 5th ed. Lewiston: Marcel Dekker Inc, 2000:459–464.

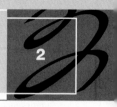

PRINCIPLES AND PRACTICE OF RADIATION THERAPY

2

Jeffrey D. Bradley, Joseph Roti Roti, and Sasa Mutic

I. **INTRODUCTION.** Optimal care of patients with malignant tumors is a multidisciplinary effort that may combine two or more of the classic disciplines: surgery, radiation therapy, and chemotherapy. Pathologists, radiologists, clinical laboratory physicians, and immunologists are integral members of the team that renders the correct diagnosis. Many professionals, including physicists, laboratory scientists, nurses, social workers, and others, are intimately involved in the care of the patient with cancer.

Radiation oncology is a clinical and scientific discipline devoted to management of patients with cancer and other diseases by ionizing radiation, alone or in combination with other modalities, investigation of the biologic and physical basis of radiation therapy, and training of professionals in the field. The aim of radiation therapy is to deliver a precisely measured dose of radiation to a defined tumor volume with as minimal as possible damage to surrounding healthy tissue, resulting in eradication of the tumor, a high quality of life, and prolongation of survival at competitive cost. In addition to curative efforts, radiation therapy plays a major role in the effective palliation or prevention of symptoms of cancer including pain, restoring luminal patency, skeletal integrity, and organ function with minimal morbidity.

The radiation oncologist, like any other physician, must assess all conditions relative to the patient and the tumor under consideration for treatment, systematically review the need for diagnostic and staging procedures, and determine the best therapeutic strategy.

II. **TYPES OF RADIATION USED IN RADIATION THERAPY.** Many types of radiation are used for treatment of both benign and malignant diseases. The most common form of irradiation is the use of external-beam photons or electrons. Photons are x-rays or γ-rays and may be considered as bundles of energy that deposit dose as they pass through matter. The term *x-ray* is used to describe radiation that is produced by machines, while γ-rays define radiation that is emitted from radioactive isotopes. Radiotherapy units used in x-ray therapy are contact (40 to 50 kilovoltage potential or kV), superficial (50 to 150 kV), orthovoltage units (150 to 500 kV), and linear accelerators (4 to 25 million volts or MV). X-rays measured in kV have a limited range and are used to treat superficial tissues such as skin or mucosa. The clinical use of kV energies for therapeutic radiation has declined within the last several years. Therefore, fewer facilities maintain active superficial or orthovoltage x-ray units. X-rays measured in MV are used when treating deeper targets (beyond 3- to 4-cm depth) and have "skin sparing" qualities. As mentioned before, γ-rays are generated from isotopes. The most common source of γ-rays for external-beam radiotherapy is cobalt 60. Most radiotherapy facilities no longer use γ-rays because of the need to replace or recalculate for decaying sources. Two exceptions are (a) the gamma knife unit used for stereotactic radiosurgery, which houses 201 cobalt 60 sources and (b) brachytherapy (described later), a subspecialty of radiation therapy that relies on placement of radioactive isotope directly inside the tumors.

Electrons or β-particles can also be used to treat patients. Similar to the distinction between x-rays and γ-rays, the term *electron* is used to describe radiation produced by machines while β-particles describe electrons emitted by radioactive isotopes. Electrons deposit their maximal energy slightly beyond the skin surface and have a sharp falloff beyond their range. Electrons are used mainly for treating skin or superficial tumors.

Other sources of external-beam radiation are protons and neutrons. Protons are charged particles that have the advantage of depositing dose at a constant rate over most of the beam, but depositing most of the dose at the end of their range, creating a Bragg peak. The advantage of protons over photons is that beyond the Bragg peak, protons fall off rapidly and avoid dose deposition beyond the target. This vastly limits radiation dose to normal tissues beyond the target. Because of the cost of protons, few radiotherapy facilities in the United States currently have proton units available for patient treatment. Protons are clearly useful in settings where tumors are adjacent to critical normal tissues such as the eye, brain, or spinal cord. Examples of these tumors include ocular melanoma, chordoma, and other base of skull tumors. As the availability of protons increases across the United States, its applications for other clinical tumors will increase as well.

Neutrons are uncharged heavy particles that are produced by a variety of mechanisms. The most common interaction producing neutrons is by accelerating protons to strike a beryllium target. Neutrons are neutral in charge and lose their energy primarily by striking protons in the cell nucleus. These nuclear events result in recoil protons and charged nuclear fragments that deposit large amounts of energy very close to the site of the initial interaction. Neutrons and protons have a relatively high relative biologic effectiveness (RBE) as compared with photons, meaning they have an efficient cell kill per unit dose. Experience with neutrons has been limited to a few centers because of the cost of producing and maintaining these radiotherapy units. Clinical trials are under way to investigate other areas in which neutrons may provide an advantage over photons. An example of depth-dose characteristics for photons, electrons, protons, and neutrons is shown in Figure 2.1.

Brachytherapy is an alternative method of irradiating targeted tissues. *Brachy* is translated from Greek, meaning short distance. In brachytherapy, sealed or unsealed radioactive sources are placed very close to or in contact with the targeted tissue. Because the absorbed dose falls off rapidly with increasing distance from the source (1/radius^2 for a point source and 1/radius for a line source), higher doses can be delivered safely to the targeted tissue over a short time. Prescribed brachytherapy doses are generally delivered in days for low-dose rate (LDR) or minutes for high-dose rate (HDR). Brachytherapy sources can be placed temporarily, as in the use of iridium

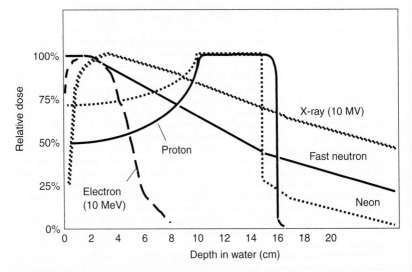

Figure 2.1. Depth–dose curves for photons (x-rays), electrons, protons, and neutrons at energies used in radiation therapy.

192 for HDR applications in cervix cancer, or permanently, as in the use iodine 125 in the treatment of prostate cancer. Unsealed sources are in the liquid state and are used in radiopharmaceutical therapy. An example is iodine 131 for thyroid cancer. Commonly used sealed brachytherapy sources include cesium 137, iridium 192, iodine 125, palladium 103, gold 198, and strontium 90. Commonly used unsealed sources include iodine 131, phosphorus 32, strontium 89, and samarium 153. Some common applications of brachytherapy include the treatment of prostate (both HDR and permanent LDR), breast (mainly HDR), and cervix (both HDR and LDR) cancers.

III. **GOALS OF RADIATION THERAPY.** The clinical use of radiation is a complex process that involves many professionals and a variety of interrelated functions. The aim of therapy should be defined at the beginning of the therapeutic intervention.

A. **Curative.** The patient has a probability of long-term survival after adequate therapy. Oncologists may be willing to risk both acute and chronic complications as a result of therapy in an attempt to eradicate the malignant disease.

B. **Palliative.** There is no hope that the patient will survive for extended periods; symptoms that produce discomfort or an impending condition that may impair the comfort or self-sufficiency of the patient require treatment.

In curative therapy, some side effects, even though undesirable, may be acceptable. However, in palliative treatment, no major side effects should be seen. In palliation of epithelial solid tumors causing complications due to mass effect or pain, relatively high doses of radiation (sometimes 75% to 80% of curative dose) are required to control the tumor for the survival period of the patient. There are some exceptions to high-dose palliative radiotherapy, including patients with lymphoma or multiple myeloma or for treatment of bleeding such as patients with cervical or endobronchial malignancies. Some disease conditions, such as low-grade lymphoma, are long-standing and incurable. These conditions also fall into the palliative category because one is generally willing to sacrifice some long-term tumor control to avoid the development of treatment-related complications.

IV. **BASIS FOR PRESCRIPTION OF RADIATION THERAPY**

A. Evaluation of tumor extent (staging), including radiographic, radioisotope, and other studies

B. Knowledge of the pathologic characteristics of the disease

C. Definition of goal of therapy (cure vs. palliation)

D. Selection of appropriate treatment modalities (irradiation alone or combined with surgery, chemotherapy, or both)

E. Determination of the optimal dose of irradiation and the volume to be treated, according to the anatomic location, histologic type, stage, potential regional nodal involvement, and other characteristics of the tumor, and the normal structures present in the region

F. Evaluation of the patient's general condition, periodic assessment of tolerance to treatment, tumor response, and status of the normal tissues treated

In addition to coordinating the patient's care with the surgical and medical oncology teams, the radiation oncologist must work closely with the physics, treatment-planning, and dosimetry staffs within the radiotherapy facility to ensure the greatest possible accuracy, practicality, and cost benefit in the design of treatment plans. The ultimate responsibility for treatment decisions and the technical execution of the therapy will always rest with the physician.

V. **RADIOBIOLOGIC PRINCIPLES**

A. **Probability of tumor control.** It is axiomatic in radiation therapy that higher doses of radiation produce better tumor control. Numerous dose–response curves for cell killing of a variety of tumors by single dose and multiple repeated-dose radiation have been published. For every increment of radiation dose, a certain fraction of cells will be killed. Therefore the total number of surviving cells will be proportional to the initial number of tumor cells present and the fraction killed with each dose (Fletcher GH. *Textbook of radiotherapy.* Philadelphia: Lea & Febiger, 1980). Therefore, various total doses will yield different probabilities of tumor control, depending on the extent of the lesion (number of clonogenic cells present) and the sensitivity to radiation. Additional factors that affect the efficacy of radiation therapy include repair of radiation damage (to DNA), the presence of hypoxic cells and their reoxygenation, cell cycle checkpoints, and tumor cell repopulation rates.

Subclinical disease has been referred to as deposits of tumor cells that are too small to be detected clinically and even microscopically but, if left untreated, may subsequently evolve into clinically apparent tumor. For subclinical disease in squamous cell carcinoma of the upper respiratory tract or for adenocarcinoma of the breast, doses of 45 to 50 Gy will result in disease control in more than 90% of patients. **Microscopic tumor,** as at the surgical margin, should not be regarded as subclinical disease; cell aggregates of 10^6/cc or greater are required for the pathologist to detect them. Therefore, these volumes must receive higher doses of radiation, in the range of 60 to 65 Gy in 6 to 7 weeks for epithelial tumors.

For **clinically palpable tumors,** doses of 60 (for T1) to 75 to 80 Gy or higher (for T4 tumors) are required (2 Gy/day, five fractions weekly). This dose range and tumor control probability (TCP) have been documented for squamous cell carcinoma and adenocarcinoma (Fletcher GH. *Textbook of radiotherapy.* Philadelphia: Lea & Febiger, 1980). Ideally, the radiation oncologist would have the ability to deliver doses in this range. However, these doses are often beyond the tolerance of normal tissues. Exceeding normal tissue tolerance may result in debilitating or life-threatening complications.

The term **boost volume** is used to describe the residual tumor volume receiving the highest dose of radiation. Baclesse (*Acta Union Int Contra Cancrum* 1959;15:1023–1026) introduced the concept of a boost to describe the additional dose given to the residual tumor after the initial subclinical dose has been delivered. The boost is designed to obtain the same probability of control as for subclinical aggregates (Fletcher GH. *Textbook of radiotherapy.* Philadelphia: Lea & Febiger, 1980). For example, the initial large volume will often receive 45 to 50 Gy, followed by a boost dose of 10 to 30 Gy through small portals.

One consequence of these concepts is the use of portals that are progressively reduced in size ("shrinking field" technique) to administer higher doses of radiation to the central portion of the tumor where more clonogenic cells (presumably hypoxic) are present, in comparison with lesser doses required to eradicate the disease in the periphery, where a lower number and better-oxygenated tumor cells are assumed to be present.

An alternative to the sequential boost (described in the preceding text) is a simultaneous boost. The use of simultaneous boosts has expanded with the use of intensity-modulated radiation therapy (IMRT) (see Section VI. C.). The concept is to deliver two different doses to two different volumes; a slightly higher dose per day to the gross tumor volume (GTV) than that to the microscopic tumor volume. An example of this would be to simultaneously deliver 2.2 Gy per fraction to a head and neck gross tumor and 1.8 Gy per fraction to volumes of possible microscopic tumor.

B. Effects of radiation on normal tissue. A variety of changes in normal tissues are induced by ionizing radiation, depending on the total dose, fractionation schedule (daily dose and time), and volume treated; these factors are closely interrelated (Fig. 2.2). For many normal tissues, the necessary dose to produce a particular sequela increases as the irradiated fraction of volume of the organ decreases (Table 2.1).

As the total dose to a particular tumor and surrounding normal tissues increases, both TCP and normal tissue complication probability (NTCP) increase. Both TCP and NTCP are sigmoidal in shape. The farther these two curves diverge, the more favorable the **therapeutic ratio** (Fig. 2.3). When the curves are close together, increases in irradiation dose will lead to exponential increases in NTCP. The TCP and NTCP curves can be separated by the use of biologic modifiers, radioprotectors, three-dimensional conformal irradiation, or IMRT. When the TCP and NTCP curves are well separated, higher doses of radiation therapy can be delivered more safely. Chemotherapy also modifies the TCP and NTCP curves, often by shifting both curves to the left. Therefore with chemoradiation, lower

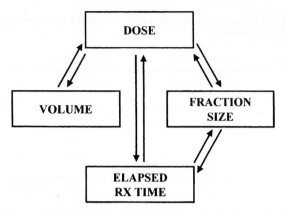

Figure 2.2. Basic dosimetric parameters determining normal tissue effects in radiation therapy. (From Perez CA, Brady LW, Roti JL. Overview. In: Perez CA, Brady LW, eds. *Principles and practice of radiation oncology,* 3rd ed. Philadelphia: Lippincott Williams & Wilkins, 1998:1–17, with permission.)

doses of radiotherapy are required to produce a given TCP/NTCP. Biologic factors can also contribute to the TCP and NTCP. Defects in DNA repair will lower the dose for both curves unless the defect is unique to the tumor. In contrast, defective apoptotic pathways tend to increase radiation resistance.

Higher tolerance doses have been observed than those initially reported for a variety of organs, which stresses the importance of updating this information in the light of more precise treatment planning and delivery of radiation and more accurate evaluation and recording of sequelae (Table 2.2) (*Int J Radiat Oncol Biol Phys* 1991;21:109–122). Burman et al. (*Int J Radiat Oncol Biol Phys* 1991;21:123–135) used these estimates to develop a series of tolerance curves for multiple organs.

Radiation causes cell death by inducing DNA double-strand breaks. The presence of DNA double-strand breaks in cells leads to lethal, sublethal, and potentially lethal damage. Lethal damage is a level of DNA damage that is too much for the cell to repair. *Sublethal damage* is defined as damage that can be repaired when a single dose of x-rays is divided into two or more fractions. Potentially lethal damage is defined as damage that can be repaired or fixed to lethal damage by modifying growth conditions (i.e., cell cycle progression) during or after a dose of x-rays. Sublethal damage repair (SLDR) and potentially lethal damage repair (PLDR) are important concepts in considering normal tissue repair. Normal tissues have a substantial capacity to recover from sublethal or potentially lethal damage induced by radiation (at tolerable dose levels). Injury to normal tissues may be caused by the radiation effect on the microvasculature or the support tissues (stromal or parenchymal cells).

The *minimal tolerance dose* is defined as $TD_{5/5}$, which represents the dose of radiation that could cause no more than a 5% severe complication rate within 5 years of treatment. An acceptable complication rate for severe injury is 5% to 10% in most curative clinical situations. Moderate sequelae are noted in varying proportions (10% to 25% of patients), depending on the dose of radiation given and the organs at risk. The $TD_{5/5}$ for various organs is listed in Table 2.2. These parameters continue to be adjusted as clinical data are obtained from conformal planning systems.

Chronologically, the effects of irradiation have been subdivided into **acute** (first 6 months), **subacute** (second 6 months), or **late,** depending on the time at which they are observed. The gross manifestations depend on the kinetic properties of the cells (slow or rapid renewal) and the dose of radiation given.

TABLE 2.1 **Possible Specific Sequelae of Therapy Discussed in Informed Consent**

Anatomic site	Acute sequelae	Late sequelae
Brain	Earache, headache, dizziness, hair loss, erythema	Hearing loss
		Damage to middle or inner ear
		Pituitary gland dysfunction
		Cataract formation
		Brain necrosis
Head and neck	Odynophagia, dysphagia, hoarseness, xerostomia, dysgeusia, weight loss	Subcutaneous fibrosis, skin ulceration, necrosis
		Thyroid dysfunction, persistent hoarseness, dysphonia, xerostomia, dysgeusia
		Cartilage necrosis
		Osteoradionecrosis of mandible
		Delayed wound healing, fistulae
		Dental decay
		Damage to middle and inner ear
		Apical pulmonary fibrosis
		Rare: myelopathy
Lung and mediastinum, or esophagus	Odynophagia, dysphagia, hoarseness, cough	Progressive fibrosis of lung, dyspnea, chronic cough
	Pneumonitis	Esophageal stricture
	Carditis	Rare: chronic pericarditis, myelopathy
Breast or chest wall	Odynophagia, dysphagia, hoarseness, cough	Fibrosis, retraction of breast
	Pneumonitis (asymptomatic)	Lung fibrosis
	Carditis	Arm edema
	Cytopenia	Chronic endocarditis, myocardial infarction
		Rare: osteonecrosis of ribs
Abdomen or pelvis	Nausea, vomiting	Proctitis, sigmoiditis
	Abdominal pain, diarrhea	Rectal or sigmoid stricture
	Urinary frequency, dysuria, nocturia	Colonic perforation or obstruction
	Cytopenia	Contracted bladder, urinary incontinence, hematuria (chronic cystitis)
		Vesicovaginal fistula
		Rectovaginal fistula
		Leg edema
		Scrotal edema, sexual impotency
		Vaginal retraction or scarring
		Sterilization
		Sexual impotence
		Damage to liver or kidneys
Extremities	Erythema, dry/moist desquamation	Subcutaneous fibrosis
		Ankylosis, edema
		Bone/soft tissue necrosis

From Perez CA, Brady LW, Roti JL, et al. Overview. In: Perez CA, Brady LW, eds. *Principles and practice of radiation oncology,* 3rd ed. Philadelphia, Lippincott Williams & Wilkins, 1998:1–78, with permission.

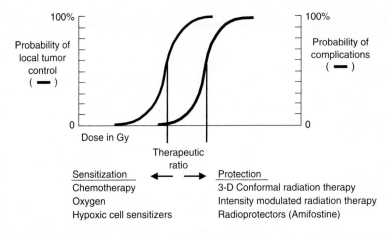

Figure 2.3. The therapeutic ratio represents the relationship between two sigmoidal curves; the tumor control probability (TCP) and the normal tissue complication probability (NTCP) curves. The further the two curves are separated, the higher the TCP and the lower the NTCP.

No correlation has been established between the incidence and severity of acute reactions and the same parameters for late effects (Karcher KH, ed. *Progress in radio-oncology II*. New York: Raven Press, 1982:287–296). This may be due to the difference in the slopes and shapes of cell-survival/dose–response curves for acute or late effects (Steel GE, Adams GE, Peckham MT, eds. *Biological basis of radiotherapy*. Amsterdam: Elsevier Science, 1983:181–194).

Combining irradiation with surgery or cytotoxic agents frequently modifies the tolerance of normal tissues and/or tumor response to a given dose of radiation, which may necessitate adjustments in treatment planning and dose prescription. For example, in curative radiation therapy for cancer of the esophagus, concurrent chemotherapy consisting of 5-fluorouracil (5-FU) and cisplatin and radiation therapy to 50 Gy result in improved local tumor control and similar esophagitis rates when compared with irradiation alone to doses of 64 Gy.

C. Dose–time factors. Dose–time considerations constitute a complex function that expresses the interdependence of total dose, time, and number of fractions in the production of a biologic effect within a given tissue volume (Fig. 2.2).

In general, fractionation of the radiation dose will spare acute reactions due to a given total dose because of SLDR and compensatory proliferation in the epithelium of the skin or the mucosa, which accelerates at 2 or 3 weeks after initiation of therapy (*Br J Radiol* 1973;54:29–35). Therefore, a prolonged course of therapy with small daily fractions will decrease early acute reactions. However, such a strategy will not reduce serious late damage to normal tissue because such effects are not proliferation dependent. Worse, extensively prolonging the treatment time will allow the growth of rapidly proliferating tumors. Therefore, prolonged treatment schedules are undesirable.

Short overall treatment times are required for tumors with rapid proliferation. For median potential doubling times of 5 days and intermediate radiosensitivity, overall times of 2.5 to 4 weeks would be optimal. More slowly proliferating tumors should be treated with longer overall times. With regard to fractionation, Fowler (Steel GE, Adams GE, Peckham MT, eds. *Biological basis of radiotherapy*. Amsterdam: Elsevier Science, 1983:181–194) stated that five fractions per week are preferable to three fractions, because there is approximately 10-fold less cell killing per week with the latter schedule.

Radiation treatments may be delivered by conventional fractionation, hypo-fractionation, hyperfractionation, or accelerated fractionation schedules. In the

| TABLE 2.2 | Normal Tissue Tolerance to Therapeutic Irradiation |

Organ	TD$_{5/5}$ Volume 1/3	2/3	Whole organ	Selected end point
Eye retina I and II	No partial volume	—	4,500	Blindness
Ear mid/external	3,000	3,000	3,000	Acute serous otitis
Ear mid/external	5,500	5,500	5,500	Chronic serous otitis
Parotid I and II	6,500	5,500	4,500	Persistent xerostomia
Larynx	7,900	7,000	7,000	Cartilage necrosis
Larynx	—	4,500	4,500	Laryngeal edema
Lung I	4,500	3,000	1,750	Pneumonitis
Lung II				
Heart	6,000	4,500	7,000	Pericarditis
Esophagus	6,000	5,800	5,500	Clinical stricture/perforation
Stomach	6,000	5,500	5,000	Ulceration, perforation
Small intestine	5,000	—	4,000	Obstruction, perforation/fistula
Colon	6,000	6,000	6,500	Obstruction, perforation/ulceration/fistula
Rectum	7,500	7,000	—	Severe proctitis/necrosis/fistular stenosis
Liver	5,000	3,500	3,000	Liver failure
Kidney	5,000	3,000	2,300	Clinical nephritis
Kidney				
Bladder	8,000	7,500	6,500	Symptomatic bladder contracture and volume loss
Bone				
Femoral head	—	—	5,200	Necrosis
T–M joint mandible	6,500	6,000	6,000	Marked limitation of joint function
Rib cage	6,000	5,500	5,000	Pathologic fracture
Skin	10 cm^2	30 cm^2	100 cm^2	Telangiectasia
	—	—	5,000	
	7,000	6,000	5,500	Necrosis, ulceration
Brain	6,000	5,500	5,500	Necrosis, infarction
Brain stem	6,000	5,500	5,500	Necrosis, infarction
Optic nerves I and II	No partial volume	—	5,000	Blindness
Chiasma	No partial volume	—	5,000	Blindness
Spinal cord	5 cm	10 cm	20 cm	Myelitis, necrosis
	5,000	5,000	4,700	
Cauda equina	No volume effect	—	6,500	Clinically apparent nerve damage
Eyes lens I and II	No partial volume	—	1,000	Cataract requiring intervention

From Emami B, Lyman J, Brown A, et al. Tolerance of normal tissue to therapeutic irradiation. *Int J Radiat Oncol Biol Phys* 1991;21:109–122.
T–M, temporomandibular; TD$_{5/5}$, minimal tolerance dose.

United States, **conventional fractionation** is defined as 30 to 40 fractions delivered once daily over a period of 7 to 8 weeks. Total doses for conventional fractionation are typically in the range of 60 to 75 Gy and are delivered in fraction sizes of 1.8 to 2.0 Gy. The other fractionation schedules are defined by overall treatment duration and total dose of radiation as compared with conventional fractionation.

Hypofractionation refers to a shorter overall treatment duration and a lower total dose designed to achieve the same TCP. For example, in the Manchester system, treatments are delivered in 16 fractions over a 3-week period. The fraction sizes are larger than conventional fractionation and are delivered once daily. Common examples of hypofractionation in the United States are palliative therapy regimens of 30 Gy in 10 fractions over a 2-week period or 10 Gy in a single fraction. The difficulty with hypofractionation is the effect of the larger dose per fraction on normal tissues. Delivering larger fractions of radiation negates the normal tissue-sparing effects of fractionation by decreasing SLDR. The basic rationale of **hyperfractionation** is that the use of small dose fractions of 1.1 to 1.2 Gy allows higher total doses to be delivered over the same treatment duration (as conventional fractionation) within the tolerance of late-responding tissues. Late-responding tissues such as bowel, spinal cord, kidney, lung, and bladder have the same probability of complications with hyperfractionation. However, the patient will experience more acute reactions as a result of the larger total dose. The typical period between daily fractions is 6 hours to allow late tissue repair. An example of hyperfractionation is 69.6 Gy total dose delivered over a 6-week period in twice-daily fractions of 1.2 Gy for head and neck or lung cancer.

The basic rationale for **accelerated fractionation** is that a reduction in overall treatment time decreases the opportunity for tumor cell regeneration during treatment and therefore increases the TCP for a given total dose. Therefore the fraction size is decreased, and the treatment duration is decreased as compared with conventional fractionation. Examples of accelerated fractionation include continuous hyperfractionated accelerated radiation therapy (CHART) delivering 54 Gy in 36 fractions over 12 days for non–small cell lung cancer or delivering 45 Gy in 30 fractions over a 3-week period in small cell lung cancer.

D. **Prolongation of overall treatment time, tumor control, and morbidity.** Treatment interruptions result in a lower TCP for the same total dose received. The total dose of irradiation to produce a given TCP must be increased when fractionation is prolonged beyond 4 weeks because of repopulation of surviving cells, which may result in improved nutrition of those cells after early shrinkage of the tumor due to the initial radiation fractions. Withers et al. (*Acta Oncol* 1988;27:131–146) estimated that the dose of radiation is to be increased by 0.6 Gy for every day of interruption of the treatment. Taylor et al. (*Radiother Oncol* 1990;17:95–102) in 473 patients with squamous cell carcinoma of the head and neck treated with irradiation, estimated an increment in isoeffect dose per day to be larger than 1 Gy (a dose consistent with the Withers estimate of 0.6 Gy).

There is the potential impact of modifying the overall time by *split course* when the daily fractions of radiation administered are higher than with conventional fractionation (administration of 2.5- to 3-Gy tumor dose for 10 fractions, 2 or 3 weeks' rest, and administration of a second course similar to the first one for a total of 50 or 60 Gy). The Radiation Therapy Oncology Group (RTOG) reported no therapeutic advantage with this technique in a variety of studies of head and neck tumors or carcinoma of the uterine cervix, lung, or urinary bladder. Tumor control and survival were comparable to those obtained with conventional fractionation. If anything, the late effects have been slightly greater in the split-course groups.

Conversely, reports published by the University of Florida of patients with carcinoma of the head and neck, uterine cervix, and prostate treated with definitive doses of radiation therapy with conventional fractionation but with a rest period halfway through the course of therapy showed that some groups of patients in the split-course regimen had lower tumor control and survival, probably as a result of the repopulation of clonogenic surviving cells in the tumor during the rest period (*Int J Radiat Oncol Biol Phys* 1980;6:1645–1652; *Int J Radiat Oncol Biol Phys*

1980;6:175–181). The split-course technique has been largely abandoned in the United States.

E. **Linear–quadratic equation (α/β ratio).** Recently formulations based on dose–survival models have been proposed to describe the radiation dose dependence of cell killing. These models are very useful in evaluating the biologic equivalence of various doses and fractionation schedules. These assumptions are based on a linear–quadratic survival curve represented by the equation

$$\ln S = \alpha D + \beta D^2 \text{ for a single dose or } \ln S = \alpha(nd) + \beta(nd)d \qquad (2.1)$$

for a fractionated dose, where n = number of fractions, d = dose/fraction and nd = total dose. In this equation, α represents the linear (i.e., first-order dose dependent) component of cell killing, and β represents the quadratic (i.e., second-order dose dependent) component of cell killing. Thus α represents the less reparable component of lethal radiation damage, i.e., damage, for which the lethality is not reduced by fractionating the radiation dose. Conversely, β represents damage that can be repaired (i.e., its lethality is reduced) when the radiation dose is fractionated. At low doses, the α (linear) component of cell killing predominates. At high doses, the β (quadratic) component of cell killing predominates. The dose at which the two components of cell killing are equal constitutes the α/β ratio. Note that neutrons produce a constant rate of cell kill as opposed to x-rays, because of the negligible contribution of sublethal damage to cell death. Therefore, for neutrons the α component is high, while the β component is close to zero.

In general, tissues reacting immediately to acute effects have a high α/β ratio (between 8 and 15 Gy), whereas tissues involved in late effects have a low α/β ratio (1 to 5 Gy). Therefore the severity of late effects changes more rapidly with a variation in the size of dose per fraction when a total dose is selected to yield equivalent acute effects. With a decreasing size of dose per fraction, the total dose required to achieve a certain isoeffect increases more for late-responding tissues than for immediately responding tissues. Therefore in hyperfractionated regimens, the tolerable dose would be increased more for late effects than for early effects. Conversely, if large doses per fraction are used, the total dose required to achieve isoeffects in late-responding tissues would be reduced more for late effects than for early effects. A biologically equivalent dose (BED) can be obtained by using the following equations, derived from the equation for cell survival after a fractionated dose:

$$\text{BED} = -\ln S/\alpha = nd[1 + d/(\alpha/\beta)] = D[1 + d/(\alpha/\beta)] \qquad (2.2)$$

To compare two treatment regimens, (with some reservations) the following formula can be used:

$$Dx = Dr[(\alpha/\beta + dx)/(\alpha/\beta + dr)] \qquad (2.3)$$

in which Dr is the known total dose (reference dose), Dx is the new total dose (with different fractionation schedule), dr is the known dose per fraction (reference), and dx is the new dose per fraction.

The following is an example of use of this formula (with some reservations!): suppose 50 Gy in 25 fractions is delivered to yield a given biologic effect. If one assumes that the subcutaneous tissue is the limiting parameter (late reaction), it is desirable to know what the total dose to be administered will be, using 4-Gy fractions. Assume α/β = 5 Gy.

Using the earlier equation

$$Dx = 50 \text{ Gy}(5 + 2)/(5 + 4) = 38 \text{ Gy} \qquad (2.4)$$

Answer: A dose of 50 Gy in 25 fractions provides the same BED as 39 Gy in 4-Gy fractions.

VI. RADIATION TREATMENT PLANNING

A. **Introduction to treatment planning.** International Commission on Radiation Units and Measurements (ICRU) No. 50 (*ICRU and 50. Prescribing, Recording, Reporting, Photon Beam Therapy*. Washington, DC: International Commission on Radiation Units and Measurements, 1994) has defined the volumes of interest in treatment planning. The delineation of tumor and target volumes is a crucial step in radiation therapy planning. GTV is all known gross disease including abnormally enlarged regional lymph nodes. When GTV is determined, it is important to use the appropriate computed tomography (CT) window and level settings that give the accurate dimension of what is considered potential gross disease. Other diagnostic imaging studies in addition to CT, such as magnetic resonance imaging (MRI) and positron emission tomography (PET), are valuable tools used by the radiation oncologist to define GTV. Clinical target volume (CTV) encompasses the GTV plus regions considered to harbor potential microscopic disease. Planning target volume (PTV) provides a margin around the CTV to allow variation in treatment setup and other anatomic motion during treatment such as respiration. The PTV does not account for treatment machine beam characteristics. Treatment portals must adequately cover all treatment volumes in addition to a margin to compensate for geometric inaccuracies during radiation exposure.

Simulation has been used in most instances to identify the tumor volume and sensitive structures accurately and to document the configuration of the portals and target volume to be irradiated. Two types of simulation units are used in most clinics. A conventional simulator consists of a table and gantry with 360 degrees of rotation as well as fluoroscopy and diagnostic x-ray capability. Most centers also have a CT simulator, in which patients are positioned for treatment with various immobilization devices; a CT scan is obtained of the area of interest, and contours are delineated (GTV, CTV, and PTV) from the CT images at a computer workstation.

Treatment aids, such as shielding blocks, molds, masks, immobilization devices, and compensators, are extremely important in treatment planning and delivery of optimal dose distribution. Simpler treatment delivery techniques that yield an acceptable dose distribution should be preferred over more costly and complex ones, in which a greater margin of error on a day-to-day treatment basis may be present. Repositioning and immobilization devices are critical because the only effective radiation is that which strikes the clonogenic tumor cells.

Quality assurance is a vital part of every radiotherapy clinic. Localization (portal) films are the primary tools for quality assurance in radiation delivery. The portal film is exposed during treatment delivery and is compared with the corresponding simulator film (reference image). Treatment delivery verification may also be accomplished with on-line imaging (electronic portal imaging) devices (*Int J Radiat Oncol Biol Phys* 1993;27:707–716). Errors detected by portal imaging can be caused by alterations in patient positioning, errors in field size and orientation, or placement and shaping of the beam apertures. Portal films are obtained during the initial treatment setup and weekly thereafter, as recommended by the American Association of Physicists in Medicine (AAPM) Task Group on Comprehensive Clinical Quality Assurance. The frequency of portal imaging may be increased by considering factors such as treatment site, patient weight, and the patient's ability to maintain a fixed position.

Various steps can be taken to decrease toxicity in normal tissues, including precise treatment planning and irradiation techniques, selective decreased volume receiving higher doses dictated by estimated cell burden, and maneuvers to exclude sensitive organs from the irradiated volume. With the emphasis on organ preservation (which is being applied to patients with tumors in the head and neck, breast, and rectosigmoid, and soft tissue sarcomas), treatment planning is critical to achieve maximal TCP and satisfactory cosmetic results.

B. Three-dimensional treatment planning. The CT simulator allows more accurate definition of tumor volume and anatomy of critical normal structures, three-dimensional (3-D) treatment planning to optimize dose distribution, and radiographic verification of volume treated, as is done with conventional simulators (*Int J Radiat Oncol Biol Phys* 1994;30:887–897). Advances in computer technology have augmented accurate and timely computation, display of 3-D radiation dose distributions, and dose–volume histograms (DVHs) (*Semin Radiat Oncol* 1992;2:246–256). These developments have stimulated sophisticated 3-D treatment-planning systems, which yield relevant information in evaluation of tumor extent, definition of target volume, delineation of normal tissues, virtual simulation of therapy, generation of digitally reconstructed radiographs, design of treatment portals and aids (e.g., compensators, blocks), calculation of 3-D dose distributions and dose optimization, and critical evaluation of the treatment plan.

In addition, DVHs are extremely useful as a means of dose display, particularly in assessing several treatment plan dose distributions. They provide a graphic summary of the entire 3-D dose matrix, showing the amount of target volume or critical structure receiving more than a specified dose level. Because they do not provide spatial dose information, they cannot replace the other methods of dose display such as room-view displays, but can only complement them. For example, the DVH may show the percentage PTV receiving the prescribed dose, but cannot locate the portion of the PTV receiving less than the prescribed dose. Treatment verification is another area in which 3-D treatment-planning systems play an important role. Digitally reconstructed radiographs of sequential CT slice data are used to generate a simulation film that can be used to aid in portal localization and comparison with the treatment portal film for verifying treatment geometry.

The increased sophistication in treatment planning requires parallel precision in patient repositioning and immobilization and portal-verification techniques (*Int J Radiat Oncol Biol Phys* 1988;14:777–786). Portal films, used for geometric/topographic verification, are generally of fair quality, making accurate identification of internal landmarks difficult. Several real-time on-line verification systems allow monitoring of the position of the area to be treated during radiation exposure.

Computer-aided integration of the data generated by 3-D radiation treatment planning with parameters used on the treatment machine, including gantry and couch position, may decrease localization errors and enhance the precision and efficiency with which radiation is administered.

Conformal radiation therapy (CRT), including the 3-D technique (3D CRT) and IMRT, represent important advances in the precise delivery of radiation therapy. 3D CRT–planning software is widely available through commercial vendors and represents the standard of care for definitive radiation therapy. 3D CRT–planning systems provide the radiation oncologist with the tools to encompass the entire tumor target, avoid marginal misses, and account for normal tissue dose–volume relations (*Int J Radiat Oncol Biol Phys* 1995;33:979–983; *Int J Radiat Oncol Biol Phys* 2000;46:3–6).

C. Intensity-modulated radiation therapy. This new approach to 3-D treatment planning and conformal therapy optimizes the delivery of radiation to irregularly shaped volumes through a process of complex inverse treatment planning and dynamic delivery of radiation that results in modulated fluence (intensity) of photon beams. By varying the fluence across multiple treatment fields, the radiation dose can be modulated to conform to irregular shapes (i.e., concave) and to design a heterogeneous dose distribution.

Several IMRT hardware and software packages are commercially available including rotational slice-by-slice, dynamic multileaf, static (step and shoot) multileaf, milled compensator, and helical tomotherapy delivery methods. Central to intensity modulation is the development of multileaf collimators (MLCs) and the concept of inverse treatment planning. MLCs are a set of shielding vanes measuring 0.5 to 1 cm wide that are located in the head of the linear accelerator and shape the radiation portal. Each vane is controlled independently and can remain static (static MLC) or move across the treatment field during "beam on" time (dynamic MLC). To understand inverse treatment planning, one must first understand traditional forward treatment planning. Under forward treatment planning, the radiation oncologist draws the radiation portals, considers the dose distribution generated by those portals, and adjusts the portals according to the desired dose distribution. Forward planning is cumbersome. Inverse planning reverses that order. The radiation oncologist contours the desired target volumes and critical structures to be avoided and prescribes an ideal dose distribution. Inverse planning starts with the ideal dose distribution and finds through mathematical optimization algorithms the beam characteristics (fluence profiles) that produce the best approximation of the ideal dose. IMRT is now in widespread clinical use and has clear advantages for treatment of many cancer sites.

The first IMRT technique, rotational slice-by-slice IMRT, was described by Carol et al. (*Int J Radiat Oncol Biol Phys* 1992;24(Suppl 1):158) with modulated photon beams that could be delivered with dynamic MLCs designed to deliver specific doses to irregularly shaped volumes. The expansion of IMRT has brought about rapid development of both IMRT delivery software and the linear accelerator equipment on which the treatments are delivered. Centers delivering IMRT are now using second- and third-generation IMRT planning and delivery systems. Recent developments in the equipment used to deliver IMRT has led to the implementation of image-guided radiation therapy (IGRT). Basically, IGRT consists of the ability to image the patient, or optimally the tumor or a surrogate in some situations, on a daily basis before treatment delivery. These daily images are used for patient positioning before treatment, greatly reducing random and systematic errors in daily localization of tumors and increasing the geographic accuracy of radiation dose delivery. The onboard imaging modality depends on the equipment, but includes ultrasonography, optical (light-based) devices, kV x-ray, kV cone-beam CT, and megavoltage computed tomographic (MVCT) imaging. The advantages of IGRT include, but are not limited to, placing the isocenter for each day's treatment and/or adjusting the treatment volume during the course of radiation therapy. Investigational trials are under way for both IMRT and IGRT. Figure 2.4 contains

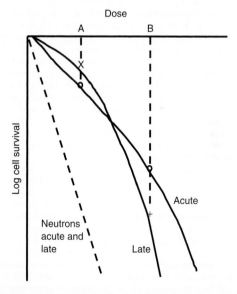

Figure 2.4. Hypothetical survival curves for the target cells for early and late effects in normal tissues exposed to x-rays or neutrons. The α/β ratio is lower for late effects than for early effects in x-irradiated tissues, resulting in a greater change in effect in late-responding tissues with change in dose. At dose A, survival of target cells is higher in late-effect than in early-effect tissues; at dose B, the reverse is true. Increasing the dose per fraction from A to B results in a relatively greater increase in late than acute injury. For neutrons, the α/β ratio is high, with no detectable influence of the quadratic function (βd^2) over the first two decades of reduction in cell survival, implying that accumulation of sublethal injury plays a negligible role in cell killing by doses of neutrons of clinical interest. (From Withers HR, Thames HD, Peters LJ. Biological basis for high RBE values for late effects of neutron irradiation. *Int J Radiat Oncol Biol Phys* 1982;8:2071, with permission.)

images showing two patients with inoperable esophagus cancer. Example A shows a 3-D CRT plan using a combination of four beams. Figure B shows a helical tomotherapy IMRT plan. Note that the high-dose region for the tomotherapy plan is much more conformal than for the more traditional 3D CRT plan.

VII. COMBINATION OF THERAPEUTIC MODALITIES

A. Irradiation and surgery. The rationale for *preoperative radiation therapy* relates to its potential ability to eradicate subclinical or microscopic disease beyond the margins of the surgical resection, to diminish tumor implantation by decreasing the number of viable cells within the operative field, to sterilize lymph node metastases outside the operative field, to decrease the potential for dissemination of clonogenic tumor cells that might produce distant metastases, and to increase the possibility of resectability. The main disadvantage of preoperative irradiation is that it may interfere with normal healing of the tissues affected by the radiation. Such interference, however, is minimal when radiation doses are less than 45 to 50 Gy in 5 weeks.

The rationale for *postoperative irradiation* is based on the fact that it is possible to eliminate any residual tumor in the operative field by destroying subclinical or microscopic foci of tumor cells after the surgical procedure by eradicating adjacent subclinical foci of cancer (including lymph node metastases) and by delivering higher doses than can be achieved with preoperative irradiation, the greater dose being directed to the volume of high-risk or known residual disease.

The potential disadvantages of postoperative irradiation are related to the delay in initiation of radiation therapy until wound healing is completed. Theoretic and experimental evidence suggests that the radiation effect may be impaired by vascular changes produced in the tumor bed by surgery.

B. Irradiation and chemotherapy. Chemotherapy and radiation therapy are combined to obtain an additive or supraadditive effect (Phillips. *Radiation oncology: technology and biology*. Philadelphia: WB Saunders, 1994:113–151). Enhancement describes any increase in effect greater than that observed with either chemotherapy or irradiation alone on the tumor or normal tissues. Calculation of the presence of additivity, supraadditivity, or subadditivity is simple when dose–response curves for irradiation and chemotherapy are linear. When chemotherapeutic agents are used, (as described by Goldie John MJ, Flam MS, et al. eds. *Chemoradiation: an integrated approach to cancer treatment*. Philadelphia: Lea & Febiger, 1993) the agents should not be scross-resistant, and each agent should be quantitatively equivalent to the other.

Chemotherapy alone or combined with irradiation may be used in several settings. **Primary chemotherapy** is used as part of the primary lesion treatment (even if later followed by other local therapy) and when the primary tumor response to the initial treatment is the key identifier of systemic effects. **Adjuvant chemotherapy** is used as an adjunct to other local modalities as part of the initial curative treatment. Frei (*J Natl Cancer Inst* 1989;80:1088–1089), proposed the term **neoadjuvant chemotherapy** when this modality is used in the initial treatment of patients with localized tumors, before surgery or irradiation.

Administration of chemotherapy **before** irradiation produces some cell killing and reduces the number of cells to be eliminated by the irradiation. Use of chemotherapy **during** radiation therapy has a strong rationale because it could interact with the local treatment (additive and even supraadditive action) and could also affect subclinical disease early in treatment. Nevertheless, the combination of modalities may enhance normal tissue toxicity.

C. Integrated multimodality cancer management. Combinations of two or all three of the classic modalities are frequently used to improve tumor control and patient survival. Steel and Peckham (Steel GG, Adams GE, Peckham MJ, eds. *The biological basis of radiotherapy*. The Netherlands: Elsevier Science, 1983:239–248) postulated the biologic basis of cancer therapy as spatial cooperation, in which an agent is active against tumor cells spatially missed by another agent; addition of antitumor effects by two or more agents; and nonoverlapping toxicity and protection of normal tissues. Figure 2.4 illustrates the selective use of a given therapeutic modality to achieve tumor control in each compartment. Large primary tumors or metastatic lymph nodes must be removed surgically or treated with definitive radiation therapy. Regional microextensions are eliminated effectively by irradiation without the anatomic and at times physiologic deficit produced by equivalent medical surgery. Chemotherapy is applied mainly to control disseminated subclinical disease, although it also has an effect on some larger tumors.

Organ preservation is being vigorously promoted, as it enhances the quality of life and psychoemotional feelings of our patients with excellent tumor control and survival, as has been demonstrated in many tumors.

VIII. FOLLOW-UP. Continued support of the patient during therapy is mandatory, with at least one weekly evaluation by the radiation oncologist to assess the effects of treatment on the tumor and the side effects of therapy. Psychological and emotional reinforcement, medications, dietetic counseling, oral cavity care, and skin care instructions are integral parts of the management of these patients and should result in better therapeutic outcome.

IX. QUALITY ASSURANCE. A comprehensive quality assurance program is critical in any radiation oncology center to ensure the best possible treatment for the individual patient and to establish and document all operating policies and procedures.

Quality assurance procedures in radiation therapy will vary, depending on whether standard treatment or a clinical trial is carried out at single or multiple institutions. Particularly in multiinstitutional studies, clear instructions and standardized parameters are needed in dosimetry procedures, treatment techniques, and treatment planning to be carried out by all participants. Many reports of the Patterns of Care Study demonstrate a definite correlation between the quality of the radiation therapy delivered at various types of institutions and the outcome of therapy.

The director of the department appoints the **Quality Assurance Committee**, which meets regularly to review the following: results of review and audit process, physics quality assurance program report, outcome studies, mortality and morbidity conference, any case of "misadministration" or error in delivery of more than 10% of the intended dose, and any chart in which an incident report is filed. Additional details can be obtained from the American College of Radiology.

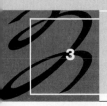

SYSTEMIC CHEMOTHERAPY: SPECIAL CONSIDERATIONS
Lindsay M. Hladnik, Angela R. Wills, and Kristan M. Augustin

I. INTRODUCTION
A. General. Antineoplastic agents have a narrow therapeutic index in which a small change in dose may result in unacceptable toxicity. Pretreatment characteristics including age, performance status, current medications, renal and hepatic function, interpatient pharmacokinetic and pharmacodynamic variability, cachexia, obesity, and other comorbidities impact the efficacy and toxicity profile of many agents administered. In addition, many of the chemotherapeutic agents are extensively metabolized by the cytochrome P-450 enzymes, resulting in the potential for drug interactions and subsequent alterations in chemotherapeutic concentrations. Drug sequencing of antineoplastics may also increase or decrease the antitumor effect or impact the severity of toxicities. Finally, calculation and manipulation of the actual dose to be administered is based on a variety of factors, including body and vial size, as well as previous response and treatment intent. With that in mind, many factors should be considered when determining a patient's chemotherapy dose.

II. CALCULATION OF DOSE
A. General. The dose of cancer chemotherapeutic agents may be based on a flat dose (e.g., imatinib), on body weight (e.g., conditioning regimens for hematopoietic stem cell transplantation), or more frequently standardized utilizing body surface area (BSA) calculations in order to provide consistent exposure of drug. Utilization of BSA is thought to be ideal due to its known relationship between body size and physiologic functions, including blood volume, cardiac output, glomerular filtration rate, and liver blood flow. The hypothesis of calculating the dose based on BSA was to reduce the patient intervariability of systemic exposure to the antineoplastic agent, and limit the toxicity exerted by the drug.

B. Formulas

1. DuBois and DuBois. This formula is the most widely accepted nomogram. It was derived in 1916 by making molds of nine nonobese individuals who varied in age, size, and shape. By trial and error, this formula was derived by using height and weight alone. However, caution should be taken when applying this formula to infants and young adults. It is considered the gold standard for BSA calculations and the basis for many nomograms.

$$BSA\ (m^2) = W^{0.425} \times H^{0.725} \times 0.007184$$
$$W = weight\ (kg) \qquad H = height\ (cm)$$

2. Gehan and George. In 1970, the DuBois and DuBois formula was validated by Gehan and George. The skin surface area of 401 individuals, including a vast number of children, was directly measured at this time. However, it was found that BSA was overestimated by 15% in 15% of the cases. In an effort to simplify the task of calculating the surface area, the authors provide tables and charts to estimate BSA from height and weight.

3. Mosteller. By modifying the equation proposed by Gehan and George, Mosteller et al. provided an equation, which is easy to remember with a slight loss of accuracy of 2%. Although the initial validation was only based on evaluations of adolescent and adult subjects, a subsequent study utilizing infants and children found it to be equally applicable.

$$\text{BSA (m}^2) = \sqrt{\frac{\text{Ht (cm)} \times \text{Wt (kg)}}{3,600}} \qquad \text{BSA (m}^2) = \sqrt{\frac{\text{Ht (in)} \times \text{Wt (lbs)}}{3,131}}$$

4. **Calvert.** Early studies of carboplatin note that the patient's pretreatment renal function impacts the severity of thrombocytopenia observed. Approximately, 70% of the drug is excreted intact and pharmacokinetics suggest that the toxicity and efficacy of carboplatin is dictated primarily by pretreatment glomerular filtration rate (GFR). On the basis of these observations, Calvert et al. validated a simple formula utilizing a targeted area under the curve (AUC) for carboplatin dose calculation in an effort to minimize the toxicity utilizing GFR.

$$\text{Dose (mg)} = \text{AUC (GFR} + 25)$$

C. **Manipulation of doses.** The final dose of cancer chemotherapy administered to a patient not only depends upon patient factors and calculation of the dose, but also upon the treating physician's practice of rounding the dose. It is not uncommon for a dose to be rounded to the nearest convenient dose to be withdrawn from the vial. In addition, rounding to the nearest vial size without impacting healthcare, while conferring a potential cost savings, has been evaluated. Overall, modification of the chemotherapy dose must be done cautiously to prevent a substantial change from the intended dose.

D. **Amputees.** The development of the above equations did not include amputees in the patient sample. Furthermore, some of the formulas found a loss in accuracy in children and short and/or obese patients, thereby questioning the accuracy of applying these same equations to amputees. Although the formulas have not been validated, it is recommended to evaluate the data provided by Colangelo et al. proposing two alternative equations for this patient population.

E. **Obesity.** It was once believed that dosing obese patients on their actual weight would result in increased toxicities secondary to the distribution of lipid soluble drugs into the adipose tissue. Therefore, ideal body weight, an adjusted body weight, or a capped BSA may have been used to calculate the dose to be administered. Although the data are limited, several reports have been published assessing this situation. Overall, it was concluded that there was no increase in toxicity observed in patients with breast, colon, or small cell lung cancer who received doses based on actual weight compared to normal weight patients. Furthermore, manipulation of the dose in obese breast cancer patients who received cyclophosphamide, doxorubicin, and 5-fluorouracil negatively impacted overall survival. Currently, there is no standard approach as to how to handle this situation and it remains a challenge in dosing.

F. **Elderly**. As a person ages, many physiologic changes may take place that influence the effects of the chemotherapy. However, these changes do not take place at the same stage of life for each individual. There are no set guidelines as to how to handle dose calculations in the elderly, but hypoalbuminemia, reduced hepatic and renal blood flow, cardiac function, and other comorbidities need to be considered when determining the treatment plan. In addition, this patient population is frequently on medications that may interact with the efficacy and safety profile of any agent(s) administered.

G. **Hepatic dysfunction.** Several chemotherapeutic agents undergo hepatic metabolism and any alteration in their clearance or the metabolic capacity of the liver may result in potential complications. Data are limited in this situation, and many take the simple approach of assessing liver function by evaluating the total bilirubin. Other laboratory values such as the transaminases, serum alkaline phosphatase and albumin, may also impact systemic exposure and the ability of the liver to handle these medications. Therefore, all hepatic function tests may need to be taken into consideration prior to deciding the final dosing of a chemotherapy regimen.

Although there is little data for combination regimens, there are some agents such as the taxanes, vinca alkaloids, anthracyclines, and irinotecan, which are known to necessitate dose adjustment based on hepatic function. To further complicate the situation, one may find that the liver dysfunction is a result of the tumor and need to determine if dose alteration should be considered at all. Currently, there are no recommendations for dosing chemotherapy drugs for tumor-related liver dysfunction.

H. Renal dysfunction. Several of the chemotherapeutic agents are eliminated through the kidneys and even minor alterations in renal function may impact their safety. Furthermore, the literature is limited to case reports and small case series with regard to end-stage renal disease and the treatment of patients with cancer. The choice and dose of the agent needs to be considered carefully, as well as the method and optimal timing of dialysis in patients with renal dysfunction to assure maximal drug exposure while minimizing toxicity.

Suggested Readings

Arriagada R, Le Chevalier T, Pignon JP, et al. Initial chemotherapeutic doses and survival in patients with limited small-cell lung cancer. *N Engl J Med* 1993;329:1848–1852.

Calvert AH, Newell DR, Gumbrell LA, et al. Carboplatin dosage: prospective evaluation of a simple formula based on renal function. *J Clin Oncol* 1989;7:1748–1756.

Colangelo PM, Welch DW, Rich DS, et al. Two methods for estimating body surface area in adult amputees. *Am J Hosp Pharm* 1984;41:2650–2655.

DuBois D, DuBois EF. A formula to estimate the approximate surface area if height and weight be known. *Arch Intern Med* 1916;17:863–871.

Eklund JW, Trifilio S, Mulcahy MF. Chemotherapy dosing in the setting of liver dysfunction. *Oncology* 2005;19:1057–1063.

Eneman JD, Philips GK. Cancer management in patients with end-stage renal disease. *Oncology* 2005;19:1199–1212.

Gehan EA, George SL. Estimation of human body surface area from height and weight. *Cancer Chemother Rep* 1970;54:225–235.

Meyerhardt JA, Catalano PJ, Haller DG, et al. Influence of body mass index on outcomes and treatment-related toxicity in patients with colon carcinoma. *Cancer* 2003;98:484–495.

Mosteller RD. Simplified calculation of body surface area. *N Engl J Med* 1987;317:1098.

Mosteller RD. More on simplified calculation of body surface area. *N Engl J Med* 1988; 318:1130.

Rosner GL, Hargis JB, Hollis DR, et al. Relationship between toxicity and obesity in women receiving adjuvant chemotherapy for breast cancer: results from Cancer and Leukemia Group B study 8541. *J Clin Oncol* 1996;14:3000–3008.

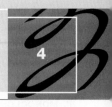

PRINCIPLES OF SYSTEMIC CANCER THERAPY: MOLECULARLY TARGETED THERAPY

Lindsay M. Hladnik, Angela R. Wills, and Kristan M. Augustin

4

I. **BACKGROUND.** Traditional cytotoxic chemotherapy generally affects both rapidly dividing normal and malignant cells. Recent advances in cancer biology have led to the identification of numerous specific molecular targets for drug therapy. These molecular targets often play a key role in the signal transduction pathways that regulate tumor cell growth, proliferation, migration, angiogenesis, and apoptosis. *Molecularly targeted therapy* is a broad term encompassing several classes of agents, including tyrosine kinase inhibitors and monoclonal antibodies (MAb).

II. **TYROSINE KINASE INHIBITORS**

A. **Tyrosine kinases.** Tyrosine kinases catalyze the transfer of γ-phosphate from adenosine triphosphate (ATP) to tyrosine residues in protein targets. They play a key role in the transduction of signals within cellular signaling cascades that are ultimately responsible for the regulation of gene transcription within the nucleus. Tyrosine kinases are further classified into receptor or nonreceptor tyrosine kinases.

1. **Receptor tyrosine kinases.** Receptor tyrosine kinases assist in the transmission of signals from extracellular ligands to the cell nucleus. They are composed of a ligand-binding extracellular domain, a lipophilic transmembrane domain, and an intracellular domain containing a catalytic site. Receptor tyrosine kinases are unphosphorylated, monomeric, and inactive without the presence of ligand.

Ligand binding to the extracellular domain induces dimerization of the tyrosine kinase. This, in turn, leads to autophosphorylation of the intracellular domain, converting the tyrosine kinase to an active state. More specifically, when the intracellular domain undergoes autophosphorylation, binding sites for signaling proteins are formed. These signaling proteins are recruited to the membrane and subsequently multiple downstream signaling cascades are activated. Signals are conveyed from the cell membrane to the nucleus, resulting in alterations of DNA synthesis and cell growth, proliferation, migration, angiogenesis, and apoptosis. Examples of receptor tyrosine kinases include epidermal growth factor receptor (EGFR) (ErbB/HER) family members, vascular endothelial growth factor receptors (VEGFR), and platelet-derived growth factor receptors α and β (PDGFR α and β).

2. **Nonreceptor tyrosine kinases.** Nonreceptor tyrosine kinases play a role in the conveyance of intracellular signals. They lack the transmembrane domain and are primarily located intracellularly. More specifically, they are found on the inner surface of the plasma membrane, cytosol, and nucleus. Inhibitory proteins and lipids and intramolecular autoinhibitory mechanisms maintain the nonreceptor tyrosine kinases in an inactive state. Activation may occur by intracellular signals causing a disassociation of the inhibitory proteins and lipids, by other kinases causing phosphorylation, or by the recruitment of the tyrosine kinase to transmembrane receptors causing subsequent oligomerization and autophosphorylation of the tyrosine kinase. Similar to receptor tyrosine kinases, the nonreceptor tyrosine kinases activate multiple signaling pathways. Examples of nonreceptor tyrosine kinases include BCR-ABL, c-KIT, and c-Src.

B. **Functional alterations of tyrosine kinases in cancer.** Within tumor cells, there is a loss of tyrosine kinase regulation. The dysregulation of tyrosine kinases within cancer cells may occur through numerous mechanisms. Proteins may be fused to tyrosine kinases resulting in constant oligomerization, autophosphorylation, and activation. This typically occurs as the result of chromosomal translocations, with

33

one of the most common examples being the formation of the BCR-ABL oncogene as a result of t(9;22) in chronic myeloid leukemia (CML). Other mechanisms described in the literature include mutations causing interruptions in the autoregulation of tyrosine kinases; abnormal expression of receptor tyrosine kinases, their associated ligands, or both; or a decrease in the processes that regulate tyrosine kinase activity, thereby causing an increase in tyrosine kinase activity. Through the action of tyrosine kinase inhibitors, unregulated tyrosine kinases and often multiple signaling pathways are inactivated, leading to a decrease in tumor cell growth, proliferation, migration, angiogenesis, and/or apoptosis.

III. MONOCLONAL ANTIBODIES

A. Background. Monoclonal antibodies (MAbs) are targeting agents that recognize cell surface proteins/receptors as antigens, particularly on the surface of tumor cells. There are three main classes of MAbs: unconjugated, conjugated, and radioimmunoconjugates.

Unconjugated MAbs directly affect signaling pathways by inhibiting ligand–receptor interactions. These are MAbs against either the receptor or its ligand. They may also indirectly stimulate host defense mechanisms, such as antibody-dependent cellular cytotoxicity (ADCC) or complement-mediated lysis, causing antitumor activity. Examples of unconjugated MAbs include rituximab, trastuzumab, cetuximab, alemtuzumab, and bevacizumab. Conjugated MAbs are MAbs combined with protein toxins or cytotoxic agents. These directly disrupt protein synthesis and cause tumor cell death. Examples of conjugated MAbs include gemtuzumab ozogamicin and denileukin diftitox. Radioimmunoconjugates are MAbs in combination with radioisotopes intended to deliver a sterilizing dose of radiation to the tumor and include ibritumomab tiuxetan and tositumomab.

Antibodies, or immunoglobulins, are Y-shaped molecules containing four chains—two identical light chains and two identical heavy chains. There is a fragment antigen binding (Fab) and a fragment crystalline (Fc) portion of the antibody. The Fab portion contains variable regions, including complementarity-determining regions (CDR), which enable the antibody to bind to a specific antigen. The Fc portion contains constant regions, which are identical in all immunoglobulins of the same isotype (i.e., IgA, IgG, IgM) and function as binding sites for leukocytes and complement.

MAbs may be manufactured from multiple sources of B lymphocytes (i.e., murine, human, primate). Murine MAbs are derived entirely from mice. Chimeric MAbs are composed of a murine variable region of the antibody with a constant region derived from humans, making approximately 65% to 90% of the agent of human origin. Humanized MAbs consist of variable and constant regions derived from humans with CDR derived from mice, making approximately 95% of the agent of human origin. Primatized MAbs contain variable regions from monkeys and constant regions from humans. Human MAbs are derived entirely from humans. MAbs are often manufactured by genetic manipulation to produce a humanized agent. Humanization of the agent decreases the immunogenicity of the MAb, thereby decreasing the production of human antimouse antibodies (HAMAs). HAMAs have the potential to inactivate and eliminate pure murine MAbs after repeated administration, decreasing the half-life of the agent. But HAMAs may also contribute to allergic reactions after the formation of antibody–HAMAs complexes. Pure murine MAbs also ineffectively stimulate host defense mechanisms, such as ADCC and complement-mediated lysis, due to differences between murine and human immune systems.

The United States Adopted Names (USAN) Council has developed guidelines for the nomenclature of MAbs for standardization purposes and to enable identification of the MAb composition for patient safety intent because of the potential for the development of source-specific antibodies. In general, the product source identifiers precede the suffix –*mab*. Also incorporated into the product name is a code syllable for the target disease state of the agent. Refer to Tables 4.1 and 4.2 for a list of product source identifiers and code syllables for the target disease states. Specific guidelines also exist for the nomenclature of radiolabeled and other conjugated MAbs.

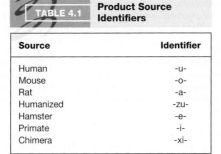

TABLE 4.1 Product Source Identifiers

Source	Identifier
Human	-u-
Mouse	-o-
Rat	-a-
Humanized	-zu-
Hamster	-e-
Primate	-i-
Chimera	-xi-

IV. MOLECULAR TARGETS IN ONCOLOGY

A. BCR-ABL tyrosine kinase inhibition. The BCR-ABL tyrosine kinase is formed by the fusion of the BCR gene on chromosome 22 and the c-ABL tyrosine kinase gene on chromosome 9. This fusion protein forms as a result of the chromosomal t(9;22), or the Philadelphia chromosome, which has been implicated in approximately 95% of adult patients with CML, 15% to 20% of adult patients with acute lymphocytic leukemia (ALL), and 5% of adult patients with acute myeloid leukemia (AML). Subsequently, there is constitutive activation of the tyrosine kinase leading to the activation of several transduction pathways resulting in dysregulated cell proliferation and an inhibition of apoptosis. Imatinib inhibits the BCR-ABL tyrosine kinase, but also has inhibitory effects on other tyrosine kinases including c-KIT and PDGFRα and β. The effects of imatinib on these other tyrosine kinases have shown efficacy in the treatment of other malignancies, including gastrointestinal stromal tumors (GISTs), most of which have mutations in c-KIT or PDGFRα. Dasatinib also has inhibitory effects on BCR-ABL as well as several other tyrosine kinases. This agent displays approximately 325-fold more potency than imatinib against ABL and has activity against imatinib-resistant BCR-ABL mutations.

1. Imatinib (Gleevec)

   a. FDA-approved indications. Philadelphia chromosome–positive CML; *c-KIT* (CD117)-positive unresectable and/or metastatic malignant GISTs.

   b. Pharmacology. Tyrosine kinase inhibitor.

   i. Mechanism. Inhibits BCR-ABL tyrosine kinase, which blocks proliferation and causes apoptosis in BCR-ABL positive cell lines; inhibits stem cell factor (SCF; *c-KIT*) receptor tyrosine kinases, which inhibit proliferation and cause apoptosis in GIST cells that express *c-KIT* mutations; inhibits PDGFRα and β tyrosine kinases.

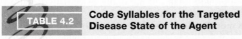

TABLE 4.2 Code Syllables for the Targeted Disease State of the Agent

Disease		Tumor	
Viral	-vir-	Colon	-col-
Bacterial	-bac-	Melanoma	-mel-
Immune	-lim-	Mammary	-mar-
Infectious Lesions	-les-	Testis	-got-
Cardiovascular	-cir-	Ovary	-gov-
		Prostate	-pr(o)-
		Miscellaneous	-tum-

ii. **Metabolism.** Hepatic metabolism through CYP 3A4 to active metabolite (N-demethylated piperazine derivative). Eliminated primarily in the feces (68%) with some urinary excretion (13%) as metabolite and unchanged drug.

c. **Toxicity**

i. **Common.** Nausea, vomiting, diarrhea, erythema multiforme rash, fluid retention/edema, fatigue, pyrexia, headache, hepatotoxicity, hemorrhage, myelosuppression, arthralgia, myalgia, cough, dyspnea.

ii. **Occasional.** Alopecia, gastrointestinal (GI) hemorrhage, ascites, increased transaminases and/or bilirubin, blurred vision, conjunctivitis, pruritus, chest pain, upper respiratory tract infection.

iii. **Rare.** Central nervous system (CNS) hemorrhage, angioedema, aplastic anemia, migraine, pulmonary fibrosis, Stevens-Johnson syndrome, syncope, electrolyte disturbances, and peripheral neuropathy.

d. **Administration**

i. **FDA-approved dose.** Chronic phase CML dose is 400 mg orally daily, may be increased to 600 mg daily. Accelerated phase or blast crisis dose is 600 mg once daily, may be increased to 800 mg daily (400 mg twice daily). Dosing for GIST is 400 to 600 mg daily.

ii. **Dose modification.** Dose adjust for hepatic impairment, hematologic and hepatotoxic adverse events, inadequate hematologic or cytogenetic response.

iii. **Supplied** as 100- and 400-mg tablets.

2. **Dasatinib (Sprycel)**

a. **FDA-approved indications.** CML in chronic, accelerated, or blast phase in patients resistant or intolerant to prior therapy including imatinib; Philadelphia chromosome-positive ALL with resistance or intolerance to prior therapy.

b. **Pharmacology.** Tyrosine kinase inhibitor.

i. **Mechanism.** Multitargeted tyrosine kinase inhibitor affecting BCR-ABL, the SRC family, c-KIT, EPHA2, and PDGFR-β kinases; binds to both active and inactive ABL kinase domains.

ii. **Metabolism.** Extensive hepatic metabolism through CYP 3A4. Primarily fecal elimination. 0.1% and 19% of the dose eliminated unchanged in the urine and feces, respectively.

c. **Toxicity**

i. **Common.** Myelosuppression, fluid retention/edema, nausea, vomiting, diarrhea, abdominal pain, headache, hemorrhage, chest pain, arrhythmia, fatigue, pyrexia, rash, pruritus, mucositis, constipation, myalgia, arthralgia, dyspnea, cough, infection, and neuropathy.

ii. **Occasional.** Congestive heart failure, pericardial effusion, pulmonary edema, ascites, febrile neutropenia, electrolyte abnormalities, elevated transaminases.

iii. **Rare.** QTc prolongation, elevated bilirubin.

d. **Administration**

i. **FDA-approved dose.** 70 mg orally twice daily (total dose of 140 mg daily) with or without food.

ii. **Dose modification.** Dose adjustment for hematologic toxicity or other nonhematologic adverse events. Consider when administered with strong CYP 3A4 enzyme inducers or inhibitors, or if inadequate hematologic or cytogenetic response.

iii. **Supplied** as 20-, 50-, and 70-mg tablets.

B. **EGFR** *targeting.* The EGFR is one of four tyrosine kinase receptors within the ErbB receptor family—ErbB1 (EGFR/HER1), ErbB2 (HER2/neu), ErbB3 (HER3), and ErbB4 (HER4). Several malignancies have been associated with an overexpression or alteration of EGFR and include head and neck, esophageal, gastric, pancreatic, colorectal, renal cell, prostate, breast, bladder, ovarian, and cervical cancers, as well as non–small cell lung cancer (NSCLC) and glioblastoma.

Activation of these receptor tyrosine kinases result in multiple downstream signaling pathways being activated including the Ras/Raf mitogen-activated protein kinase (MAPK) pathway, the phosphatidylinositol 3'-kinase (PI3K)/Akt pathway, the protein kinase C pathway, and the Janus kinase (JAK)/signal transducer and activator of transcription (STAT) pathway. These pathways affect cell proliferation, migration, differentiation, and inhibit apoptosis. The activation of EGFR also causes an upregulation of vascular endothelial growth factor (VEGF) expression, leading to an increase in angiogenesis.

EGFR tyrosine kinase inhibitors are small molecules that bind to the ATP-binding site on the tyrosine kinase domain of the receptor and inhibit the catalytic activity of the kinase or they may inhibit fusion tyrosine kinases by blocking dimerization. The available EGFR tyrosine kinase inhibitors include erlotinib and gefitinib. The EGFR-targeting MAb available, cetuximab, inhibits ligand binding to the receptor.

1. **Erlotinib (Tarceva)**
   a. **FDA-approved indications.** Refractory locally advanced or metastatic NSCLC; in combination with gemcitabine for locally advanced, unresectable, or metastatic pancreatic cancer.
   b. **Pharmacology.** Tyrosine kinase inhibitor.
      i. **Mechanism.** Inhibits intracellular phosphorylation of the EGFR tyrosine kinase.
      ii. **Metabolism.** Extensive hepatic metabolism primarily through CYP 3A4. Eliminated primarily by feces (83%) with a small amount in the urine (8%).
   c. **Toxicity**
      i. **Common.** GI upset (diarrhea, nausea, vomiting, anorexia), mucositis, dermatologic toxicity (acneform rash, erythematous rash, maculopapular dermatitis, dry skin, pruritus), fatigue, headache, depression, dizziness, insomnia, dyspnea, cough, infection, edema, eye irritation/conjunctivitis, elevated hepatic transaminases and/or bilirubin.
      ii. **Occasional.** Deep vein thrombosis, myocardial infarction/ischemia, cerebrovascular events, ileus, pancreatitis.
      iii. **Rare.** Corneal ulcerations, epistaxis, GI bleeding, interstitial lung disease–like events, and hemolytic anemia.
   d. **Administration**
      i. **FDA-approved dose.** Dose for NSCLC is 150 mg orally once daily. Dose for pancreatic cancer is 100 mg orally once daily in combination with gemcitabine. Administer at least 1 hour before or 2 hours after food.
      ii. **Dose modification.** No adjustment for renal impairment. May need to dose adjust if severe liver impairment exists. Dose modifications may be made for intolerance or concomitant CYP 3A4 inhibitor or inducer administration.
      iii. **Supplied** as 25-mg, 100-mg, 150-mg tablets.
2. **Gefitinib (Iressa)**
   a. **FDA-approved indications.** Locally advanced or metastatic NSCLC after failure of both platinum-based and docetaxel therapies. Clinical trials have failed to demonstrate a survival benefit with gefitinib. Physicians are encouraged to use other agents. Gefitinib is only available through a risk-management plan known as the IRESSA Access Program. Its use is limited to patients who have received and benefited from, or are currently receiving and benefiting from the drug; patients previously enrolled or new patients in non-Investigational New Drug (non-IND) clinical trials involving gefitinib if the protocol was approved by an Institutional Review Board (IRB) prior to June 15, 2005; or new patients if the manufacturer makes gefitinib available under an investigational new drug (IND) and the patients meet the criteria for enrollment under the IND.

    b. Pharmacology. Tyrosine kinase inhibitor.
      i. Mechanism. Inhibits intracellular phosphorylation of EGFR tyrosine kinases.
      ii. Metabolism. Extensive hepatic metabolism through CYP 3A4 to five metabolites (only active metabolite is O-desmethyl gefitinib). Excreted primarily by the feces (86%) with minimal renal elimination (<4%).
    c. Toxicity
      i. Common. Acneform rash, erythema multiforme rash, dry skin, GI upset (diarrhea, nausea, vomiting, anorexia), and pruritus.
      ii. Occasional. Amblyopia, conjunctivitis, dyspnea, interstitial lung disease, weight loss, increased transaminases and alkaline phosphatase, and edema.
      iii. Rare. Hypersensitivity reactions (angioedema, urticaria), corneal erosion/ulceration sometimes in association with aberrant eyelash growth, corneal membrane sloughing, toxic epidermal necrosis, pancreatitis, ocular ischemia and/or hemorrhage.
    d. Administration
      i. FDA-approved dose. 250 mg orally once daily with or without food.
      ii. Dose modification. Interruption of therapy may be necessary if pulmonary decompensation, diarrhea, adverse skin reaction, eye pain, or hepatic injury occurs. No adjustment is necessary for renal and/or hepatic impairment. May need to increase dose to 500 mg orally once daily in patients receiving CYP3A4 inducers (rifampin, phenytoin).
      iii. Supplied as 250-mg tablets.
  3. Cetuximab (Erbitux)
    a. FDA-approved indications. Metastatic colorectal cancer; squamous cell carcinoma of the head and neck.
    b. Pharmacology. Chimeric MAb.
      i. Mechanism. Binds to the extracellular domain of the EGFR inhibiting the binding of endothelial growth factor (EGF) to the receptor; inhibits cell growth and metastasis, induces apoptosis, inhibits VEGF production, causes ADCC, and downregulates EGFR.
      ii. Metabolism. Elimination through EGFR binding/internalization.
    c. Toxicity
      i. Common. Dermatologic toxicities (acneform rash, skin drying and fissuring, inflammatory/infectious reactions), malaise, fever, hypomagnesemia, nausea, constipation, abdominal pain, diarrhea, headache, weakness, cough, peripheral edema, alopecia, and anemia.
      ii. Occasional. Sepsis, pulmonary embolism, kidney failure, dehydration, conjunctivitis, infusion-related reactions, and cardiopulmonary arrest.
      iii. Rare. Interstitial lung disease, leukopenia.
    d. Administration
      i. FDA-approved dose. Initial loading dose: 400 mg/m^2 intravenously on day 1. Maintenance dose: 250 mg/m^2 intravenously once a week starting on day 8.
      ii. Dose modification. Dose adjustment for toxicities. No adjustment needed for renal or hepatic impairment.
      iii. Supplied as 100-mg vials.
C. HER2 targeting. The human epidermal growth factor receptor 2 (HER2) is a member of the ErbB receptor family, which includes ErbB1/EGFR/HER1, ErbB3/HER3, and ErbB4/HER4. HER2 is the only one out of the four ErbB receptors that does not have a known ligand. Interactions between the other HER-family members and the extracellular domain of HER2 result in the formation of heterodimer complexes after ligand binding. Therefore, the primary role of HER2 is as a coreceptor, facilitating signal transduction after ligand binding to other HER family members. Activation of HER2 may also occur by homodimerization. The HER2 intracellular domain displays tyrosine kinase activity upon activation and regulates cell growth, differentiation, and migration. Amplification of the *HER2/neu* oncogene results in overexpression

of HER2, which occurs in approximately 20% to 30% of breast cancer tumors. HER2-overexpressing breast cancers generally have a worse prognosis than nonoverexpressing breast tumors. Trastuzumab is a humanized MAb against HER2.

1. **Trastuzumab (Herceptin)**
   a. **FDA-approved indications.** Metastatic breast cancer whose tumors overexpress the HER-2/*neu* protein.
   b. **Pharmacology.** Humanized MAb.
      i. **Mechanism.** Binds to the extracellular domain of the HER2/*neu* protein. It mediates several intracellular effects including internalization of the HER2 receptor and downregulation of surface HER2 expression; alters downstream signaling pathways and leads to a decrease in cell proliferation and VEGF production, induces apoptosis, and potentiates chemotherapy. It also causes several extracellular effects including interference with homodimer and heterodimer formation between HER-family receptors and induces antibody-dependent cellular toxicity against cells that overproduce HER2.
      ii. **Metabolism.** Elimination through internalization after receptor binding.
   c. **Toxicity**
      i. **Common.** Infusion-related reactions (fever, chills), rash, headache, diarrhea, myelosuppression, and infections.
      ii. **Occasional.** Left ventricular dysfunction, cardiomyopathy, congestive heart failure, and arthralgia.
      iii. **Rare.** Severe hypersensitivity reactions (anaphylaxis, urticaria, bronchospasm, angioedema, and/or hypotension), severe infusion-related reactions (fever, chills, nausea, vomiting, pain at the tumor site, headache, dizziness, dyspnea, hypotension, rash, asthenia), pulmonary events (dyspnea, pulmonary infiltrates, pleural effusions, noncardiogenic pulmonary edema, pulmonary insufficiency and hypoxia, acute respiratory distress syndrome (ARDS), pneumonitis, and pulmonary fibrosis).
   d. **Administration**
      i. **FDA-approved dose.** Initial loading dose is 4 mg/kg intravenously on day 1. Maintenance dose is 2 mg/kg intravenously once weekly starting on day 8.
      ii. **Dose modification.** None recommended.
      iii. **Supplied** as a 440-mg vial.
D. **VEGF** *targeting.* VEGF is a member of the PDGF family. Several ligands for VEGFRs exist including VEGF-A through -E and placenta growth factor. These ligands are capable of binding to various VEGFRs that are expressed on vascular endothelial cells. Binding to VEGFR-1 (Flt-1; Fms-like tyrosine kinase-1) induces endothelial cell migration. Binding to VEGFR-2 (KDR) stimulates endothelial cell proliferation, antiapoptotic effects, and vascular permeability. This receptor is primarily responsible for the activation of the tyrosine kinase domains once ligands are bound.

Binding to VEGFR-3 (Flt-4) induces lymphangiogenesis. VEGF also plays a key role in the induction of angiogenesis, or the growth of new blood vessels from existing vasculature, which helps sustain tumor growth and survival by supplying nutrients and oxygen. The overexpression of VEGF occurs in various tumor types including colorectal, breast, cervical, endometrial, gastric, renal, pancreatic, and hepatic cancers, and NSCLC, melanoma, glioblastoma, and AML. Several factors may upregulate VEGF expression including hypoxia, acidosis, embryogenesis, endometriosis, wound healing and various growth factors (PDGF, fibroblast growth factor [FGF], epidermal growth factor [EGF], tumor necrosis factor [TNF], transforming growth factor beta, interleukin 1 [IL-1]). Within tumor cells, hypoxia is the key mediator of VEGF overexpression. Agents with effects on VEGF/VEGFRs include sunitinib and bevacizumab.

1. **Sunitinib (Sutent)**
   a. **FDA-approved indications.** GIST after disease progression on or intolerance to imatinib; advanced renal cell cancer.

   b. Pharmacology. Tyrosine kinase inhibitor.
   i. Mechanism. Inhibits multiple tyrosine kinases including VEGFR 1, 2, and 3; SCF receptor (*c-KIT*); PDGFR α and β; and Fms-like tyrosine kinase-3 (Flt-3).
   ii. Metabolism. Hepatic through CYP 3A4 to the active *N*-desethyl metabolite SU12662. Primarily excreted in the feces (61%) with a small amount excreted renally (16%).
   c. Toxicity
   i. Common. Hypertension, rash, hand-foot syndrome, alopecia, skin discoloration (yellow-orange), hair pigmentation changes, dry skin, diarrhea, nausea, vomiting, mucositis/stomatitis, constipation, dyspepsia, dyspnea, cough, edema, fever, fatigue, hyperuricemia, increased liver function tests (LFTs), increased amylase/lipase, myelosuppression, arthralgia, myalgia, increased serum creatinine, decreased left ventricular ejection fraction (LVEF), and hemorrhage.
   ii. Occasional. Electrolyte disturbances, hypothyroidism, oral pain, thromboembolism, myocardial ischemia/infarction, anorexia, and peripheral neuropathy.
   iii. Rare. Febrile neutropenia, pancreatitis, reversible posterior leukoencephalopathy syndrome, and seizure.
   d. Administration
   i. FDA-approved dose. 50 mg orally once daily with or without food for 4 weeks in a 6-week treatment cycle (4 weeks on, 2 weeks off).
   ii. Dose modification. Dose reductions to 37.5 mg daily should be considered with concomitant use of strong CYP 3A4 inhibitors. Dosage increases to 87.5 mg daily should be considered with concomitant use of strong CYP 3A4 inducers.
   iii. Supplied as 12.5-, 25-, and 50-mg capsules.
2. Bevacizumab (Avastin)
   a. FDA-approved indications. Treatment of metastatic colorectal cancer (in combination with fluorouracil).
   b. Pharmacology. Humanized MAb.
   i. Mechanism. Recombinant, humanized MAb that binds to and neutralizes VEGF.
   c. Toxicity
   i. Common. Hypertension, headache, abdominal pain, nausea, vomiting, diarrhea, anorexia, constipation, proteinuria, leukopenia, weakness, exfoliative dermatitis, stomatitis, epistaxis, dyspnea, upper respiratory infection, and wound healing.
   ii. Occasional. Venous thromboembolic events, hemorrhagic events, GI perforation, arterial thromboembolic events, left ventricular dysfunction, and infusion-related reactions.
   iii. Rare. CNS hemorrhage, nephrotic syndrome.
   d. Administration
   i. FDA-approved dose. 5 mg/kg intravenously every 2 weeks (in combination with bolus-IFL); 10 mg/kg intravenously every 2 weeks (in combination with FOLFOX4).
   ii. Dose modification. Temporary suspension of therapy is warranted in patients with moderate or severe proteinuria or severe, uncontrolled hypertension. Permanent discontinuation is recommended for wound dehiscence requiring intervention, GI perforation, hypertensive crisis, serious bleeding, severe arterial thromboembolic events, or nephrotic syndrome.
   iii. Supplied as 100- and 400-mg vials.
E. Raf tyrosine kinase inhibition. The Raf/mitogen extracellular kinase (MEK)/extracellular signal-related kinase (ERK) signal transduction pathway is overactivated in different cancers including thyroid, hepatocellular, pancreatic, colorectal, ovarian, prostate, breast, and kidney tumors, as well as in NSCLC, AML, and melanoma. Once extracellular ligands such as transforming growth factor alpha (TGF-α),

EGF, VEGF, and PDGF-β bind to their respective receptors, the Raf/MEK/ERK pathway is activated. The pathway transmits signals from the cell surface through autophosphorylation to the nucleus. The Raf/MEK/ERK pathway is involved in the regulation of proliferation, differentiation, survival, angiogenesis, metastasis, and adhesion. Various Raf isoforms exist and sorafenib has shown inhibitory effects on several of the Raf kinases.

1. **Sorafenib (Nexavar)**
   a. **FDA-approved indication.** Advanced renal cell carcinoma.
   b. **Pharmacology.** Multitargeted tyrosine kinase inhibitor.
      i. **Mechanism.** Inhibits several intracellular Raf kinases including C-Raf, wild-type B-Raf, and mutant B-Raf. Also inhibits several cell surface kinases including VEGFR2 and 3, PDGFR-β, c-KIT, and Flt-3. These inhibitory effects decrease tumor cell proliferation and angiogenesis.
      ii. **Metabolism.** Hepatic metabolism primarily through CYP 3A4 and glucuronidation by UGT1A9. Elimination occurs primarily by the fecal route (77%; 51% as unchanged drug); 19% of the dose undergoes urinary excretion.
   c. **Toxicity**
      i. **Common.** Rash, hand-foot syndrome, diarrhea, hypertension, elevations in amylase/lipase, bleeding events, fatigue, hypophosphatemia, alopecia, pruritus, dry skin, diarrhea, nausea, vomiting, constipation, dyspnea, cough, myelosuppression, and neuropathy.
      ii. **Occasional.** Cardiac ischemia/infarction, mucositis/stomatitis, and dyspepsia.
      iii. **Rare.** GI perforation, thromboembolism.
   d. **Administration**
      i. **FDA-approved dose.** 400 mg by mouth twice daily (total daily dose of 800 mg) without food.
      ii. **Dose modification.** Modifications recommended for skin toxicities. No adjustments in mild or moderate renal impairment; not studied in severe renal dysfunction or dialysis. No adjustments necessary for Child-Pugh Class A or B hepatic dysfunction; not studied in Child-Pugh Class C.
      iii. **Supplied** as 200-mg tablets.

V. *Other targets*
   A. **Unconjugated monoclonal antibodies**
      1. **Alemtuzumab (Campath)**
         a. **FDA-approved indication.** B-cell chronic lymphocytic leukemia (CLL).
         b. **Pharmacology.** Humanized MAb.
            i. **Mechanism.** Binds to CD52 resulting in complement-mediated and/or antibody-dependent cellular cytotoxicity.
            ii. **Metabolism.** Initial half-life is 11 hours but increases to 6 days after repeated dosing (due to depletion of CD52-positive cells).
         c. **Toxicity**
            i. **Common.** Hypotension, fever, chills, headache, rash, nausea, vomiting, diarrhea, rigors, chest pain, dyspnea, pharyngitis, infection, neutropenia, thrombocytopenia, and anemia.
            ii. **Occasional.** Pancytopenia, autoimmune idiopathic thrombocytopenia, and hemolytic anemia.
            iii. **Rare.** Pulmonary fibrosis, bone fracture, tumor lysis syndrome, and electrolyte disturbances.
         d. **Administration**
            i. **FDA-approved dose.** Initial dose is 3 mg intravenously once daily, which is then increased to 10 mg intravenously once daily as tolerated. Once the 10-mg dose is tolerated, the dose is increased to 30 mg intravenously once daily. Most patients can tolerate dose escalation in 4 to 7 days. The maintenance dose is 30 mg intravenously once daily, three times per week, on alternate days for a duration of 12 weeks. If therapy is

interrupted for more than 7 days, dose escalation should gradually be reinitiated.

   ii. Dose modification. Hematologic toxicities.

   iii. Supplied as 30-mg vials.

2. Rituximab (Rituxan)

   a. FDA-approved indications. Relapsed or refractory low-grade or follicular CD20-positive, B-cell non-Hodgkin's lymphoma (NHL); diffuse large B-cell CD20-positive NHL.

   b. Pharmacology. Chimeric murine/human MAb.

      i. Mechanism. Binds to CD20, which regulates cell cycle initiation. Rituximab induces complement-dependent cytotoxicity and antibody-dependent cell mediated cytotoxicity.

      ii. Metabolism. Not appreciably metabolized. Elimination is uncertain, but it may undergo phagocytosis by the reticuloendothelial system.

   c. Toxicity

      i. Common. Cytokine release syndrome (fever, chills, dyspnea, bronchospasm, hypoxia, hypotension, urticaria, angioedema), headache, GI upset (nausea, vomiting, diarrhea), myelosuppression, weakness, cough, rhinitis, infusion-related reactions (hypotension, angioedema, hypoxia, bronchospasm), infections, rash, arthralgia, myalgia, and hypersensitivity reactions (hypotension, angioedema, bronchospasm).

      ii. Occasional. Edema, hypertension, dyspnea, sinusitis, and tumor lysis syndrome.

      iii. Rare. Severe infusion-related reactions (pulmonary infiltrates, ARDS, myocardial infarct, ventricular fibrillation, cardiogenic shock), optic neuritis, serum sickness, severe mucocutaneous reactions (paraneoplastic pemphigus, Stevens-Johnson syndrome, lichenoid dermatitis, vesiculobullous dermatitis, toxic epidermal necrolysis), and acute renal failure.

   d. Administration

      i. FDA-approved dose. Refer to individual protocols. Usual dose is 375 mg/m^2 intravenously once weekly for four or eight doses.

      ii. Dose modification. No specific recommendations.

      iii. Supplied as 100- and 500-mg vials.

B. Conjugated monoclonal antibodies

   1. Denileukin Diftitox (Ontak)

      a. FDA-approved indication. Treatment of persistent or recurrent cutaneous T-cell lymphoma whose malignant cells express the CD25 component of the IL-2 receptor.

      b. Pharmacology

         i. Mechanism. Recombinant fusion protein designed to deliver a cytotoxic dose of diphtheria toxin directly to targeted cells. It interacts with the IL-2 receptor on malignant cells and inhibits protein synthesis, which leads to cell death.

         ii. Metabolism. Through proteolytic degradation pathways.

      c. Toxicity

         i. Common. Vascular leak syndrome (hypotension, edema, hypoalbuminemia), headache, hypocalcemia, anemia, lymphopenia, increased transaminases, flulike illness (fever, chills, asthenia, myalgias, arthralgias, digestive symptoms), hypersensitivity (hypotension, dyspnea, vasodilation, rash, chest pain, tachycardia, syncope), nausea, vomiting, diarrhea, rash, and infections.

         ii. Occasional. Hypertension, thrombotic events, leukopenia, thrombocytopenia, myocardial infarction (MI), acute renal insufficiency, thyroid dysfunction, and pancreatitis.

         iii. Rare. Visual loss

      d. Administration

         i. FDA-approved dose. 9 or 18 μg/kg/day intravenously on days 1 through 5 every 21 days.

ii. **Dose modification.** None recommended.

iii. **Supplied** as 300-μg vials.

2. **Gemtuzumab ozogamicin (Mylotarg)**

a. **FDA-approved indication.** Relapsed CD33-positive AML in patients aged 60 years or more. Indicated for patients who cannot receive cytotoxic chemotherapy.

b. **Pharmacology.** Humanized MAb.

i. **Mechanism.** MAb conjugated to a cytotoxic antitumor antibiotic, calicheamicin. Binding to the CD33 antigen on myeloid cells results in internalization of the antigen–antibody complex. Subsequently, the calicheamicin derivative is released in the cell resulting in double strand breaks in DNA and cell death.

ii. **Metabolism.** Not well defined.

c. **Toxicity**

i. **Common.** Infusion-related reactions (fever, chills, rigors, hypotension/ hypertension, dyspnea, nausea, vomiting, headache), peripheral edema, tachycardia, myelosuppression, abnormal LFTs, sepsis, pneumonia, herpes simplex infections, neutropenic fever, and mucositis/stomatitis.

ii. **Occasional.** Cerebral hemorrhage, epistaxis, electrolyte disturbances, rhinitis, myalgia, and veno-occlusive disease.

iii. **Rare.** Hepatic failure, jaundice, hepatosplenomegaly, GI hemorrhage, pulmonary hemorrhage, and ARDS.

d. **Administration**

i. **FDA-approved dose.** 9 mg/m^2 intravenously on days 1 and 15. Full hematologic recovery is not required for administration on day 15.

ii. **Dose modification.** No recommendation for renal and/or hepatic impairment.

iii. **Supplied** as 5-mg vials.

C. **Radioimmunoconjugates**

1. **Ibritumomab tiuxetan (Zevalin)**

a. **FDA-approved indications.** Relapsed or refractory low-grade, follicular, or transformed B-cell NHL.

b. **Pharmacology.** Radioimmunoconjugated MAb.

i. **Mechanism.** Ibritumomab is joined through covalent bonds to tiuxetan, a chelating agent. The chelator tightly binds to the radioisotopes indium 111 (^{111}In) or yttrium 90 (^{90}Y). Ibritumomab binds to the CD20 antigen found on normal and malignant B cells while allowing the emission of radiation against the target and neighboring cells. The agent causes antibody-dependent and complement-mediated cytotoxicity and induces apoptosis.

ii. **Metabolism.** Primarily eliminated from circulation by binding to the tumor and metabolized through radioactive decay. The product of the radioactive decay of ^{90}Y is zirconium 90 (nonradioactive); ^{111}In decays to cadmium 111 (nonradioactive). Approximately 7% of the radiolabeled activity undergoes urinary excretion over 7 days.

c. **Toxicity**

i. **Common.** Chills, fever, GI upset (nausea, vomiting, abdominal pain), myelosuppression, weakness, infection, headache, dizziness, dyspnea, and cough.

ii. **Occasional.** Hypotension, diarrhea, constipation, insomnia, anxiety, arthralgia, myalgia, epistaxis, allergic reactions, pruritus, rash, peripheral edema, and secondary malignancies.

iii. **Rare.** Arthritis, encephalopathy, pulmonary edema, hemorrhagic stroke, angioedema, and pulmonary embolus.

d. **Administration**

i. **FDA-approved dose.** Step 1: inject ^{111}In ibritumomab tiuxetan 5 mCi (1.6-mg total antibody dose) over 10 minutes after rituximab infusion of 250 mg/m^2. Biodistribution is then assessed with a first image taken

2 to 24 hours after ^{111}In ibritumomab tiuxetan, a second image 48 to 72 hours after the infusion, and an optional third image 90 to 120 hours after the infusion. If biodistribution is considered acceptable, proceed to step 2. Step 2 (initiated 7 to 9 days after step 1): rituximab infusion 250 mg/m^2 followed by ^{90}Y ibritumomab tiuxetan 0.4 mCi/kg over 10 minutes (if platelet count >150,000) or 0.3 mCi/kg (if platelet count between 100,000–149,000). Ibritumomab should not be administered if platelet count is less than 100,000 cells/mm^3 and the maximum allowable whole-body dose should not exceed 32 mCi regardless of patient's weight.

    ii. Dose modification. No dosage modifications recommended for renal and/or hepatic impairment.

    iii. Supplied as ibritumomab 3.2-mg vials.

2. Tositumomab (Bexxar)

  a. FDA-approved indications. Relapsed or refractory low-grade, follicular, or transformed CD20-positive NHL.

  b. Pharmacology. Radioimmunoconjugated MAb.

    i. Mechanism. Tositumomab is covalently bonded to iodine-131 (^{131}I), forming the radioiodinated derivative, ^{131}I tositumomab. Tositumomab is a murine MAb that binds to CD20, which is found on normal and malignant B lymphocytes, while emitting ionizing radiation locally. The radiation that is emitted is cytotoxic over 1 to 2 mm distances causing the death of antigen-negative tumor cells. Therefore, cell death occurs by apoptosis, ADCC, complement-mediated cytotoxicity, and the ionizing radiation from the radioisotope.

    ii. Metabolism. Elimination of ^{131}I occurs by radioactive decay and renal excretion. Renal excretion accounts for approximately 98% of the total-body clearance. Whole-body clearance was 67% of the dose after approximately 5 days.

  c. Toxicity

    i. Common. Myelosuppression, hemorrhagic events, infections, GI events (nausea, vomiting, abdominal pain, diarrhea), infusion reactions (fever, rigors/chills, sweating), asthenia, headache, myalgia, arthralgia, rash, pruritus, and HAMAs seropositivity.

    ii. Occasional. Secondary malignancies, hypersensitivity reactions, hypothyroidism, peripheral edema, and pneumonia.

  d. Administration

    i. FDA-approved dose. Phase 1: trace-labeled dosimetric dose is administered for dosimetry studies. Unlabeled tositumomab 450 mg is administered over 60 minutes ("cold" dose) on day 0 followed by 5 mCi (millicurie) of ^{131}I tositumomab 35 mg ("hot"dose) administered over 20 minutes. Three whole body gamma counts are obtained on day 0; on day 2, 3, or 4; and on day 6 or 7. The patient specific dose is calculated based on the residence time of the antibody. The desired total-body dose for patients with platelet counts of 150,000 or greater is 75 cGy and for patients with platelet counts of 100,000 to 149,000 it is 65 cGy. Phase 2: therapeutic dose is administered between days 7 and 14. It should not be administered if there is altered biodistribution. Unlabeled tositumomab 450 mg over 60 minutes ("cold" dose) is administered, followed by a patient-specific therapeutic mCi dose of ^{131}I tositumomab 35 mg over 20 minutes ("hot" dose). Important note: oral thyroid-blocking agents (i.e., saturated solution of potassium iodide) should be initiated 24 hours before the dosimetric infusion and continued for 2 weeks following the administration of the therapeutic dose to prevent ^{131}I uptake by the thyroid gland.

    ii. Dose modification. None recommended. Excretion occurs primarily by the kidneys, and renal function impairment may decrease the rate of excretion of the radiolabeled iodine and increase exposure to the radioactive component.

    iii. Supplied as tositumomab 35- and 225-mg vials.

D. Proteasome inhibition. The 26S proteasome is a protein complex that degrades ubiquitinated proteins. The role of the ubiquitin–proteasome pathway is to regulate intracellular concentrations of specific proteins and maintain cellular homeostasis as it relates to cell cycle and transcriptional regulation, cell signaling, and apoptosis. Bortezomib reversibly inhibits the activity of the 26S proteasome, preventing proteolysis and affecting multiple signaling cascades within cells, which leads to cell cycle arrest and apoptosis.

1. Bortezomib (Velcade)

    a. FDA-approved indications. Multiple myeloma in patients refractory to other treatments.

    b. Pharmacology. Proteasome inhibitor.

        i. Mechanism. Selective, reversible inhibitor of the 26S proteasome.

        ii. Metabolism. Primarily hepatic through CYP 1A2, 2C19, and 3A4 with minor metabolism through CYP 2D6 and 2C9 to inactive metabolites. Elimination pathways in humans are unknown.

    c. Toxicity

        i. Common. Peripheral neuropathy, hypotension, thrombocytopenia, anemia, neutropenia, nausea, vomiting, diarrhea, constipation, pyrexia, psychiatric disorders, decreased appetite, asthenia, paresthesia, dysesthesia, anemia, headache, cough, dyspnea, rash, pain, insomnia, lower respiratory tract infections, arthralgia, myalgia, dizziness, herpes zoster, lower limb edema, blurred vision, and pneumonia.

        ii. Occasional. Heart failure events (acute pulmonary edema, cardiac failure, congestive cardiac failure, cardiogenic shock, pulmonary edema).

        iii. Rare. QT-interval prolongation, pneumonitis, interstitial pneumonia, lung infiltration, ARDS, cardiac tamponade, ischemic colitis, encephalopathy, disseminated intravascular coagulation, hepatitis, pancreatitis, and toxic epidermal necrolysis.

    d. Administration

        i. FDA-approved dose. Administer 1.3 mg/m^2 intravenously twice weekly for 2 weeks on days 1, 4, 8, and 11 in a 21-day cycle. Doses given consecutively should be separated by at least 72 hours.

        ii. Dose modification. Clinical studies included patients with creatinine clearance (CrCl) greater than 13 mL/hour. No pharmacokinetic studies have been conducted on patients with CrCl less than 13 mL/hour, on hemodialysis, or in hepatic impairment. Monitor closely for toxicity.

        iii. Supplied as 3.5-mg vials.

Suggested Readings

Arora A, Scholar EM. Role of tyrosine kinase inhibitors in cancer therapy. *J Pharmacol Exp Ther* 2005;315(3):971–979.

Balmer CM, Valley AW, Iannucci A. Cancer treatment and chemotherapy. In: DiPiro JT, Talbert RL, Yee GC, et al. eds. *Pharmacotherapy: a pathophysiologic approach*, 6th ed. New York: McGraw-Hill, 2005:2279–2328.

Carmeliet P. VEGF as a key mediator of angiogenesis in cancer. *Oncology* 2005;69 (Suppl 3):4–10.

Ferrara N. VEGF as a therapeutic target in cancer. *Oncology* 2005;69(Suppl 3):11–16.

Finley RS. Overview of targeted therapies for cancer. *Am J Health Syst Pharm* 2003;60(9): S4–10.

Gollob JA, Wilhelm S, Carter C, et al. Role of Raf kinase in cancer: therapeutic potential of targeting the Raf/MEK/ERK signal transduction pathway. *Semin Oncol* 2006;33:392–406.

Harari PM. Epidermal growth factor receptor inhibition strategies in oncology. *Endocr Relat Cancer* 2004;11:689–708.

Harris M. Monoclonal antibodies as therapeutic agents for cancer. *Lancet Oncol* 2004;5: 292–302.

Krause DS, Van Etten RA. Tyrosine kinases as targets for cancer therapy. *N Engl J Med* 2005;353:172–187.

Mendelsohn J, Baselga J. Epidermal growth factor receptor targeting in cancer. *Semin Oncol* 2006;33(4):369–385.

O'Brien S, Albitar M, Giles FJ. Monoclonal antibodies in the treatment of leukemia. *Curr Mol Med* 2005;5:663–675.

Rotea W, Saad E. Targeted drugs in oncology: new names, new mechanisms, new paradigm. *Am J Health Syst Pharm* 2003;60:1233–1243.

Stern M, Herrmann R. Overview of monoclonal antibodies in cancer therapy: present and promise. *Crit Rev Oncol Hematol* 2005;54:11–29.

The United States Adopted Names (USAN) Council. *Nomenclature for biologic products: monoclonal antibodies.* www.ama-assn.org/ama/pub/category/13280.html. Accessed Sep. 23, 2006.

Vlahovic G, Crawford J. Activation of tyrosine kinases in cancer. *Oncologist* 2003;8: 531–538.

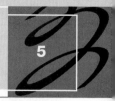

PRINCIPLES OF HEMATOPOIETIC STEM CELL TRANSPLANTATION

5

Geoffrey L. Uy, Bruno Nervi, and John F. DiPersio

I. INTRODUCTION. Hematopoietic stem cell transplantation (HSCT) involves the administration of dose-intense chemotherapy and/or radiation followed by the infusion of either autologous or allogeneic (donor-derived) hematopoietic stem cells (HSCs). More than 40,000 HSCTs are performed annually worldwide to treat patients with life-threatening malignant and nonmalignant diseases. This chapter summarizes the underlying principles and clinical aspects of both autologous and allogeneic HSCT.

II. TYPES OF TRANSPLANTS. Stem cell transplants may be classified by the source of donor cells as either (a) autologous, (b) allogeneic, or (c) syngeneic.

  A. Autologous transplantation. In an autologous transplant, a patient's own HSCs are harvested and cryopreserved. The autologous stem cells are then reinfused after the administration of high-dose chemotherapy and/or radiation therapy. Autologous transplantation allows the delivery of higher doses of drugs to maximize tumor-kill in situations where myelosuppression would otherwise be dose limiting.

  B. Allogeneic transplantation. Allogeneic transplantation is the infusion of HSCs from a human leukocyte antigens (HLA)-compatible or HLA-mismatched individual, either from a sibling or an unrelated donor source. In addition to permitting myeloablative doses of chemotherapy and/or radiation therapy to be administered, an allogeneic transplant allows for a potent immunologic effect mediated by donor lymphocytes, known as the graft-versus-tumor effect. In the pediatric setting, allogeneic transplants are also used to correct congenital conditions of the immune system and some inborn errors of metabolism.

  C. Syngeneic transplantation. Transplantation from an identical twin is similar to an autologous transplant with the benefit of providing a "clean" graft or stem cells that are free of contaminating malignant cells. In addition, syngeneic transplants are not associated with either the graft-versus-host or graft-versus-disease effect of an allogeneic transplant and does not require post-transplant immunosuppression.

III. PATIENT SELECTION

  A. Indications for transplantation. Stem cell transplantation has been successfully used in the treatment of a number of malignant and nonmalignant conditions (Table 5.1). The choice of autologous-versus-allogeneic transplantation largely depends on the disease being treated and the availability of a compatible donor. Currently, multiple myeloma and lymphoma (non-Hodgkin's and Hodgkin's) are the most frequent indications for autologous transplant whereas acute leukemia and myelodysplastic syndromes are the most frequent for allogeneic transplant. Guidelines for transplant referrals in adult patients have been published by the American Society for Blood and Marrow Transplantation (ASBMT, Table 5.2).

  B. Pretransplant evaluation of candidates for hematopoietic stem cell transplantation. Pretransplant evaluation of patients considered for HSCT is required to identify candidates with comorbid conditions that may preclude the administration of high-dose therapy with their associated toxicity. Although the risk of transplant-related complications increases with advancing age, age alone is not be considered an absolute contraindication, but rather one of many factors affecting the overall suitability of a patient for HSCT. Guidelines for pretransplant evaluations are listed in Table 5.3.

IV. DONOR SELECTION

  A. HLA typing. For allogeneic transplants, donors are selected on the basis of their histocompatibility with the recipient. The major histocompatibility complex (MHC) encodes class I and class II HLA which allow the immune recognition of

TABLE 5.1	Diseases Treatable with Hematopoietic Stem-Cell Transplantation

Autologous transplantation
Multiple myeloma
Hodgkin's and non-Hodgkin's lymphoma
Acute myeloid leukemia
Neuroblastoma
Germ-cell tumors
Allogeneic transplantation
Acute and chronic myeloid leukemia
Acute and chronic lymphocytic leukemia
Myelodysplastic and myeloproliferative syndromes
Hodgkin's and non-Hodgkin's lymphoma
Multiple myeloma
Aplastic anemia and other bone marrow failure disorders
Hemoglobinopathies: thalassemia major and sickle cell anemia
Immunodeficiency syndromes: severe combined immunodeficiency, Wiskott-Aldrich
Inborn errors of metabolism: Hurler's syndrome, adrenoleukodystrophy

foreign antigens. In hematopoietic and solid organ transplantation, HLA molecules function as alloantigens that can trigger immune recognition and graft rejection in mismatched recipients.

1. **HLA alleles.** HLA are defined serologically by testing for reactivity against a panel of monoclonal antibodies. DNA-based testing has largely replaced serologic testing and utilizes sequence-specific DNA primers and probes which define HLA alleles. DNA testing permits precise HLA matching between donors and transplant patients, which has resulted in improved patient outcomes. Because the MHC complex is tightly clustered on chromosome 6, HLA alleles are inherited as a set also referred to as the patient's *haplotype*. The chance of any individual sibling being HLA-matched is 25% whereas the probability of having a fully HLA-matched sibling donor is $1-(3/4)^n$, where n is the number of full siblings.

2. **HLA matching of unrelated donor transplants.** In individuals who do not have an HLA-identical sibling, selection of an unrelated donor is required. Typing of HLA-A, -B, -C and, -DR (DRB1) is routinely used to select unrelated donors. In addition, other class II loci HLA-DQB1, -DPB1, and -DRB3/4/5 are often tested although there is no established association with patient outcomes. In the United States, unrelated donor transplants are coordinated by the National Marrow Donor Program (NMDP). NMDP donations require, at a minimum, a low-resolution or antigen level match (at first two digits) of at least five of six HLA at HLA-A, -B, and -DR for marrow or peripheral blood stem cell (PBSC) transplants and at least four of six for umbilical cord blood transplants. The NMDP Registry includes more than 9 million potential marrow or PBSC donors and more than 50,000 cord blood units. The likelihood of finding an unrelated donor for a given patient depends upon the frequency of the patient's HLA haplotype in the general population. For all patients, the likelihood of finding a potential unrelated marrow or PBSC donor in the donor registries is approximately 85% for Caucasians, 60% for African Americans, and 30% to 35% for Hispanics.

B. **Non-HLA factors.** Other factors are often considered when donors are selected, including cytomegalovirus (CMV)—negative serology (for patients with CMV-negative serology), male sex, younger age, ABO compatibility, larger body weight, and matched race. Multiparous female donors are associated with a higher risk of chronic graft-versus-host disease (cGVHD), but with no effect overall survival.

TABLE 5.2   **Recommended Timing for Transplant Consultation**

AML
High-risk AML
  Antecedent hematologic disease (e.g., myelodysplasia)
  Treatment related leukemia
  Induction failure
CR1 with poor risk cytogenetics
CR2 and beyond

ALL
High-risk ALL
  Poor risk cytogenetics (e.g., t(9;22), abnormalities of 11q23)
  High WBC (>30,000–50,000) at diagnosis
  CNS or testicular leukemia
  No CR within 4 wk of initial treatment
  Induction failure
CR2 and beyond

MDS
Intermediate-1, intermediate-2 or high IPSS score which includes either:
  >5% marrow blasts
  Other than good risk cytogenetic response
  >1 lineage cytopenia

CML
No hematologic or minor cytogenetic response 3 mo postimatinib initiation
No complete cytogenetic response 6 to 12 mo postimatinib initiation
Disease progression, accelerated phase, blast crisis

Non-Hodgkin's lymphomas
Follicular
  Poor response to initial treatment
  Initial remission duration <12 mo
  Second relapse
  Transformation to diffuse large B cell lymphoma
Diffuse large B cell
  At first or subsequent relapse
  CR1 for patients with high or high-intermediate IPI risk
  No CR with initial treatment
Mantle cell
  Following initial therapy

Hodgkin's lymphoma
  No initial CR
  First or subsequent relapse

Multiple myeloma
  After initiation of therapy
  At first progression

AML, acute mylogenous leukemia; ALL, acute lymphoblastic leukemia; WBC, white blood corpuscles; CNS, central nervous system; CR, complete remission; MDS, myelodisplastic syndromes; IPSS, International Prognostic Scoring System; CML, chronic myelogenous leukemia; IPI, International Prognostic Index.

TABLE 5.3 Pretransplant Evaluation

Test	Comment
History and physical examination	Assess: performance status, active infection, significant organ system dysfunction
Review of tissue samples	Confirmation of diagnosis
Review of initial staging and restaging tests	Assess responsiveness to therapy and current disease status
Bone marrow biopsy/aspirate	
Confirmatory donor and recipient HLA and ABO Rh blood typing (allogeneic HSCT candidates)	
Serum chemistry panel (electrolytes, creatinine, bilirubin, AST, ALT, alkaline phosphatase, LDH)	Creatinine >2 may result in altered metabolism of drugs commonly used in HSCT (certain antibiotics, methorexate); AST, ALT, bilirubin >2 times normal increases the risk of venoocclusive disease
Radioventriculogram or echocardiogram	LVEF >40%–45% desirable
ECG	Evaluate for underlying cardiovascular disease
Chest radiograph	Evaluate for underlying pulmonary disease or infection
Pulmonary function tests	FEV_1, FVC, DLCO >50% predicted
Viral serologies (CMV, HSV, HIV, HTLV-I, hepatitis A, hepatitis B core antigen and surface antibody, hepatitis C)	HSV seropositivity requires antiviral prophylaxis; hepatitis seropositivity without evidence of active disease increases the risk of venoocclusive disease, but is not a contraindication to HSCT
Radiation oncology evaluation	TBI conditioning regimen candidates
Nutrition evaluation	
Pregnancy test (premenopausal women)	
Sperm/oocyte banking	

HLA, human leukocyte antigen; HSCT, hematopoietic stem cell transplant; AST, aspartate aminotransferase; ALT, alanine aminotransferase; LDH, lactate dehydrogenase; LVEF, left ventricular ejection fraction; ECG, electrocardiogram; FEV_1, forced expiratory volume in the first second; FVC, forced vital capacity; DLCO, carbon dioxide diffusion in the lung; CMV, cytomegalovirus; HSV, herpes simplex virus; HIV, human immunodeficiency virus; HTLV-I, human T-cell lymphoma virus type 1; TBI, total-body irradiation.

V. SOURCES OF HEMATOPOIETIC STEM CELLS

A. Bone marrow. Historically, bone marrow was used as the sole source of HSCs in transplantation. Bone marrow is collected from the posterior iliac crest by performing repeated aspirations while the donor is under general or regional anesthesia. The volume collected varies but generally ranges from 10 to 15 mL/kg of donor weight. Improved survival has been correlated with higher transplanted cell dose with more robust engraftment and fewer infectious complications. A dose of approximately 2×10^8 nucleated cells/kg is considered adequate to proceed to transplantation. Side effects of marrow collection include fatigue and pain at the collection site and effects related to general anesthesia such as nausea and vomiting.

B. Peripheral blood stem cells. HSCs normally circulate in low levels in the peripheral circulation but can be recruited into the peripheral blood from the marrow in response to stressors such as inflammation or infection. In addition, the exogenous administration of hematopoietic growth factors can increase the numbers of peripheral blood stem cells by 40- to 80-fold in a process termed *stem cell mobilization*. These mobilized PBSCs can then be harvested and used for HSCT. The use of these PBSCs for transplantation has grown dramatically over the last 10 years with currently, more than 95% of autologous transplants and most of the adult allogeneic transplants performed using PBSC.

1. **Stem cell mobilization.** Although a number of cytokines and cytokine combinations can mobilize HSCs, only granulocyte-stimulating factor (G-CSF) (filgrastim, 10 to 16 μg/kg) and granulocyte-macrophage colony-stimulating factor (GM-CSF) (sargramostim) have been approved by the FDA for use as mobilizing agents. Donors may experience myalgia, bone pain, headache, nausea, and fever with G-CSF. Splenic rupture due to extramedullary hematopoiesis has been reported as a rare complication.

   HSCs also increase in the peripheral circulation during neutrophil recovery after the administration of chemotherapy. For autologous stem cell collection, high-dose cyclophosphamide may be used to mobilize PBSC and can be augmented with the administration of G-CSF or GM-CSF to increase the stem cell yield.

   AMD3100 is a CXCR4 antagonist used for the mobilization of stem cells. CXCR4 is a receptor for the chemokine CXCL12 (stromal-derived factor-1 [SDF-1]) produced by marrow stromal cells and is critical for the homing and retention of HSCs in the marrow. By disrupting the CXCR4/CXCL12 axis, AMD3100 has been shown to be effective for the mobilization of stem cells either alone or in combination with G-CSF.

2. **PBSC harvesting.** Following mobilization, PBSCs are collected by large volume apheresis (up to 20 L) through the antecubital veins or a central venous catheter. The mononuclear fraction containing the PBSC is retained and the remainder is reinfused into the patient. Hypocalcemia from the anticoagulation with acid-citrate-dextrose solution used during apheresis may cause perioral numbness, parasthesias, and carpopedal spasm and is treated with calcium supplementation. A minimum of 2×10^6 CD34$^+$/kg recipient weight is required for an autologous transplant whereas a goal of 5×10^6 CD34/kg increases the probability of early platelet recovery. Most normal donors require only a single apheresis session to collect adequate numbers of stem cells while autologous donors may require multiple (five or more) sessions depending on their degree of exposure to previous chemotherapy.

   Compared to marrow, PBSC contain higher numbers of CD34$^+$ cells than bone marrow and are associated with faster neutrophil and platelet recovery. In addition, PBSCs have approximately, a tenfold higher numbers of T lymphocytes in the graft, which are associated with higher rates of cGVHD but without an effect on overall survival.

C. **Umbilical cord blood.** Blood present in the umbilical cord and placenta following childbirth is a rich source of HSCs. After delivery of the placenta, the umbilical cord is clamped and approximately 50 to 100 mL remaining in the placenta and umbilical cord is drained and cryopreserved. Cord blood typically contains about a 10- to 20-fold smaller dose of nucleated and CD34$^+$ cells than an adult bone marrow. Because of the limitations in stem cell dose, cord blood transplants have been primarily performed in pediatric populations with a minimum of 2.0×10^7 mononuclear cells/kg typically required for successful transplant and greater than 3.0×10^7 mononuclear cells/kg for optimal results. In the adult population, two or more cord units may be pooled for a single recipient, which can result in a more rapid hematopoietic revovery. Of interest, in double-cord allogeneic HSCT, one of the two cord units dominates hematopoiesis over the long term.

   Cord blood transplants are associated with lower risks of acute and cGVHD and can be performed successfully with a greater degree HLA-mismatching than adult stem cell sources. In addition, cord blood units are much more readily available than stem cells from adult donors and are associated with lower rates of viral transmission. Cord blood registries unlike adult donor registries do not suffer from the loss of the donor pool due to advancing age or difficulties in locating potential donors. Disadvantages include the inability to collect additional donor HSC for patients experiencing graft failure and the unavailability of donor lymphocytes for recipients who relapse after initial allografting.

VI. CONDITIONING REGIMENS

A. Myeloablative conditioning. Traditional conditioning regimens used in HSCT use myeloablative doses of alkylating agents (cyclophosphamide, busulfan, melphalan) with or without total body irradiation (TBI) before transplant to (a) eliminate residual disease and to (b) suppress immune function to allow engraftment of donor stem cells. Standard conditioning regimens vary by disease with a list of commonly used regimens listed in Table 5.4. In addition to severe myelosuppression, agents used in HSCT are typically associated with side effects such as mucositis, alopecia, nausea, and may cause significant organ damage including hepatic or pulmonary dysfunction.

B. Reduced intensity conditioning. In the allogeneic setting, nonmyeloablative or reduced intensity conditioning (RIC) regimens were designed to reduce the toxicity associated with high dose therapy. These regimens do not attempt to completely eliminate malignant cells before transplant, but instead provide enough

 TABLE 5.4   **Myeloablative Conditioning Regimens in Hematopoietic Stem Cell Transplant**

Allogeneic regimens		
Regimen	**Total dose**	**Daily dose**
Cy/TBI		
TBI	1,225 cGy	175 cGy b.i.d. d-6/-5/-4, 175 cGy d-3
Cyclophosphamide	120 mg/kg	60 mg/kg/d i.v. × 2, d-3/-2
MESNA	120 mg/kg	60 mg/kg CIVI over 24 h × 2, d-3/-2
Bu/Cy		
Busulfan	16 mg/kg	1 mg/kg p.o. q6h, d-7/-6/-5/-4
Cyclophosphamide	120 mg/kg	60 mg/kg/d i.v. × 2, d-3/-2
MESNA	120 mg/kg	60 mg/kg CIVI over 24 h × 2, d-3/-2
Autologous regimens		
Regimen	**Total dose**	**Daily dose**
Multiple myeloma		
Mel-200		
Melphalan	200 mg/m^2	100 mg/m^2 i.v. × 2, d-3/-2
Lymphoma		
BEAM		
BCNU	450 mg/m^2	450 mg/m^2, d, d-8
Etoposide	800 mg/m^2	100 mg/m^2 i.v. b.i.d. × 4, d-7/-6/-5/-4
Ara-C	800 mg/m^2	100 mg/m^2 i.v. b.i.d. × 4, d-7/-6/-5/-4
Melphalan	140 mg/m^2	140 mg/m^2, d-3
Solid tumors		
MEC		
Etoposide	1,200 mg/m^2	300 mg/m^2 × 4, d-6/-5/-4/-3
Carboplatinum	1,400 mg/m^2	700 mg/m^2 × 2, d-4/-3
Melphalan	140 mg/m^2	140 mg/m^2, d-2

TBI, total-body irradiation; MESNA, [sodium-2]-mercaptoethane sulfonate; VP, vincristine/prednisone; CIVI, continuous intravenous infusion; BCNU, 1,3- bis-(2-chloroethyl)-1-nitrosourea; Ara-C, acytosine arabinose.

TABLE 5.5	Nonmyeloablative Conditioning Regimens	
Regimen	**Total dose**	**Daily dose**
Flu/Cy		
Cyclophosphamide	120 mg/kg	60 mg/kg/d × 2, d-7/-6
Fludarabine	125 mg/m²	25 mg/m² × 5, d-5/-4/-3/-2/-1
MESNA	120 mg/kg	60 mg/kg CIVI over 24 h × 2, d-4/-3
Cy/ATG/thymic RT		
Cyclophosphamide	200 mg/kg	50 mg/kg/d × 4, d-6/-5/-4/-3
Thymic RT	700 cGy	d-1
ATG	45–90 mg/kg	15–30 mg/kg × 3, d-2/-1/ + 1
MESNA	200 mg/kg	50 mg/kg CIVI over 24 h × 4, d-6/-5/-4/-3
Flu/Bu ± ATG		
Busulfan (oral)	8 mg/kg	4 mg/kg/d × 2, d-6/-5
Fludarabine	150 mg/m²	30 mg/m²/d × 5, d-10/-9/-8/-7/-6/-5
ATG	40 mg/kg	10 mg/kg/d × 4, d-4/-3/-2/-1

RT, reverse transcription; ATG, antithymocyte globulin.

immunosuppression to allow donor engraftment and rely upon a graft-versus-tumor effect mediated by donor-derived T cells to achieve their therapeutic goal. Although there is no established definition for RIC, commonly used regimens are listed in Table 5.5.

RIC regimens have expanded the number of patients eligible for HSCT and in particular, the elderly and those patients with significant comorbid conditions. In retrospective analyses conducted in myeloid malignancies, RIC regimens are associated with lower treatment-related mortality but with higher relapse rates and no change in overall survival. Rates of acute and cGVHD after reduced incidence of relapse (RIR) are comparable to those observed in standard high-dose transplants, but the onset of graft-versus-host disease (GVHD) is often delayed by weeks to months. Due to the increased risk of relapse, these regimens are best suited to patients who are in remission at the time of transplant.

VII. **STEM CELL INFUSIONS.** Stem cells collected for autologous transplant are cryopreserved in the liquid or vapor phase of liquid nitrogen with 10% dimethyl sulfoxide (DMSO) used as a cryoprotectant. Before reinfusion of stem cells, a bicarbonate infusion is used to alkalinize the urine to protect against renal injury caused by the hemolysis of contaminating red cells. Stem cells products are rapidly thawed at 37-degree water bath and typically infused over a 15-minute period as longer infusion times subject the HSCs to DMSO toxicity. Side effects associated with DMSO include flushing, unpleasant taste, nausea, and vomiting with rare hypotension, atrial arrhythmias, and anaphylactic reactions. Allogeneic stem cells are usually infused fresh, with patients monitored for any hypersensitivity reactions. Large volume bone marrow products should be infused over the period of 3 to 4 hours and the patient monitored for fluid overload.

VIII. **POSTTRANSPLANT CARE AND COMPLICATIONS**

A. **Hematopoietic**

1. **Engraftment.** Following HSCT, stem and progenitor cells home to the marrow microenvironment through interactions between adhesion molecules and their receptors expressed on hematopoietic cells and the marrow stroma. These cells must then proliferate and differentiate to repopulate the peripheral blood with mature blood cells in a process termed *engraftment*. Neutrophil engraftment (ANC greater than 500/mm³) typically occurs between 10 and 15 days' post-transplant with PBSC transplants and slightly longer in bone marrow transplants. The administration of colony-stimulating factors, either G-CSF or

GM-CSF, post-transplant have been demonstrated to lessen the duration of neutropenia. Platelet recovery tends to be much more variable post-transplant.

Donor/recipient chimerism is evaluated post-HSCT by analyzing either peripheral blood or bone marrow for differences in allele types between at variable number tandem repeat loci. The differences in the allele pattern of the two cell sources (graft donor and recipient) distinguish between donor and patient DNA and the ratio of these two cell populations. In the case of sex-mismatched transplantation, chimerism can be analyzed by the ratio of sex chromosomes by fluorescence in situ hybridization (FISH).

2. **Transfusion support.** Transfusions of red blood cells and platelets are common in HSCT. Although transfusion parameters are arbitrary, it is reasonable to maintain hemoglobin levels greater than 8 to 9 g/dL, platelets greater than 10,000/mm^3. To reduce the risk of transfusion-associated GVHD, all blood products should be irradiated with 2,500 cGy before administration.

3. **ABO incompatibility.** Because stem cell products are matched based on HLA compatibility, ABO incompatible HSCTs frequently occur. Red cell incompatibility is classified according to whether donor isoagglutinins, isoantigens, or both are incompatible with those of the recipient. Major incompatibility occurs when the recipient has antibodies directed against donor red blood cell antigens (e.g., A donor, O recipient); minor incompatibility occurs when donor plasma contains antibodies directed against patient red cells (e.g., O donor, A recipient). Reds cells are typically reduced from the HSC component in major incompatible bone marrow transplantation to reduce the risk of clinically significant hemolysis of large quantities of red cells contained in the stem cell product. Immune-mediated hemolysis is indicated by a positive direct antiglobulin test (direct Coombs) in the setting of other markers of hemolysis such as an elevated lactate dehydrogenase (LDH) or indirect bilirubin. In cases of mild hemolysis, RBC transfusion support is adequate. In more severe cases, plasma exchange may be used. In contrast, patients receiving minor incompatible transplants have a risk of immediate hemolysis from the infusion of incompatible plasma. Immediate hemolysis can be prevented by removal of plasma from the bone marrow grafts by centrifugation. In PBSC transplants, apheresis used to collect the stem cell product effectively removes most of the donor plasma.

4. **Graft failure.** Rejection of the donor hematopoietic cells by the immune system of the recipient is termed *graft failure* and may be classified as primary (defined as failure of the absolute neutrophil count to reach 2×10^6/dL by day 28 after transplant) or secondary (transient donor hematopoiesis). Causes for graft failure include HLA disparity at major and minor loci, inadequate conditioning of the host, inadequate number of donor stem cells, T-cell depletion of the donor graft, inadequate immunosuppression, and allosensitization to donor antigens by transfusion from the donor before transplantation. Therapeutic options include more intensive immunosuppression, the administration of hematopoietic growth factors, donor lymphocyte infusions (DLIs), and even a second HSCT.

B. **Acute graft-versus-host disease (aGVHD)**

1. **Pathogenesis.** The pathogenesis of GVHD begins with issue damage from either the conditioning regimen or infections. The damage releases inflammatory cytokines which activate donor-derived lymphocytes. These donor-derived T cells within the stem cell graft recognize the recipient tissues as foreign resulting in an inflammatory disease that can affect multiple organs. GVHD can be severe in the setting of a major MHC class mismatch but also occurs because of disparities in minor histocompatibility antigens.

2. **Clinical manifestations.** aGVHD typically manifests itself at the time of neutrophil engraftment with the most commonly involved organs being the skin, liver and gut. The first clinical manifestation of aGVHD is usually a mild maculopapular rash. Liver involvement is commonly seen with a conjugated hyperbilirubinemia and elevation of the alkaline phosphatase. Lower gastrointestinal (GI) involvement typically presents as diarrhea and

TABLE 5.6   Glucksberg Acute Graft-versus-Host Disease (aGVHD) Grading

Clinical grading of aGVHD

Stage	Skin	Liver	Gut	Functional Impairment
0	0	0	0	0
I	1+ −2+	0	0	0
II	1+ −3+	1+	1+	1+
III	2+ −3+	2+ −3+	2+	2+
IV	2+ −4+	2+ −4+	3+	3+

Clinical staging of aGVHD

Stage	Skin	Liver	Gut
1+	Maculapapular rash <25% body surface	Bilirubin 2–3 mg/dL	Diarrhea 500–1,000 mL/d; persistent nausea
2+	Maculapapular rash 25%–50% body surface	Bilirubin 3–6 mg/dL	Diarrhea 1,000–1,500 mL/d
3+	Generalized erythroderma	Bilirubin 3–6 mg/dL	Diarrhea >1,500 mL/d
4+	Desquamation and bullae	Bilirubin >15 mg/dL	Pain ± ileus

abdominal cramping while upper GI involvement usually presents as nausea and vomiting.

Although several scoring systems are used to grade GVHD, most are based on the original Glucksberg criteria with those having stage II and IV disease having a significantly poorer outcome (Table 5.6). Grade II–IV GVHD occurs in approximately 35% of the patients undergoing HLA-matched transplants with 15% developing severe grade IV disease.

3. **GVHD prophylaxis**

   a. **Pharmacologic prophylaxis.** Because of the high morbidity and mortality associated with the development of aGVHD, routine prophylaxis against GVHD is required in all patients undergoing allogeneic transplant. Although a number of different pharmacologic agents can be used, a typical regimen uses methotrexate (10 mg/m^2) on days 1, 3, 6, and 11 post-transplant with a calcineurin inhibitor, either cyclosporine or tacrolimus. Immunosuppression is generally continued until day 100 post-transplant and gradually tapered in the absence of GVHD or disease relapse.

   b. **T cell depletion.** T cell depletion may be used as either an alternative or adjuvant to pharmacologic prophylaxis for GVHD. As donor-derived T cells are central to the pathogenesis of aGVHD, T cell depletion of the donor graft can effectively reduce the incidence of GVHD. A number of methods for T cell depletion have been used and include physical adsorption of T cells to proteins such as lectins, elutriation, or depletion with T cell or lymphocyte specific antibodies. A loss of donor T cells is associated however, with higher rates of graft rejection mediated by residual host T cells and a disease relapse due to partial loss of the graft-versus-tumor effect. In addition, T cell depletion results in delayed immune reconstitution in recipients leading to higher rates of viral infections and in particular, cytomegalovirus (CMV) and Epstein-Barr virus (EBV).

4. **Treatment.** Corticosteroids are the primary treatment for aGVHD. For mild (grade I) GVHD of the skin, topical steroids may be sufficient. For grade II or higher disease, prednisone or methylprednisolone 1 to 2 mg/kg/day is usually initiated. Steroid doses are then generally tapered gradually after clinical

improvement. For patients with steroid refractory disease, a number of agents have been used with modest success. These include agents such as mycophenolate mofetil, cyclosporine, tacrolimus, sirolimus, pentostatin, thalidomide, and monoclonal antibodies including daclizumab and infliximab.

C. Infections

1. **Timing of infectious complications.** HSCT recipients are at increased risk for opportunistic infections. The risk for developing specific types of infections seen in stem cell transplant recipients vary by the type of transplant (autologous or allogeneic) and the length of time since undergoing transplant. Before neutrophil engraftment, patients are at increased risk for infection due to neutropenia caused by the conditioning regimen and breaks in mucosal barriers from chemotherapy or indwelling vascular access devices. During this period, febrile neutropenia caused from both gram-positive and gram-negative organisms are common. In addition, Candida infections and herpes simplex virus (HSV) reactivation may occur. The postengraftment period (day 30 to 100) is characterized by impaired cell mediated immunity. After engraftment, the herpes viruses, particularly CMV, are major pathogens. Other dominant pathogens during this phase include *Pneumocystis carinii* and *Aspergillus* species.

2. **Prophylaxis and management of specific infections**
   a. **CMV.** CMV infections in HSCT recipients most commonly present as fever or interstitial pneumonitis. Other clinical manifestations include bone marrow suppression, retinitis, or diarrhea. Patients at risk for developing CMV infection include those undergoing allogeneic HSCT where either the donor or recipient is CMV positive. Prevention of CMV disease in allogeneic transplant can be accomplished using either a prophylactic or pre-emptive strategy. A prophylactic strategy of ganciclovir through day +100 post-transplant is effective at preventing CMV disease but may result in drug induced marrow suppression and prevent reconstitution of CMV-specific T-cell immunity, resulting in late occurrences of CMV disease. A preemptive strategy uses sensitive PCR techniques to detect viremia and initiates therapy with ganciclovir before to the development of overt disease. For patients with resistant disease, foscarnet or cidofovir may be used.

   To reduce the risk of transfusion acquired CMV infection, all donors and recipients are screened for their CMV serostatus. CMV antibody negative blood products should be given to CMV-negative recipients. Alternatively leukofiltration to reduce the white cell fraction in the transfused produce may be used as an alternative if no CMV-negative products are available.

   b. **HSV and VZV.** Routine prophylaxis with either acyclovir 400 mg t.i.d. or valacyclovir 500 mg qd. to prevent reactivation of HSV and varicella zoster virus (VZV) is given to patients until neutrophil engraftment in autologous transplant patients and immunosuppression is discontinued in allogeneic transplant patients.

   c. **PCP prophylaxis.** Prophylaxis with TMP-SMX one DS tablet b.i.d. 2× a week, dapsone 100 mg day or aerosolized pentamidine should be given to all patients undergoing allogeneic transplant and selected patients undergoing autologous transplant. PCP prophylaxis is continued while patients remain on immunosuppressive medications.

D. Veno-occlusive disease of the liver.

Veno-occlusive disease (VOD) of the liver is a clinical diagnosis based on the presence of hyperbilirubinemia associated with fluid retention and painful hepatomegaly. Histologically, VOD is associated with central vein occlusion, centrilobular hepatocyte necrosis and sinusoidal fibrosis. Ultrasonography may reveal reversal of flow in the portal and hepatic veins. The etiology of VOD is believed to arise from damage to the hepatic endothelium secondary to high-dose chemotherapy and/or radiation.

Risk factors for VOD include pre-existing hepatic disease (e.g., viral hepatitis, cirrhosis), high dose radiation as part of the conditioning, mismatched or unrelated donor HSCT, and the use of cyclosporine and methotrexate for GVHD prophylaxis. Spontaneous resolution of VOD is observed in approximately 70% of cases but can frequently evolve into fatal multisystem organ failure. Low-dose heparin or ursodeoxycholic acid may provide some protection when used in a prophylactic manner. Supportive care measures are the mainstay of treatment for VOD with attention to fluid and electrolyte management. Other agents used for the treatment of VOD include defibrotide, alteplase and high dose methylprednisolone although the evidence supporting their use is mixed.

E. Management of relapsed disease. For relapsed disease following allogeneic transplant, maneuvers which attempt to maximize the graft-versus-leukemia effect of the allograft may be useful. Withdrawal of immunosuppression is usually attempted first. If no effect is seen, a DLI can augment the immunologic effect of the allograft. DLI can result in significant toxicity including acute and cGVHD and severe pancytopenia. Responses are seen more frequently in diseases thought to be most sensitive to a graft-versus-disease effect such as chronic myeloid leukemia (CML) and in those patients who develop GVHD.

IX. LATE COMPLICATIONS OF ALLOGENEIC TRANSPLANTATION
A. cGVHD
1. Clinical manifestations. The clinical manifestations of cGVHD are heterogeneous in terms of the organ systems involved, the disease severity, and clinical course. By convention, GVHD is classified as chronic when it occurs after day +100 post-HSCT although this distinction is somewhat arbitrary (Table 5.7). The most frequently affected organs in cGVHD include the skin, liver, GI tract and lungs. Epidermal involvement is characterized as an erythematous rash which may appear papular, lichen planus-like, papulosquamous, or poikiloderma. Dermal and subcutaneous involvement is characterized by sclerosis, fasciitis and ulcerations. Oral manifestations of cGVHD include erythema, lichenoid hyperkeratosis, ulcerations or mucocoeles. Lacrimal gland dysfunction frequently results in keratoconjunctivitis sicca also known as the dry eye syndrome and can manifest as burning irritation, pain, blurred vision, and photophobia. GI symptoms include nausea, vomiting, anorexia, and unexplained weight loss. Liver involvement is characterized by rising bilirubin and transaminases. Pulmonary cGVHD can result in a debilitating bronchiolitis obliterans syndrome with pulmonary function testing often demonstrating decreases in the FEV_1 and the diffusing capacity of the lung for carbon monoxide (DLCO).

2. Diagnosis and treatment. The diagnosis of cGVHD can often be made based on classical features of skin involvement, manifestations of gastrointestinal involvement, and a rising serum bilirubin concentration. Often the diagnosis is less clear in which case histologic confirmation may be desirable.

 TABLE 5.7 **Clinicopathologic Classification of Chronic Graft-versus-Host Disease (cGVHD)**

Limited cGVHD
Either or both
    1. Localized skin involvement
    2. Hepatic dysfunction due to cGVHD
Extensive cGVHD
Either
    1. Generalized skin involvement or
    2. Localized skin involvement and/or hepatic dysfunction due to cGVHD
Plus
    3a. Liver histology showing chronic aggressive hepatitis, bridging necrosis, or cirrhosis
    3b. Involvement of eye (Schirmer's test with <5-mm wetting), or
    3c. Involvement of minor salivary glands or oral mucosa demonstrated on labial biopsy, or
    3d. Involvement of any other target organ

TABLE 5.8	Ancillary and Supportive Care of Chronic Graft-versus-Host Disease (cGVHD)

Organ system	Intervention

Skin and appendages	Prevention
	    Photoprotection. Surveillance for malignancy
	Treatment
	    For intact skin — Topical emollients, corticosteroids, antipruritic agents, and others (e.g., psoralen–UV-A, calcineurin inhibitors)
	    For erosions/ulcerations — microbiologic cultures, topical antimicrobials, protective films or other dressings, debridement, hyperbaric oxygen, wound care specialist consultation

Mouth and oral cavity	Prevention
	    Maintain good oral/dental hygiene. Consider routine dental cleaning and endocarditis prophylaxis
	    Surveillance for infection and malignancy
	Treatment
	    Topical high and ultra-high potency corticosteroids and analgesics. Therapy for oral dryness

Eyes	Prevention
	    Photoprotection. Surveillance for infection, cataract formation, and increased intraocular pressure
	Treatment
	    Artificial tears, ocular ointments, topical corticosteroids or cyclosporine, punctal occlusion, humidified environment, occlusive eye wear, moisture chamber eyeglasses, cevimeline, pilocarpine, tarsorrhaphy, gas-permeable scleral contact lens, autologous serum, microbiologic cultures, topical antimicrobials, doxycycline

Vulva and vagina	Prevention
	    Surveillance for estrogen deficiency, infection (herpes simplex virus, human papilloma virus, yeast, bacteria), malignancy
	Treatment
	    Water-based lubricants, topical estrogens, topical corticosteroids or calcineurin inhibitors, dilators, surgery, for extensive synechiae/obliteration, early gynecologic consultation

Gastrointestinal tract and liver	Prevention
	    Surveillance for infection (viral, fungal)
	Treatment
	    Eliminate other potential etiologies. Dietary modification, enzyme supplementation for malabsorption, gastroesophageal reflux management, esophageal dilatation, ursodeoxycholic acid

Lungs	Prevention
	    Surveillance for infection (*Pneumocystis carinii*, viral, fungal, bacterial)
	Treatment
	    Eliminate other potential etiologies (e.g., infection, gastroesophageal reflux) Inhaled corticosteroids, bronchodilators, supplementary oxygen, pulmonary rehabilitation. Consideration of lung transplantation in appropriate candidates

Hematopoietic	Prevention
	    Surveillance for infection (cytomegalovirus, parvovirus)
	Treatment
	    Eliminate other potential etiologies (e.g., drug toxicity, infection) Hematopoietic growth factors, immunoglobulin for immune cytopenias

TABLE 5.8   *(Continued)*

Organ system	Intervention
Neurologic	Prevention Calcineurin drug-level monitoring. Seizure prophylaxis including blood pressure control, electrolyte replacement, anticonvulsants Treatment Occupational and physical therapies, treatment of neuropathic syndromes with tricyclic antidepressants, selective serotonin reuptake inhibitors, or anticonvulsants
Immunologic and infectious diseases	Prevention Immunizations and prophylaxis against *P. carinii,* varicella zoster virus, and encapsulated bacteria based on guideline of the Centers for Disease Control. Consider immunoglobulin replacement based on levels and recurrent infections. No current evidence supports the use of mold-active agents. Surveillance for infection (viral, bacterial, fungal, atypical) Treatment Organism-specific antimicrobial agents. Empiric parenteral broad-spectrum antibacterial coverage for fever
Musculoskeletal	Prevention Surveillance for decreased range of motion, bone densitometry, calcium levels and 25-OH vitamin D. Physical therapy, calcium, vitamin D, bisphosphonates Treatment Physical therapy, bisphosphonates for osteopenia and osteoporosis

Systemic immunosuppression with corticosteroids and other agents are often required to treat cGVHD. In addition, ancillary and supportive care measures tailored to the organ system involved are critical for the management of cGVHD and in many circumstances reduce or eliminate the need for systemic immunosuppression. Recommendations from the National Institutes of Health Consensus Development Project for cGVHD are summarized in Table 5.8.

B. Late infections. Autologous HSCT patients have a more rapid recovery of immune function and a lower risk of opportunistic infections than allogeneic HSCT patients. Because of cell mediated and humoral immunity defects and impaired functioning of the reticuloendothelial system, allogeneic HSCT patients with cGVHD are at risk for various infections during this phase. Late infections include EBV–related post-transplant lymphoproliferative disease, community-acquired respiratory virus infection, and infections with encapsulated bacteria. In addition, fungal infections with Aspergillus species and zygomycoses can be seen in the late period, particularly, in patients with cGVHD.

C. Secondary malignancies. Patients undergoing both autologous and allogeneic are at risk either for the development of treatment-related myelodysplastic syndromes (MDS) or acute myelogenous leukemia (AML) due to the high-dose alkylators and irradiation typically used as part of the conditioning regimens. Exposure to radiation and the photosensitizing effects of many commonly used transplantation related medications increase the risk of skin cancers among recipients. Post-transplant lymphoproliferative disorders due to EBV can be observed particularly in patients receiving T cell depleted grafts.

D. Other complications. Although stem cell transplantation can result in long-term survival with an excellent quality of life, late sequelae of the transplantation can result in significant morbidity. For example, TBI is associated with hypothyroidism and development of cataracts. Patients receiving prolonged corticosteroids can develop muscle weakness and bone loss. Recommendations for screening and preventative practices for long term survivors of HSCT have been published.

Suggested Readings

Alyea EP, Kim HT, Ho V, et al. Comparative outcome of nonmyeloablative and myeloablative allogeneic hematopoietic cell transplantation for patients older than 50 years of age. *Blood* 2005;105(4):1810–1814.

Couban S, Simpson DR, Barnett DJ, et al. A randomized multicenter comparison of bone marrow and peripheral blood in recipients of matched sibling allogeneic transplants for myeloid malignancies. *Blood* 2002;100(5):1525–1531.

Dykewicz S. Guidelines for preventing opportunistic infections among hematopoietic stem cell transplant recipients: focus on community respiratory virus infections. *Biol Blood Marrow Transplant* 2001;7(7 Suppl):19S–22S.

Flowers ME, Parker PM, Johnston LJ, et al. Comparison of chronic graft-versus-host disease after transplantation of peripheral blood stem cells versus bone marrow in allogeneic recipients: long-term follow-up of a randomized trial. *Blood* 2002;100(2):415–419.

Grewal SS, Barker JN, Davies SM, et al. Unrelated donor hematopoietic cell transplantation: marrow or umbilical cord blood? *Blood* 2003;101(11):4233–4244.

Hurley CK, Baxter Lowe LW, Logan B, et al. National Marrow Donor Program HLA-matching guidelines for unrelated marrow transplants. *Biol Blood Marrow Transplant* 2003;9(10):610–615.

Kolb HJ, Schattenberg A, Goldman JM, et al. Graft-versus-leukemia effect of donor lymphocyte transfusions in marrow grafted patients. *Blood* 1995;86(5):2041–2050.

Pavletic SZ, Martin P, Lee SJ, et al. Measuring therapeutic response in chronic graft-versus-host disease: National Institutes of Health consensus development project on criteria for clinical trials in chronic graft-versus-host disease: IV. Response Criteria Working Group report. *Biol Blood Marrow Transplant* 2006;12(3):252–266.

Rizzo JD, Wingard JR, Tichelli A, et al. Recommended screening and preventive practices for long-term survivors after hematopoietic cell transplantation: joint recommendations of the European Group for Blood and Marrow Transplantation, the Center for International Blood and Marrow Transplant Research, and the American Society of Blood and Marrow Transplantation. *Biol Blood Marrow Transplant* 2006;12(2):138–151.

Rowley SD. Hematopoietic stem cell transplantation between red cell incompatible donor-recipient pairs. *Bone Marrow Transplant* 2001;28(4):315–321.

Sorror ML, Maris MB, Storb R, et al. Hematopoietic cell transplantation (HCT)-specific comorbidity index: a new tool for risk assessment before allogeneic HCT. *Blood* 2005;106(8):2912–2919.

BIOSTATISTICS 101 AS APPLIED TO ONCOLOGY

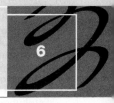

6

Kathryn M. Trinkaus, Feng Gao, and J. Philip Miller

I. INTRODUCTION. Statistics is the mathematical science of estimation in the presence of uncertainty. Its strengths are identifying patterns and teasing out relations in complex data, comparing information from multiple sources, quantifying similarities or differences, and estimating the degree of uncertainty or level of confidence with which to regard the results. Statistics includes an extensive toolbox of solutions for practical problems, with a well-established mathematical foundation. Statistics is more than just tricks, tests, and theorems, however. In a broader sense, it is an efficient, systematic, and reproducible means of investigating patterns and relations in complex data. It is a framework for organized thinking about the issues that generate these data.

A. A few words about data. The **hypotheses** of a study state the scientific ideas being tested, the **objectives** state the tasks required to test those hypotheses, and the **endpoints** are the quantities that will be measured while carrying out the tests. A good endpoint is clearly related to the biological or behavioral process that it measures, ascertainable with minimal error, and readily reproducible.

If an endpoint cannot be directly observed, a related quantity may be substituted as a **surrogate**. Surrogates are ethically preferable if the true endpoint requires invasive procedures or otherwise puts the patient at additional risk. They may be more efficient if the true endpoint takes a long time to observe or is costly to obtain. To be valid, a surrogate must provide the same conclusion as a test of the true endpoint, so it must respond to disease and treatment in the same manner as the true endpoint. Association alone is not sufficient, nor is availability of a more precise measurement. A surrogate endpoint will produce useless or misleading results if it is more precise at the expense of accurately capturing the quantity of interest.

A useful endpoint is consistently observable and easy to record accurately as **missing data** put a study at risk of failure. **Primary endpoints** are used to achieve the primary objectives, so every missing value of a primary endpoint is the loss of a participant. **Systematic data loss** is the absence of most endpoints from individuals or from most individuals for a single endpoint. Dropping variables or individuals with missing data may substantially influence, or **bias**, results by narrowing the scope of the study or reducing the power of the study to identify patterns and differences accurately. Including only patients with nonmissing values means that each conclusion will be based on a different subsample of patients. An alternative is substitution of values for those that are missing, or **imputation**. Numerous methods of imputation exist, all of which are controversial as they can substantially alter the conclusions of a study.

Missing data may be important indicators that a study is encountering logistic, administrative, or procedural difficulties. The best solution is to monitor data loss and address the underlying problems as promptly as possible. A study is only as successful as its data are accurate, precise, and consistently recorded. Good experimental design and data analysis strategies can help with the complex realities of biomedical and clinical research, but they are no substitute for good data.

II. A SHORT INTRODUCTION TO PROBABILITY. Probabilities are used to describe discrete events, such as "response to therapy," as well as the likelihood that a continuous measurement, such as serum creatinine or blood pressure, will take on a specific value. For brevity, both are referred to as *events*. The individuals to whom results of a clinical study will be generalized make up the **target population**. The probability that an event will occur can be defined as the frequency with which the event or value occurs in the target population; this definition is referred to as "**frequentist**." A clinical study usually estimates frequencies in a **sample** from the target population. The **sample size** is large enough to include all relevant features of the target population. The selection process is designed so that all members of the target population have the same (or a predefined) probability of being chosen for the sample; that is, the sample is **randomly chosen**. Randomness helps ensure that no characteristic of the target population is over- or underrepresented, so the selection process does not bias the conclusions of the study.

The frequency of all possible events in the target population is their **probability distribution**. Hypotheses are tested, inferences drawn, and conclusions based on comparison of observed frequencies with those expected from the probability distribution in the target population. A well-defined target population is necessary for sound frequentist statistical analysis. The frequentist approach has great intuitive clarity. However, clearly defining the target population can be difficult, as can identifying a reasonable probability distribution.

An alternative is to use existing knowledge, beliefs, or assumptions to define a **prior (probability) distribution**. A mathematical function is stated, describing the likelihood of the observed data given the characteristics of the prior distribution. The prior distribution and the **likelihood function** are then combined to generate a revised probability distribution, the **posterior distribution**, for the measure of interest. This chain of reasoning is based on a theorem about conditional probabilities first stated by Thomas Bayes, hence the term "**Bayesian**" **statistics**. Bayesian approaches are particularly suited to iterative decision making, as in dose finding studies, because the posterior distribution provides a new prior for the next stage of data collection. The prior has a substantial effect on the conclusions, even a so-called "neutral" prior. This element of subjectivity has weighed against Bayesian statistics where human well-being is involved. Frequentist and Bayesian approaches make different use of a common mathematical foundation, and most standard analyses can be carried out using either method.

Independence is a critical concept in probability theory. Generally speaking, two events are independent if the occurrence of one provides no information about the probability of occurrence of the second. In most cases, observations taken on separate and unrelated biological organisms are considered to be independent, whereas repeated observations taken from the same biological organism are dependent. Some common sources of dependence are association in space (e.g., expression levels of two proteins from a single individual), time (e.g., measures at time of treatment and subsequent weekly intervals), function (e.g., blood pressure and heart rate of the same individual), or inheritance (e.g., genetic studies of family members). Dependence is a matter of degree and can be modeled.

Repeated observations may be incorporated into the experimental design and the methods of analysis to be used. **Replication** of a measure within an individual helps to better estimate within-subject differences, whereas taking measurements on additional individuals helps to better estimate differences between subjects. Repeating an experiment with the same samples already analyzed (**technical replication**) is primarily useful for quality control and adds little to any conclusion drawn about the study sample or target population.

In general, the effective sample size is the number of independent observations taken, not the number of events or measurements. The more complex or variable a quantity is, the larger the number of independent measurements needed to adequately describe it.

III. MEASUREMENT WITH ERROR. Random error occurs by chance alone and is a part of essentially every measurement in a clinical study. Over a large series of measurements, random error has an average value of zero, so it can be reduced by replication. **Systematic error** is a more serious problem as it is due to some aspect of the biological phenomenon of interest, the sample being studied, or the measurement process. Systematic error has an average value greater or less than zero in the long run, so it shifts (biases) estimates away from the true value of the quantities being observed. It may be amplified by replication rather than reduced. A study can be designed to minimize identified sources of systematic error to improve its estimates of the quantities of interest. **Biological variability** contributes to the overall variability of observations. If, of interest to the study, then it is considered "signal," if not of interest to the study, then it is "noise." The study design is used to maximize the capture of signal and minimize the capture of noise.

Most clinical measurements are **random variables (RV)**, measurements that take on a different value for each experimental subject with each value having a specific probability distribution. Discrete RVs fall into unordered (nominal) or ordered (ordinal) categories. The probability distributions of discrete RVs are often known, such as the binomial or multinomial for probability of falling into two or more categories, respectively. Counts, especially relatively rare events per unit time, may approximate a Poisson distribution. **Continuous RVs** are measured on a real or complex number scale with or without upper or lower boundaries. The values that completely describe a continuous distribution are its **parameters**. The parameters of a distribution are usually related to its mean (location of the center) or variance (the spread). Common **parametric** distributions are generalizations from observation of natural processes, not merely mathematical abstractions, and many are related to one another. For a large number of observations of a relatively rare event, the binomial is a good approximation of the Poisson. For a large number of observations, both the binomial and Poisson approach the Gaussian distribution.

If the parameters of a distribution can be estimated, so can the probability that the random variable will take on any given value. If it is very improbable that two sets of observations could have been drawn from a distribution with a single set of parameters, then we have evidence that the groups differ with respect to the measurement. This chain of reasoning is the basis of most frequentist tests of whether a given set of observations is consistent with a hypothesized relation. It also explains the large role of estimating means and variances in statistical analysis.

If the observations do not seem to fit any known distribution, some eccentricities of shape can be adjusted by analyzing the data on an alternative scale, in effect, transforming the data to a recognizable shape. **Transformation** alters the intervals between observations, not their order, so it does not alter conclusions drawn from hypothesis tests. A log transform, for example, makes a multiplicative relationship additive, a useful feature if additive models such as regression are to be used. **Taking ratios** is a way of adjusting each measurement with respect to a baseline or denominator. Mild eccentricity, such as skewness without a large number of duplicate measurements, can also be analyzed with **robust, nonparametric**, or **semiparametric** methods. These methods are less strongly influenced by a few unusual values (**outliers**) and make fewer, weaker assumptions about the distribution from which observed values are drawn.

More highly eccentric distributions, such as those with multiple peaks, abrupt descents, and reascents ("singularities"), large numbers of single values (e.g., a "floor" at zero or a "ceiling" at the detection limit of the measuring instrument), or a combination of discrete and continuous elements are not adequately characterized by a few parameters. With some loss of information, the values can be **categorized** and discrete methods used. Another alternative is **resampling,** which is a form of simulation using probability ("**Monte Carlo**") methods to draw repeated samples from observed data. The repeated samples can be used to estimate parameters or confidence intervals ("**bootstrap**") or test hypotheses (e.g., **permutation tests**) regardless of the underlying distribution of the data. If the data are too complex to be dealt with as a whole, piecewise methods, such as **locally weighted regression** and **splines,** may be preferable. These analyze the data in segments, carrying out the estimation process over a small region rather than trying to find an analysis appropriate for the observations as a whole.

IV. **VIEWING THE DATA.** Given the complexity of biological phenomena, a preliminary overview is essential before diving into analysis. Plots, charts, lists, and frequency tables provide a comprehensive, visual representation of pattern, distribution, and difference. They highlight unusual data points, help with error checking, summarize the shape of individual variables, and illustrate relations between sets of variables.

Visual summaries are so important for understanding data that it is essential to have a software program with good graphics capability.

For continuous, interval or ordinal variables, **dot plots** and **stem-and-leaf plots** contain a symbol for each data point, stacking the occurrences of each value. The location of most common values, symmetry or skewness, and presence of unusual values (**outliers**) are readily seen. **Histograms** summarize counts or proportions in a solid column rather than representing each data value separately. Relative numbers or proportions in nominal or ordinal categories are easily identified. **Bivariate scatter plots** are useful for examining relations between two or more continuous variables, as well as finding the center(s) of the distribution and the location and distance to outlying values. **Box plots** represent the distribution of a continuous variable in each of one or more categories. The "box" represents the middle of the distribution, e.g., the 25th to 75th percentiles. Lines extending outward from the ends of the box and plot symbols represent the spread of the data. A **trellis plot** is a matrix of scatter plots, one for each pair of a set of variables. Trellis plots make it very easy to scan a relatively large number of variables at a glance; for example, for a first look at a set of variables to be used in a multivariable analysis. **Robust smoothing methods** draw a curve through the bulk of data points, giving more weight to nearby observations than to more distant ones.

A useful plot highlights patterns by suppressing detail. In general, it is more illuminating to compare several kinds of plots than to add information to a single plot. Whatever method is used, the human eye is extraordinarily good at finding patterns where there may be none. Random scatters may falsely appear patterned, especially when few data points are available. Plots are a starting point but they do not replace a more rigorous statistical examination.

V. DIMENSION REDUCTION. Measurement devices such as questionnaires, imaging methods, microarrays, and mass spectroscopy or gel-based protein expression measurements collect a large number of dependent, and partly redundant, information from individual subjects. Finding a smaller subset of observations that contains a high proportion of the information in the full data set is **dimension reduction.** Commonly used techniques include **principal components analysis**, which identifies a linear combination of variables that represent as much as possible of the information in the full set. **Factor analysis** defines underlying dimensions of the data using the correlations or covariances between variables. **Discriminant analysis** generates a mathematical (discriminant) function or a linear combination of independent variables that assigns observations to groups. **Cluster analysis** performs a similar task by splitting the data set one observation, or set of observations, at a time until relatively homogeneous clusters are identified. Tree-based methods, such as classification and regression trees (**CART**), are sets of instructions (algorithms) for using data from multiple dimensions to group observations and define their relations. Each of these families of methods has distinctive properties and data requirements. All of them tend to impose structure on the data according to their particular algorithm. As descriptive and exploratory tools, they can be informative when used with their requirements in mind.

VI. MAKING INFERENCES ABOUT DATA. The goal of most clinical studies is to improve clinical decision-making and patient outcomes, so the study data will be used for making inferences and testing hypotheses. Hypothesis testing, whether frequentist or Bayesian, is a well-defined, repeatable methodology for answering questions about observed data using probability models. Traditionally, hypothesis tests require a null hypothesis, which describes the background against which research results will be interpreted, and an alternative hypothesis, stating the expected result or difference. These differences are expresseed as a measure of interest and its probability distribution given that the null hypothesis is true. Finally, a definition is needed of the values that are compatible with the null hypothesis, the critical region, as opposed to those that are extreme or atypical when the null hypothesis is true.

Samples are drawn from a well-defined target population, with randomization to reduce selection bias, and the measure of interest is observed. If the measure falls within the critical region, there is no evidence that the null hypothesis is false. If the measure falls outside the critical area, the result is not compatible with the null hypothesis, and the alternative is chosen instead. There are two correct decisions: to accept the alternative when the null hypothesis is false or to fail to reject the null hypothesis when it is true. The corresponding errors are to reject the null hypothesis when it is true (**a false-positive** or **type I error**) or to fail to reject the null hypothesis when it is false (a **false-negative or type II error**). No probability is attached to the results, only whether it falls inside or outside the critical region.

In practice, a ***p*-value** is usually calculated, expressing the probability of results that are as extreme as or more extreme than the observed results, assuming that the observations are drawn from the probability distribution specified by the null hypothesis. "More extreme than" refers to values far from the center of the distribution, or in the "tails" of the distribution. If the alternative hypothesis is concerned with any difference from the null hypothesis, then the *p*-value measures the probability of falling into either tail of the distribution, a **two-tailed test**. If the alternative is concerned only with values greater than, or only values less than, the critical value, then the *p*-value measures the probability of falling into a single tail, a **one-tailed test**. Two-tailed tests are more demanding as the area in each tail is smaller and are generally preferred unless there is a strong reason for a one-tailed test.

Studies are designed to minimize the probability of a false positive (the **significance level,** or α) while maximizing the probability of a correct positive (the **study power**). Conventional significance levels are 0.01 and 0.05, whereas power is usually no less than 0.8. Calculating study power is a routine part of designing any clinical trial using inferential procedures. Calculating power requires information about the expected values of endpoints under standard conditions (the null hypothesis) and the study treatment (the alternative hypothesis) as well as the expected variability and precision of measurement. If some of this information is not available, the maximum detectable difference can be calculated for a given null hypothesis and a specified study power. In the absence of any preliminary evidence, no inferential procedures can be planned, so only an observational trial is possible. If the preliminary information is weak or of uncertain relevance, a review of study power can be built into the study design to ensure that the entire study does not rest on a shaky foundation. There is no useful information to be had from a power calculation carried out after observations have been made, a ***post hoc* power calculation**.

Estimates of study power generally refer to single tests. If many tests are to be carried out, then some positive results may be observed purely by chance. A significance level of 0.05 implies that any result that is expected to occur less frequently than 5 in 100 times, or 1 in 20 times, is considered "unlikely." In a large series of similar tests, then, one falsely significant result can be expected among every 20 tests. There are many methods for taking into account the effect of **multiple testing**. Most were developed for moderate numbers of tests in a single analysis or model. Their usefulness for combining results from several types of analyses on related data or from multiple studies (**meta-analyses**) is unclear. Genomic and proteomic studies, which may involve tens of thousands of tests, are also not well served by traditional multiple testing correction methods. Multiple testing corrections are more useful in confirmatory studies, where the goal is to avoid a false-positive result, than in discovery studies, where overcorrection may prevent recognition of interesting results. Results from discovery studies usually require validation in fully independent studies.

If the conditions of a hypothesis test are too difficult to meet or if a more information-rich result is needed, then a Bayesian procedure may be preferable. These make more efficient and comprehensive use of prior information. The *caveat* is that prior data must be substantially accurate if a reliable prior distribution is to be found.

VII. MODELING RELATIONS. Modeling provides a richer, more nuanced approach to data analysis than simple hypothesis testing. Traditional single or multiple linear models describe the relation between independent variables and Gaussian-distributed dependent variables. The effect of each independent variable is adjusted for the effect of the others, so the model describes the joint effect of several covariates on the outcome. Models may be stratified, allowing different curves to be fit to subsets of the data and their distinctness tested. **Generalized linear, nonlinear,** and

time-to-event modeling allow the same strategies to be applied to non-Gaussian, dependent nonlinear, or censored data. **Mixed models** have extended the linear framework to **random effects**; that is, independent variables that represent a sample of the values to which conclusions will be generalized, rather than a complete set. **Hierarchical models** allow inclusion of multiple levels of dependence, such as multiple observations taken from each individual and at several time points. **Robust** methods can accommodate some forms of eccentrically distributed data by modeling a curve or surface in segments, estimating the value of the dependent variable based on nearby observations. **Splines** take a similar piece-wise approach in a more formal way, fitting a model to each segment. Artificial **neural networks** are nonlinear models of complex relations incorporating substantial redundancy.

The complexity of relations being modeled is both a strength and a weakness of the modeling process. **Confounding** describes two or more independent variables that are related to one another as well as to the outcome. Confounding can exaggerate or mask the effect of any single covariate on the outcome, and it is best dealt with in the study design. A related problem is **colinearity**, a situation in which two or more covariates provide redundant information about the outcome. One or more will appear less strongly related to the outcome than is actually the case, presenting a counterintuitive or apparently nonsensical result. If it is important to estimate the effect of each covariate, several models will have to be created.

The joint effect of several covariates may be quite different than their individual effects, or **main effects**. When the effect of a covariate differs depending on the presence or level of another covariate, an **interaction** is present. In this case, there is no simple way to describe the effect of any single covariate, so it is important to avoid attempting to interpret main effects when interactions are present.

The outstanding effects in a model are usually easy to identify. If there are few observations to work with, then only large effects are likely to be identified even if the sample is a good representation of the target population. Some real effects may not be measurable with a given sample, and a difficult choice of covariates is usually necessary. The p-values indicate whether a covariate contributes to a model, but they are not sensitive measures of how much information is provided. Measures of information or tests, such as likelihood ratio tests, are better indicators of how much information is gained or lost with each independent variable. If a model is based on most of the variation in the input data, with few anomalies and little ignored information, then it is said to fit well. Any change in the model can alter its fit, so the fit must be reexamined at each step. Diagnostic tools such as **residuals** measure unexplained variability, while tests for **goodness-of-fit** estimate how closely the model fits the input data. **Outliers** occur where model's estimation of the outcome value differ from the observed value for a specific set of covariates. **Influential points** are closely approximated by the model, although at the expense of a substantial number of the remaining observations. Any of these may distort the model and render its conclusions inaccurate or misleading. To fit a sound model and interpret it correctly, the analyst must know the input data well, understand the model being used, test the fit with care, and examine the output results in detail.

VIII. **CONCLUSION.** A basic knowledge of statistics allows one to investigate data at first hand in a systematic and organized manner as well as to collaborate more effectively with a statistician when more extensive analyses are needed.

   A. **How to learn more.** Statistics is most interesting when it is helping to do something important, so learning statistics is more effective and more fun with good software at hand. **JMP** (www.jmp.com), **SPSS** (www.spss.com) and **NCSS** (www.ncss.com) provide immediate access with good graphics and user-friendly, menu-driven interfaces. JMP and NCSS include genomic data analysis methods, as well as power and sample size calculators. **Spotfire** (www.spotfire.com) provides extensive data visualization tools with a flexible, menu-driven user interface. For more complex or customized analyses, **SAS** (www.sas.com), **S-Plus** (www.insightful.com), and **R** (www.r-project.org) are powerful programming languages that require some study to be used effectively. **R** is open source and can be used without charge. The others require a license.

Suggested Readings

General Interest

Hacking I. *The Emergence of Probability*. Cambridge: Cambridge University Press, 1984.

Salsburg D. *The Lady Tasting Tea: How Statistics Revolutionized Science in the Twentieth Century*. New York: Henry Holt, 2002.

Stigler S. *Statistics on the Table: A History of Statistical Concepts and Methods*. Cambridge: Harvard University Press, 2002.

Basics

Altman D. *Practical Statistics for Medical Research*. New York: CRC Press, 1990.

Gonick L, Smith W. *The Cartoon Guide to Statistics*. New York: HarperCollins, 1994.

Huff D. *How to Lie with Statistics*. New York: W.W. Norton & Co, 1993.

Motulsky H. *Intuitive Biostatistics*. London: Oxford University Press, 1995.

Newton H, Harvill J. *StatConcepts: A Visual Tour of Statistical Ideas*. Boston: Duxbury Press, 1997.

Rosner B. *Fundamentals of Biostatistics*. Boston: Duxbury Press, 2005.

Salkind N. *Statistics for People Who (Think They) Hate Statistics*. Thousand Oaks: Sage Publications Inc, 2003.

Van Belle G, Fisher L. *Biostatistics: A Methodology for the Health Sciences*. New York: Wiley-Interscience, 1996.

Software-Guided Learning

Cody R, Smith J. *Applied Statistics and the SAS Programming Language*, 5th ed. New York: Prentice Hall, 2005.

Field A. *Discovering Statistics Using SPSS*. Thousand Oaks: Sage Publications, 2005.

Heiberger R, Holland B. *Statistical Analysis and Data Display: An Intermediate Course, with Examples in S-Plus, R, and SAS*. New York: Springer-Verlag, 2004.

Lehamn A, O'Rourke N, Hatcher L, et al. *JMP for Basic Univariate and Multivariate Statistics: A Step-by-Step Guide*. Cary NC: SAS Publishing, 2005.

Maindonald J, Braun J. *Data Analysis and Graphics Using R: An Example-Based Approach*, 2nd ed. Cambridge: Cambridge University Press, 2007.

Venables W, Ripley B. *Modern Applied Statistics with S-Plus*. New York: Springer, 2002.

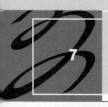

PRINCIPLES OF CLINICAL RESEARCH
Feng Gao, Kathryn M. Trinkaus, and J. Philip Miller

I. **WHAT IS CLINICAL RESEARCH?** Broadly speaking, clinical research is an activity involving people having or suspected of having a disease—what causes human disease and how it can be prevented and treated. It is a patient-oriented, systematic investigation of human disease including its mechanisms, diagnosis, therapeutic interventions, and prevention, with intent to develop or contribute to generalizable knowledge. It is the "generalizable knowledge" component that differentiates a daily clinical practice, where information is sought for diagnosis or treatment of an individual patient, from a research activity, where data is collected among a sample of patients with the intention of drawing conclusions applicable to a larger population.

II. **BIOSTATISTICAL ELEMENTS BEHIND CLINICAL RESEARCH.** Biostatistics is a body of methods for learning from experience. It applies probability theory and statistical techniques for collecting, describing, analyzing, and interpreting health data. Statistical thinking has become an integral part in designing a modern clinical research, especially for preventing potential bias and confounding, increasing the efficiency in data collection, conducting quality control (QC) to ensure the integrity of the research process, and determining the size of sample. The following are some statistics-related questions frequently asked in initiating a clinical research protocol.

A. **What are the research questions being asked?** Most clinical research is hypothesis-driven. For example, comparisons are made to determine whether there is a difference between treatments, or between treatment and control, with respect to a hypothesized null value. The first steps in designing a clinical research are identification of the scientific questions to be addressed, formulation of research hypotheses, and definition of study objectives. Two complementary hypotheses are involved—the **null hypothesis** represents a theory that has been put forward as a basis for argument while the **alternative hypothesis** is a statement of what a statistical test intends to establish. The usual research objective is to demonstrate that a new treatment is superior to an existing therapy, where the null hypothesis is that the two treatments are the same. By contrast, in an **equivalence study** designed to show that a new treatment is the same as an existing therapy, the null hypothesis is amended such that the treatments differ by more than a defined amount. Every clinical research should have a primary hypothesis (the most important question) that can be answered with less ambiguity.

B. **How will the questions be answered?** This determines the overall design of a research. An efficient study design obtains the fullest information possible about study endpoints from the fewest possible study participants over the shortest possible time. A variety of formal designs are available to increase the efficiency in data collection, control confounding effects, or manage the impact of missing data. Clinical researches can be classified in several ways. Depending on whether interventions are imposed or not, a study can be **experimental** or **observational**. An experimental study usually involves some sort of intervention and the investigators have some control on the experimental conditions. By contrast, an observational study aims for solely observation without altering or influencing the subjects being studied. Depending on the time sequence, a study can be retrospective, prospective, or cross-sectional. A retrospective study collects data that already exists. A prospective study follows up participants and measures outcomes over time course, whereas a cross-sectional study gathers such information simultaneously during a brief interval. A study may be classified based on its research intent, for example, a **screening study** focuses on means of early detection while a **therapeutic study** intends to alleviate or cure a preexisting disease. A study may also be classified based on how the design is constructed. Participants in a **parallel study** receive a single treatment before their results are compared, whereas participants in a **crossover study** receive two or more treatments in sequence. Note that all these classifications are not mutually exclusive. A study can include both retrospective and prospective components and/or with a combination of diagnostic and therapeutic aims. Section III lists the features of some most frequently used designs.

C. **Who will benefit from the study?** The purpose of clinical research is to draw conclusion about a population based on a sample taken from the population. Therefore, it is important to identify a proper **target population**, which is that part of the human population to which the results will be applicable in a clinical setting. The **sampling frame** is that part of the target population from which the study sample will be drawn. The process by which study participants are identified and recruited is the **sampling strategy**. A sound sampling strategy ensures that endpoints are represented fully in the study sample so that the results may be generalized to the population that may benefit from them. The research hypotheses and sampling frame are used to identify characteristics of participants who may benefit from the treatment and the eligibility criteria for the trial. Characteristics of participants who are unlikely to benefit or who may be at an unusually high risk if enrolled define the excylusion criteria. Eligibility and exclusion criteria are usually specific to the condition and treatment under study, although the presence of unknown or poorly estimable risks (e.g., pregnant or breast-feeding women and their offspring) may also be a reason for exclusion. Participants should never be included or excluded automatically (e.g., by age, gender, or race/ethnicity) or as a matter of convenience. A consecutive series of participants from a single clinic or practice, even if they represent "all-comers," is biased by the nature of the clinic, its location, the mechanisms of referral, and many other factors. Such a single-institution sample may not be easily generalized to the target population, and any results may require subsequent confirmation before they are accepted.

D. **What are the endpoints being studied?** Once the objectives are clearly stated and the target populations are properly identified, the next step is to choose measurements of the effects of interest, or **endpoints**. If these cannot be measured directly, then careful consideration is needed to find the best available surrogates. Informative study endpoints are clearly related to the study hypotheses and objectives, unambiguously measurable with minimal error, and available within a reasonable period. Information-rich measures are preferable, those that finely discriminate between degrees or states of the phenomena of interest. For example, Table 7.1 shows some endpoints, primarily for comparative treatment studies, in cancer drug approval by the U.S. Food and Drug Administration (FDA) (*http://www.fda.gov/cder/guidance/6592dft.htm*).

E. **What are the confounding variables?** Study hypotheses and objectives will usually make clear which characteristics of the participants, their environment, or the condition of interest may have effects on the endpoints. These **covariates** often include demographic and clinical characteristics of the participants, aspects of the disease process under study, and any striking features of past or current treatments received. The study hypotheses define how covariates will be included in the analysis and interpretation of study results. A **confounding variable**, or confounder, is an extraneous factor that wholly or partially accounts for the observed effect. The existence of such a confounding effect may distort the true relation between the outcome and the factor of primary interest (i.e., treatment)—either causing a relationship to falsely appear or masking the true relation. If the study arms contain very unequal numbers of participants with differing disease-related characteristics, then it may be impossible to separate the effect of treatment from the effect of the characteristics. For example, if a pulmonary function study contains one treatment group composed largely of smokers and another of nonsmokers, the effect of treatment will be difficult to separate from the effect of smoking status. The term *confounding* also refers to the inability to separate effects of two or more covariates on an endpoint. The confounding effects must be considered and controlled, at

TABLE 7.1 A Comparison of Some Important Cancer Approval Endpoints

Endpoint	Assessment	Advantages	Disadvantages
OS	Randomized studies needed Blinding not essential	Direct measure of benefit Easily and precisely measured	Requires larger studies; requires longer studies; potentially affected by cross-over therapy; does not capture symptom benefit; includes noncancer deaths
DFS	Randomized studies needed Blinding preferred	Considered as clinical benefit Needs fewer patients than OS	Not a validated survival surrogate in most settings; not precisely measured and subject to assessment bias; various definitions exist
ORR	Single-arm or randomized studies Blinding preferred in comparative study	Can be assessed in single-arm studies	Not a direct measure of benefit; usually reflects drug activity in a minority of patients; data moderately complex compared to survival
CR	Single-arm or randomized studies can be used Blinding preferred	Obvious benefit in some setting Assessable in single-arm studies	Few drugs produce high rates of CR; data moderately complex compared to survival
PFS	Randomized studies needed Blinding preferred Blinded review recommended	Measured in responding and stable tumors Usually assessed before change in therapy Less missing data Assessed earlier and in smaller studies compared with survival	Various definitions exist; not a direct measure of benefit; not a validated survival surrogate; not precisely measured & subject to assessment bias; frequent radiologic studies are needed; data are voluminous and complex compared to survival
Symptom endpoints	Usually needs randomized blinded studies (unless endpoints have an objective component and effects are large)	Direct measure of benefit	Blinding is often difficult in oncology trials; missing data are common; few instruments are validated for measuring cancer-specific symptoms; data are voluminous and complex compared to survival

OS, overall survival; DFS, disease-free survival; ORR, objective response rate; CR, complete response; PFS, progression-free survival.

design stage and/or at the subsequent data analysis stage. In case–control studies, for example, confounding is frequently dealt with by **matching** so that the comparison groups have similar values of confounding variables (e.g., age, gender, history of treatment). The subsequent data analysis must account for the matching design. In experimental studies, **randomization** is the most effective way to control potential confounders. It helps to create treatment groups that are balanced on both known and unknown baseline characteristics, and thereby to ensure that the statistically significant differences between treatment groups are solely due to treatment effect. A **stratified randomization** will specifically make each treatment group containing approximately equal numbers of participants with each characteristic (e.g., in a two-arm study, stratified by gender approximately half the number of men and half the number of women will be randomized to each treatment group). In summary, whether covariates are effects of interest or factors to be adjusted, their definition and role need careful planning.

F. **What are the potential biases?** Bias represents the difference between an estimated value and the true value of the quantity being measured. It can arise at any stage and must be minimized as far as possible. For example, **selection or allocation bias** will arise if the investigators know the assignment of treatment and are tempted to give new treatment to patients who have failed on previous therapy. An **observer bias** arises if the investigators know which treatment a subject is taking and tend to give a more optimistic score in measuring the efficacy of the new treatment. A subjective endpoint (e.g., the assessment of pain) is more likely to suffer from a **measurement bias**. **Publication bias**, a tendency to only report results that are statistically significant, may be present at the stage of reporting a clinical research. Using a control group, randomization, and blinding of endpoints are ways to avoid bias, especially in designing prospective comparative studies. Inclusion of a **concurrent control** (either parallel or sequential) is helpful in reducing the bias of so-called placebo effect. **Randomization** creates more comparable treatment groups that are balanced on both known and unknown baseline characteristics, and is therefore capable of eliminating various sources of bias. Blinding is a way to restrict knowledge of individual treatment assignments to participants, investigators or biostatisticians. In an **unblinded, unmasked, or open-label** study, assignments are known to study participants, treating physicians, and other study personnel. In a **single-blind** study, either the study participant or the investigator is unaware of study group assignments. If both study participants and investigators do not know which treatment is being received, the study is **double blind**. To maintain a double blind, it is usually necessary to extend the blind to other clinical personnel involved with participant treatment, data collection, and data management. Data analysts may also be blinded. Care must be taken to design treatments and controls to be as nearly indistinguishable as possible.

G. **How will the data be analyzed?** Once the study hypotheses and endpoints are defined, a data analysis plan will be developed to identify the possible confounders and to specify the detailed modeling procedures for primary analysis as well as secondary or exploratory analyses, if any. The purpose of statistical testing is to make a decision about a population parameter by examining a sample from that population. That is, the decision is not about the particular subjects observed in the study, but rather about the larger population from which the patients were drawn. The strength of the statistical evidence will be expressed as *p* **values**. In a loose sense, the *p* value measures surprise under the null hypothesis. The smaller the *p* value, the more surprising the results if the null hypothesis is true. Common comparisons among treatment and control groups include tests for difference of proportions (e.g., response rates), mean or median values (e.g., temperature, blood pressure), counts (e.g., episodes of toxicity), and distribution of events (e.g., time to death, disease progression, or recurrence). Unlike rates, means, or counts that are observed for all participants at specific times, events may occur after the follow-up period has ended. The time to event will be unknown for some participants (e.g., survival time for patients alive at end of study). Such values are referred to as **censored data** and require analytic techniques such as Kaplan–Meier or Cox proportional hazards modeling. The primary analysis is usually carried out on the **intent-to-treat** principle, in which each participant's results are included in estimation of the effect in the treatment group to which they were assigned, regardless of whether they actually received that, or any, treatment. Subsequent analyses may estimate effects by using only participants who actually received each treatment. Such analyses must always be interpreted with reference to intent-to-treat analyses to establish that their results are not dependent on conscious or unconscious selection of participants based on their outcomes. Further analyses suggested by study results (for example, analysis of subsets of the study population) may be carried out to explore directions for future research. Results of such **post hoc data analyses** are regarded as hypothesis generating (supplying questions to ask in future trials) rather than definitive, regardless of the level of statistical significance or their clinical interest.

H. **How many subjects will be needed?** Once the study design is clear, the study power and sample size can be determined. **Power** is the probability of rejecting the null hypothesis when the alternative hypothesis is true, or the ability to detect the effects of interest if they do exist. The complement of power (1−power) is the probability of failing to find an effect of a particular size when one does exist, a **type II error**. Common values for type II error are 0.2 (or 1 in 5) and 0.1 (or 1 in 10), which correspond to a power of 0.8 and 0.9, respectively. The study **significance level** is the probability of detecting an apparent effect when none exists and differences observed are the result of chance, a type I error. Common values for **type I error** are 0.05 (1 in 20) and 0.01 (1 in 100). Too small a sample will have less power to detect any significant difference. Too large a sample wastes resources, extends the study duration, and exposes participants unnecessarily to the risks associated with the trial. It may also detect differences that are statistically significant but too small to be clinically important. To calculate sample size, the investigator must know the desired power, type I error, and expected magnitude of the effect to be observed based on the best information available at the outset of the trial. Sample size and power also depend on the "side-ness" of a significance test. In a **two-sided test**, the null hypothesis will be rejected if the observed value is greater or less than the null value (i.e., if any difference is observed). By contrast, a **one-sided test** only determines whether a treatment increases (decreases) the endpoint. One-sided hypotheses will have greater power and require smaller numbers of observations. This is not surprising because the one-sided study is designed based on more prior knowledge—the direction of treatment effect is assumed to be known. At present, the two-sided tests are more commonly used, to be conservative. Sample size and power calculations are specific for a particular statistical hypothesis test. In an **equivalence test**, to show that the new treatment is not significantly worse than the standard therapy, for example, the type I error (the error of falsely claiming a significant difference) will be less serious because such an error, if occurred, will take us to the standard therapy. As a consequence, the power calculation can be based on a less restrictive type I error (i.e., 0.1 or even 0.2) with a one-sided test.

III. **FREQUENTLY USED TYPES OF DESIGNS**
A. **Case report and case series study.** This study describes experience about a single patient or of a small group of patients with the same diagnosis. The object of this design is to make observations about the patient(s) with defined characteristics. This study is useful in learning the natural history of a disease, enriching clinical experience, and generating hypotheses for future studies. It is a simple descriptive study and there is no hypothesis to test.
B. **Prevalence survey or cross-sectional study.** The objective of this design is to make observations about the prevalence of a disease, and/or to assess the associations a set of covariates (i.e., hypothesized risk factors) to the disease outcomes. A distinct feature of this study is that it is a "snapshot" of health experience, i.e., the information regarding covariates and disease is obtained at a single time point. Since a cross-sectional study cannot usually determine whether the covariates precede the occurrence of disease, it is useful for generating but not for testing the hypothesis about causal relations.

C. Case–control study. The objective of a case–control study is to identify the possible causal relations between the hypothesized risk factors and the disease of interest. One distinct feature of this study is that the data regarding risk factors are collected retrospectively. In a case–control study, cases (who have developed a disease of interest) and controls (who do not have the disease) are first identified and then the frequency or levels of potential risk factors are compared between the two groups. Case–control studies provide a cheaper and quicker tool for studying possible causal relationship, especially efficient for rare diseases. In addition, case–control studies allow investigators to explore multiple etiologic factors in a single study. However, case–control studies are very likely to suffer from bias. Another limitation is that each case–control study can only investigate one disease outcome. (This is because cases and controls are sampled separately based on the definition of the disease, and different diseases would produce totally different study groups.) Extreme care must be taken in the selection of cases and controls. Cases should be representative of all patients who develop the disease while controls are representative of patients who do not develop the disease but are drawn from the same population at risk for the disease. **Matching design** may be used so that cases and controls have similar values of potential confounding variables (i.e., age, gender, smoking status, etc.) or other already known risk factors. The simplest matching is where each case is matched with a single control (**1:1 matching** or **paired matching**). A **1:k matching**, where one case is matched to k controls, can be applied to improve efficiency if there are more controls available than cases. Unlike the aforementioned individual matching, a **frequency matching** is to ensure that the control sample has a similar overall makeup of the matching variables to the case sample. Sometimes a close matching may reduce the number of participants, as appropriate matches become difficult to find. Equally important in a case–control design is that the information from cases and controls should be collected in the same way. However, this can be practically difficult because the disease status is usually known to investigators before data collection.

D. Longitudinal cohort study. A cohort study has the same research objective as a case–control study, except that the data regarding hypothesized risk factors are collected before the occurrence of disease outcomes. In a **concurrent cohort study**, the research population is defined at the time the study is initiated and then followed prospectively for the disease outcomes. By contrast, **a retrospective cohort study** records the information of risk factors at some time point in the past, and the disease outcomes are determined at the time of study initiation (an approach that is most frequently seen in **clinical chart review studies**). Compared to case–control studies, cohort studies have fewer potential sources of bias and can provide an explicit temporal relationship between risk factors and outcomes. However, a prospective cohort can require a rather large sample size and long study duration, and sometimes such a follow-up study can be prohibitively expensive. **Nested case–control studies** are proposed to combine the features of case–control and cohort studies. At first, cases of a disease that occur in a defined cohort are identified. Then, for each case, a number of matched controls are selected from among those in the cohort who have not yet developed the disease. Compared to the traditional cohort design, such a nested case–control approach potentially offers impressive reductions in the costs on data collection and analysis, while resulting in a relatively minor loss in statistical efficiency.

E. Clinical trials. Clinical trials are true experiments on human beings to assess one or more potentially beneficial therapies. Heavily influenced by drug development (especially cytotoxic agents) for oncology studies, clinical trails are usually classified as phase I, II, III and IV.

    1. Phase I or dose-finding trial. In a typical phase I trial, a small cohort of patients (usually three to six patients) is treated with a small dose (e.g., 10% of the dose [in mg/kg] that is lethal in rats) of the drug being studied. This cohort is observed for toxicity. If no unacceptable or dose-limiting toxicities are observed in the first cohort, then another cohort of patients may be treated with a higher dose. This process is continued until toxicity is demonstrated. If only one patient demonstrates toxicity in a cohort, then that group may be expanded and additional patients treated before escalating the dose further. Once dose-limiting toxicity is demonstrated in more than one patient in a cohort, then the trial is completed, and the next lowest dose is considered the maximal tolerable dose (**MTD**). The MTD is recommended for further testing. Although efficacy is not a traditional endpoint of a phase I trial, patient responses, if observed, may indicate directions for further testing. One problem with the traditional phase I design described here is that too many patients may be treated at low doses, wasting resources by needlessly enlarging the trial and treating patients with subtherapeutic doses. This has led to increasing use of novel phase I designs with more rapid dose escalation. Examples include the **continuous reassessment method** (**CRM**) proposed by O'Quigley et al. and the dose **escalation with overdose control** (**EWOC**) by Babb et al., both of which take a Bayesian strategy and use MTD as a parameter in the model. Instead of treating MTD as a fixed quantity, CRM and EWOC will continuously update the estimated MTD as data accumulates. Studies of toxicity, absorption, activity, and clearance of the drug (**safety, pharmacokinetics, and bioavailability**) are also carried out as phase I trials. In an oncology phase I trial (i.e., on cytotoxic agents), the participants are usually cancer patients with terminal disease for whom no standard therapy or salvage treatment exists, whereas healthy volunteers are often used in the phase I trials in other branches of medicine.

2. **Phase II trials.** Once the dose and schedule of an agent has been set as a result of a phase I trial, the regimen is ready for a phase II trial where the primary goal is to screen new regimens based on the efficacy. Unlike a phase I trial where a problem of estimation is addressed, a phase II trial inherently deals with a problem of hypothesis testing although there is usually no control arm in the trial. Approximately 20 to 40 participants will be enrolled to investigate the drug's **efficacy** as well as **toxicity** profile. A phase II trail is frequently implemented in a two-stage approach. Study results are analyzed before the trial is complete (**interim analysis**) for an early termination of trials due to lack of benefit and/or unacceptable toxicity. A typical phase II trial considers an **objective response rate** (**ORR**, which is based on tumor shrinkage) as the solely primary endpoint. Recently, some innovative designs have been proposed to assess toxicity and efficacy simultaneously, while some other designs intend to distinguish the relative importance of **complete response** (CR) versus **partial response** (PR). Some investigators further classify phase II trials into subclasses of IIA and IIB. Usually a phase IIA trial is performed on a single agent and the typical objective is to determine whether the experimental regimen has any antidisease activity as measured by ORR. In contrast, phase IIB trials are conducted on combination regimens to determine whether the antidisease activity is sufficiently high to warrant further evaluation by a phase III study, and some survival-based endpoints such as progression-free survival (PFS) or disease-free survival (DFS) also need to be considered. In recent years, an increasing number of phase II trials have been implemented as randomized studies. However, the design of a randomized phase II trial is quite different from that of a phase III study. The purpose of a phase II trial is to select a promising treatment for further evaluation. In this framework, the study is not designed to ensure that the best treatment is definitely selected (such a decision would be more appropriate for a phase III trial). Rather, the design is to ensure that an inferior treatment would have a very low probability to be selected. To this end, a randomized phase II trial can have a rather large type I error. In such a **selection design** approach (i.e., to pick up the winner among competing candidates regardless of the magnitude of improvement), each group will require fewer patients than conventional single-arm phase II designs.

3. **Phase III trials.** If the results in the phase II trials are encouraging, larger, multicenter, controlled, randomized phase III trials will compare treatment effects with standard therapy. Both for ethical reasons and for the purpose of allocating limited resources, recently there has been an increasing interest to incorporate the concepts of **adaptive design** (also known as **sample size re-estimation [SSR]**) and **sequential design** to phase III trials. In an adaptive design, the interim data

is evaluated for scientific reasons to update the knowledge based on accumulated data and thereby to readjust the study design if necessary. In a sequential design, on the other hand, interim data is mainly examined for ethical reasons to seek an early stopping due to either excess toxicity or overwhelming evidence of efficacy.

4. **Phase IV trials.** After a new drug application (**NDA**) has been approved and a drug released by the FDA, additional post marketing phase IV trials may be carried out to observe treatment effects with long-term follow-up in a broader clinical setting to examine issues of cost-effectiveness, quality of life, new indication/new formulation, or simply for marketing purpose.

5. **More comments on clinical trials**

   a. **Phase I trials on therapeutic cancer vaccines.** The classification given earlier is largely based on the oncology study of cytotoxic agents that work by killing tumor cells. However, a quite different developmental strategy, especially at early phases, can be taken for biologic agents that work through modulating tumor environments and/or delaying tumor progression. In **therapeutic cancer vaccine studies**, for example, the boundary lines between phase I and II trials become blurred. Even in a phase I trial to identify the optimal dose, it is equally important to quantify the therapeutic efficacy. Compared to trials on cytotoxic agents, a phase I trial on cancer vaccines can be quite different in patient selection, the endpoints, as well as the overall design construction. First, due to lack of intact immune systems, patients who are in the end stage of the disease are less likely to benefit from a cancer vaccine. Normal volunteers or less advanced cancer patients who have intact immune systems will be a more appropriate target population. Second, the response based on tumor shrinkage is no longer the best efficacy endpoint, and immunologic endpoints or clinical benefit endpoints such as time to tumor progression are frequently considered in cancer vaccine studies. Finally, dose-escalation design is rarely used in phase I vaccine trials. Rather, the study usually works on fixed dose levels that are determined by preclinical studies, preferably as a randomized design with 10 to 15 patients per dose level.

   b. **Special issues with trials on medical devices or surgical procedures.** Though most of the aforementioned principles are still applicable, trials on medical devices or surgical procedures can raise some special issues that deserve careful considerations. For example, blinding is rarely implemented on such trials and extra care should be taken to avoid the potential sources of bias. In addition, the success or failure of the therapy is not only based on the device/procedure itself, but also highly associated with the technical skills of the clinicians.

IV. DATA COLLECTION, QC, AND DATA MANAGEMENT

A. **Data collection.** Once the endpoints and study design are defined, data collection forms can be created. Well-designed forms smooth the daily operation of the study, save time and effort, and produce complete, clean, and unambiguous data for subsequent analysis. A comparatively small investment in planning at this stage saves a great deal of time and effort later. Any discrete encounter with a participant that produces study data should have a form. Information collected at different times is kept on separate forms, so that forms are not routinely left partly blank. All forms containing information to be gathered at a particular stage of the study are gathered together into a discrete packet. Forms should be printed ahead of time, kept up-to-date with any changes in data collection, and made readily accessible to those who use them. Their content is determined largely by the study design. The format and organization are best worked out collaboratively with staff members experienced in data collection, entry, and analysis. If the study requires that a specific script is followed when asking questions or presenting information to participants, then the text is included at the appropriate point on the form. Individual data items are presented as clearly as possible, offering selection lists and check boxes rather than free-text fields when possible. The format and units of dates and numbers are printed on the form to avoid confusion later. Required data fields are printed in bold or otherwise clearly identified. Data items are presented as nearly as possible in the order in which they will be recorded, so that data fields are not routinely skipped. Data fields are never routinely left blank. Codes or check boxes are used to indicate why values are missing to make clear that data collection has been completed. The person filling out a form initials and dates each one, in case questions arise later about the information on the form. Completed forms are sorted by participant and stage of the project and kept in locked filing cabinets in a secure area to preserve **confidentiality** of participant information.

B. QC. QC includes periodic operational checks throughout the research to verify that clinical data are generated, collected, handled, analyzed, and reported according to protocol, **standard operating procedures** (SOP, or manual of procedures), and **good clinical practice guidelines** (GCPs). It should be emphasized that QC is a very personnel-focused process. Educational courses in QC in clinical practice are invaluable and all the training activities should be documented in case of an inspection. All members of the study team must have the credentials, training, and experience that are relevant to their role in the research to be conducted. For example, study coordinators need to understand the protocol, with an emphasis on the inclusion and exclusion criteria, the known side effects, anticipated study events, and prohibited medications. For statistical staff, the randomization process must be documented as part of the trial and the assignment needs to be kept in sealed envelopes or be available from a randomization center. In a blinded study, unblinded personnel must be discrete in discussing study-related information with those who are blinded and any document linking individuals with treatments must be inaccessible to all blinded study members. For studies involving multiple institutions, data should be collected and submitted at the indicated time to the data coordinating center where the submitted forms are checked for their completeness, consistency, and accuracy. A rigorous review of the protocol by the Institutional Review Board (IRB) and obtaining **Informed Consent** are also prerequisites for insuring the quality of the given trial at high scientific level.

C. Data management. A data management plan and an agreement on means of protecting **participant confidentiality** follow development of data collection forms. The process of converting written records into electronic data files is specified. Issues to consider are who will be responsible for data entry, what resources they will use, which format and software will be used for data storage, what processing or manipulation is needed before analysis, how the data will be converted into one or more files for the planned analyses, and how any personal information is to be stored.

   1. Participant confidentiality must be protected at the time of enrollment, including any information gathered from persons who decide against participation. Confidentiality is also maintained during data collection, transfer, analysis, processing, and storage. Increasing use of Internet-based enrollment and data entry requires **encryption** as data are transferred over the web and stored on **secure servers**. Once data are stored in encrypted form, the means to access data files must be available to at least two study members, usually including the data manager or data analyst and the principal investigator. If lost, this information is not easily retrieved, so data files may become permanently inaccessible. A clear plan for long-term storage and emergency accessibility of passwords and encryption keys is needed, especially during the absence of critical study personnel. Confidentiality is also maintained by storing source documents in locked file cabinets, protecting passwords, maintaining discretion in communicating study results or individual case information, and carefully disseminating reports. In multicenter trials, centers usually have access only to their own data as the trial progresses. Secure, off-site storage is also recommended for up-to-date backup copies of data files, copies of keys to essential storage areas, passwords, and encryption keys.

   2. The informed consent is the most important form. This form is reviewed and approved by the IRB before being put to use. Approval is normally given for up to 1 year and must be kept up to date. The form cannot contain any explicit or implied waiver of the participant's legal rights or any release of the investigator(s), sponsor, supporting institution, or their agents from responsibility for negligence.

An essential ingredient to obtaining the informed consent is making certain that the participant is fully aware of the risks and benefits of participating in the study and has a clear understanding of what is expected of the participant. A legal representative may sign the form if the participant is unable to understand the contents of the form because of youth or impaired cognitive function. A legal representative may also sign the form if the participant is able to understand the conditions of the trial but is unable to read or sign and date the form because of noncognitive impairment. In the latter case, the signature of an impartial witness is also required. There is ongoing discussion concerning an appropriate means of obtaining consent when it is difficult to ensure an absence of restraint or coercion, as is the case when enrolling prisoners.

3. **Source documents.** Original documents, data forms, and other records are the source of all information produced by the trial. Source documents are filed at the participating institutions and made available as needed for monitoring or auditing. The supporting institutions may make, or delegate, periodic checks to ensure that the study protocol is being followed. Sponsors may require auditing by their own independent personnel. The auditors review the progress, procedures, and results of the trial, relying heavily on source documentation.

4. **Reporting adverse events.** Any medical occurrence during a trial that causes the death of a participant, is considered life threatening, requires hospitalization or extension of existing hospitalization, or results in significant or prolonged disability or loss of capacity is a **serious adverse event (SAE)**. All SAEs must be reported to participating institutions and sponsors within a fixed period, often 24 hours. A means of observing, documenting, and communicating SAEs is established as the trial is planned. If toxicities, drug reactions, or other negative health-related occurrences (adverse events) are anticipated, a **Data Safety and Monitoring Board** or Independent Data Monitoring Committee is established. The monitoring committee is charged with providing an independent review of the progress of the trial and the safety and efficacy of its treatments. After review, the monitoring committee may recommend that the protocol be altered or the trial stopped in the participants' best interests. Efficient data collection and processing are needed to provide timely and accurate information for review. Committee members must make decisions without conflict of interest if the monitoring process is to be effective.

V. **STATISTICAL CONSIDERATIONS ON REPORTING A CLINICAL RESEARCH.** The following 15 statistical guidelines on preparing a manuscript for biomedical journals were initially proposed by the International Committee of Medical Journal Editors (NEJM 1991) and have been widely adopted. The same principles are also applicable in creating a general report for a clinical research.

1). Describe statistical methods with enough detail to enable a knowledge reader with access to the original data to verify the reported results. **2).** When possible, quantify findings and present them with appropriate indicators of measurement error or uncertainty. **3).** Avoid sole reliance on statistical hypothesis testing, such as use of p values, which fails to convey important quantitative information. Discuss the eligibility of experimental subjects. **4).** Give details about randomization. Describe the methods for, and success of, any blinding of observations. **5).** Report treatment complications. **6).** Give number of observations. **7).** Report loss to observations (such as dropout from a clinical trial). **8).** References for study design and statistical methods should be to standard works (with pages stated) when possible, rather than to papers where designs or methods were originally reported. **9).** Specify any general-use computer programs used. **10).** Put general descriptions of methods in the Methods section. **11).** When data are summarized in the Results section, specify the statistical methods used to analyze them. **12).** Restrict tables and figures to those needed to explain the argument of the paper and to assess its support. **13).** Use graphs as an alternative to tables with many entries; do not duplicate data in graphs and tables. **14).** Avoid nontechnical uses of technical terms in statistics, such as "random" (which implies a randomizing device), "normal", "significant", "correlation" and "sample". **15).** Define statistical terms, abbreviations and most symbols.

Suggested Readings

Armitage P, Colton T, eds. *Encyclopedia of biostatistics*. New York: John Wiley and Sons, 1998.

Bailar JC, Mosteller F, eds. *Medical uses of statistics*. Massachssetts Medical Society, 1992.

Chow S-C, ed. *Encyclopedia of biopharmaceutical statistics*. New York: Marcel Dekker Inc, 2000.

International Committee of Medical Journal Editors. Uniform requirement for manuscripts submitted to biomedical journals. *N Engl J Med* 1991;324:424–428.

Kolman J, Hafier H, Meng P, et al. *Good clinical practice: standard operating procedures for clinical researchers*. New York: John Wiley and Sons, 1998.

Meinert C, Tonascia S. *Clinical trials: design, conduct and analysis*. Oxford: Oxford University Press, 1986.

Piantadosi S. *Clinical trials: a methodological approach*. New York: John Wiley and Sons, 1997.

Spilker B. *Guide to clinical trials*. New York: Raven Press, 1991.

BASICS OF MOLECULAR ONCOGENESIS

John D. Pfeifer

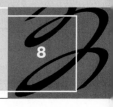

I. SOURCES OF DNA DAMAGE

A. Endogenous sources of DNA damage. There are several constant, unavoidable sources of background DNA damage.

1. **Reactive oxygen species (ROS).** ROS are produced by normal cellular metabolism, ionizing radiation, infection, and reperfusion of ischemic tissue. The most common ROS include ·OH, NO·, and peroxides. DNA damage produced by ROS is collectively referred to as *oxidative damage*, and includes sugar and base modifications, DNA–DNA and DNA–protein crosslinks, and DNA strand breaks.

2. **Spontaneous chemical reactions.** The most common spontaneous chemical changes that alter the structure of DNA are deamination and depurination reactions, but spontaneous hydrolysis, alkylation, and adduction reactions also occur. The mutagenic potential of the different types of reactions varies.

3. **Metal ions.** Although the evidence for DNA damage by endogenous metals is especially strong for iron and copper, nickel, chromium, magnesium, and cadmium are also well-established human carcinogens. Oxidative damage through metal-catalyzed ROS generation is by far the most important mechanism of DNA damage, although metal-catalyzed reactions also produce metabolites of a variety of organic compounds that form DNA adducts. Metals such as arsenic, cadmium, lead, and nickel also directly inhibit DNA repair, which augments the mutagenic potential of the DNA damage they cause.

B. Exogenous sources of DNA damage

1. **Chemicals.** Although virtually an infinite number of chemicals can damage DNA, a few families of environmental and therapeutic compounds illustrate the general mechanisms involved.

   a. **Polycyclic aromatic hydrocarbons and related compounds.** These molecules are converted into reactive intermediate metabolites by the normal physiologic action of cytochrome P-450, a process termed *metabolic activation*. It is the reactive intermediates that mediate DNA damage through the formation of DNA adducts. Variation in the balance between metabolic activation and detoxification influences cancer rates, providing a rationale for pharmacogenomic analysis of the relevant enzymatic pathways in individual patients. Cigarette smoke is a particularly rich source of compounds that mediate DNA damage through the formation of DNA adducts.

   b. **Antineoplastic agents.** Drugs such as cisplatin act primarily by causing intrastrand and interstrand crosslinks. However, cytotoxic alkylating agents such as cyclophosphamide, busulfan, nitrogen mustard, nitrosourea, and thiotepa damage DNA through the formation of covalent linkages that produce alkylated nucleotides, DNA–DNA crosslinks, DNA–protein crosslinks, and DNA strand breaks.

2. **Radiation.** DNA damage caused by radiation can be classified into damage caused by ultraviolet radiation (UV light) and damage caused by ionizing radiation.

   a. **UV light.** UVB radiation from sunlight (wavelength 280–315 nm) produces cyclobutane pyrimidine dimers (due to covalent bonds between adjacent thymine residues in the same strand of DNA) as well as pyrimidine (6–4) pyrimidone photoproducts (due to covalent bonds between TC or CC dimers in the same strand of DNA). Damage caused by UVA radiation (wavelength 315–400 nm) is usually due to ROS-mediated mechanisms.

b. Ionizing radiation. A broad spectrum of DNA damage is caused by ionizing radiation, including individual base lesions, crosslinks, and single- and double-strand breaks. Low linear energy transfer (LET) radiation (x-rays, γ-rays, electrons, and β-particles have a typical LET less than 10 keV/μm) and high-LET radiation (protons and neutrons have a typical LET of 10 to 100 keV/μm, whereas α-particles have an LET greater than 175 keV/μm) each produce a characteristic pattern of damage.

II. TYPES OF DNA ALTERATIONS

A. Single base pair (bp) substitutions. This class of mutations is among the most common. Single bp substitutions are the end result of a number of different processes, including errors in DNA replication, spontaneous chemical reactions, ROS damage, chemical mutagenesis, and ionizing radiation. Coding and noncoding regions are almost equally susceptible to this type of mutation.

A single bp substitution in the coding sequence of a gene can cause a significant change in the encoded amino acid, but will not cause a shift in the translational reading frame. Single bp substitutions in coding DNA are classified into synonymous mutations (result in a different codon that still specifies the same amino acid), and nonsynonymous mutations of which there are two types, missense mutations (result in a codon that specifies a different amino acid) and nonsense mutations (result in a stop codon).

Single bp substitutions that occur outside the coding region of a gene can still be deleterious. Substitutions in the 5′ regulatory region of a gene can alter the pattern of gene expression, and substitutions in introns, exons, or untranslated regions of a gene can affect RNA processing.

B. Gross gene deletions. There are two types of recombination events that give rise to gross gene deletions. Homologous unequal recombination occurs at either related gene sequences or repetitive sequence elements, and involves the cleavage and rejoining of homologous but nonallelic DNA sequences; repetitive DNA sequences are especially prone to unequal crossovers and are the site of many large-scale deletions, as well as insertions, duplications, inversions, and translocations. Nonhomologous recombination (or illegitimate recombination) occurs between DNA loci that have minimal or no sequence homology.

C. Gene conversion. This type of mutation is a nonreciprocal transfer of sequence information between a pair of loci. One of the pair of interacting sequences (the donor or source) remains unchanged whereas the other sequence (the target or acceptor) is altered by partial or total replacement by the donor sequence. Gene families with tandem repeats and clusters are prone to gene conversion.

D. Short gene deletions. The mutation rate at some microsatellites is remarkably high. Because the mutant alleles differ from the wild type by a single repeat unit without exchange of flanking markers, the proposed mechanism involves misalignment of the short direct repeats during DNA replication (known as the *polymerase slippage hypothesis*).

E. Insertions. The polymerase slippage hypothesis can account for short insertions just as it can for short deletions. Homologous unequal recombination between repetitive sequence elements provides a mechanism for the generation of larger insertions (which may actually be gene duplications). Active transposition of repetitive DNA elements can also produce larger insertions.

F. Expansion of unstable repeat sequences. A small subset of tandem trinucleotide repeats, as well as a very limited number of longer repeats, shows anomalous behavior that causes abnormal gene expression. Repeats above a certain threshold length become extremely unstable and are virtually never transmitted unchanged from parent to child. Genes containing unstable expanding trinucleotide repeats can be grouped into two major classes; one includes genes that show very large expansions of repeats outside coding sequences, while the other class consists of genes that show modest expansion of repeats within coding sequences.

G. Inversions. A high degree of sequence similarity between repeats on the same chromosome may predispose to inversions by a mechanism that involves bending back of the chromatid upon itself in a process that is essentially homologous intrachromosomal recombination. Inversions not associated with significant sequence homology are apparently the result of nonhomologous recombination events.

H. Illegitimate recombination. The RAG enzyme, responsible for the double-stranded DNA breaks that underlie the V(D)J recombination of antigen receptor genes, occasionally cuts DNA at unrelated loci that have complementary recombination signals, producing a translocation.

I. Mitochondrial DNA damage and mutations. Mitochondrial DNA (mtDNA) is damaged by the same processes that damage nuclear DNA. ROS are an especially important source of damage, given the proximity of mtDNA to the reactive intermediates produced by the electron transport/oxidative phosphorylation of the respiratory chain. Although the types of mtDNA mutation are similar to those of nuclear DNA, the unique features of mitochondrial genetics result in an entirely different pattern of phenotype–genotype correlations.

III. DNA REPAIR. DNA repair rarely involves simple chemical reversal of the damage, but instead usually entails excision of the stretch of DNA harboring the alteration, followed by resynthesis of DNA to fill the gap. However, it is important to emphasize that some classes of DNA alterations, such as insertions and deletions, duplications, inversions, and translocations, are not targeted by cellular DNA repair pathways and so are highly mutagenic.

A. Direct repair. Human cells produce only a few enzymes that directly reverse DNA damage. One of the few is O^6-methylguanine methyltransferase, an enzyme that removes the non-native methyl group from O^6-methylguanine; this dealkylation reaction is important because the altered base pairs with either C or T and hence is highly mutagenic. Another set of recently discovered enzymes catalyze the oxidative demethylation of 1-methyladenine and 3-methylcytosine.

B. Base excision repair (BER). Small chemical alterations are the type of DNA damage repaired by BER. For example, BER is responsible for repair of oxidized bases, alkylated bases, and spontaneously formed bases, and is also responsible for repair of spontaneous depurination events, single-strand breaks, and some mismatched bases. Because the lesions repaired by BER are especially prone to produce mutations (they are the most common types of DNA damage and do not typically impede transcription or DNA replication), BER is important for maintaining the integrity of the genome.

C. Nucleotide excision repair (NER). This is the most flexible DNA repair pathway and is responsible for correction of various structurally unrelated lesions. The common denominator of damage repaired by NER seems to be a significant DNA helix distortion with interference of normal base pairing.

D. Transcription-coupled repair. NER and BER inefficiently repair damage to the transcribed DNA strand of actively expressed loci because RNA polymerase II stalls at the site of the damage and sterically inhibits repair. Because the stalled RNA polymerase effectively inactivates the gene, independent of whether the DNA damage would cause a mutation affecting gene function, transcription-coupled repair not only corrects DNA damage but also restores gene expression.

E. Mismatch repair. The mismatch repair system removes nucleotides mispaired by DNA polymerases. The repair system also removes insertion/deletion loops 1 to 10 bp long that result from polymerase slippage during replication of repetitive sequences or that arise during recombination. Cells defective in mismatch repair have mutation rates up to a 1,000 times higher than normal, with a particular tendency for replication slippage at short tandem repeats or homopolymeric stretches. Defective mismatch repair facilitates malignant transformation through the production of mutations in genes that harbor microsatellites in their coding regions, some of which have critical roles in the regulation of cell growth and apoptosis (e.g., the *TGFBR2* gene, which encodes the transforming growth factor β receptor II, and the *BAX* gene, which encodes a proapoptotic protein).

F. Translesion synthesis. The polymerases primarily responsible for replication of nuclear DNA are hampered when they encounter a chemically altered base. Translesion synthesis, which occurs through replacement of the conventional polymerase in the vicinity of the DNA lesion by one (or several) of a group of specialized polymerases that have the ability to replicate damaged DNA, is the mechanism by which cells manage to replicate damaged nuclear DNA templates despite the almost limitless diversity of DNA lesions. However, translesion synthesis polymerases display low fidelity replication of nondamaged templates, lack a proofreading function, and have flexible (and even alternative) base-pairing properties. Hence, the capability of replicating damaged DNA comes at the expense of a high error rate.

G. **Recombinatorial repair.** The two main double-strand break repair mechanisms are homologous recombination and nonhomologous end joining. Both activate a cascade of kinase reactions that not only recruit repair factors to the site of the break, but also delay or stop the cell cycle through DNA damage checkpoint control. The mechanism of crosslink repair in human cells remains unknown.

H. **Defective DNA damage repair.** Some of the most striking examples of hereditary cancer syndromes are due to mutations affecting genes involved in DNA repair, which emphasizes the fundamental role of repair pathways in oncogenesis.

1. **Defective BER.** Other than germline mutations in the gene *MYH*, a glycosylase that removes adenine mispaired with 8-oxoguanine or guanine and is associated with recessive inheritance of multiple colorectal adenomas, no other mutations in the core BER pathway that cause diseases have been described.

2. **Defective NER.** Inborn defects in NER are associated with the autosomal recessive photosensitivity syndrome xeroderma pigmentosum, the photosensitive form of the brittle hair disorder trichothiodystrophy, and a clinical disorder that combines features of both xeroderma pigmentosum and Cockayne syndrome.

3. **Defective transcription-coupled repair.** Inborn defects in transcription-coupled repair are associated with Cockayne syndrome.

4. **Defective mismatch repair.** Defects in mismatch repair genes are responsible for hereditary nonpolyposis colorectal carcinoma (HNPCC). However, it is important to recognize that although microsatellite instability can be demonstrated in a variety of malignancies, in most cases the phenotype is due to somatic rather than germline mutations at mismatch repair loci.

5. **Defective translesion synthesis.** Defective replication of damaged DNA due to inherited mutations in one of the translesion polymerases is responsible for xeroderma pigmentosum variant.

6. **Defective double-strand break and crosslink repair.** Diseases associated with impaired double-strand break repair by homologous recombination include ataxia telangiectasia, ataxia telangiectasia–like disorder, Nijmegen breakage syndrome, Fanconi anemia, familial breast and ovarian cancer syndromes, Werner syndrome, Bloom syndrome, and Rothmund-Thomson syndrome. Not unexpectedly, the diseases share radiosensitivity, genome instability, cancer susceptibility, and immunodeficiency as prominent clinical features.

IV. **VIRUSES.** Several RNA and DNA viruses have been associated with the development of malignancies.

A. **RNA viruses.** Three RNA viruses that have been associated with the development of malignancies are the retroviruses human T-lymphotrophic virus (HTLV-1) and human immunodeficiency virus (HIV), and the flavivirus hepatitis C virus (HCV).

1. **Retroviruses.** In general, there are four mechanisms by which retroviruses are oncogenic. Slowly transforming viruses are oncogenic as a result of insertional mutagenesis, which occurs when the random integration of the provirus occurs within or adjacent to a cellular proto-oncogene. Acutely transforming retroviruses harbor viral oncogenes that are derived from cellular oncogenes. Transacting retroviruses (of which HTLV-1 is an example) directly alter the expression or function of proteins involved in cell growth or differentiation. Retroviruses that cause immunodeficiency (of which HIV is an example) apparently promote oncogenesis only indirectly, most likely as a consequence of the immunosuppression associated with infection.

2. **Flaviviruses.** HCV is indirectly oncogenic. Hepatocellular carcinoma is thought to develop as a result of the increased cellular turnover caused by long-term

hepatocyte necrosis and regeneration, fibrosis, and inflammation associated with infection.

B. DNA viruses. DNA viruses from several different families have oncogenic properties.

   1. Hepadnaviruses. Hepatitis B virus (HBV) encodes a protein (known as *HBx*) involved in transcriptional activation and signal transduction that has been implicated in tumorigenesis. The virus is also oncogenic through insertional mutagenesis. However, HBV primarily promotes hepatocellular carcinogenesis indirectly, likely through the increased cellular turnover caused by long-term hepatocyte necrosis and regeneration, fibrosis, and inflammation associated with infection.

   2. Herpesviruses. Epstein-Barr virus (EBV) is associated with the oncogenesis of lymphoid malignancies (including Burkitt's lymphoma and Hodgkin's disease), gastric cancer, and nasopharyngeal carcinoma. The viral genome encodes several proteins that play a direct role in cellular transformation.

   Kaposi's sarcoma–associated herpesvirus (KSHV), also known as human herpes virus-8 (HHV-8), is associated with the development of Kaposi's sarcoma, primary effusion lymphoma, and multicentric Castleman's disease. The oncogenic mechanisms of the virus remain unclear.

   3. Papillomaviruses. The high-risk, cancer-associated serotypes of human papillomavirus (HPV) harbor two principal transforming genes, *E6* and *E7*. The E6 protein inactivates p53, and the E7 protein interacts with the retinoblastoma (*RB1*) gene product. However, *E6* and *E7* alone are insufficient for carcinogenesis; development of a fully transformed cellular phenotype requires derangements in a number of cellular pathways. It remains unclear why only a subset of patients infected with high-risk HPV serotypes eventually develop malignant disease.

V. INDIVIDUAL GENES THAT ARE TARGETS OF ONCOGENIC MUTATIONS. According to the clonal model of carcinogenesis, a malignant tumor arises from a single cell. This founder cell acquires an initial mutation that provides its progeny with a selective growth advantage, and from within this expanded population another single cell acquires a second mutation that provides an additional growth advantage, and so on, until a fully transformed, malignant tumor emerges. Tumor suppressor genes and oncogenes are frequent targets of mutation in this multi-step process of tumor evolution.

A. Tumor suppressor genes. Proteins encoded by tumor suppressor genes are involved in a wide range of cellular functions, including regulation of the cell cycle, differentiation, apoptosis, and maintenance of genome integrity. Over 20 tumor suppressor genes have been identified, and at least 10 other candidates have been described. Tumor suppressor genes have been broadly divided into two classes, gatekeepers and caretakers.

   1. Gatekeepers. This group of tumor suppressors directly regulates cell growth by inhibiting cellular proliferation or promoting apoptosis; familiar examples include the products of the *RB1*, *TP53*, *APC*, *NF1*, *NF2*, *WT1*, *MEN1*, and *VHL* genes. Because the functions of the proteins encoded by gatekeeper genes are rate-limiting for tumor growth, tumor development occurs only when both copies of the gene are inactivated; individuals with an autosomal dominant cancer susceptibility syndrome inherit one damaged copy, and so require only one somatic mutation to inactivate the remaining wild-type allele and initiate tumor formation. Nonetheless, inactivating mutations of both alleles of a gatekeeper are still insufficient for acquisition of a fully transformed malignant phenotype. Gatekeepers vary with tissue type, and so germline inactivation of a particular gatekeeper gene leads to only specific forms of cancer predisposition.

   2. Caretakers. Inactivation of a caretaker gene leads to genetic instability that indirectly promotes tumorigenesis by causing an increased rate of mutation. Genes that encode proteins involved in DNA repair are the classic examples of caretakers, including *MSH2*, *MLH1*, *PMS1*, *ATM*, *XPA* through *XPG*, and *FANCA* through *FNACL*.

B. Oncogenes. Proto-oncogenes encode proteins that regulate cell growth and differentiation. More than 75 proto-oncogenes have been identified, and their products include extracellular cytokines and growth factors (e.g., int-1 and int-2), transmembrane growth factor receptors (e.g., c-erb2/EGFR, HER2/neu, src, c-abl, c-ret, H-ras, K-ras, and N-ras), cytoplasmic kinases (e.g., b-raf), and nuclear proteins involved in the control of DNA replication (e.g., c-myc, N-myc, L-myc, c-myb).

Oncogenes are mutated forms of proto-oncogenes that cause neoplastic transformation. Despite their variety, oncogenes can be divided into two general groups based on the mechanism of their action. One group induces continuous or unregulated cell proliferation by inactivation of growth inhibitory signals, or by activation of growth-promoting genes, growth factors, receptors, intracellular signaling pathways, or nuclear oncoproteins. The other group immortalizes cells by rescuing them from senescence and apoptosis. Accumulated evidence from human malignancies and transgenic animal models indicates that mutation of a single oncogene is insufficient for acquisition of a fully transformed, malignant phenotype.

Only a few inherited cancer syndromes are due to germline mutations in oncogenes. Instead, most oncogene mutations are somatic and therefore associated with sporadic malignancies. For many tumor types, the involved oncogene and the type of mutation are characteristic.

VI. INTRACELLULAR PATHWAYS THAT ARE TARGETS OF ONCOGENIC MUTATIONS

A. Signal transduction. In the context of oncology, the important signal transduction pathways are those that regulate cellular proliferation, differentiation, and death, often through regulation of gene transcription. Signal transduction pathways make it possible for the cell to produce and integrate responses to an enormous variety of stimuli. Many of the genes involved in signal transduction are classified as tumor suppressor genes or oncogenes.

1. **Ligands.** The various types of ligands include soluble, cell-bound, and matrix proteins; individual amino acids; lipids; gases; and soluble and polymerized nucleotides.

2. **Receptors.** Examples of cell surface receptors include receptor tyrosine kinases, serine kinases, and phosphotyrosine phosphatases; members of the Notch family; and G protein-coupled receptors. The guanylate cyclase family of receptors provides an example of related receptors that can be either membrane bound or soluble. The transcription factors that bind glucocorticoids, thyroxine, and vitamin D are examples of receptors that are located in the nucleus.

3. **Signal propagation.** Many ligand–receptor interactions transmit a signal through a relatively small set of second messengers, including cyclic adenosine monophosphate (cAMP), phospholipases (that generate inositol triphosphate and diacylglycerol), Ca^{2+}, and eicosanoids.

B. Regulation of the cell cycle. Cell proliferation is rigorously controlled in both development and adult life. Many signal transduction pathways specifically regulate promitogenic and antimitogenic proteins that control the cell cycle including the A-, B-, D-, and E-type cyclins, cyclin-dependent kinases (CDKs), and the SCF and APC/C families of protein-ubiquitin ligases. Not surprisingly, many of genes involved in regulation of the cell cycle are commonly mutated or show an altered pattern of expression in a variety of human malignancies.

C. Cell cycle checkpoints. Since progression through the cell cycle before DNA damage has been repaired is potentially harmful, a number of cell cycle checkpoints delay the cell cycle pending DNA repair. These DNA damage checkpoints occur before S phase entry, during S phase, and before M phase entry. Other cell cycle checkpoints include a replication checkpoint (that ensures that replication is complete before entry into M phase), a spindle integrity checkpoint (that blocks initiation of anaphase until all chromosomes are correctly attached to a bipolar spindle), and a restriction checkpoint (that blocks cell cycle progression in mid-G1 phase in the absence of essential growth factors or nutrients). Loss of function at one or more checkpoints is a characteristic feature of many malignancies.

D. Apoptosis. Signal transduction pathways control not only cell proliferation but also programmed cell death. Control of apoptosis is achieved through regulation of the proapoptotic proteins BAX and BAK and antiapoptotic proteins BCL-2, BCL-X_L, and MCL-1. The activity of inhibitors of apoptosis (IAPs), including XIAP, c-IAP1, and c-IAP2, is also tightly regulated (IAPs block the function of the various caspases that are the final effectors of the apoptotic pathway). Not surprisingly, there is substantial cross-talk between cellular proliferation and apoptosis pathways, often focused at the various cell cycle checkpoints. Mutations or alterations in the level of expression of pro- and antiapoptotic proteins are characteristic of many human malignancies, and various proteins in the apoptotic pathways have received attention as possible targets for therapeutic intervention.

E. Telomere metabolism. The telomere is the nucleoprotein complex present at the ends of each chromosome. The enzyme telomerase catalyzes the unique reaction by which the long TTAGGG tandem repeat arrays of the telomere are synthesized. Telomerase activity is tightly controlled, although the details of the different regulatory mechanisms are not fully understood. Dysfunctions of telomere maintenance have an important role in tumorigenesis as well as in genomic instability, since chromosomes lacking a telomere are unstable and tend to fuse with other broken chromosomes, undergo recombination, or be degraded.

F. RNA interference. Several classes of short double-stranded or single-stranded RNA molecules also have a role in regulation of gene expression, including short interfering RNA (siRNA), micro-RNA (miRNA), and small modulatory RNA (smRNA). Also referred to as *RNA interference* (RNAi), RNA-mediated control of gene expression has been shown to be abnormal in several malignancies. The potential of RNAi-based therapeutic approaches has been demonstrated in several model systems.

VII. EXTRACELLULAR PATHWAYS THAT ARE TARGETS OF ONCOGENIC MUTATIONS

A. Angiogenesis. Tumor growth requires the development of an adequate blood supply, known as *angiogenesis*. Two types of angiogenesis have been described. Sprouting angiogenesis occurs through branching of new capillaries from preexisting capillaries, a process that includes degradation of the basement membrane, migration of endothelial cells in the direction of the angiogenic stimulus, endothelial cell proliferation, and capillary tube formation. Nonsprouting angiogenesis occurs through proliferation of endothelial cells within preexisting vessels, with subsequent lumen enlargement, splitting, or fusion. It has been calculated that any increase in tumor size beyond a diameter of 0.5 mm requires angiogenesis, and consequently angiogenic pathways are the targets of many drug therapies.

Angiogenesis involves alteration of the balance between proangiogenic and antiangiogenic molecules in the local tissue environment. The proangiogenic and antiangiogenic factors are produced by tumor cells, inflammatory cells, and adjacent normal tissue cells, and their levels are regulated by interdependent stimuli such as tissue hypoxia (mediated through the hypoxia-inducible factor-1 (HIF-1) pathway), tissue pH, and other growth factors. Proangiogenic molecules bind to specific receptors on endothelial cells, smooth muscle cells, and pericytes, and include members of the vascular endothelial growth factor (VEGF) family, members of the angiopoietin (Ang) family, members of the fibroblast growth factor (FGF) family, epidermal growth factor (EGF), platelet derived growth factor (PDGF), and various chemokines.

B. Invasion and metastasis. Metastasis is the spread of transformed cells from the primary tumor site and consists of a series of interrelated steps known as the *metastatic cascade*. The metastatic cascade includes detachment of a tumor cell (or cells) from the primary tumor mass; movement across the basement membrane and into the lumen of a capillary, venule, or lymphatic; intravascular survival; arrest in a capillary bed, with subsequent adherence to the capillary wall and extravasation into the adjacent tissue; and proliferation with associated angiogenesis and evasion of host defenses. The metastatic cascade is dependent on alterations in tumor cell motility, cell migration, protease expression, and autocrine and paracrine growth factor expression.

1. **Cell motility.** A number of stimuli increase cell motility, including tumor-secreted molecules, local tissue microenvironment-derived factors, and growth factors. Tumor-secreted molecules usually function in autocrine loops, such as autocrine motility factor (AMF) and antotoxin (ATX) produced by melanoma cells.

2. **Cell migration.** Changes in the repertoire of cell surface adhesion molecules produce an altered pattern of tumor cell interaction with the intercellular matrix and non-neoplastic cells. Important adhesion molecules include members of the cadherin family, members of the Ig superfamily (especially VCAM-1 and NCAM), and integrins.

3. **Proteases.** Tumor cells must produce a number of difference proteases in order to migrate through the interstitial matrix and connective tissue barriers such as vascular basement membranes. The group of proteases that has been most extensively studied is the matrix metalloproteinases (MMPs), which are inhibited by the appropriately named tissue inhibitors of metalloproteinases (TIMPs). Over 25 MMPs and 4 TIMPs have been characterized to date. The biologic activity of several MMPs apparently extends beyond simple destruction of structural barriers to invasion, since some of the degradation products of MMP proteolysis have a role in chemotaxis and angiogenesis.

4. **Autocrine and paracrine growth factors.** Growth factors produced by transformed cells as well as non-neoplastic cells are required for many steps in the metastatic cascade. The role of non-neoplastic cells in the local tissue microenvironment is increasingly recognized as an important source of the various growth factors that play a significant role in the metastatic cascade.

Suggested Readings

Barik S. Silence of the transcripts: RNA interference in medicine. *J Mol Med* 2005;83: 764–773.

Bhowmick NA, Neilson EG, Moses HL. Stromal fibroblasts in cancer initiation and pregression. *Nature* 2004;432:332–337.

Fearon ER. Tumor-suppressor genes. In: Vogelstein B, Kinzler KW, eds. *The genetic basis of human cancer*. New York: McGraw-Hill, 2002:197–206.

Park M. Oncogenes. In: Vogelstein B, Kinzler KW, eds. *The genetic basis of human cancer*. New York: McGraw-Hill, 2002:177–196.

Pearson CE, Edamura KN, Cleary JD. Repeat instability: mechanisms of dynamic mutations. *Nat Rev Genet* 2005;6:729–742.

Pfeifer JD. DNA damage, mutations, and repair. In: *Molecular genetic testing in surgical pathology*. Philadelphia: Lippincott Williams & Wilkins, 2006:29–57.

Rodriguez-Antona C, Ingelman-Sundberg M. Cytochrome P450 pharmacogenetics and cancer. *Oncogene* 2006;25:1679–1691.

Schultz DR, Harrington WJ Jr. Apoptosis: programmed cell death at a molecular level. *Semin Arthritis Rheum* 2003;32:345–369.

Strachan T, Read AP, eds. *Human molecular genetics 3*, 3rd ed. London: Garland Science Publishers, 2004.

Weinberg RA. *Biology of cancer*. London: Taylor and Francis, Inc, 2006.

Zeviani M, Carelli V. Mitochondrial disorders. *Curr Opin Neurol* 2003;16:585–594.

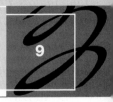

PHARMACOGENOMICS

Richard A. Walgren and Howard L. McLeod

9

I. THE ROLE OF PHARMACOGENOMICS. For most malignancies, cancer cells are heterogeneous with multiple histologic and pathologic appearances. However, even within the same tissue type differences are observed in presentation, treatment response, and outcomes. Although traditional methods of cancer classification have been useful in facilitating identification of subgroups for prognostic, predictive, and treatment selection purposes, these methods have not achieved an optimal degree of therapeutic success. The use of targeted or rational therapy has furthered the success of oncology, allowing therapeutic modification of the biologic activity of a specific "targeted" protein with abnormal function in malignant cells. Until recently, the number of biologic targets, metabolizing enzymes, and transporters was relatively small, but in a short period of time, genomic tools have developed such that every gene product must now be considered.

This has certainly not diminished the difficulties facing clinicians in deciding which drug in which dose or regimen is the best for an individual patient. Optimization of therapy must also not neglect to consider patient-specific safety concerns including interindividual genetic variability in pharmacokinetic and pharmacodynamic biology. Currently, there are a number of active drug regimens available for most common malignancies. However, administration of the same dose of a given anticancer drug to a population of patients can be expected to have a varied effect on any given individual in that population with regard to both treatment outcome, ranging from success to tumor progression, and treatment-associated toxicity, ranging from no effect to a lethal event (Fig. 9.1).

The idea that genetic inheritance contributes to variations in drug response is not new, and there are many known examples of pharmacogenetic traits influencing the pharmacokinetics of drugs (e.g., variation in *N*-acetyltransferase activity, thiopurine *S*-methyltransferase activity, and the activity of cytochrome P-450 isoforms). Genetic polymorphisms in drug targets have also been identified which result in altered pharmacodynamics. For example, mutations in epidermal growth factor receptor (EGFR) alter the response to gefitinib, an EGFR tyrosine kinase inhibitor, and polymorphisms in the promoter of the thymidylate synthase gene result in a diminished responsiveness to preoperative 5-fluorouracil–based chemoradiation therapy.

Unfortunately, for most therapeutic agents it is not currently possible to prospectively identify patients who are likely to benefit the most, based on their genetic profile, nor is it possible to identify those individuals who are likely to experience either no benefit or a severe adverse reaction. Clearly the identification and understanding of these factors has the potential to allow clinicians to appropriately select therapeutic agents, adjust dose and administration regimens to favor successful outcomes, and avoid therapy that could be harmful. Additionally, the ability to preselect individuals who would not benefit from a first-line therapy and steer them to a therapy that would be more beneficial has obvious advantages.

This chapter uses recent clinical examples to illustrate the ways that pharmacogenomics will be applied in clinical oncology.

II. APPROACHES TO PHARMACOGENOMIC STUDIES. The field of pharmacogenomics has grown out of an effort to explore and define the relationships of genomics, pathology, and pharmacology. Pharmacogenomic studies can be linked back to pharmacogenetic studies that attempted to associate a pattern of inheritance to a particular pharmacodynamic or pharmacokinetic phenotype. In the era of genomics, these genetic techniques have largely been replaced by gene-based or candidate gene approaches and by genome-wide approaches.

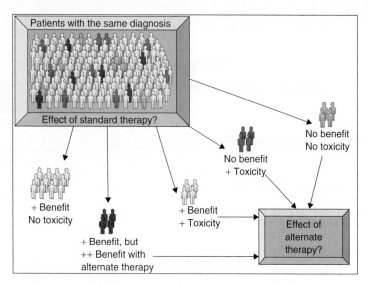

Figure 9.1. The Utility of Pharmacogenomic Testing.
Currently many patient populations are treated as if they are homogenous, when in fact they are not. For an increasing number of situations, it is becoming clear that these populations can be segregated further. Pharmacogenomic testing may allow categorization based on therapeutic benefit and toxicologic risk. This ability to identify subpopulations will drive clinical research to develop and introduce individualized therapy.

A candidate gene approach employs *a priori* knowledge of pathology and pharmacology to identify genes for which expression may impact therapeutic response. Often candidate genes are selected based on signaling and metabolic pathways and use of this approach yields a narrow list of biologic targets which are deemed to have a stronger potential chance of affecting therapeutic outcome. Candidate gene lists are often limited to a few dozen up to a few 100 genes. Examination of this number of genes is more manageable, but it remains costly and labor intensive. Therefore, lists of candidate genes are often credentialed or further ranked so that stronger candidates can be tested first. Candidate gene approaches offer the advantage of a potential cost saving if the initial gene list proves sufficient to explain the observed interindividual variation. In addition, the smaller number of starting genes reduces the risk of false-positive findings, which could occur in a genome-wide approach. A major risk of this approach is the potential exclusion of unknown or unsuspected genes that may turn out to be important.

Whole genome approaches are framed in such a way as to allow the experiment, rather than the investigators, to identify genes that play a significant role in a phenotype. The clear strength of this strategy is the ability to screen in a manner that can reveal not only genes that could be anticipated to be involved, but also genes which may not, at first, be expected to play a significant role, potentially adding new insight into pathophysiology or pharmacology. Key challenges faced in genome-wide strategies include controlling for the influence of the environment on a trait, gaining access to relevant populations, obtaining adequate sample sizes, and the associated cost. To reduce the often prohibitive costs associated with genome-wide studies, these experiments can be performed at reduced resolutions. For example, resolution can be reduced by selecting functionally interesting single nucleotide polymorphisms (SNPs) or haplotype-tagging SNPs to represent a gene. Studies examining thousands of genes pose additional problems through the generation of a significant number of false positives.

A. Mechanistic studies. Candidate gene strategies are well suited to mechanistic studies to answer questions about the involvement of a gene product in a particular biological function. For most widely used chemotherapeutic agents, a proposed mechanism of action is available. Additionally, most drugs are already known to interact with a number of gene products (i.e., receptors, metabolic enzymes, drug transporters). Therefore, for each of these agents a list of candidate genes is available. Systematic evaluation of these candidate genes for polymorphisms can readily be explored to allow for identification of polymorphisms that are relevant for predicting patient response to chemotherapy. The prediction of cancer treatment outcome based on gene polymorphisms is becoming possible for a number of chemotherapeutic agents and classes, including irinotecan, a topoisomerase I inhibitor.

Irinotecan has regulatory approval for the treatment of advanced colorectal cancer and has been shown to be active in the treatment of a wide variety of solid tumors. Irinotecan is a prodrug, which is converted by carboxylesterase to its active metabolite, SN-38. Clearance of SN-38 is primarily dependent on intrahepatic glucuronidation by UDP-glucuronosyltransferase 1A1 (UGT1A1), resulting in the polar and inactive SN-38 glucuronide which is subsequently excreted in the bile and urine. Diarrhea and leucopenia, the two significant dose-limiting toxicities of irinotecan, have been attributed to elevated levels of unconjugated SN-38. Expression of UGT1A1 is highly variable, with up to a 50-fold interpatient variability in the rate of SN-38 glucuronidation. Expression of UGT1A1 is inversely related to the number of thymine-adenine (TA) repeats in the gene promoter region. Within the general population the UGT1A1 promoter region contains between five and eight TA repeats, and a six-repeat allele is the most common variant. The presence of seven repeats, instead of the wild-type number of six, results in the variant allele UGT1A1*28. SN-38 glucuronidation in liver microsomes from individuals homozygous for 6 repeats was 3.85-fold higher than that observed in microsomes from individuals homozygous for seven repeats (UGT1A1*28 homozygotes).

In clinical studies, the presence of the UGT1A1*28 allele leads to significantly increased amounts of the active metabolite SN-38, and an increased chance of developing diarrhea and leukopenia during irinotecan therapy. In a retrospective study of 118 cancer patients treated with irinotecan, 26 patients experienced severe diarrhea (grade 3 or worse) or neutropenia (grade 4) and 12 of these patients were found to have at least one UGT1A1*28 allele. Four of the seven patients (57%) in the study who were found to be homozygous for UGT1A1*28 experienced severe toxicity, as did 8 of the 18 patients (44%) in the study who were heterozygous for UGT1A1*28. Among the 92 patients without toxicity, only 3% were UGT1A1*28 homozygotes and 11% were UGT1A1*28 heterozygotes. These studies provided the first clear demonstration that determination of UGT1A1 genotypes may be clinically important for the prediction of irinotecan toxicity, and laid the groundwork for the prospective study by Innocenti et al. in which irinotecan was administered at a dose of 350 mg/m^2 over 90 minutes to 63 patients (*J Clin Oncol* 2004;22:1382–1388). UGT1A1 genotype and haplotype were then correlated with SN-38 pharmacology and incidence of severe toxicity. Three of the six patients identified as homozygous for UGT1A1*28 were among the six patients who experienced grade 4 neutropenia. The remaining three patients who experienced grade 4 neutropenia were identified as heterozygous for the seven-repeat allele. Patients with the 7/7 genotype (UGT1A1*28 homozygous) had a 9.3-fold greater risk of grade 4 neutropenia compared with the patients with a 6/6 or 6/7 genotype. This study was the first prospective trial with sufficient statistical power to demonstrate that patients with a UGT1A1*28 allele are at a higher risk of grade 4 neutropenia.

Collectively this data suggests that the determination of the UGT1A1 genotypes may be clinically useful for predicting severe toxicity to irinotecan. By excluding patients who are homozygous for the UGT1A1*28 genotype from receiving the standard dose of irinotecan, the incidence of grade 4 neutropenia would have been cut in approximately half in the study by Innocenti et al., and the incidence would drop still further if all patients with a UGT1A1*28 allele were excluded.

This data has also now been reviewed by the U.S. Food and Drug Administration (FDA) and data on UGT1A1 pharmacogenetics have been added to the package insert. However, the application of UGT1A1 testing remains challenging.

There appear to be at least three key settings where testing is beneficial. First, irinotecan dose testing is most beneficial with doses greater than 150 mg/m^2. Second, testing can guide dose selection and aid in minimizing toxicity in concomitant therapy involving the coadministration of another myelotoxic agent. In addition, for patients where the anticipated benefit of therapy with irinotecan is less clear-cut (i.e., advanced-line palliative treatment), an assessment of a patient's cumulative risk including UGT1A1 testing is likely to be of greater utility and will assist in the overall risk to benefit analysis.

B. **In vitro discovery approaches.** Traditional familial genetic methods in chemotherapy studies are simply not possible for a number of reasons. First, it is obviously very rare to observe the simultaneous occurrence of a specific tumor type among family members and second, the inherent nature and toxicity of chemotherapeutic agents precludes the administration of these agents to healthy, volunteer subjects. The identification of a need for cell line–based assays which would enable family-based linkage analysis and tests for association led to the development of the Centre d'Etude du Polymorphisme Humain (CEPH) pedigree cell lines (*Genomics* 1990;6:575–577). CEPH pedigrees are Epstein-Barr virus–transformed lymphoblastoid cell lines derived from individuals in a number of multigenerational families. The CEPH multigenerational families are easily accessible and microsatellite and SNP genotype data are widely and freely available. Recent studies have highlighted the use of phenotype generation in these pedigrees as a means of conducting linkage analysis to discover genes that are associated with drug effect.

As a novel discovery model for evaluating the interaction of genes and chemotherapeutic drugs, Watters et al. used an *ex vivo* familial genetics strategy in which CEPH pedigrees were used to quantify the impact of genetic variation on cytotoxicity for docetaxel and 5-fluorouracil (*Proc Natl Acad Sci U S A* 2004;101:11809–11814).

With this system, the authors were able to demonstrate a heritable pattern for cytotoxicity after exposure of chemotherapeutic agent. Narrow sense heritability estimates for docetaxel, varying by dose, ranged from 0.21 to 0.70 whereas the heritability estimates for 5-fluorouracil ranged from 0.26 to 0.65. Therefore, the heritability of cytotoxicity observed in this system is similar to or greater than that of several common phenotypes such as plasma triglyceride levels (0.19 to 0.55), body mass index (0.32 to 0.59), and asthma (0.06 to 0.52). The mean IC$_{50}$ for both docetaxel and 5-fluorouracil observed in the CEPH population was similar to IC$_{50}$ values observed across the NCI60 panel of human tumor cell lines (http://dtp.nci.nih.gov). In addition, docetaxel- and 5-fluorouracil-induced cell death is mediated by caspase-3 cleavage, similar to that observed in tumor cells. These data are encouraging for the use of CEPH pedigrees as a discovery tool.

A genome-wide linkage analysis was used to identify regions likely to contain the genes important for the observed differences in response to docetaxel and 5-fluorouracil. The effects of 5-fluorouracil were mapped to chromosome 9q13-q22 and those of docetaxel were mapped to chromosomes 5q11-21 and 9q13-q22. High-resolution SNP genotype data is available for a subset of CEPH individuals, through the efforts of the International Haplotype Map Project (www.hapmap.org). These data are helping to fine-map the region and narrow the candidate gene list. Further studies are under way to determine the specifically involved genes within the mapped QTL regions, but this method has narrowed the search for the causative genes from the entire genome to a significantly smaller and more manageable subset.

1. **Murine in vivo comparative studies.** Interindividual variation in drug response is a complex trait, and it is safe to assume that for most drugs, multiple genes contribute, with varying degrees, to any given phenotype. Therefore, for technical, economic, and ethical reasons, pharmacogenomic studies in humans have been limited to a small number of candidate genes which are expected to have a relatively large influence on drug response. In contrast, there are a number of features that favor the use of well-characterized laboratory animals with validated similarities in pathophysiology and anatomy such as the mouse. Use of a murine system allows control of diet and other environmental factors

such that observed phenotypic differences between groups are most likely of a genetic origin. Whole-genome association studies analyze the differences in the frequency of genetic variants between two groups of unrelated subjects (i.e., case and control groups) in comparison to phenotypic differences. With a murine approach it is possible to create rather large family pedigrees by cross breeding populations from distinct well-defined inbred mouse strains. The short generation time of the mouse yields statistical strength in numbers while the more than 20 generations of inbreeding has served to reduce genetic complexity by segregating and fixing genetic factors.

In an attempt to identify genes that influence bleomycin-dependent susceptibility to pulmonary fibrosis, Haston et al. applied a genome-wide screening approach to compare phenotypically extreme mice derived from susceptible (C57BL/6J(B6)) and resistant (C3Hf/Kam) strains. Two loci were identified as having highly significant linkage, one on chromosome 17 and the other on chromosome 11, and were named bleomycin-induced pulmonary fibrosis 1 (Blmpf1) and bleomycin-induced pulmonary fibrosis 2 (Blmpf2). The Blmpf1 loci accounted for approximately 20% of the observed phenotypic variation in both males and females, while Blmpf2 accounted for approximately 9% of the phenotypic variation in males only. The existence and sex specificity of Blmpf2 was confirmed in a chromosome substitution strain and the presence of Blmpf2 was associated with a reduction in pulmonary fibrosis. Although the precision of the mapping did not allow identification of a single associated gene for each region, the authors were able to narrow the linkage region for Blmpf1 to a 2.7 cM region between markers D17Mit175 and D17Mit148 within the major histocompatibility complex (MHC). Further studies will be needed to examine the influence of the candidate genes from these loci on the bleomycin-induced phenotypic response.

As an alternative to generating and characterizing cross-bred populations, many groups have begun to identify and catalog genetic variations across the genomes of recognized inbred strains. Lists of inbred strains and their known phenotypic characteristics are accessible on the web (http://www.informatics.jax.org; Mouse Genome Informatics) along with detailed murine genealogies. This collection of information has the potential to rapidly detail how the strains are related and could serve to speed up quantitative trait loci (QTL) mapping by focusing efforts on genomic intervals that have been previously shown to differ between strains Studies in murine models will never completely recapitulate the pharmacogenomic relationships in humans, but these studies may provide sufficient insights to better select candidate markers for clinical evaluations.

2. **Pharmacogenomics as a prognostic and predictive tool.** Examination of tissues specimens by both genome-wide and candidate gene approaches has been utilized in the search for better prognostic and predictive tools. Tumor specimens are routinely obtained for many types of cancer at the time of initial diagnosis and staging. Pathologic evaluation of these samples and assessment of local or metastatic spread form the basis of current staging systems. However, even with the most rigorous initial evaluations, individuals within a particular staging group will not behave identically. For example, even after definitive surgical treatment approximately one-fourth of individuals with Dukes' B colorectal cancer will die from recurrent disease and using current prognostic techniques, it is unclear if adjuvant chemotherapy is of benefit. Recognizing the complexity of disease progression, Wang et al. employed a DNA microarray-based gene expression profiling strategy to systematically search in a combinatorial manner for molecular markers of cancer classification and outcome prediction in patients with Dukes' B colon cancer (*J Clin Oncol* 2004;22:1564–1571). This effort generated a gene expression–based algorithm with a 23-gene signature that was able to identify patients among a homogeneously classified Dukes' B group who had an increased probability of recurrence. Validation of the signature in independent patients demonstrated a performance accuracy of 78%, correctly identifying 13 of 18 relapse patients and 15 of 18 disease-free patients, with an odds ratio of 13 for recurrence (95% CI, 2.6 to 65; p 0.003).

Similar studies of the simultaneous analysis of large numbers of genes in other cancers suggest that this approach may develop into a powerful clinical tool that will greatly complement current staging methods. In a genome-wide search, van't Veer et al. examined fresh, frozen tumor tissue from 78 lymph node negative sporadic breast cancers from patients who were younger than 55 years old at the time of diagnosis. RNA was isolated and examined on gene microarrays in which DNA sequences complementary to sequences of interest for approximately 25,000 human genes were arrayed on a solid surface (*Nature* 2002;415:530–536). From the training set, 5,000 genes were identified which varied significantly across the samples. From this list, a 70-gene prognostic signature was identified.

This 70-gene prognostic signature was then tested in a validation study, which examined stored fresh frozen tissue banked at the Netherlands Cancer Institute from 295 consecutively treated patients younger than 53 years of age (*N Engl J Med* 2002;347:1999–2009). This population included 151 node-negative patients (10 treated with adjuvant therapy) and 144 node-positive patients (120 treated with adjuvant therapy) with a median follow-up of 6.7 years. Patients who were identified as having a good prognostic genetic signature were observed to have an 85%, 10-year distant metastases-free survival and a 95%, 10-year overall survival compared to 51%, 10-year distant metastases-free survival and 55%, 10-year overall survival in those women who were identified to have a poor prognostic genetic signature (log-rank $p < 0.001$). This discrimination held true when patients were subdivided into node-negative and node-positive groups.

The European Organization for the Research and Treatment of Cancer (EORTC) has begun a trial with early stage breast cancer patients younger than 55 which will further test this 70-gene array. In the Microarray for Node Negative Disease may Avoid Chemotherapy (MINDACT) study, patients who are deemed to be at low risk based on clinical assessment or gene array will receive either endocrine therapy or no therapy whereas patients who are considered to have an average or high risk will receive either chemotherapy alone or combination with hormone therapy.

In another research effort employing a candidate gene approach, breast cancer tumor gene expression was associated with prediction of distant disease-free survival. After examining a list of 250 candidate genes in 3 different data sets, 16 genes were identified as being strongly associated with disease recurrence. These genes were grouped based on function, correlated expression, or both (Table 9.1). An algorithm was developed to yield a recurrence score that helps to quantify risk for distant disease recurrence based on the expression of these 16 genes and 5 reference genes. Evaluation of these genes was initially undertaken on a chip platform but was subsequently transferred and reevaluated with a reverse transcriptase-polymerase chain reaction (RT-PCR) technique which is now commercially available as the OncotypeDX assay (Genomic Health, Inc.).

TABLE 9.1   21-Gene Panel of the OncotypeDX Assay

Proliferation	Estrogen	Invasion	Miscellaneous	Reference
Ki67	ER	MMP11 (stromolysin 3)	GSTM	ACTB
STK15	PGR	CTSL2 (cathepsin L2)	CD68	GAPDH
Survivin	BCL2		BAG1	RPLPO
CCNB1(cyclin B1)	SCUBE2			GUS
MYBL2				TFRC

The recurrence score ranges from 0 to 100, and scores are categorized as low-risk if less than 18, high-risk if greater than 30, and intermediated for 19 to 30. The National Surgical Adjuvant Breast and Bowel Project (NSABP) B-14 trial examined whether patients with a low recurrence score indeed had a better outcome than those with a high recurrence score. Those with a low-risk recurrence score (approximately one half of the patients studied) had a 6.8% (95% CI, 4.0 to 9.6) risk of distant recurrence at 10-years of follow-up. By comparison, the risk of recurrence was 14.3% (95% CI, 8.3 to 20.3) for those with an intermediate-risk and 30.5% (95% CI, 23.6 to 37.4) for those with a high-risk score

Recurrence scores were evaluated in tumors from the NSABP B20 trial. Participants in this trial had previously been randomly assigned to treatment with tamoxifen alone or in combination with cyclophosphamide-methotrexate-5-fluorouracil (CMF) or melphalan, fluorouracil (MF). Recurrence scores were assessable in 227 patients in the tamoxifen-only arm and 424 patients who had received combination therapy. Patients whose tumors yielded a high-risk score (greater than 30) were observed to have an absolute decrease in 10-year distant recurrence rate after chemotherapy of 27.6% [standard error (SE) 8%]. Patients with a low-risk score (less than 18) were observed to have minimal benefit from chemotherapy with an absolute decrease in 10-year distant recurrence rate after chemotherapy of −1.1% (SE 2.2%). From these retrospective analyses, the 21-gene breast cancer recurrence score appears to be useful in quantifying the risk of recurrence in women with node-negative, estrogen receptor-positive breast cancer and may also assist in predicting the magnitude of benefit these women may have from chemotherapy.

Similar efforts have been undertaken in a number of tumor types including lung and lymphoma. These collected efforts suggest that this approach is a powerful clinical tool that will greatly complement current staging methods. Aside from serving as a diagnostic tool, the identified sets of genes from these approaches may help to direct novel research into the biology of treatment failures, recurrences, and metastasis. This utility is further illustrated by several exciting pharmacologic observations involving childhood acute lymphocytic leukemia (ALL).

Although pediatric ALL is considered curable, approximately one fifth of patients will have a treatment failure, and little is known about the genetic basis of this resistance. Two recent studies have assessed the genome-wide expression patterns in pediatric patients diagnosed with ALL in an attempt to identify genes that influence the response to treatment. In a comparison study of leukemia cells from 173 newly diagnosed ALL patients for *in vitro* sensitivity to prednisolone, vincristine, asparginase, and daunorubicin, gene expression was evaluated with a 14,500 probe set. Sets of differentially expressed genes were identified in B-lineage ALL that were sensitive or resistant to the four chemotherapeutic agents. A combined gene-expression score of resistance to all four agents was significantly related to treatment outcome ($p = 0.027$) and was confirmed in an independent cohort of 98 patients ($p = 0.003$). Of the 124 differentially expressed genes identified, only 3 had been previously associated with resistance to any of the four agents investigated.

In a second study from the same group, Lugthart et al., using a similar genome-wide differential expression approach, identified 45 genes which contribute to cross-resistance to prednisolone, vincristine, asparginase, and daunorubicin in ALL (*Cancer Cell* 2005;7:375–386). Genes included in the list were involved in nucleic acid metabolism, transcription, nucleic acid processing, and DNA repair. Of the genes associated with multidrug resistance, only 16 of the genes overlapped with the genes that the group had previously found to be associated with single agent resistance. Expression of the 45 multidrug resistance genes was found to identify a subset of patients with poorer treatment outcome in two independent patient cohorts. Collectively these two studies have used genome-wide approaches to provide novel insights into the biology of treatment resistance, illuminating novel potential therapeutic targets. Additionally, they have provided tools to identify patients predisposed to treatment failure, which may help to redirect early intervention with chemotherapy. The sheer number of genes involved in identifying and segregating this polygenetic phenotype is also staggering evidence for the power of genome-wide approaches.

III. CONCLUSIONS. Genetic inheritance plays a significant role in interindividual variability of drug response. Likewise the genetic makeup of any given tumor contributes significantly to the observed heterogeneity of malignancy. Pharmacogenomics offers a chance to improve individualization of care by providing research tools for gaining a greater understanding of the genome-dependent biology of malignancy and clinical tools for selection of therapy based on an individual's genetic inheritance. Our current technology is well suited to the development of tools which are effective guides for improved utilization of currently available therapies. Available techniques are also suitable for the development and validation of therapeutically relevant prognostic and predictive classifiers. Properly developing these tools will be challenging and costlier than traditional clinical laboratory and pathology tools and will require paradigm shifts in clinical trial design. Already these changes are beginning to be implemented. If properly developed, these tools will offer significant advantages to patients in terms of morbidity and mortality. It is also hoped that these advances will be able to help curtail the spiraling costs of oncology care by helping to direct appropriate care while avoiding treatments that are unnecessary, ineffective, or potentially toxic on an individual basis. As we grapple with genomic data and new discoveries in biology, pharmacogenomic approaches will demonstrate utility in the identification of novel therapeutic targets. Although current resolution limitations yield broad candidate gene lists, in the foreseeable future, advances in and refinements to technology will allow narrowing of these lists and more efficient selection of target genes. There will continue to be many nongenetic variables that prove to be useful in achieving individualized therapy. However, genomic markers must augment or replace currently used clinical variable in order for cost-effective application of therapy to occur.

Suggested Readings

Evans WE, McLeod HL. Pharmacogenomics—drug disposition, drug targets, and side effects. *N Engl J Med* 2003;348:538–539.

Evans WE, Relling MV. Pharmacogenomics: translating functional genomics into rational therapeutics. *Science* 1999;286:487–491.

Kalow W. *Pharmacogenetics: Heredity and the Response to Drugs.* Philadelphia and London: WB Saunders, 1962.

Watters JW, McLeod HL. Cancer pharmacogenomics: current and future applications. *Biochim Biophys Acta* 2003;1603:99–111.

MOLECULAR DIAGNOSTICS

Barbara A. Zehnbauer and John D. Pfeifer

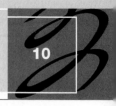

10

I. ROLE OF MOLECULAR DIAGNOSTICS. Clinical application of insights derived from molecular genetic research studies has become increasingly important in patient care. Clinical molecular diagnostic methods have been integrated into many laboratory disciplines, and published guidelines and recommendations from both professional societies and regulatory agencies have been developed to assist in the development and performance of clinical molecular pathology testing. Molecular analysis is useful for diagnosis, for predicting prognosis or response to various treatment options, for monitoring minimal residual disease (treatment efficacy), for identifying predisposition to disease, and for detection of therapeutic targets in gene-specific therapy.

In one sense, molecular testing has been practiced for several decades in surgical pathology in the context of immunohistochemistry, in which antibodies are used to detect and quantify the expression of specific proteins of diagnostic, prognostic, or therapeutic importance. However, in current common usage, *molecular diagnostics* refers to the analysis of changes in nucleic acids, either DNA or RNA, and most frequently implies direct mutation testing. Genetic testing protocols can be designed to detect heritable DNA variations or, as is usually the case in neoplastic diseases, somatic or acquired DNA variations limited to specific cells of the disease process.

At the interface of genetic disorders and acquired mutations in sporadic cancers are familial cancer syndromes. Familial cancer syndromes are inherited disorders that cause patients to be predisposed to increased risk for developing particular types of tumors. These syndromes are frequently distinguished from the sporadic tumor of the same types by several clinical features: earlier age of onset, bilateral or multifocal tumors, occurrence in multiple family members, and occurrence in more than one generation of a family. The carriers of the increased risk inherit a genetic predisposition for tumor formation as an autosomal dominant trait; this risk factor is a gene-specific germline mutation that may be screened for in DNA isolated from circulating lymphocytes of affected individuals rather than primary tumor tissue. The characterization of the specific genes underlying familial cancer syndromes has provided important insights into the nature of many tumor suppressor genes and oncogenes. Many examples of genes that confer a hereditary predisposition to cancer have been described and include *RB1* (retinoblastoma, osteosarcoma, leukemia, and lymphoma), *TP53* (Li-Fraumeni syndrome; bone and soft tissue sarcomas, breast cancer, leukemia, and brain tumors), *BRCA1* and *BRCA2* (breast, ovarian, colon, and prostate cancers), *APC* (adenomatous polyposis coli, colon carcinoma, and osteomas), *MSH2, MLH1,* and *MSH6* (hereditary nonpolyposis colon carcinoma; colon, endometrium, ovary, and stomach cancers), *RET* (MEN2 and FMTC; medullary thyroid carcinoma and pheochromocytoma), *VHL* (von Hippel-Lindau disease; renal carcinoma, and pheochromocytoma), *NF1* (neurofibromatosis; neurofibroma and optic gliomas), and many others. A subset of sporadic tumors also carries mutations in these genes.

A. Specimens. Specimen requirements are dictated by disease pathology, including the type of tissue, amount of tissue, type of sample (fresh/frozen tissue, formalin-fixed paraffin-embedded (FFPE) tissue, cytology specimen, etc.), and the extent of the disease in the sample. Since most (but not all) molecular diagnostic techniques are currently based on polymerase chain reaction (PCR) amplification, the amount of tissue required is relatively small, and so many routine pathology specimens can be analyzed effectively.

Regardless of specimen type, two general features of the tissue sample influence molecular pathology assays. First, there must be a sufficient quantity of

95

the specific target cell, and therefore target DNA or RNA, in the sample. If testing involves a clonal tumor admixed with normal cells, or a heterogeneous tissue specimen with many different gene expression patterns, a detection threshold must be defined. Second, since the size of the nucleic acid molecules after isolation from the tissue can dramatically affect the sensitivity of the detection of specific alterations, degradation (whether due to enzymatic, heat, pH, or mechanical forces) can reduce the utility of testing.

1. **Tissue types.** Fresh peripheral blood, bone marrow, solid tissue biopsies, and enriched cell populations (e.g., from flow cytometry) are all adequate substrates for molecular analysis. They should be collected and transported to the molecular pathology laboratory using aseptic techniques. Transport on ice reduces cell lysis, minimize nuclease activity, and reduces nucleic acid degradation.

2. **Tissue quality.** Appropriate handling of the tissue postexcision and pretesting maximizes detection limits. Prompt preservation of solid tissue samples by freezing or fixation will minimize degradation and loss of nucleic acid integrity. Hematologic specimens (peripheral blood, bone marrow) should be collected in the presence of an anticoagulant, preferably ethylenediaminetetraacetic acid (EDTA) or acid citrate dextrose (ACD), but not heparin because heparin carry-over after nucleic acid isolation may inhibit subsequent PCR steps.

   Freezing solid tissue specimens after excision also yields good preservation of nucleic acids. However, frozen whole blood or bone marrow presents distinct obstacles to the preparation of good quality nucleic acid and should be generally avoided.

   FFPE tissue sections are also suitable substrates for molecular analysis. Fixed tissue has several advantages; fixation suspends the degradation of nucleic acids, and fixed specimens can be easily stored and transported. However, a significant limitation of fixed tissue is that the quality of the extracted nucleic acids is extremely variable (due to the fact that all fixatives, including formalin, chemically degrade nucleic acids to a greater or lesser extent).

3. **Tissue quantity.** Minimum sample requirements are determined by the assay methodology and extent of target cell involvement in the tissue submitted for analysis. Genomic Southern hybridization requires approximately 10 μg of DNA (approximately 10^6 cells) per enzymatic digest for detection of single copy genomic DNA targets; hybridization signals to detect smaller molecular weight DNA fragments (less than 1 kb in length) may require more DNA. PCR amplification has significantly reduced DNA requirements, and typically only 20 to 200 ng of DNA (approximately 10^3 to 10^4 cells) is needed per reaction for many applications; multiplexed PCR may require a bit more DNA in order to equally represent all targets. The sensitivity of PCR for detection of a few target molecules in a large background of unaltered DNA molecules (1 in 10^5) is one of the principle strengths of this methodology in molecular pathology.

B. **Technical versus diagnostic aspects of testing.** The analytical sensitivity and specificity of a molecular genetic test may be unrelated to its diagnostic sensitivity and specificity. Since only a subset of cases of a specific tumor may harbor a characteristic mutation, more than one genetic abnormality may be associated with a specific tumor, or more than one tumor may share the same mutation, a molecular genetic method with perfect analytic performance can have a lower sensitivity and specificity when used for diagnostic or prognostic testing of patient samples. Differences between the analytical and diagnostic levels of analysis are often overlooked even though they account for many of the confusing or seemingly conflicting results regarding the utility of diagnostic molecular genetic testing in clinical practice.

1. **Reported estimates of test performance.** The experimental design of published studies regarding the utility of molecular diagnosis varies considerably. Many studies of test performance are complicated by the presence of selection bias (also called verification bias, post-test referral bias, and work-up bias) or discrepant analysis (also known as discordant analysis or review bias), which hinders interpretation of the test results in the setting of routine clinical practice.

2. **Discordant cases.** Cases arise in which there is a lack of concordance between the diagnosis suggested by molecular genetic findings and the morphologic diagnosis. The debate over the best approach to resolve the ambiguity presented by these cases, especially those that are presumed false positives, reflects the fundamental impact of molecular genetics on the classification of disease as well as the power of morphology as the historic standard of pathologic diagnosis by which new methods of classification are measured. Rather than arbitrarily assuming that genetic testing or morphology is superior in all cases, the most reasonable way to handle discordant cases is to acknowledge the presence of the discrepancy, and to reappraise all the clinical data, pathologic findings, and therapeutic implications. For those cases in which the diagnosis suggested by morphology and genetic testing are different, prospective clinical trials are required to assess whether stage, prognosis, and response to treatment are more accurately predicted by the molecular test than by the morphologic findings on which current staging and treatment protocols are based. Although it is often assumed that molecular testing can provide a more objective basis for diagnosis or therapy in those cases in which there is a disagreement with traditional morphology, it is important to recognize that there are no formal prospective, randomized studies that have demonstrated that this is true.

II. **CYTOGENETICS.** A number of specific cytogenetic abnormalities uniquely characterize morphologically and clinically distinct subsets of hematopoietic malignancies and solid tumors.

A. **Traditional karyotype analysis.** Metaphase chromosome analysis can be performed on many different cell types, although different sample and handling procedures may be required. Inappropriate handling, as well as delay between specimen collection and culture initiation, can markedly decrease the likelihood that the sample will grow *in vitro*. Communication and coordination with the cytogenetics laboratory are essential.

Traditional karyotype analysis utilizes a period of *in vitro* cell culture of the tissue sample, followed by arrest of cell division in metaphase, cell lysis, fixation, and staining to produce banded chromosomes that can be visualized by light microscopy. The most widely used staining techniques, termed *G-, Q-, and R-banding*, produce 350 to 550 bands per haploid set of chromosomes. The final step in cytogenetic analysis is the production of a karyotype, which is the chromosomal complement of the cell displayed in a standard sequence on the basis of size, centromere location, and banding pattern.

1. **Advantages.** The power of conventional cytogenetic analysis lies in its ability to provide simultaneous analysis of the entire genome without any foreknowledge of the chromosomal regions involved in the disease process. In most cases, the type and/or location of the identified chromosomal abnormalities can be used to establish a diagnosis or to direct additional testing.

2. **Limitations.** The clinical utility of traditional cytogenetic analysis is restricted by two general features of the method. First, from a technical standpoint, analysis can be performed only on viable tissue specimens that contain proliferating cells. Second, from a sensitivity standpoint, analysis has a resolution of only approximately 3 to 4 million base pairs (Mb) at an 850-band level, and only approximately 7 to 8 Mb at a 400-band level. Consequently, traditional cytogenetic analysis is only suited for detection of numerical abnormalities and gross structural rearrangements; the method does not have the sensitivity to detect mutations such as small deletions and insertions, single base-pair substitutions, and so on.

B. **Metaphase fluorescence *in situ* hybridization (FISH).** Virtually all metaphase FISH is performed using nucleic acid probes labeled with fluorophores. Most metaphase FISH probes fall into one of three general categories. Repetitive sequence probes hybridize to sequences that are present in hundreds to thousands of copies, and so produce strong signals; the most widely used probes of this type bind to α-satellite sequences of centromeres. Unique sequence probes detect sequences that are present only once in the genome or at most at only one copy per chromosome;

they are used to detect changes in the copy number of a specific locus, to confirm the presence of rearrangements involving a specific locus, or to detect so-called cryptic rearrangements that cannot be identified by routine banding methods. Whole chromosome probes, also known as chromosome painting probes or chromosome libraries, consist of thousands of overlapping probes that recognize unique and moderately repetitive sequences along the entire length of individual chromosomes; they are used to confirm the interpretation of aberrations identified by traditional karyotype analysis, or to establish the chromosomal origin of rearrangements that are difficult to evaluate by other approaches.

C. **Multiplex metaphase FISH and spectral karyotyping.** These two related techniques make it possible to hybridize metaphase chromosome spreads with a combination of probes. Both techniques are useful for detection of aneuploidy as well as chromosome rearrangements; in many cases, the techniques can establish the chromosomal origin of rearrangements that cannot be defined on the basis of traditional karyotype analysis.

III. **TISSUE *IN SITU* HYBRIDIZATION.** This technique makes it possible to detect target DNA and mRNA sequences in histologic sections of fresh tissue or FFPE tissue, and so permits direct correlation of the morphology of individual cells with the presence or absence of the target sequence or mutations.

A. **Tissue interphase FISH.** Use of nucleic acid probes labeled with fluorophores and visualized through fluorescence microscopy has revolutionized tissue *in situ* hybridization for detection of abnormalities in chromosome number and chromosome structure. Since interphase FISH analysis eliminates the need for *in vitro* cell culture, the technique can be used to study a broader range of cell and tissue types (and therefore a broader range of tumors) than can be evaluated by traditional karyotype analysis. The higher sensitivity of interphase FISH also makes it useful for uncovering small rearrangements not detectable in standard karyotypes.

1. **Advantages.** Both repetitive sequence probes and unique sequence probes can be used for interphase FISH; concurrent hybridization with a combination of probes labeled with different fluorophores permits simultaneous detection of two or more DNA regions of interest. Methodologic advances have made it possible to detect low copy number gene sequences as small as 500 base pairs in length, although the efficiency of interphase FISH with small probes is quite low.

2. **Limitations.** Even with optimized probes, interphase FISH lacks the resolution in routine use to detect small chromosomal aberrations less than several kb in size. Consequently, the technique cannot be used to evaluate some classes of mutations that are characteristic of many sporadic tumors and familial cancer syndromes, such as single base-pair substitutions, or small insertions or deletions.

B. **Tissue interphase analysis of mRNA.** Tissue *in situ* hybridization for mRNA is a versatile technique, although the method is technically demanding. The approach can be used to correlate the expression level of a specific gene with tissue changes characteristic of a disease, with a tumor's phenotype, or to monitor transgene expression in gene therapy regimens. However, even when optimized, the technique's sensitivity is below that of PCR-based methods.

IV. **SOUTHERN AND NORTHERN BLOT HYBRIDIZATION.** These two filter hybridization methods are similar in principle. Purified nucleic acids (DNA after digestion by a restriction endonuclease for Southern blots, RNA for northern blots) are size fractionated by gel electrophoresis, transferred and immobilized on a synthetic membrane made of nitrocellulose or nylon, and then hybridized to a specific nucleic acid probe. The probe is visualized by either radioisotopic or nonisotopic methods, and the location of the probe indicates not only the presence of the target sequence, but also the size of the enzyme-digested DNA fragment or RNA molecule in which it is contained.

A. **Southern blot hybridization.** This method is most often used to detect genomic rearrangements characteristic of specific tumor types, but can also be used to detect different alleles of the same gene, point mutations, deletions, and insertions. Since the method is quantitative, it may provide information about gene copy number. Southern blot hybridization is a reliable and versatile method for sequence-specific DNA analysis, but requires at least 10 mm^3 of fresh or frozen tissue in which there has been limited DNA degradation. Although the technique was widely used for molecular analysis of tissue specimens for several decades, PCR-based methods have replaced the routine use of Southern blot hybridization for many assays because PCR-based methods have similar reliability but have increased sensitivity, are usually more rapid and less cumbersome, require less tissue, and can be performed on FFPE tissue.

B. Northern blot hybridization. This method is most often employed to detect abnormal gene expression in the absence of gross karyotypic abnormalities. Northern blotting, although technically demanding, simultaneously provides information about both mRNA transcript abundance and structure, including the utilization of alternative transcript initiation or termination sites, alternative splicing patterns, and mutations. The method is quantitative and so can be used to indicate the relative abundance of different transcript types.

Northern blot analysis is technically demanding and requires a large sample of fresh tissue. Consequently, routine use of northern blot hybridization has been replaced by reverse transcriptase-polymerase chain reaction (RT-PCR)–based methods that have similar reliability but are more sensitive, quicker, less cumbersome to perform, require less tissue, and can be performed on FFPE tissue.

V. POLYMERASE CHAIN REACTION (PCR). PCR makes it possible to detect a broad range of chromosomal abnormalities, from gross structural alterations such as translocations and deletions, to single base-pair mutations in individual genes. PCR can be performed on areas of tumor (or even individual cells) microdissected from routinely prepared tissue or cytology slides, or separated by flow cytometry, and therefore PCR methods make it possible to correlate tissue morphology with genetic abnormalities of specific regions of tumor, specific cell populations, or even individual cells. The clinical utility of PCR is due to the wide range of template DNA that can be amplified, the technique's intrinsic extreme sensitivity, and the wide range of variations of the basic method that can be performed.

A. Basic PCR. A PCR mixture includes the DNA sample to be assayed, a thermostable DNA polymerase, the four deoxynucleotide triphosphates, and short oligonucleotide primers specifically designed to be complementary to the regions that flank the DNA sequence of interest. With each PCR cycle, the DNA region of interest is enriched twofold, and the target region is therefore exponentially amplified by the successive cycles of resynthesis.

1. Advantages. Basic PCR (and the variations described in the subsequent text) have many advantages over the techniques of Southern and northern blot hybridization that have traditionally been used to analyze specific regions of DNA and mRNA. PCR-based analysis is more rapid (may be performed in only a few hours rather than days); can be applied to a wider range of tissues (including fresh, frozen, or fixed tissue); is far more sensitive (requires much less tissue) and specific (target DNA or RNA is detectable even when present within a background of a vast excess of nontarget sequence); and is very versatile.

2. Limitations. When optimized, PCR can detect one abnormal cell in a background of 10^5 normal cells, and can detect single copy genes from individual cells. However, many technical factors conspire to lower the clinical sensitivity of PCR; the most important practical limitation is degradation of target DNA or mRNA, especially when extracted from fixed tissue.

The extreme sensitivity of PCR demands constant attention to laboratory organization and test design to avoid specimen contamination, the most troublesome technical issue. Contamination can be largely avoided by careful laboratory technique and maintenance, physical separation and containment of the various stages of the PCR procedure, and regular UV irradiation of laboratory workspaces and instruments to degrade any transient uncontained DNA.

PCR only analyzes the chromosomal region amplified by the primers employed, and therefore, unlike conventional cytogenetics, does not survey the entire genome. Similarly, RT-PCR only analyzes the target mRNA, and provides no information about the presence of mutations or level of transcription of other related genes.

    B. **Reverse transcriptase PCR (RT-PCR).** mRNA extracted from the sample is reverse transcribed into complementary DNA (cDNA); this cDNA then serves as the template in the subsequent PCR amplification. The use of RT-PCR permits straightforward amplification of the coding region of multi-exon DNA sequences.

    C. **Multiplex PCR.** This approach involves the simultaneous amplification of multiple target sequences in a single PCR through the use of multiple primer pairs for distant and diverse DNA targets. It is used to evaluate a number of different sites for the presence of a mutation in a single reaction, and is therefore a practical screening method.

    D. **Methylation-specific PCR.** Pretreatment of the DNA sample with sodium bisulfite makes it possible to evaluate the methylation status of individual CpG sites. This approach is used in tests to characterize specific gene silencing patterns that are correlated with tumor subgroups that are likely to respond to specific chemotherapeutic regimens.

    E. **Quantitative PCR.** Also referred to as real-time PCR, this method permits more reliable quantification of the amount of input DNA than is possible by simple endpoint measurement of the DNA product. Since the PCR product is quantified as the reaction progresses (i.e., in real-time) rather than after PCR completion, it avoids the potential artifacts of amplification efficiency. Many different reaction chemistries have been developed that allow the detection of gene copy number that may have prognostic or therapeutic implications. When mRNA is the substrate, quantitative RT-PCR can be used to correlate changes in gene expression with the clinical features of a disease or a specific tumor type. Quantitative PCR often provides more precise measurements of DNA or mRNA than can be achieved by filter hybridization or microarray based methods.

VI. DNA SEQUENCE ANALYSIS

    A. **Direct methods of sequence analysis.** Virtually all routine direct DNA sequence analysis is automated and performed on templates generated by the enzymatic chain termination method using the methodology known as *cycle sequencing.* Even though cycle sequencing reactions require a very low quantity of template DNA to generate enough product for subsequent automated DNA sequence analysis, the amount of DNA present in most patient specimens is frequently not sufficient for analysis without a preliminary amplification step, usually PCR.

    B. **Indirect methods of sequence analysis.** Once normal and mutant alleles at a specific locus have been characterized by direct DNA sequence analysis, indirect methods can often provide enough sequence information to be of clinical utility. These indirect techniques include allelic discrimination by size, restriction fragment length polymorphism analysis, allele-specific PCR, single strand conformational polymorphism analysis, heteroduplex analysis, denaturing gradient gel electrophoresis, cleavage of mismatched nucleotides, ligase chain reaction, the protein truncation test, and numerous variants, used either alone or in combination. These indirect methods are based on PCR and may be applied to a broad range of clinical specimens. In addition, many of the indirect methods are quicker and less expensive than direct sequence analysis, and are ideally suited for screening large numbers of samples from patients.

    C. **Sequence analysis by microarray technology.** High-density DNA microarrays have found their greatest use in hybridization-based evaluation of gene expression (discussed in the subsequent text), but chip-based hybridization analysis is also a promising technology for sequence analysis.

VII. MICROARRAY-BASED GENE EXPRESSION PROFILING. The morphologic features of disease are essentially reflections of altered gene expression within diseased cells. Characterization of disease-specific alterations in gene expression is therefore an area of intense interest. Given the limitations of Northern blot hybridization, a variety of new methodologies have been developed to identify differentially expressed genes, of which microarray technology is the most widely used.

Microarray technology is based on the principle of nucleic acid hybridization, and makes it possible to perform rapid analysis of the expression level of thousands of genes in parallel. Fundamentally, a DNA microarray (or gene chip) employs multiple sets of DNAs or oligonucleotides complementary to the thousands of genes to be investigated, each attached at a known location on a glass or nylon membrane substrate the size of a computer chip. Fluorophore-labeled test (or target) nucleic acids derived from the specimen are hybridized to the chip, and the emissions produced by laser scanning allow for quantitation of gene expression of even low-abundance transcripts.

A. Applications. Microarray-based techniques, although still largely experimental, are increasingly being used in clinical settings to demonstrate specific and reproducible differences in gene expression profiles that are of diagnostic utility, or that can be used to predict prognosis or response to specific therapeutic regimens.

B. Limitations. Microarray-based gene expression technology is currently applicable only to fresh or frozen tissue, and cannot be reproducibly applied to FFPE samples. Another major challenge facing microarray-based expression profiling (as well as the other genomewide techniques discussed subsequently) is interpretation of the massive quantity of data generated by each sample tested.

VIII. EMERGING TECHNIQUES. Despite the fact that molecular analysis of single markers has established clinical value for many neoplasms, testing focused on individual loci is a reflection of the immaturity of molecular diagnostics rather than an optimized testing paradigm. Analysis of multiple loci will likely provide more accurate diagnostic, prognostic, and therapeutic information, and consequently clinical use of microarray technologies that make it possible to evaluate thousands of markers from individual tumor specimens will likely expand. Several microarray technologies other than gene expression profiling (discussed earlier) hold particular promise.

A. Pharmacogenetics. In addition to tumor-specific genetic abnormalities, genetic variation has been estimated to account for 20% to 95% of variability in the metabolism, disposition, and effect of the drugs used to treat patients with cancer. Pharmacogenetics offers the opportunity not only to optimize the efficacy of therapy, but also to minimize toxicity. Many centers are now using prospective genotyping of a few targeted genes to guide antineoplastic treatment and dosing choices. These include thiopurine methyltransferase (*TPMT*) point mutations in mercaptopurine therapy for acute leukemia, thymidylate synthase enhancer region (*TSER*) polymorphisms in 5-fluorouracil therapy for colorectal cancer, and UDP glucuronosyl transferase (*UGT1A1*) promoter region variants in irinotecan therapy for metastatic colorectal cancer. Genomewide analysis of the role of genetic variation to predict an individual patient's response to treatment with a specific drug is known as *pharmacogenomics*.

B. Single nucleotide polymorphism (SNP) analysis. SNPs are common in the human genome, and once a set of SNPs is linked with an increased susceptibility to a certain disease, prognosis, or response to therapy, focused analysis of the SNPs (also known as haplotype analysis) may circumvent the need for more extensive DNA sequence analysis. Genomewide analysis is still too expensive for clinical use, but increased automation and more refined SNP catalogs will likely make systematic analysis of SNPs an important clinical tool.

C. Analysis of epigenetic modifications. Techniques for quantitative detection of the methylation status of every human gene individually have been developed. Given the effect of epigenetic changes on gene expression, it is reasonable to anticipate that the pattern of methylation at defined sets of loci may eventually become a component of the pathologic evaluation of individual tumors.

D. Comparative genomic hybridization (CGH). Essentially a modification of *in situ* hybridization (ISH), CGH makes it possible to survey the genome of even fixed tissue for chromosomal deletions and amplifications. The resolution of array CGH is in theory limited only by the number and length of the DNA sequences in the array; arrays are currently available that yield approximately 5 kb resolution.

E. Proteomics. This technique is focused on the analysis of patterns of protein expression rather than the analysis of nucleic acids. Methods for high sensitivity, high throughput evaluation of protein expression profiles have been developed—methods that make it possible to identify patterns that correlate with specific malignancies, underlying mutations, epigenetic changes, transcriptional profiles, response to drug therapy, and so on.

F. Analysis of RNA interference. It has recently become clear that several classes of short single-stranded or double-stranded RNA molecules that are responsible for RNA interference (RNAi) have a profound role in the regulation of gene expression. The demonstration that the profile of miRNAs (one class of small RNAs that mediate RNAi) is different in normal and neoplastic tissue, that alterations in miRNA are oncogenic, and that RNAi-based approaches can have therapeutic benefit all suggest that analysis of specific small RNA molecules, either individually or on a genomewide basis, will likely have an important role in the molecular evaluation of tumors.

Suggested Readings

Barik S. Silence of the transcripts: RNA interference in medicine. *J Mol Med* 2005;83: 764–773.

Bossuyt PM, Reitsma JB, Bruns DE, et al. Towards complete and accurate reporting of studies of diagnostic accuracy: the STARD initiative. *Ann Intern Med* 2003;138:40–44.

Dieffenbach CW, Dveksler GS. *PCR primer*. Cold Spring Harbor: Cold Spring Harbor Laboratory Press, 2003.

The International HapMap Consortium. A haplotype map of the human genome. *Nature* 2005;437:1299–1320.

Keagle MB, Gersen SL. *Principles of clinical cytogenetics*, 2nd ed. Totowa: Humana Press, 2005:63–79.

Ladanyi M, Gerald WL, eds. *Expression profiling of human tumors: diagnostic and research applications*. Washington, DC: AACC Press, 2003.

Lewin J, Schmitt AO, Adorjan P, et al. Quantitative DNA methylation analysis based on four-dye trace data from direct sequencing of PCR amplicates. *Bioinformatics* 2004;20:3005–3012.

Marsh S, McLeod HL Pharmacogenomics: from bedside to clinical practice *Hum Mol Genet* 2006;15:R89–R93.

Misek DE, Imafuku Y, Hanash SM. Application of proteomic technologies to tumor analysis. *Pharmacogenomics* 2004;5:1129–1137.

Pfeifer JD. *Molecular genetic testing in surgical pathology*. Philadelphia: Lippincott Williams & Wilkins, 2006.

Pfeifer JD, Hill DA, O'Sullivan MJ, et al. Diagnostic gold standard for soft tissue tumours: morphology or molecular genetics? *Histopathol* 2000;37:485–500.

Vogelstein B, Kinzler KW, eds. *The genetic basis of human cancer*, 2nd ed. New York: McGraw-Hill, 2002.

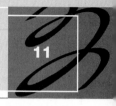

NEURO-ONCOLOGY

Dennis Rivet, Michael R. Chicoine, Gerald P. Linette,
and Joseph R. Simpson

11

I. APPROACH TO THE PATIENT WITH TUMORS OF THE CENTRAL NERVOUS SYSTEM

A. General. Tumors of the central nervous system (CNS) include a variety of diseases with highly variable presentation and natural histories. These rare tumors occur in both pediatric and adult populations. The histologic types are varied, but gliomas are the most frequent.

B. Presentation. Most patients have signs or symptoms from one of three general categories: a progressive neurologic deficit, headaches, or seizure.

1. Localized brain dysfunction due to the presence of a tumor results in a pattern of deficits relating to the specific location. This may result from physical compression or invasion of adjacent brain parenchyma by tumor. Deficits such as hemiparesis or altered mentation and/or consciousness may resemble a stroke or transient ischemic attack. A widely variable time course of symptoms often results in a delay in diagnosis of slow-growing tumors (e.g., meningiomas or well-differentiated gliomas).

2. Headaches may result from mass effect itself or obstructive hydrocephalus. The classic pattern of being worse in the morning may be related to hypoventilation during sleep, causing hypercapnia and vasodilation, which increases the intracranial pressure. Posterior fossa tumors may produce hydrocephalus and severe headaches accompanied by nausea, vomiting, lethargy, and visual problems. Emesis often yields temporary relief.

3. Seizures are another common first manifestation of brain tumors. An idiopathic seizure for the first time after age 18 should prompt aggressive investigation for a tumor. Locations such as the temporal lobe or cerebral hemisphere are more likely to develop seizures, whereas pituitary and posterior fossa are unlikely to do so.

4. Spinal neoplasms also vary widely in their presentation based on their nature and location. The most common presenting symptom is pain, often worse when lying supine and localized to the region of the tumor. Other common manifestations include numbness, weakness, paresthesias, and bowel or bladder dysfunction.

5. Physical examination of the patient with a CNS tumor should begin with a careful neurologic examination, assessment of the cranial nerves, motor and sensory examination, and assessment of reflexes and coordination. Fundoscopic examination is used to assess for papilledema, a sign of increased intracranial pressure. A general physical examination and assessment of performance status is important for determining the overall health of the patient, comorbid conditions, potential sources of metastatic spread to the CNS, and functional status. The use of tests such as the Mini-Mental Status Examination, interpretation of proverbs, and the ability of the patient to follow commands may assess higher function.

6. Diagnosis and evaluation

a. Radiographic imaging. Since the inception of computed tomographic (CT) scanning in 1973 and magnetic resonance imaging (MRI) in the mid-1980s, imaging of the nervous system has been revolutionized. Part of the increased incidence of neurologic malignancies has been ascribed to common use of these imaging techniques. The initial evaluation of patients suspected of having a brain neoplasm should consist of an **MRI** with and without the

103

administration of gadolinium contrast. **MRI** is more sensitive than CT and provides multiplanar imaging. CT remains a useful tool for evaluation in the setting of bony involvement of tumors and an acute neurologic deterioration, and to assess the degree of calcification. Ultrasound may be useful for the initial evaluation of the infant and for surgical planning. Positron emission tomography (PET) is often used to differentiate tumor progression from radionecrosis. Imaging modalities that are linked to the metabolic activity of tumors, such as functional magnetic resonance imaging (MRI) are being refined and are useful in the depiction of the primary motor, sensory, and language cortex. Magnetic resonance spectroscopy is a developing technique that is currently being used to help differentiate between primary CNS tumors and metastases.

b. **Classification.** Tumors can be divided based on location, cell type of origin, histologic appearance, or the age group they affect.

   i. **Grading** of **tumors**. Many different grading and classification schemes have been used over the years. The World Health Organization (WHO) grading scale is commonly used in diagnostic and treatment protocols. Table 11.1 lists the most common tumors with their typical WHO grade in the WHO classification scheme. Tumors are arranged by cell type and malignancy potential or grade.

   ii. **A tumor's "Malignancy" describes a tendency toward an aggressive growth rate** and infiltrative nature. The "benign" or lower-grade tumor suggests only slow growth, and these tumors may still have rare malignant transformation. A low-grade or indolent lesion may be incurable or cause severe morbidity, even death, because of its location. In

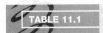

| **TABLE 11.1** | WHO Classification of Common Tumors |

Most common tumors	WHO grade
Pilocytic astrocytoma	1
Diffuse astrocytoma	2
Anaplastic astrocytoma	3
Glioblastoma	4
Anaplastic (malignant) astrocytoma	3-4
Glioblastoma	4
Oligodendroglioma	1-2
Anaplastic oligodendroglioma	3-4
Oligodendroglioma	2
Anaplastic oligodendroglioma	3
Ependymoma	1-2
Anaplastic (malignant) ependymoma	3-4
Primitive neuroectodermal tumor (PNET)	4
Medulloblastoma	
Cerebral or spinal PNET	
Schwannoma	1
Neurofibroma	1
Meningioma	1
Atypical meningioma	2
Anaplastic (malignant) meningioma	3
Primary malignant lymphoma	3-4
Pituitary adenoma	1

From World Health Organization. *AJCC cancer staging manual,* 5th ed. Philadelphia: Lippincott-Raven, 1997:282, with permission.

certain cases, medulloblastomas, ependymomas, and, less commonly, other gliomas disseminate to other locations, usually restricted to the neuraxis.

iii. **Location.** The tentorium divides the intracranial space into infratentorial and supratentorial compartments. This anatomic distribution serves to separate both age incidence and typical clinical manifestations. Approximately 60% of pediatric intracranial malignancies occur in the posterior fossa or infratentorial location. They often have severe headache, vomiting, ataxia, and nystagmus or Parinaud syndrome (paralysis of upward gaze and convergence, rotatory nystagmus).

7. **General guidelines of treatment.** The specific role that surgery, radiation, and chemotherapy may play in the management of CNS tumors is dependent on tumor type and classification. Some general principles of treatment are broadly applicable.

a. **Surgery.** The goals of surgical treatment for tumors of the CNS are relief of symptoms, tissue diagnosis, and cytoreduction. Examples of symptoms that may be relieved after resection are seizures, headaches, and neurologic dysfunction related to mass effect from a tumor. Options for obtaining a tissue diagnosis include a resection of the tumor after a biopsy. Biopsy can be done by using a stereotactically guided needle technique or an open biopsy in situations in which the tumor cannot be safely or easily accessed with needle techniques. In general, surgical resection offers the greatest magnitude of cytoreduction and, although it is usually not curative for intrinsic gliomas, may cure many lower-grade CNS tumors. In all cases, consideration must be given to patient age, functional status, medical condition, neurologic status, likely diagnosis, prior treatments, and possible complications to determine when surgery is most appropriate.

b. **Radiation** plays a significant role in the management of both primary and metastatic CNS tumors. The degree of success is determined by the responsiveness of such tumors to the doses of radiation therapy, tolerated by normal brain tissue. When used as a definitive therapy, irradiation is given over a multiweek course of daily or occasionally twice-daily fractionations to a total dose expected to produce long-term tumor control or even cure. When used in a palliative sense, radiation courses are shorter, with a higher dose being delivered per fraction, and the aim being temporary relief of symptoms, although such relief can last for a year or more.

i. **The tolerance of CNS** to fractionated radiation therapy depends on volume treated, fraction size, and total dose. Typically, 5,400 to 6,000 cGy delivered at 180 to 200 cGy/day is considered tolerance for the nervous system, with the expectation that approximately 5% of patients so treated would develop symptoms of radiation injury within a 5-year period. These doses are adequate for rather durable control of tumors such as childhood medulloblastoma, certain low-grade astrocytomas, and a proportion of anaplastic oligodendrogliomas or ependymomas. An effective dose producing durable long-term control for anaplastic astrocytomas and glioblastomas has not been found and remains limited by normal tissue tolerance at present.

ii. **Attempts to increase the radiation dose** above 60 to 70 Gy to restricted volumes have yielded results that suggest that an alternation in relapse pattern may be achieved by focal escalation of dose by means of brachytherapy or radiosurgery. However, a major need is for development of agents that will either selectively sensitize tumor cells or alternatively protect the normal glial, neuronal, and vascular tissues incidentally exposed to radiation.

iii. **When palliative treatment is given,** for example, for multiple metastases to the brain, or for spinal cord compression, the treatment course is usually approximately 2.5 to 3 weeks, with 250 to 300 cGy delivered daily. When a significant mass effect is exerted in either organ, steroids are generally begun before therapy, and are tapered as tolerated.

iv. **Certain specialized radiotherapy treatments** are particularly useful for primary or metastatic brain tumors. These include radiosurgery, the use of a large single dose of irradiation with the Gamma Knife, or a modified linear accelerator (Linac) and intensity-modulated radiation therapy (IMRT). These techniques, where available, have the advantage of distributing radiation doses more precisely within a radiographically defined tumor with maximal sparing of surrounding normal brain tissue in either a single fraction or multiple fractions. These techniques are finding additional usefulness in primary tumors as well as in the management of patients with recurrence of CNS tumors.

v. **Whole-brain radiotherapy (WBRT)** is used mainly in three situations.

One is in the definitive treatment of medulloblastoma where craniospinal irradiation is used. Another is in the instance of multiple brain metastases when more focal treatment would be inadequate. Third is in the case of meningeal carcinomatosis, along with intrathecal chemotherapy. In nearly all other situations, partial brain irradiation, preferably with three-dimensional conformal radiotherapy techniques, is used. This is to spare the maximal amount of normal brain tissue from the potentially deleterious late effects of irradiation.

vi. **Stereotactic radiosurgery** represents the other extreme in terms of size, dose and number of treatments in radiation therapy of the CNS. This can be done with either a linear accelerator or the Gamma Knife. The principle here is to focus a very large single dose of radiation on one target or a small number of tumor targets, with minimal dose to the surrounding normal tissue because of very steep dose fall-off of 10% to 14% per mm. This technique can be used as a boost after partial brain irradiation for certain locally progressing gliomas or for retreatment of a small number of metastases. The doses typically used range from 1,400 to 2,400 cGy to the target border in a single fraction. This is in contrast to the usual daily dose for conventional radiation therapy of 180 to 200 cGy for definitive treatment or of 250 to 300 cGy for palliative whole-brain irradiation. In certain situations, radiosurgery alone is the treatment of choice (e.g., for acoustic neuromas, small inoperable meningiomas, and recurrent metastasis). The juvenile pilocytic astrocytoma in childhood and adolescence is a particularly focal type of glioma for which radiosurgery has been used in addition to partial surgical resection. In cases where long-term survival is likely and CNS disease is not infiltrative, radiosurgery may be the sole useful modality.

c. **Chemotherapy** has a limited role in the treatment of solid tumor CNS metastasis. Most commonly used chemotherapeutic agents are limited by their inability to cross the blood–brain barrier and have low activity against intracranial solid tumor metastases. In contrast, chemotherapy is now preferred as initial treatment of primary CNS lymphoma. Chemotherapy for malignant glioma has evolved, especially with the approval of temozolomide for recurrent anaplastic astrocytoma and for the newly diagnosed glioblastoma multiforme (GBM). Clinical trials evaluating additional chemotherapeutic agents and newer targeted agents are viewed as a high priority.

i. **Active agents** against malignant glioma include temozolomide and the nitrosoureas, carmustine (BCNU) and lomustine (CCNU). Platinum compounds, etoposide and irinotecan, do show modest activity and are considered active agents. Older chemotherapeutic drugs such as procarbazine and vincristine have minimal activity against malignant gliomas. High-dose methotrexate (3.5 to 8 g/m^2 i.v.) has significant activity in PCNSL.

ii. **Temozolomide** is a newer oral alkylating agent with excellent CNS penetration. It is an imidazotetrazine derivative of dacarbazine with 100% bioavailability and promotes methylation of the O^6 position on guanine. Major toxicities include nausea and myelosuppression—often thrombocytopenia. An oral 5-HT$_3$ antagonist (i.e., ondansetron 8 mg p.o.) should be given 30 to 60 minutes prior to each dose. Temozolomide has had a significant impact on the treatment of malignant gliomas since the initial U.S. Food and Drug Administration (FDA) approval in 1999.

iii. **Nitrosoureas** are associated with a delayed myelosuppression and are typically given on a schedule every 6 to 8 weeks. Single-agent BCNU is most often used as second line in the treatment of GBM after progression on temozolomide.

iv. **Procarbazine, CCNU, and vincristine (PCV)** are used in the treatment of anaplastic astrocytomas and oligodendrogliomas. Procarbazine is a monoamine oxidase inhibitor and may be associated with hypertensive crisis in response to certain foods. Patients should he advised to avoid foods containing tyramine, including aged cheeses, red wine, and nuts. Allergies to procarbazine are also common. CCNU, an oral nitrosourea, may also cause delayed myelosuppression and is associated with nausea, vomiting, and rash. Pulmonary fibrosis is a rare complication. Vincristine is a vinca alkaloid (binds to tubulin) and is associated with a syndrome of jaw pain associated with the first dose, and may cause peripheral neuropathy.

v. **Other agents.** Gliadel wafers are an implantable depot form of BCNU that can be placed in the resection cavity of patients with recurrent or newly diagnosed GBM. Methotrexate, given at high dose with leucovorin rescue or given intrathecally, is used in leukemia and lymphoma. Cytarabine also can be given intrathecally in hematologic malignancies. A liposomal formulation also is available for intrathecal therapy of lymphomatous meningitis.

d. **Corticosteroids** are used in both primary and metastatic tumors of the CNS to control symptoms related to edema surrounding these tumors. Dexamethasone is most commonly used with initial doses of 4 to 10 mg i.v. or p.o. every 6 hours. This dose may be tapered over several weeks, as long as symptoms due to the tumor do not worsen. Steroids may be started before radiation therapy for control of reactive edema during treatment. Generally, patients should be maintained on the lowest dose that controls symptoms, and a requirement for increasing doses may indicate progression of disease, whereas a decreasing steroid requirement is associated with response.

II. BRAIN METASTASES

A. **Brain metastases** from primary tumors that originate outside the CNS are overwhelmingly the most common intracranial tumors in adults. Autopsy studies have revealed the presence of intracranial metastasis in 24% of cancer patients. In those older than 65 years, the rate of CNS metastases increases to 42.7% per 100,000 population. More than 75% will originate from a primary tumor in the breast, lung, or melanoma in adults. In approximately 10% to 15% of cases, there may be no known primary tumor at the time of diagnosis. In the pediatric population, sarcomas and germ cell tumors are the most common primary malignancies.

B. **Presenting signs and symptoms** for intracranial metastases are similar to those of most brain neoplasms (i.e., focal neurologic deficit, headaches, and seizures). Tumors such as melanoma, choriocarcinoma, and renal cell carcinoma often occur with a symptomatic hemorrhage. Metastases may be single or multiple, and tend to be located at the grey–white junction. They are usually well circumscribed, demonstrate peripheral enhancement with the administration of contrast agents on CT or MRI, and often have a significant amount of associated edema. The finding of multiple lesions strongly supports the diagnosis of metastasis and is helpful in differentiating from primary tumors, infections, and other lesions. In a patient in whom a brain mass is discovered and no primary is known, the evaluation should focus on the lungs, as 66% of these patients will have a lesion on the chest radiograph that represents primary lung cancer or pulmonary metastasis from systemic disease.

C. Treatment of metastatic disease should involve corticosteroids and, where appropriate, surgery and/or radiotherapy. Prognosis is related to age, Karnofsky performance score (KPS), number of metastases, response to therapy, and progression of systemic disease. In older series, the median survival in untreated patients was 1 month. The addition of corticosteroids alone, typically dexamethasone (see earlier), prolongs survival to 2 months. WBRT combined with steroids increases the median survival to 3 to 6 months. Chemotherapy is seldom used and is usually reserved for asymptomatic, chemosensitive tumors (*Neurosurgery* 2005;57(5 Suppl):S54–S65).

1. **Solitary brain metastasis.** The current treatment of choice for solitary lesions in patients who are candidates for surgery is surgical excision combined with radiotherapy. Several randomized, prospective trials have demonstrated a survival benefit to resection plus WBRT over WBRT alone. Life expectancy increases to 12 to 14 months with combined surgery and radiation in well-selected patients. Alternatively, many patients are treated with stereotactic radiosurgery, if they have surgically inaccessible lesions or poorly controlled systemic disease. Several studies of radiosurgery have demonstrated survival benefit comparable to that with surgery. Current studies and areas of controversy are focusing on the role of surgery in multiple metastases, the need for postoperative WBRT versus stereotactic radiosurgery, and the role of stereotactic radiosurgery versus surgery in patients with small (less than 3 cm), accessible lesions.

2. Certain types of tumors originate in the CNS but may still metastasize, both within the CNS and systemically. Medulloblastoma, ependymoma, and hemangiopericytoma are all examples. Common systemic sites are bone and lung.

III. GLIOMAS

A. Glial tumors as a whole account for more than 50% of all primary brain tumors across all age groups. Glioma is a broad classification for tumors that derive from any of the glial cell types, mainly astrocytoma, oligodendroglioma, and ependymoma. Fifty to sixty percent of gliomas are GBM, the most malignant variety.

B. Astrocytomas are divided into four grades in the WHO classification, I to IV, each with distinctive behaviors. Grade II–IV tumors are infiltrative and variably lethal.

1. **Grade I** tumors consist primarily of pilocytic astrocytomas, although other tumors of glial origin such as gangliocytoma and subependymoma are classified as grade I, indolent lesions. Pilocytic astrocytomas are slow growing, circumscribed, often cystic lesions that occur in children and young adults. They tend to occur in the cerebellum, anterior optic pathways, and brain stem, and occur with chronic signs of neurologic dysfunction related to location, obstruction of cerebrospinal fluid (CSF) pathways causing hydrocephalus, and rarely, seizures. The clinical course is one of indolent growth or even regression, although frequently they recur after resection. When location allows, complete surgical excision is the preferred treatment and allows 80% to 100% 10-year survival. Long-term follow-up with serial imaging is warranted even when total resection has been performed, as it is not possible to predict which lesions might recur.

2. **Grade II** tumors are often classified as diffuse or low-grade astrocytomas. They have a wider range of histologic appearance and clinical behavior than do other astrocytomas. A high percentage of these tumors ultimately progress to higher grades, although the dynamics of progression are difficult to predict. Mean age at diagnosis is in the 30- to 40-year range with a slight male predominance. Seizure is a common presentation along with chronic neurologic changes such as personality change, speech difficulties, or visual disturbances. MRI often shows a lesion with decreased T_1 signal, increased T_2 signal, and no enhancement. These lesions usually occur in supratentorial locations, may be

deep, diffuse, or relatively circumscribed, and are often difficult to differentiate from surrounding edematous brain. Treatment for these tumors is controversial because of the widely variable clinical course and lack of prospective studies. A period of observation in a patient with a low-grade glioma may be reasonable; however, close neurologic and radiologic monitoring is appropriate. In addition, survival and time to recurrence have shown statistically significant improvement in retrospective studies looking at the role of surgical resection. The role of biopsy, aggressive surgical resection, and radiotherapy must be tailored to the individual patient. Median survival time is approximately 5 years, with a wide range of variability.

3. **Grade III** tumors are clinically more aggressive than diffuse tumors. Mean age at onset is also slightly older, usually 40 to 50 years. Several tumor types other than pure anaplastic astrocytoma are given this grade, including mixed tumors, which are composed of both astrocytic and oligodendroglial components. These tumors may arise from preexisting low-grade tumors or be discovered *de novo*, and also can progress to GBM. The predominant location is the cerebral hemispheres, and there is usually a similar but more rapid clinical presentation as in the lower-grade lesions. Radiographically, they resemble low-grade astrocytomas but may demonstrate contrast enhancement. In terms of treatment, these tumors are grouped with GBM and treated similarly *(see* later). Short-term prognosis is better, however. Patient age, histologic criteria, and KPS all individually influence survival. Treated with a combination of surgery, radiation, and chemotherapy, patients with anaplastic astrocytoma have a 60% to 70% 1-year survival and a 40% to 50% 2-year survival, (*Cancer* 1985;56:1106–1111) as compared with the UCSF (University of California, San Francisco) series: median progression-free survival (PFS) 24 months with an overall median survival of 36 months.

4. **Grade IV.** GBM is the most common primary brain tumor and makes up most tumors classified to be high grade or malignant. They are similarly believed to originate both *de novo* and by progression of lower-grade tumors. These are often designated primary and secondary tumors, respectively, with distinctive molecular genetic pathways of development (*Neurooncology* 1999;1:44–51). The location of GBM tends to favor the subcortical white matter of the cerebral hemispheres, and the mean age at onset is 65 years. There is often a rapid onset of symptoms. These tumors typically demonstrate a prominent, ring-like enhancement pattern on MRI. Despite many advances and an improved understanding of their genetic composition, prognosis remains poor when patients are aggressively treated with surgery and adjuvant therapy; median survival is 12 months with a 2-year survival of 10%. Age and KPS remain significant independent predictors of survival.

Surgery, radiation, and chemotherapy are all used routinely in the treatment of high-grade astrocytomas. Surgery alone is not curative but does improve the quality and duration of life in selected patients. Although no prospective, randomized trials have been performed to evaluate the role of aggressive resection, retrospective series have supported a survival advantage to complete resection. Radiation therapy is the mainstay of treatment in high-grade astrocytomas, demonstrating survival benefit regardless of the extent of resection. The role of chemotherapy is now established and provides clear benefit. A randomized, controlled cooperative group (EORTC 22981, *N Engl J Med* 2005;352:987–996), study concluded that addition of temozolomide to radiation followed by 6 months of high-dose adjuvant temozolomide confers a significant relapse-free survival (RFS) and overall survival (OS) benefit to patients with newly diagnosed GBM. For example, patients receiving radiotherapy and temozolomide had improved overall survival as compared to patients who received radiotherapy alone (14.6 months vs. 12.1 months, hazard ratio 0.63, *p* less than 0.001). The 2-year survival rate was also significantly better in the temozolomide arm (26.5% vs. 10.4%, adjusted hazard ratio 0.62). Concurrent temozolomide is administered daily at 75 mg/m^2 p.o. during the entire radiation period, which is generally 6 weeks. After a 4-week break, additional temozolomide is given at 150 to 200 mg/m^2 p.o. qd for 5 consecutive days every 28 days. On the basis of the EORTC 22981 study results, treatment is provided for 6 months to patients; however, many practitioners now recommend 12 months of treatment on the basis of the favorable side-effect profile and activity. In patients with either clinical or clear radiographic progression, temozolomide should be discontinued and new therapeutic options for recurrent/refractory disease provided. As part of the multidisciplinary management of recurrent high-grade gliomas, options include further surgery, reirradiation, systemic chemotherapy, and clinical trial participation. Most patients are not eligible for further surgery or reirradiation, so clinical trial participation is the best option for most. Chemotherapy options (all given as single agents) for recurrent high-grade gliomas include BCNU, carboplatin, irinotecan, and etoposide. Exciting preliminary data from phase I and phase II clinical trials support continued development of antiangiogenesis agents, epidermal growth factor receptor (EGFR) antagonists, and mammalian target of rapamycin (mTOR) inhibitors. In addition, investigational approaches using convection-enhanced delivery are being studied at various major centers.

C. **Oligodendrogliomas** are a subtype of diffusely infiltrating, well-differentiated gliomas that compose 5% to 15% of all intracranial gliomas. They correspond to WHO grade II, with the more aggressive anaplastic variety being grade III. An oligodendroglial component may be present in mixed gliomas and predicts a more favorable outcome, as compared with that of pure astrocytoma. Oligodendrogliomas have a predilection for the frontal lobes in 50% to 60% of cases and are rare in the cerebellum and spinal cord. Other characteristic features are a tendency to occur with seizures and the presence of calcification on diagnostic imaging. Prognosis is influenced by histologic features, age, and completeness of surgical resection. Most tumors will respond to chemotherapy, with the most experience being with PCV (procarbazine, CCNU, and vincristine); however, temozolomide should be considered. The most frequent genetic alterations found in these tumors are loss of heterozygosity on chromosomes 19q and 1 p. These deletions also have been shown to correlate with increased chemosensitivity (*J Natl Cancer Inst* 1998;90:1473–1479) and radiosensitivity (*Int J Radiat Oncol Biol Phys* 2000;48:825–830).

D. **Ependymoma** This subset of glial tumors comprises 5% to 8% of CNS neoplasms and originates from the cells lining the ventricular system. They may occur throughout the neural axis but predominate in an infratentorial location (two-thirds of cases) in the pediatric population. In children younger than 3 years, they make up 30% of intracranial tumors. In the spinal cord, they make up 50% to 60% of gliomas.

1. **Most ependymomas are WHO grade II,** with an anaplastic ependymoma receiving a histologic designation of grade III. MRI appearance is heterogeneous with mixed areas of cystic regions, areas of old hemorrhage, and calcifications. They often track along CSF pathways into the cisterns and originate in the floor of the forth ventricle. At the time of diagnosis, 12% will have seeded the spinal column with "drop metastases."

2. **Presenting symptoms** depend on location, but infratentorial tumors tend to occur with headache, vomiting, cranial nerve palsies, and ataxia. In all patients with ependymoma, extent of surgical resection is an important prognostic factor, and complete surgical removal will cure a small percentage of cases. A complete resection is often not possible because of location, and radiation to the remaining tumor, or to the neural axis in cases of disseminated tumor, may offer some survival benefit. Overall, children have a poorer prognosis than adults, possibly related to an infratentorial predominance. Subtotal resection, age younger than 3 years, and anaplastic features are all associated with a poorer prognosis. Recurrence favors the original tumor site and usually remains a similar grade, although progression can occur. Overall, 5-year survival ranges are 30% to 40% in children and 40% to 50% in adults.

3. **Myxopapillary ependymoma,** a separate clinical and histologic entity, occurs in the conus medullaris–cauda equina region in young adults. They are WHO grade I lesions and carry a favorable prognosis after surgical excision.

IV. MENINGIOMA

A. **Meningiomas are benign,** slow-growing, extra-axial tumors that are attached to the dura mater and arise from arachnoidal cap cells. They represent 15% to 20% of primary intracranial tumors and are a common incidental finding at autopsy. Advances in cranial imaging have increased the number of incidentally discovered asymptomatic lesions. They may occur in almost any location but favor the falx cerebri, over the cerebral convexity, along the skull base at the sphenoid bone, olfactory groove, or parasellar region, along the tentorium cerebelli, within the ventricles, or along the spinal canal.

1. **The peak age incidence** is 45 years and with a female predominance of almost 2:1. In particular, this female predominance increases to almost 10:1 in spinal meningiomas. They are rare in children, except in association with either neurofibromatosis-1 (NF1) or -2 (NF2). Many histologic variants have been described and are not useful for predicting clinical behavior, except in determining grade. Approximately 95% of meningiomas are WHO grade I. On the basis of histologic criteria, 4% to 6% are called atypical and WHO grade II and approximately 1% are anaplastic WHO grade III. Most express progesterone receptors, although the role they may play in formation and possibly in therapy is not clear.

2. **Most meningiomas cause symptoms *by* compression** of adjacent neural structures, and may be present for many years because of their slow rate of growth. They may also come to attention by causing seizures or in the evaluation of headaches. On imaging, they frequently demonstrate calcifications and have a typical extra-axial location. MRI usually demonstrates isointensity before contrast administration with homogeneous gadolinium enhancement. An attachment to adjacent dura may be visualized on the MRI (a "dural tail") and significant edema in the surrounding brain parenchyma may be seen.

3. **Treatment.** The decision about whether to treat an asymptomatic tumor is often difficult and requires consideration of multiple factors including location, patient age, general medical condition, and operative morbidity. Expectant management with serial imaging is often reasonable for incidentally discovered lesions. Surgical removal offers the greatest chance of cure for symptomatic lesions and is usually feasible, depending on the location. Recent advances in radiotherapy techniques make this an option for treatment both in nonoperative cases and as adjuvant therapy. The chance of recurrence, even after complete extirpation, is significant and occurs as long as 20 years after treatment. Extent of resection and grade of tumor predict recurrence rates. Overall, the prognosis for patients with meningiomas remains good, with a 5-year survival of 90% to 95%. Typical grade I meningiomas have a 10% to 20% recurrence rate, whereas atypical tumors recur in 30% to 40% of cases; anaplastic tumors have nearly an 80% recurrence rate and a median survival less than 2 years.

V. PITUITARY ADENOMA

A. **The anterior pituitary gland** (adenohypophysis) is the site of origin for 10% of all intracranial tumors collectively referred to as *pituitary adenomas*. These are generally benign tumors, affect men and woman equally, and are incidentally found in as many as 20% of adults at autopsy. Incidence is increased in multiply endocrine neoplasia (MEN) type 1. Many classifications exist based on cell of origin, endocrine status, or histologic appearance. The tumors may be divided into micro- (less than 1 cm) or macro- (more than 1 cm) tumors.

B. **Functional adenomas.** It is useful to divide tumors clinically as functioning and nonfunctioning, on the basis of whether they secrete active endocrine hormones. This may include the hypersecretion of adrenocorticotropic hormone (ACTH), prolactin, growth hormone (GH), luteinizing hormone (LH), follicle-stimulating hormone (FSH), or rarely, thyroid-stimulating hormone (TSH).

1. **The clinical presentation** may be endocrine disturbance, such as Cushing's disease (ACTH secretion) and acromegaly (GH secretion); amenorrhea or galactorrhea; symptoms from mass effect on surrounding structures, such as the bitemporal visual loss from optic chiasm compression; or even pituitary apoplexy caused by tumor hemorrhage. Frequently, these tumors are identified during an evaluation for headaches.

2. **In nonfunctioning tumors** or in tumors secreting inactive substances, the tumors are usually larger at the time of diagnosis. Compression of the surrounding pituitary gland may produce the insidious loss of function of other pituitary hormones or even an increase in the level of prolactin due to interference with the pathway through which dopamine provides negative regulation. This is known as *stalk effect* and may help differentiate prolactinomas from other tumor types.

C. **Radiographically** these tumors are demonstrated on MRI as masses in the region of the sella that may extend laterally into the region of the cavernous sinus or superiorly toward the optic apparatus. Enhancement is variable, and many microadenomas are too small to visualize on imaging. Angiography may rarely be necessary to help localize a tumor or determine the relation to the carotid arteries. The sella may be enlarged on skull radiographs.

D. **Treatment** depends on the clinical presentation and therefore on the cell type of origin. Overall management may include observation with serial imaging, medical treatment, surgery, and radiotherapy. All patients suspected of having a pituitary tumor require a thorough endocrine evaluation and, depending on tumor size, ophthalmologic evaluation.

Cushing's disease, acromegaly, nonfunctioning tumors, and all macroadenomas are usually managed with surgery, possibly combined with various adjuvant therapies. Options include a transcranial or trans-sphenoidal sinus approach and depend on tumor size and anatomy. Treatment of prolactinomas is more variable, as often these tumors may initially be managed medically with dopamine agonists (e.g., bromocriptine) until definitive therapy with surgery or radiation therapy is completed. Radiotherapy, including stereotactic radiosurgery, plays a role in treatment of recurrences or in certain subtotally resected tumors. Prognosis also depends on tumor type and size. For nonfunctioning tumors and prolactinomas, in most (more than 80%) cases, the growth of the tumor can be controlled through the life of the patient. Cushing's disease can be controlled with surgery in 93% of microadenomas and 50% of macroadenomas. In cases of acromegaly, transsphenoidal surgery alone results in cure in 85% of microadenomas and 30% to 40% of macroadenomas. Results are improved with adjuvant therapies such as treatment with somatostatin and radiotherapy.

VI. PRIMARY CENTRAL NERVOUS SYSTEM LYMPHOMA

A. **Primary central nervous system lymphoma (PCNSL)** is an unusual, aggressive form of non-Hodgkin's lymphoma that does not represent spread from systemic disease. In most cases, it is a tumor of B-cell origin and is staged I_E. The differentiation between spread of systemic lymphoma and PCNSL is not always clear and can make staging controversial. Although it was previously considered a rare tumor, the incidence has been increasing, as a result of the increased prevalence of human immunodeficiency virus (HIV) and also in immunocompetent individuals. Patients receiving long-term immunosuppression and individuals with an inherited immunodeficiency also have an increased incidence. The median age at diagnosis is 52 years in immunocompetent patients and 34 years in immunosuppressed patients. The tumors may occur anywhere but are common in the frontal lobes, deep, periventricular regions, and in the posterior fossa. PCNSL favors an intraparenchymal location, whereas secondary lymphoma tends to occur in the leptomeninges. In all patients, the lesions may be multiple, with 70% to 80% of immunocompromised patients having more than one lesion. Ocular disease, in the form of lymphoma or uveitis, may accompany as many as 20% of all cases. The clinical presentation is usually a focal neurologic deficit or symptoms related to increased intracranial pressure, such as headache, nausea, and vomiting. Seizures are not common.

B. Imaging with MRI often demonstrates multiple, iso- to hyperdense lesions, with dense or ring-like enhancement, and generally a limited amount of surrounding edema. Positron emission tomography (PET) or single-photon emission computed tomography (SPECT) scan may be useful in differentiating ring-enhancing lesions in immunosuppressed patients as lymphoma or nonneoplastic entities, such as toxoplasmosis.

C. Staging. Recommended studies include brain MRI with gadolinium, lumbar puncture for CSF studies (cell count, cytology, total protein, and β2-microglobulin), bone marrow biopsy, CT scan of the chest, abdomen, and pelvis, slit lamp examination, and HIV serology.

D. Treatment. Many tumors have a rapid and lytic response to corticosteroid treatment so it should be withheld until a diagnostic biopsy has been performed, unless there is severe mass effect. There is no benefit to surgical resection, and stereotactic biopsy is the preferred method for obtaining a tissue diagnosis.

   1. Radiation therapy. These tumors are quite radiosensitive; however, the role of radiotherapy is changing. Most experts do not recommend whole-brain radiation as initial treatment for PCNSL unless there is a contraindication to chemotherapy. Radiation can be given as consolidation therapy (after induction chemotherapy), or in many cases, reserved for progressive PCNSL that is refractory to chemotherapy.

   2. Chemotherapy has gained an increasingly important role in the treatment of PCNSL. High-dose methotrexate (3.5 g/m$_2$ or more given i.v.) is considered the most active single agent. The optimal combination of methotrexate-based chemotherapy is not yet defined; however, clinical trials are currently pursuing this question (*Curr Oncol Rep* 2005;7:47–54).

   3. HIV-associated PCNSL is associated with a particularly poor prognosis. A negative toxoplasmosis immunoglobulin G (IgG) serology helps eliminate the diagnosis of CNS toxoplasmosis. The institution of highly active antiretroviral therapy (HAART) may prolong survival, as opportunistic infection remains a leading cause of death in these patients. Please refer to Chapter 31, HIV and Cancer, for treatment options.

   4. CNS toxicity, including progressive memory loss and ataxia, may result from radiotherapy, especially from use of radiation therapy in older patients. Initial therapy with chemotherapy and delaying or withholding radiation therapy until relapse in elderly patients are strategies for limiting these toxicities.

VII. EMBRYONAL

   A. Embryonal tumors encompass a wide variety of clinically important, mainly pediatric tumors that do not have a universally accepted classification scheme based on histopathologic criteria. They may demonstrate many different patterns of histologic differentiation. Some tumors included in this class are medulloblastoma, ependymoblastoma, medulloepithelioma, atypical teratoid/rhabdoid tumors, and all other tumors known as *primitive neuroectodermal tumors* (PNETs). As a group, they represent aggressive, malignant tumors and, with the exception of medulloblastoma, are rare. All are WHO grade IV tumors. Because medulloblastoma accounts for almost a fourth of all pediatric brain tumors and is the most common malignant brain tumor of childhood, it is considered in detail.

   B. Medulloblastoma occurs primarily in children, 70% before age 16, with a peak incidence from ages 5 to 7 years. In adults, they very rarely occur after age 50. They are also uncommon before age 1, and 65% occur in boys. They are located in the vermis of the cerebellum, arising in the roof of the fourth ventricle in most cases. As the age of the patient increases, they tend to occur more laterally, in the cerebellar hemisphere. It has not been established from what cell these tumors arise. In one-third of patients, there is dissemination through the CSF pathways, and up to 5% may have systemic spread, usually to bone or lung.

   1. Presentation. Most patients have symptoms of hydrocephalus or cerebellar symptoms such as ataxia, lethargy, headache, and vomiting. Radiographic features are of a midline, well-demarcated, densely enhancing mass that is often hyperdense on noncontrast **CT** scan. Obstructive hydrocephalus is a common feature, and **MRI** may demonstrate foci of leptomeningeal dissemination.

2. **Treatment strategies** use a combined-modality approach. Surgical goals are to perform gross total resection when safe, as this improves survival. Invasion of the brain stem often limits resection. Additionally, CSF diversion (temporary ventricular drainage, ventricular shunt, or third ventriculostomy) is often necessary. In 30% to 40% of cases, permanent CSF diversion will be necessary. These tumors are also fairly radiosensitive, and craniospinal radiation is combined with surgery, except in children younger than 3 years, in whom chemotherapy is a preferable and efficacious alternative. Chemosensitivity is variable, and a variety of protocols are used with disease progression. Unfavorable prognostic factors are age less than 3 years, subtotal resection, and dissemination at the time of diagnosis. In the last 30 years, outcomes have improved, with the current 5-year survival ranging from 50% to 70%.

C. **Neuronal tumors.** This group of tumors is varied in location and histology but shares some degree of differentiation into neuronal cell types. All of these tumors are unusual and relatively benign. All are WHO grade I or II and are almost always controlled with surgical excision.

1. **Gangliogliomas and gangliocytomas** are benign tumors of either ganglion cells and glial cells, or ganglion cells alone. Gangliogliomas may occur anywhere in the CNS but have a tendency to occur in the temporal lobe, where they are a frequent cause of medically intractable epilepsy. Rarely, the glial component may demonstrate anaplastic or malignant features and designate the tumor as high grade. Surgery is usually curative.

2. **Dysembryoplastic infantile astrocytoma/gangliogliomas** are large, recently defined, cystic tumors of the cerebral cortex and, often involving the leptomeninges, composed of poorly differentiated cells mixed with either neoplastic astrocytes or a neuronal component. They are often large, and typically cause macrocephaly in the affected infant.

3. **Dysembryoplastic neuroepithelial tumors** are hamartomata-like lesions that have been described in children and young adults, with a male predominance, and are found during resection of lesions for treatment of refractory epilepsy. They are usually supratentorial, retain a cortical topography, and may deform the overlying skull. They also may be associated with areas of cortical dysplasia.

4. **Central neurocytoma** is a tumor of young adults that characteristically occurs in the lateral and third ventricles in the region of the foramen of Monro. They histologically resemble ependymomas or oligodendrogliomas and are designated WHO grade II. Typically they cause obstructive hydrocephalus and occur with resulting headache, visual changes, or lethargy. In cases in which total resection cannot be performed, postoperative radiotherapy may be considered, although experience is limited.

VIII. **TUMOR OF SPECIAL LOCATION**

A. **Cranial nerves or extra-axial locations** may give rise to schwannomas, neurofibromas, and hemangiopericytomas.

1. **Schwannomas** are benign tumor arising from the Schwann cells located in a variety of places including the head and neck, peripheral nerves, and spinal nerves. They are well encapsulated, tend to favor sensory nerves, and very rarely undergo malignant change. Incidence peaks in the fourth through sixth decades and symptoms invariably relate to compression of surrounding neural structures. Schwannomas make up 29% of primary intraspinal tumors and, along with acoustic neuromas, make up the predominance of cases that require treatment.

2. **Acoustic neuromas** are technically schwannomas of the vestibular nerve and represent 5% to 7% of intracranial tumors, but 80% of tumors in the cerebellopontine angle (CPA). They are slightly more common in women and are increased in the neurofibromatosis type (NF2), for which they are pathognomonic when bilateral. Both in sporadic and NF2-associated cases, these tumors arise from a mutation that causes the lack of expression of the protein

merlin, the product of NF2 gene on the long arm of chromosome 22. Although they are histologically benign and are WHO grade I tumors, they may cause significant morbidity because of proximity to the brain stem and adherence to the cranial nerves. Symptoms include hearing loss, tinnitus, and dysequilibrium. MRI evaluation demonstrates a rounded, enhancing mass extending into the internal auditory canal. CT imaging of the temporal bone often shows expansion of the internal auditory meatus. Evaluation of individuals must also include audiometric testing to assess hearing quantitatively.

The management of these tumors entails balancing the risks of surgery or radiosurgery to treat these lesions, with the natural history of continued observation. Both surgery and radiosurgery are options to control disease. Decisions regarding intervention consider the age and general medical condition of the patient, hearing status, patient symptoms, and the size of the tumor. Several surgical approaches exist, each with inherent advantages and disadvantages. Management decisions depend on these factors and are probably best made by a collaborative team including neurosurgeons, radiation oncologists, neuro-otologists, and neuroradiologists. Observation should include both serial audiograms and MRI evaluations. Decision making is further complicated in the patient with NF2 and bilateral vestibular schwannomas, as these patients tend to be first seen at a younger age and have a higher morbidity associated with resection.

3. **Neurofibromas** are also benign (WHO grade I) tumors associated with peripheral nerves that are infiltrative or intraneural in location and consist of a mixture of cells including Schwann cells, fibroblasts, and perineurial-like cells. They can occur as solitary nodules associated with a peripheral nerve, often in a cutaneous location, or may be multiple. Patients with NF1 tend to have multiple lesions, which may involve spinal roots, and may have plexiform involvement of a major nerve. Neurofibromas are most often treated expectantly, unless there is suspicion of degeneration into a malignant peripheral nerve sheath tumor (MPNST).

4. **Malignant peripheral nerve sheath tumor.** In 3% to 5% of cases, usually when there is proximal major nerve or plexiform involvement, neurofibromas can develop into an MPNST. These are rare, aggressive tumors (WHO grade III or IV) and can develop sporadically. They may develop from neurofibromas, often in the setting of NF1. The goal of treatment is a total resection with negative margins to prevent systemic metastases. They are generally chemo- and radioresistant. Prognosis is poor overall, with a 34% 5-year survival rate.

5. **Hemangiopericytomas** are rare tumors making up less than 1% of all intracranial tumors. Previously classified as angioblastic meningiomas, these tumors arise from pericapillary mesenchymal cells known as *pericytes of Zimmerman*. They are indistinguishable from those that occur extracranially and are usually found attached to the leptomeninges when they occur in the CNS. A tendency to metastasize systemically is well documented. They occur predominantly supratentorially, may affect children or infants in 10% of cases, and appear clinically like meningiomas with a more rapid onset. They are richly vascular and can be associated with significant intraoperative blood loss. The goal of treatment is gross total resection before systemic spread. Several studies have demonstrated a survival benefit to postoperative radiotherapy. In one series, 5-year and 10-year survival rates were 67% and 40% respectively.

B. **Pineal region tumors.** Several tumor types commonly occur in the pineal region and are therefore considered as a group under this heading.

1. **Germ cell tumors.** Intracranial germ cell tumors generally occur in the midline, more often in the pineal region in men or the suprasellar region in women. Over half of the tumors that occur in the pineal region are germ cell tumors, and most of these are germinomas. These tumors are predominantly pediatric tumors, are unusual after young adulthood, and are predominate in boys. They have an increased incidence in individuals with Klinefelter (XXY) syndrome

and are more common in Asia, where it may make up as much as 15% of pediatric tumor series in Japan. They commonly occur with obstructive hydrocephalus because of their location and often cause Parinaud syndrome. Radiologic appearance is somewhat nonspecific, but generally these tumors appear as homogeneous, isodense lesions that enhance in the region of the pineal gland, sella turcica, and third ventricle. They often have a distinctive relation to the calcifications of the pineal gland parenchyma. The evaluation of someone with a suspected germ cell tumor includes serum and CSF markers such as human chorionic gonadotropin (HCG), alpha-fetoprotein (AFP), and placental alkaline phosphatase (PLAP). These markers are suggestive of certain histologies and are useful in determining prognosis and response to treatment. As many as 35% of germ cell tumors may show metastasis throughout the CNS at the time of discovery, and therefore, with the exception of mature teratomas, most are considered malignant neoplasms.

    a. Germinomas are the most common type of germ cell tumors, and 30% will consist of a mixture of cell types. Germinomas make up 60% to 70% of germ cell tumors. They typically demonstrate positivity for PLAP, although NCG may also be present, as they are known to contain elements of syncytiotrophoblastic cells. These are distinct from choriocarcinoma tumors that are positive for HCG, but histologically have evidence of both cytotrophoblastic and syncytiotrophoblastic elements. Choriocarcinoma may commonly occur with intracranial hemorrhage, both when it occurs as a primary intracranial lesion and in cases of metastatic spread. Germinomas are exceptionally radiosensitive, and this fact is used as an adjunct to diagnosis. Response to a course of empiric radiation in a characteristic lesion and in the markers is often enough evidence to warrant further treatment as a germinoma.

    b. The remainder of germ cell tumors consist of teratomas, mature and immature, embryonal carcinomas, and yolk sac tumors. Positivity for AFP helps distinguish teratomas and yolk sac tumors. Embryonal carcinoma may express PLAP, although this is inconsistent.

2. **Pineal parenchymal tumors.** The cells that make up the pineal gland perform a diverse array of neuroendocrine functions, and when neoplasia occur, a spectrum of differentiation from primitive to relatively terminal pineocytes is found. Tumors are classified as pineocytomas, pineoblastomas, or some intermediate forms, and make up 15% of tumors in the region of the pineal gland. All are classified as WHO grade IV lesions, with the exception of pineocytomas, which are WHO grade I. They appear similar to other tumor types in this area, and no serum markers are available. Pineocytomas tend to occur in adults, are slow growing, and may show a variety of phenotypes such as neuronal or glial lesions. Pineoblastomas are more aggressive lesions that often disseminate throughout the CNS and resemble primitive neuroectodermal tumors histologically.

3. **Primitive neuroectodermal tumors.** These tumors compose 10% to 15% of pineal region tumors and are derived mostly from tumors of glial origin, such as ependymomas or astrocytomas. They occur in the third and fourth decades, have no gender predominance, and have no CSF markers.

4. **The remainder of pineal region tumors** consist of small numbers of miscellaneous tumor types such as meningiomas, craniopharyngiomas, and hemangiomas.

5. **Treatment** of all these lesions is multidisciplinary and somewhat controversial. The pineal region remains a difficult region to access surgically, although an aggressive approach has been advocated by centers with more experience in lesions of this region. Some tumors that are benign may be more amenable to aggressive surgical resection, such as meningioma, epidermoid, and mature teratoma. Stereotactic biopsy is generally safe, although it also carries risk for morbidity and the chance for sampling error because of the mixed nature of many lesions. Several series have demonstrated the usefulness and safety of

stereotactic biopsy in initial management of pineal tumors and cysts. The role of radiotherapy including stereotactic radiosurgery and chemotherapy in these tumors is significant.

IX. BACKGROUND

A. **Epidemiology.** Over 30,000 new brain tumors are diagnosed each year in adults in the United States. Their annual incidence is 12 per 100,000, with half of these cases being malignant gliomas. In the pediatric population, brain tumors represent the most common solid tumor and have an incidence of 2 to 5 cases per 100,000. This comprises 40% to 50% of all tumors in children and 25% of cancer-related deaths.

The overall average age at onset is 53 years for all brain tumors, although there is considerable variability by site of origin and histologic type. Across multiple epidemiologic surveys, gliomas are slightly more common in men, whereas meningiomas favor women (2:1).

Some known associations and predisposing syndromes have helped shed light on the role of tumor suppressor genes in hereditary syndromes. Examples include the hereditary retinoblastoma (RB) syndrome, in which there is mutation of the *RB* tumor suppressor gene. The neurocutaneous syndromes include NF1, NF2, tuberous sclerosis (TS), and von Hippel-Lindau (VHL) syndrome. Other syndromes associated with CNS tumors are Li-Fraumeni syndrome (mutation of *p53*), Turcot syndrome, Gorlin syndrome (also known as basal cell nevus syndrome), and Cowden syndrome.

B. **Future directions** include investigation of gene therapy, immunotherapy, antiangiogenesis agents as well as newer targeted agents that inhibit receptor tyrosine kinases. Studies have been carried out by the Radiation Therapy Oncology Group (RTOG) evaluating the role of radiosurgery in the management of one to three brain metastases, as well as boost treatment for GBM. Radiosurgery given in this manner did not improve the outcome in patients with GBM. Similarly, radiation sensitization with chemotherapy or other agents has been tested, with equivocal results so far. An RTOG intergroup (0525) study comparing concurrent and adjuvant standard dose with concurrent and dose intense adjuvant temozolomide is currently ongoing. Clearly, there is a need to develop more and better chemotherapeutic regimens that can penetrate the CNS.

Suggested Readings

Batchelor T, Loeffler JS. Primary CNS lymphoma. *J Clin Oncol* 2006;24(8):1281–1288.

van den Bent MJ, Afra D, de Witte O, et al. EORTC Radiotherapy and Brain Tumor Groups and the UK Medical Research Council. Long-term efficacy of early versus delayed radiotherapy for low-grade astrocytoma and oligodendroglioma in adults: the EORTC 22845 randomised trial. *Lancet* 2005;366(9490):985–990.

Butowski NA, Sneed PK, Chang SM. Diagnosis and treatment of recurrent high-grade astrocytoma. *J Clin Oncol* 2006;24(8):1273–1280.

Green MR, Chowdhary S, Lombardi KM, et al. Clinical utility and pharmacology of high-dose methotrexate in the treatment of primary CNS lymphoma. *Expert Rev Neurother* 2006;6(5):635–652.

Hegi ME, Diserens AC, Gorlia T, et al. MGMT gene silencing and benefit from temozolomide in glioblastoma. *N Engl J Med* 2005;352(10):997–1003.

Nguyen PL, Chakravarti A, Finkelstein DM, et al. Results of whole-brain radiation as salvage of methotrexate failure for immunocompetent patients with primary CNS lymphoma. *J Clin Oncol* 2005;23(7):1507–1513.

Reardon DA, Rich JN, Friedman HS, et al. Recent advances in the treatment of malignant astrocytoma. *J Clin Oncol* 2006;24(8):1253–1265.

Richards GM, Khuntia D, Mehta MP. Therapeutic management of metastatic brain tumors. *Crit Rev Oncol Hematol* 2007;61:70–80.

Shah GD, DeAngelis LM. Treatment of primary central nervous system lymphoma. *Hematol Oncol Clin North Am* 2005;19(4):611–627.

Stupp R, Mason WP, van den Bent MJ, et al. Radiotherapy plus concomitant and adjuvant temozolomide for glioblastoma. *N Engl J Med* 2005;352(10):987–996.

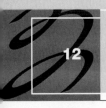

HEAD AND NECK CANCER

12

David Kuperman, Matthew Arquette,
and Douglas Adkins

I. **APPROACH TO THE HEAD AND NECK CANCER PATIENT.** As the late head and neck medical oncologist Dr. Matthew Arquette so eloquently stated, "the poignancy of head and neck cancer is difficult to underestimate; in the face, we recognize an individual, and through speech, we communicate." Although there are many similarities between head and neck cancers arising from different sites, there are particular differences in anatomy, natural history, and functional consequence that present unique treatment challenges for each site. In addition, these patients frequently have comorbid illnesses related to the effects of alcohol and tobacco use that may further complicate therapy.

II. **BACKGROUND**

A. **Squamous cell cancer** of the head and neck is an example of the multistep process of carcinogenesis with accumulated genetic mutations that result in changes ranging from hyperplasia to dysplasia to carcinoma *in situ* to invasive cancer. A number of frequent genetic mutations have been identified, whereas others remain under investigation. Loss of tumor suppressor genes, including *p16*, *p53*, and *RB*, are frequent, and amplification of the proto-oncogene cyclin D1 and expression of the epidermal growth factor receptor (EGFR) occurs.

B. **Risk factors.** For most patients, tobacco, often augmented by ethanol, is the source of carcinogens that result in these mutations. The incidence of new cancers of the head and neck is estimated at 45,000 in the United States in 2006, most of which are smoking-related. These figures underscore the importance of educating patients about smoking cessation. The male-to-female ratio is approximately 3:1. Among nonsmokers, viruses, including human papilloma virus (HPV) and Epstein-Barr virus (EBV), are implicated.

III. **OVERVIEW OF THERAPY FOR CANCERS OF THE HEAD AND NECK**

A. **General considerations.** Care of patients with cancers of the head and neck requires a multidisciplinary team that includes specialists in surgery, radiation, chemotherapy, and supportive treatments. Nutritional support often plays an essential role in the care of these patients because swallowing may be impaired either by the disease or as a consequence of therapy. Placement of a gastrostomy tube is often needed. The functional status of the patient and location of the tumor play a key role in determining the management of the patient.

The following overview deals with the most common cancer of the head and neck, squamous cell cancer (SCCHN). Variation in therapy does occur depending on site and these variations will be discussed in their appropriate sections.

B. **Management of early-stage cancers (Stage I to II).** Early-stage SCCHN is managed with either surgery or definitive radiation. Both of these approaches have similar cure rates. Advantages of surgery include a shorter treatment time and avoidance of radiation toxicity (xerostomia, dental caries, and mucositis). The disadvantages are that some patients are not able to tolerate the surgical procedure and complete surgical resection may have an unacceptable effect on speech or swallowing. Radiation therapy has the advantage of allowing the patient to avoid a resection that would result in unacceptable morbidities and allows cure of patients who could not tolerate a major operation. Disadvantages of radiation include a prolonged treatment time (approximately 7 weeks of radiation and several months of recuperation) and long-term radiation toxicity.

C. Management of locally advanced, nonmetastatic disease (III to IVB)
   1. Surgery. Surgery to resect gross tumor completely may be used as the initial therapy for locally advanced cancers of the head and neck. Current approaches to surgery increasingly involve procedures such as transoral CO_2 laser resection, selective neck dissection, and/or flap reconstruction. These newer approaches to surgery lower the morbidity of the procedure and improve the likelihood of postoperative function. Following complete resection, adjuvant radiation-based therapy is usually recommended to most of these patients. In some patients, a biopsy of the primary tumor and suspicious regional nodes is performed by the surgeon for diagnosis, after which the patient is referred for definitive radiation-based therapy.
   2. Adjuvant Therapy following surgery. Following gross tumor resection, adjuvant therapy with postoperative radiation or concurrent chemoradiation is usually recommended in patients with locally advanced disease. Adjuvant therapy is required when there is involvement of one or more cervical lymph nodes, perineural involvement, lymphovascular invasion, and/or a positive surgical margin at the site of primary tumor resection. The total radiation dose in this setting is usually 60 Gy administered to the primary and involved lymph nodes and 50 Gy to lower-risk nodal stations in the neck. The duration of radiation therapy is 6 to 7 weeks, with treatment optimally starting 3 to 6 weeks postoperatively. The exact fractionation schema, portals, and use of boost-dose radiation are determined by site and are subject to controversy. Concurrent chemoradiation versus radiation alone is recommended for tumors with high risk features: multiple positive lymph nodes, cervical lymph nodes with extranodal extension, or positive surgical margins. Some also include tumors with perineural and lymphovascular invasion but the National Comprehensive Cancer Network (NCCN) currently does not.
   3. Chemoradiation. Definitive concurrent chemoradiation is the standard of care for the nonsurgical management of locally advanced cancers of the head and neck in patients who are candidates to tolerate such therapy (good performance status and few or no comorbidities). Several meta-analyses have consistently demonstrated a significant survival benefit with concurrent chemoradiation over radiation alone. The magnitude of that survival benefit is 8% at 5 years with concurrent chemoradiation. The morbidity of concurrent chemoradiotherapy, however, is clearly greater than that of radiation alone, which may explain why the survival benefit of chemoradiation is limited to patients with good performance status who are under the age of 60.
      Several chemotherapeutic agents have been combined with radiation; however, the most commonly used agents include cisplatin given alone or in combination with 5-fluorouracil (5-FU). Recently, the EGFR inhibitor cetuximab has been shown to benefit patients when given concurrently with definitive radiation.
      Cisplatin has been given concurrently with radiation in many trials. Al-Sarraf et al. administered cisplatin 100 mg/m^2 on days 1, 22, and 43 of a 7-week course of 70 Gy of radiation for 124 patients with locally advanced, unresectable SCCHN. Sixty-nine percent of patients achieved a complete response. Toxicities associated with this regimen included significant mucositis, xerostomia, skin irritation, and anemia. Despite the toxicities, 60% of patients were able to complete all of the therapy (*Cancer* 1987;59:259).
      Cetuximab, an EGFR antibody, has also been given concurrently with radiation. Bonner et al. recently published the results of a multicenter randomized phase III trial of concurrent cetuximab and radiation versus radiation alone for definitive treatment of locally advanced squamous cell cancer of the oropharynx, larynx, and hypopharynx. Two hundred and thirteen patients were assigned to radiation alone and 211 were assigned to radiation and concurrent weekly cetuximab. In those treated with cetuximab, a 400 mg/m^2 dose was given the week before radiation, followed by 250 mg/m^2 weekly for the duration of the radiation (total of eight doses given). Median survival was increased

from 29.3 months in the radiation alone arm to 49.0 months in the cetuximab plus radiation arm ($p = 0.006$). Survival at 3 years favored the cetuximab and radiation arm (55% vs. 45%, $p = 0.05$). The toxicities were similar between the two arms with the exception of a greater risk of skin toxicities (acneform rash) and infusion reactions in the cetuximab arm. In contrast to a significantly higher risk of mucositis observed with concurrent cisplatin and radiation, the risk of mucositis with concurrent cetuximab and radiation was similar to that with radiation alone (*N Engl J Med* 2006;354:567).

4. **Salvage surgery following definitive chemoradiation.** If a complete tumor response is not achieved following definitive chemoradiation, salvage surgical resection may result in long-term survival in a significant fraction of patients.

5. **Induction chemotherapy before definitive chemoradiation.** Several randomized trials of induction chemotherapy have shown mixed results. A survival benefit was not consistently observed with induction chemotherapy except in the subset of patients given cisplatin and 5-FU (PF). However, recently Possner et al. presented the results of the TAX 324 trial, which compared two different induction regimens (TPF vs. PF) before definitive chemoradiation. TPF (docetaxel 75 mg/m^2 on day 1, cisplatin 100 mg/m^2 on day 1, and 5-FU 1,000 mg/m^2 c.i.v.i. daily on days 1 to 4 every 3 weeks) was compared with PF (cisplatin 100 mg/m^2 on day 1 and 5-FU 1000 mg/m^2 c.i.v.i. daily on days 1 to 5 every 3 weeks) before definitive chemoradiation. Both TPF and PF were given for three cycles before chemoradiation. The median overall survival (OS) was significantly longer in the TPF arm compared to that in the PF arm (70.6 months vs. 30.1 months; $p = 0.0058$). Given that one induction regimen (TPF) showed improved survival over another (PF), this would imply that at least the TPF induction regimen would have a survival benefit over concurrent chemoradiation alone (results presented at a special session of the 2006 American Society of Clinical Oncology [ASCO] meeting in Atlanta, GA). There are currently three randomized clinical trials evaluating the effect on OS of induction chemotherapy followed by definitive chemoradiation over definitive chemoradiation alone. All three of these trials are using TPF.

Induction chemotherapy may also be used as a method to predict tumor response to chemoradiation. Earlier trials have shown that if the primary tumor response to induction chemotherapy is less than partial, it is unlikely that the patient's cancer will be cured by subsequent concurrent chemoradiation alone. Such patients are usually treated by surgery followed by postoperative radiation or chemoradiation.

D. **Management of locally recurrent disease.** Patients with locoregional recurrence only should be evaluated for potential salvage surgery or radiation therapy. If salvage surgery is not possible, and radiation therapy has previously been administered, concurrent chemotherapy with repeat irradiation may be effective in some patients; however, tissue tolerance, the extent of earlier radiation, and significant morbidity may limit this approach. Patients who are not candidates for local therapies may be treated with palliative chemotherapy.

E. **Management of metastatic disease.** Median survival of patients with metastatic SCCHN is 6 to 8 months in most series. Lung, bone, and liver are the most common sites of distant disease. Several standard chemotherapeutic agents have significant activity against SSCHN and can provide palliation of symptoms. These include cisplatin, carboplatin, 5-FU, paclitaxel, docetaxel, methotrexate, ifosfamide, gemcitabine, and bleomycin. The most commonly used first-line therapy is a platinum agent combined with a second agent, usually a taxane or 5-FU. First-line therapy typically has a tumor response rate of approximately 20% to 30%. In patients with platinum-refractory SCCHN, the tumor response rate of alternative standard chemotherapy is low (less than 5%) (*Proc Am Clin Oncol* 2005;23:16s).

Because of the poor tumor response rate to second-line chemotherapies, interest has developed in targeted therapies. Cetuximab has activity in platinum-refractory SCCHN. Trigo et al. presented the results of a phase II trial of cetuximab as a single agent in 103 patients with recurrent or metastatic platinum-refractory SCCHN. Tumor response occurred in 17% of patients, with five complete responses. Stable disease occurred in 38% of these patients. Median time to progression (TTP) and survival were 85 and 175 days, respectively (*Proc Am Soc Clin Oncol* 2004;23:487a). In a study by Baselga, et al. patients with locally advanced or metastatic SCCHN, whose disease had progressed after platinum-based cytotoxic chemotherapy, had cetuximab added to their regimen. Ten percent of these patients had a partial tumor response to the addition of cetuximab. Also, 43% of patients had stable disease with a TTP of 85 days and median OS of 183 days (*J Clin Oncol* 2005;24:5568). Cetuximab alone or its combination with a platinum agent are reasonable therapeutic options for patients with platinum-refractory SCCHN.

Erlotinib and gefitinib are EGFR tyrosine kinase inhibitors that have also been used to treat SCCHN. In a phase II trial, erlotinib resulted in a tumor response rate of 4%, a disease control rate (CR + PR + stable disease) of 38%, and a median overall survival of approximately 6 months (*J Clin Oncol* 2004;22:77). Similar outcome data was seen with gefitinib. Both drugs are generally well tolerated, with the most common side effects being fatigue, rash, and diarrhea. Erlotinib or gefitinib may be reasonable options for those patients with metastatic SCCHN who have chemotherapy-refractory disease or a poor performance status that would exclude use of other chemotherapeutic agents.

F. Complications of disease

1. Aspiration with risk of pneumonia should be considered in the patient with fever or cough. Weight loss or risk of aspiration may require placement of feeding gastrostomy tubes. Some patients will avoid aspiration with certain postures (chin tuck maneuver) or food consistencies, and consultation with a speech pathologist is often helpful in rehabilitation. Shortness of breath should prompt evaluation of the airway and the potential need for tracheostomy.

2. Fungating tumors may ulcerate and bleed. Invasion of the carotid artery by tumor may be a terminal event and may be heralded by an episode of sentinel bleeding.

3. Pain control. Inability to swallow may limit narcotic analgesic choices. Transdermal fentanyl patches or methadone elixir may allow longer pain relief with concentrated opiate elixirs for breakthrough pain. Opiate doses should be titrated to achieve pain control. Tumors invading nerves at the skull base may produce neuropathic pain syndromes that are helped by coanalgesics such as amitriptyline or gabapentin.

4. Paraneoplastic syndromes may include hypercalcemia and syndrome of inappropriate secretion of antidiuretic hormone (SIADH).

G. Complications of treatment

1. Complications of surgery may affect cosmesis, intelligibility of speech, and ability to swallow. Reconstructive flap techniques and prosthetics may minimize this. Neck dissection may result in shoulder weakness with resection of the 11th cranial nerve. After total laryngectomy, a tracheoesophageal puncture (TEP) may allow speech by diverting expired air into the esophagus to vibrate the cricopharyngeus muscle as a "pseudovocal cord." An electrolarynx, a handheld device that serves as a vibratory source for phonation, may also be used to allow communication following laryngectomy.

2. Acute radiation toxicity may include severe mucositis with pain and inability to swallow. Oral candidiasis complicating mucositis may be treated with topical agents (nystatin or clotrimazole) or systemic agents (e.g., fluconazole). A cocktail of equal volumes of diphenhydramine suspension, nystatin, viscous lidocaine, and aluminum hydroxide/magnesium hydroxide suspension may be used as a topical oral swish solution for mucositis. Some patients may prefer a solution of one teaspoon of baking soda and 1/2 teaspoon of salt in a quart of water for milder mucositis. Opiates are indicated for more severe pain. Skin toxicity in the radiation port should be treated with emollients (e.g., Aquaphor, Biafine) and wound dressings as appropriate.

3. **Late radiation effects include xerostomia,** which may be addressed by frequent access to water, or pilocarpine. Pilocarpine may cause uncomfortable sweats, especially at higher doses. Artificial saliva is available but poorly accepted by most patients. Dental caries is a chronic toxicity that may lead to tooth loss. Good dental care and use of fluoride preparations may minimize this. Osteoradionecrosis may be treated conservatively with antibiotics, surgical debridement, or hyperbaric oxygen therapy. Fibrosis of the neck tissues may result in trismus, lymphedema, and loss of range of motion. Exercises may be helpful in preventing trismus. Impaired swallowing due to weakness of pharyngeal constrictor muscles and aspiration may occur. Laryngeal edema may require tracheostomy for management and should prompt consideration of possible disease recurrence.

4. **Chemotherapy toxicities** vary according to the agents used. Used concurrently with radiation, they may increase the severity of mucositis. Cisplatin is associated with significant nausea, nephrotoxicity, peripheral neuropathy, ototoxicity, and myelosuppression. 5-FU may cause myelosuppression and mucositis. Taxanes are associated with alopecia, myelosuppression, myalgias, and allergic reactions. Cetuximab is associated with acneform rash, diarrhea, and hypersensitivity infusion reactions. Minocycline or other acne treatments may be helpful in managing the rash.

IV. LIP AND ORAL CAVITY

A. **Anatomy.** Cancer of the lip and oral cavity is the most common site of malignancy in the head and neck representing 30% of total cancers. Sites contained within this group are cancers originating from the lip, floor of mouth, anterior two-thirds of the tongue, buccal mucosa, gingival, hard palate, and retromolar trigone.

B. **Presentation.** Although this region is easily accessible, patients often delay presentation. As a result, many patients are first seen with advanced disease. Patients often present with symptoms including nonhealing lesions in their mouth, pain in the mouth or ear, trismus, weight loss, and "hot potato speech." When a patient does present, it is important to perform a thorough history and physical examination. A pertinent history should include tobacco use including smokeless tobacco and alcohol consumption. Dental history and history of chronic irritation should also be noted. As with any cancer patient, determination of functional status is essential.

On physical examination, complete evaluation of the nares, oral cavity, oropharynx, hypopharynx, and larynx should be examined by laryngoscopy. Evaluation for trismus (the mouth should permit the entry of three fingers vertically) and tongue movement is also important. Fixation of the tongue (ankyloglossia) may suggest a more advanced lesion. Palpation with a gloved finger should be used to inspect the base of tongue, retromolar trigone, and floor of mouth. The state of the patient's dentition should also be noted. Cranial nerve evaluation should also be performed. The neck should be evaluated for lymphadenopathy.

C. **Staging.** In addition to the history and physical examination, the staging evaluation should include an examination under anesthesia, dental examination, and radiographic imaging. CT or magnetic resonance imaging (MRI) of the head and neck is necessary to obtain a better anatomical understanding of the extent of the cancer. A CT scan may show better details of bone involvement. MRI gives a better view of soft tissues. Often these techniques are complimentary. A panorex may also be necessary to examine for mandibular bony involvement. CT scan of the chest should be performed to rule out pulmonary metastasis. Positron emission tomography (PET)/CT has an increasing role in the staging of this cancer and is ordered routinely in some centers. The American Joint Committee on Cancer (AJCC) staging system for lip and oral carcinoma can be found in Table 12.1, lymph node staging is found in Table 12.2, and AJCC stage grouping is found in Table 12.3.

D. **Pathology.** Squamous cell carcinoma is the leading histology of lip and oral cancers. Adverse pathologic features include depth of invasion, infiltrative borders, poorly differentiated tumors, and perineural and perivascular invasion. Sarcomatoid and baseloid features may also portend a worse prognosis. Less common histologies

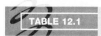

TABLE 12.1   AJCC Staging of Lip and Oral Cavity Cancer: Primary Tumor (T)

Stage	Description
Tumor (T) TX	Primary tumor cannot be assessed
T0	No evidence of primary tumor
Tis	Carcinoma *in situ*
T1	Tumor ≤2 cm in greatest dimension
T2	Tumor >2 cm but ≤4 cm in greatest dimension
T3	Tumor >4 cm in greatest dimension
T4 (lip)	Tumor invades adjacent structures (e.g., through cortical bone, inferior alveolar nerve, floor of mouth, skin of face)
T4a (oral cavity)	Tumor invades adjacent structures (e.g., through cortical bone, into deep [extrinsic] muscle of tongue, maxillary sinus, skin. Superficial erosion alone of bone/tooth socket by gingival primary is not sufficient to classify as T4)
T4b (oral cavity)	Tumor invades masticator space, pterygoid plates, or skull base and/or encases internal carotid artery

American Joint Committee on Cancer. *AJCC cancer staging manual,* 6th ed. New York: Springer-Verlag, 2002, with permission.

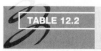

TABLE 12.2   AJCC Staging of Lip and Oral Cavity Cancer, Oropharynx, Hypopharynx, and Larynx: Regional Lymph Nodes (N), Distant Metastasis (M)

Stage	Description
NX	Regional lymph nodes cannot be assessed
N0	No regional lymph node metastasis
N1	Metastasis in a single ipsilateral lymph node, ≤3 cm in greatest dimension
N2	Metastasis in a single ipsilateral lymph node, >3 cm but not ≤6 cm in greatest dimension; or in multiple ipsilateral lymph nodes, none >6 cm in greatest dimension; or in bilateral or contralateral lymph nodes, none >6 cm in greatest dimension
N2a	Metastasis in a single ipsilateral lymph node >3 cm but not ≤6 cm in greatest dimension
N2b	Metastasis in multiple ipsilateral lymph nodes, none >6 cm in greatest dimension
N2c	Metastasis in bilateral or contralateral lymph nodes, none >6 cm in greatest dimension
N3	Metastasis in a lymph node >6 cm in greatest dimension
MX	Distant metastasis cannot be assessed
M0	No distant metastasis
M1	Distant metastasis

American Joint Committee on Cancer. *AJCC cancer staging manual,* 6th ed. New York: Springer-Verlag, 2002, with permission.

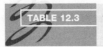

Stage	Tumor (T)	Node (N)	Metastasis (M)
Stage 0	Tis	N0	M0
Stage I	T1	N0	M0
Stage II	T2	N0	M0
Stage III	T3	N0	M0
	T1–T3	N1	M0
Stage IVA	T4a	N0–N1	M0
	Any T	N2	M0
Stage IVB	Any T	N3	M0
	T4b	Any N	M0
Stage IVC	Any T	Any N	M1

American Joint Committee on Cancer. *AJCC cancer staging manual*, 6th ed. New York: Springer-Verlag, 2002, with permission.

include adenoid cystic carcinoma and mucoepidermoid cancer of the minor salivary glands. These will be discussed in more detail later in this chapter.

E. Natural history of disease. Squamous cell cancer of the lip and oral cavity is predominantly a locoregional disease with relatively late spread to distant sites in most patients. This is important for the success of the local modalities of surgery and radiation therapy in treating these patients.

   1. Field cancerization is an important concept in the natural history of head and neck cancer, especially oral cavity tumors. Because the exposure of the mucosa to carcinogens in tobacco is diffuse across the aerodigestive tract, tumors may be surrounded by areas of dysplasia or carcinoma *in situ*. Patients with head and neck cancer are at an increased risk of development of new primary tumors in the head and neck, lung, and esophagus. The risk is approximately 3% to 4% per year.

   2. Leukoplakia and erythroleukoplakia are premalignant lesions of the oral mucosa, related to the epithelial injury due to tobacco and ethanol. Leukoplakia is a white patch of mucosa that cannot be scraped off and shows hyperkeratosis on biopsy. Erythroleukoplakia may appear red and velvety and may demonstrate dysplasia or carcinoma *in situ* on biopsy. The risk of malignant transformation increases with duration of observation and is higher with erythroleukoplakia.

   Treatment may include careful observation or surgical resection if the area involved makes this feasible. Retinoids such as isotretinoin (13 *cis*-retinoic acid) have shown promising results in the treatment of leukoplakia, but treatment is associated with cheilitis, skin irritation, dry eyes, and a risk of birth defects in patients with reproductive potential. In a trial, an isotretinoin dose of 1.5 mg/kg/day by mouth for 3 months followed by a maintenance dose of 0.5 mg/kg/day produced a response rate of 55%, with most patients maintaining their response over the course of 1 year (*N Engl J Med* 1986;315:1501).

V. OROPHARYNX

   A. Anatomy. Cancer of the oropharynx includes sites in the soft palate, tonsils, posterior and lateral oropharyngeal walls, and the base of tongue. Its borders include the junction of the hard and soft palate, the tonsillar arch, and the circumvallate papillae on the tongue.

   B. Presentation. Many of the features described earlier for cancers of the oral cavity also apply to cancers of the oropharynx.

   1. Pertinent history should include a history of tobacco and ethanol use and comorbid diseases. Bleeding from the mouth, alterations in speech, difficulty or pain with swallowing, and weight loss should also be noted.

2. **The physical examination** includes an assessment of performance status, complete evaluation of the nares, oral cavity, oropharynx, hypopharynx and larynx (with indirect or fiberoptic laryngoscopy), and neck. Assessment should include the cranial nerves. Evaluate for trismus, status of dentition, and tongue movement and atrophy. Palpation of the tongue base with a gloved finger is very useful. Lymph nodes in the neck should be palpated with measurements of palpable nodes, noting their size, level, and whether they are fixed to underlying tissue.

C. **Staging.** Along with history and physical examination, the staging evaluation of patients with oropharynx cancers includes diagnostic imaging, triple endoscopy with biopsy of the primary lesion, and evaluation for distant metastasis and synchronous primaries. CT or MRI imaging of the primary site and neck and chest radiograph or CT should be performed. The staging of oropharynx cancer is defined by the size and extension of the primary and extent of nodal disease or distant metastasis (Tables 12.2 to 12.4).

D. **Pathology. Squamous cell carcinoma** is the histology found in more than 90% of cancers of the oropharynx. Less common pathologies include lymphomas involving Waldeyer's ring of lymphoid tissue (tonsils, lingual tonsils, and adenoids), mucosal melanomas, and tumors arising in the minor salivary glands that lie in the mucosa (including adenocarcinomas, adenoid cystic carcinomas, and mucoepidermoid carcinomas). Distinction should be made between well-differentiated and poorly differentiated squamous cell carcinomas. Adverse pathologic features include increasing depth of invasion, infiltrative borders, poorly differentiated tumors, and perineural and lymphovascular invasion. Sarcomatoid differentiation or basaloid features may also portend a worse prognosis. Lymphoepithelioma represents squamous cell carcinoma with extensive infiltration of lymphocytes that usually arises in Waldeyer's ring or the nasopharynx and may be confused with non-Hodgkin's lymphoma. Immunostaining for clonal lymphoid populations may be necessary for correct identification of these entities with critical treatment implications.

A growing number of cancers of the oropharynx are found in younger patients who are not users of tobacco or alcohol. These are typically nonkeratnizing and have been found to be linked to the human papillomavirus (HPV).

E. **Natural history of disease.** Squamous cell cancer of the oropharynx is, as in oral cavity cancer, predominantly a disease of locoregional control. Vertical growth may occur early where tissue planes permit, as in base of tongue and tonsil, and this may explain why tumors here represent a significant proportion of unknown primaries

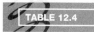

TABLE 12.4	AJCC Staging of Oropharynx Cancer: Primary Tumor (T)
Stage	**Description**
Tumor (T) TX	Primary tumor cannot be assessed
T0	No evidence of primary tumor
Tis	Carcinoma *in situ*
T1	Tumor ≤2 cm in greatest dimension
T2	Tumor >2 cm but ≤4 cm in greatest dimension
T3	Tumor >4 cm in greatest dimension
T4a	Tumor invades the larynx, deep/extrinsic muscle of tongue, medial pterygoid, hard palate, or mandible.
T4b	Tumor invades lateral pterygoid muscle, pterygoid plates, lateral nasopharynx, or skull base or encases carotid artery.

American Joint Committee on Cancer. *AJCC cancer staging manual,* 6th ed. New York: Springer-Verlag, 2002, with permission.

found on blind biopsies in patients who present with cervical metastases. The effects of tobacco and alcohol on the mucosa explain the risk of second primaries and field cancerization. Patients with advanced or recurrent disease are prone to poor lymphatic or venous drainage, and edema of the face and head may develop, which gets worse after lying supine. The effects of earlier treatment with neck dissection or radiation fibrosis in the neck may exacerbate this. Corticosteroids may help some patients, and upright posture should be encouraged. These patients may be at risk for airway obstruction that may benefit from tracheostomy.

VI. LARYNX AND HYPOPHARYNX

A. **Anatomy.** Cancers of the larynx and hypopharynx represent challenges in treatment because of their intimate involvement with speech and swallowing. As such, these sites have been associated with the most research on organ preservation, attempts to avoid laryngectomy, while maintaining the best chance for cure. The boundaries of the hypopharynx are the level of the hyoid bone superiorly and the lower border of the cricoid inferiorly. Tumors in this area may be divided into those arising from the pyriform sinuses, the posterior wall of the hypopharynx, and the postcricoid area. Tumors of the larynx may be divided into those located predominantly above the true vocal cords (supraglottic), those arising from the true vocal cords (glottic), or those below the true vocal cords (subglottic).

B. **Presentation.** The presentation of cancers of the hypopharynx and larynx varies greatly with their primary site. Tumors of the supraglottic region or the pyriform sinus may be diagnosed only after cervical metastasis develop because of their greater access to rich lymphatics and vague symptoms of dysphagia that may not become significant until the tumors are quite large. Conversely, glottic carcinomas are associated with symptoms of hoarseness, often despite a small size, and the tumors may remain localized until cartilage invasion takes place.

1. **Pertinent history** should include a history of tobacco and ethanol use, comorbid diseases, and symptoms of dysphagia, odynophagia, weight loss, dyspnea, and hoarseness. Unilateral paralysis of a vocal cord may result in speech that deteriorates with longer use of the voice and improves with rest. Patients may also become dyspneic with speech. Symptoms of aspiration should be sought. The patient's use of the voice in his or her occupation and a history of gastroesophageal reflux should be noted. Symptoms of pain, trismus, altered speech, and weight loss should be included, along with the duration of symptoms.

2. **Physical examination** includes assessment of performance status, complete evaluation of the oral cavity, oropharynx, hypopharynx, and larynx with indirect or fiberoptic laryngoscopy, testing of cranial nerves, and palpation of the neck. Palpation and visualization of the base of tongue should be done to note whether there is extension of the tumor to this site. Pooling of saliva in the hypopharynx may interfere with the office examination and requires better visualization at the time of endoscopy and biopsy. Fixation of the true vocal cords should be noted, as this affects staging, and diagrams of the extent of the lesion are helpful.

C. **Staging.** The staging of cancers in the hypopharynx and larynx uses examination with laryngoscopic biopsy to determine the extent of the lesion and search for nodal disease and synchronous primaries. Triple endoscopy is usually done at the time of biopsy. CT or MRI imaging is included to look at the extension of the primary and cervical nodes. Chest radiograph or CT is used to assess for distant metastases and second primary tumors. The tendency of the thyroid cartilage to display irregular calcification should be noted, as it may result in overestimating cartilage invasion on staging. In addition to using size criteria, many of the staging criteria for the primary (T stage) include whether adjacent subsites of the hypopharynx (pyriform sinus, pharyngeal wall, and postcricoid region) or supraglottic larynx (suprahyoid epiglottis, infrahyoid epiglottis, aryepiglottic folds, arytenoids, and false vocal cords) are involved (Tables 12.2, 12.3, 12.5, and 12.6).

D. **Pathology.** Squamous cell carcinoma, or one of its variants, is the histologic description of more than 95% of tumors arising in the hypopharynx and larynx. Tumors of minor salivary gland histology (adenoid cystic, adenocarcinoma, and

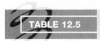

TABLE 12.5   AJCC Staging Hypopharynx Cancer: Primary Tumor (T)

Stage	Description
TX	Primary tumor cannot be assessed
T0	No evidence of primary tumor
Tis	Carcinoma *in situ*
T1	Tumor limited to one subsite of hypopharynx and ≤2 cm in greatest dimension
T2	Tumor involves more than one subsite of hypopharynx or an adjacent site, or measures >2 cm but ≤4 cm in greatest dimension without fixation of hemilarynx
T3	Tumor measures >4 cm in greatest dimension or with fixation of hemilarynx
T4a	Tumor invades thyroid/cricoid cartilage, hyoid bone, thyroid gland, esophagus, prelaryngeal strap muscles, or subcutaneous fat
T4b	Tumor invades prevertebral fascia, encases carotid artery, or involves mediastinal structures.

American Joint Committee on Cancer. *AJCC cancer staging manual,* 6th ed. New York: Springer-Verlag, 2002, with permission.

mucoepidermoid carcinoma) occur infrequently. The supraglottic larynx may be the site for neuroendocrine small cell carcinomas and should be recognized because of their tendency for distant spread and sensitivity to chemotherapy and radiation.

E. **Stage-directed approach to therapy**

1. **Early-stage disease (Stage I to II)** is most likely to be encountered in laryngeal carcinomas. The primary approach may consist of surgical resection or radiation therapy with generally equivalent cure rates. In many cases, the patient may be able to undergo a larynx-conservation surgery, such as a supraglottic or hemilaryngectomy, in which one or both vocal cords are preserved to allow speech.

2. **Advanced-stage disease (Stage III to IVB).** Tumors of the pyriform sinus are usually advanced at the time of diagnosis. Tumors of the posterior pharyngeal wall may remain exophytic and superficial, allowing surgical resection if there is no invasion of the prevertebral fascia and muscle. The traditional approach to advanced tumors of larynx and hypopharynx has been surgical resection with laryngectomy or laryngopharyngectomy, as appropriate, to achieve a complete resection, with postoperative radiation therapy. Over the last 15 years, however, chemoradiation has been shown to be very effective and to allow preservation of speech and swallowing.

Interest in larynx conservation has led to trials of chemotherapy and radiation in an attempt to avoid laryngectomy and preserve anatomy and function. The Veterans Administration (VA) Larynx Trial compared laryngectomy and postoperative adjuvant radiation with induction chemotherapy followed by definitive radiation therapy for those patients whose tumors responded favorably to chemotherapy (*N Engl J Med* 1991;324:1685). Cisplatin and 5-FU (PF) were administered every 3 weeks, with primary tumor response assessed after the second cycle. Patients with responsive tumors received a total of three cycles of chemotherapy followed by radiation, whereas patients whose tumor did not respond to chemotherapy or who had persistent disease after radiation underwent laryngectomy. This induction chemotherapy approach resulted in equivalent OS as compared with up-front surgery followed by postoperative radiation and allowed 64% of patients to retain their larynx.

A European Organization for the Research and Treatment of Cancer (EORTC) trial in cancers of the pyriform sinus compared the results of surgical resection and postoperative radiation therapy with a similar experimental arm (*J Natl Cancer Inst* 1996;8:890). Patients were randomized between surgery and adjuvant radiation or induction chemotherapy with PF followed

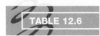

TABLE 12.6 | **AJCC Staging Larynx Cancer: Primary Tumor (T)**

Stage	Description
Tumor (T) TX	Primary tumor cannot be assessed
T0	No evidence of primary tumor
Tis	Carcinoma *in situ*
T1 Supraglottis	Tumor limited to one subsite of supraglottis with normal vocal cord mobility
T1 Glottis	Tumor limited to vocal cord(s) (may involve anterior or posterior commissure) with normal mobility
T1a	Tumor limited to one vocal cord
T1b	Tumor involves both vocal cords
T1 Subglottis	Tumor limited to the subglottis
T2 Supraglottis	Tumor invades mucosa of more than one adjacent subsite of supraglottis or glottis or region outside the supraglottis (e.g., mucosa of base of tongue, vallecula, medial wall of pyriform sinus) without fixation of the larynx
T2 Glottis	Tumor extends to supraglottis and/or subglottis, and/or with impaired vocal cord mobility
T2 Subglottis	Tumor extends to vocal cord(s) with normal or impaired mobility
T3 Supraglottis	Tumor limited to larynx with vocal cord fixation and/or invades any of the following: postcricoid area, preepiglottic tissues
T3 Glottis	Tumor limited to the larynx with vocal cord fixation
T3 Subglottis	Tumor limited to the larynx with vocal cord fixation
T4a Supraglottis	Tumor invades through the thyroid cartilage, and/or extends into soft tissues of the neck, thyroid, and/or esophagus
T4a Glottis	Tumor invades through the thyroid cartilage, and/or to other tissues beyond the larynx (e.g., trachea, soft tissues of neck, including thyroid, pharynx)
T4a Subglottis	Tumor invades through cricoid or thyroid cartilage, and/or extends to other tissues beyond the larynx (e.g., trachea, soft tissues of neck, including thyroid, esophagus)
T4b Supraglottis	Tumor invades prevertebral space, encases carotid artery, or invades mediastinal structures.
T4b Glottis	Tumor invades prevertebral space, encases carotid artery, or invades mediastinal structures.
T4b Subglottis	Tumor invades prevertebral space, encases carotid artery, or invades mediastinal structures.

American Joint Committee on Cancer. *AJCC cancer staging manual,* 6th ed. New York: Springer-Verlag, 2002, with permission.

by definitive radiation. Patients with chemosensitive tumors as assessed after cycle 1 received a total of three cycles of chemotherapy followed by definitive radiation with surgery used as salvage for nonresponders to chemotherapy or in persistent disease following definitive radiation. As in the VA larynx trial, OS was equivalent between these two treatment approaches, and functional larynx conservation at 3 years was achieved in 42% (95% CI, 31% to 53%) of patients on the chemoradiation arm.

In a follow-up trial study, an intergroup, three-arm randomized trial compared induction chemotherapy with PF followed by definitive radiation, as given in the VA trial, with concurrent cisplatin during radiation versus radiation therapy alone. The concurrent cisplatin and radiation arm scheduled three cycles of cisplatin given every 21 days, during radiation therapy. Eligible patients included patients with stage III to IV laryngeal cancer who would require total laryngectomy as surgical management. Patients with T4 primaries were excluded if they had more than minimal thyroid cartilage invasion or more than 1-cm extension onto the base of tongue. The ability to preserve the larynx was significantly better with the concurrent chemoradiotherapy arm versus the induction followed by radiotherapy arm and the radiation-only arm (83.6% vs. 70.5% vs. 65.7%, respectively). There was no significant difference in 5-year survival between the three arms (approximately 55%) (*N Engl J Med* 2003;349:2091; *Proc Am Soc Clin Oncol* 2006;25:284s). Together, these trials demonstrate the feasibility of organ preservation in most cases of locally advanced cancers of the larynx and hypopharynx without adversely effecting survival.

F. Natural history of disease. Locoregional control is the major challenge in the treatment in patients with cancer of the hypopharynx and larynx, but these sites demonstrate the variable natural history of squamous cell cancer arising in adjacent structures. The lack of symptoms in early pyriform sinus cancers can be contrasted with the frequent development of symptoms (hoarseness) with early glottic cancer. The effect of anatomy with confinement of many laryngeal cancers to the primary site due to surrounding thyroid cartilage contrasts with the advanced disease typically seen in hypopharynx cancers to demonstrate these differences. Although most recurrences of head and neck cancers occur within the first 2 to 3 years after treatment, continued vigilance is warranted for the development of metachronous primaries, and all patients should be counseled about the benefits of smoking cessation. Patients with cancer of the larynx are at significant risk for lung cancer.

VII. NASOPHARYNX CANCER

A. Anatomy. The borders of the nasopharynx include the choanae (anterior), the soft palate (inferior), and lateral walls, including the fossae of Rosenmuller and the eustachian tube orifices. Its sloping roof along the skull base (superior and posterior) lies in close proximity to the foramen lacerum and the carotid artery as it enters the cavernous sinus. Tumors may extend through the foramen ovale to access the middle cranial fossa and the cavernous sinus with access to the oculomotor (CN III), trochlear (CN IV), trigeminal (CN V), and abducens (CN VI) nerves. Optic nerve (CN II) and orbital invasion is possible in advanced cases. There is a rich lymphatic supply with retropharyngeal nodes, including the lateral retropharyngeal nodes (of Rouvière), representing an important route of spread.

B. Presentation. The presentation of nasopharyngeal cancer has many unique features. Symptoms at diagnosis may be related to the primary site, disease in the neck, or distant metastases. The epidemiology of this cancer is different from that of other head and neck sites, with a separate set of risk factors.

1. Pertinent history may include genetic and environmental factors. The highest incidence of nasopharyngeal cancers is found in southern China and Southeast Asia. Places that have significant immigrant populations from these countries have a higher incidence, and a history of travel to these parts of the world may convey a higher risk of cancer among North American whites. This risk may be related to strains of Epstein–Barr virus (EBV), as viral titers for EBV are often elevated among patients with this disease. Genetic factors related to host response may explain the increased risk among people of Asian ancestry. Other risk factors have been implicated, including diet (consumption of salted fish, low intake of fresh fruits and vegetables) and smoking. Symptoms may include a painless neck mass, nasal obstruction, epistaxis, dysphagia, odynophagia, eustachian tube obstruction with otitis media, or cranial neuropathies. Trismus may indicate invasion of the pterygoid region. Other symptoms may include headache, referred pain to the ear or neck, and weight loss.

2. A thorough physical examination includes assessment of performance status, complete evaluation of the nares and oral cavity, and a thorough evaluation of the cranial nerves. Proptosis may indicate orbital invasion. Evaluation of the nasopharynx with fiberoptic endoscopy or examination under anesthesia with biopsy is appropriate. The status of dentition should be noted, as any needed restoration or extractions should precede the initiation of radiation therapy.

Lymph nodes in the neck should be palpated, with measurements of palpable nodes.

C. Staging. Along with history and physical examination, the staging evaluation of patients with nasopharynx cancers includes diagnostic imaging, including MRI or CT from the base of skull to clavicles, endoscopy, and chest radiograph or CT to look for distant metastases. Nuclear medicine bone scan should be considered in any patient with unexplained bone pain. The staging of nasopharynx cancer is shown in Tables 12.7 and 12.8.

D. Pathology. Carcinomas represent 85% of nasopharynx tumors (less common are lymphoma, adenocarcinoma, melanoma, plasmacytoma, rhabdomyosarcoma, and others). Nasopharyngeal carcinoma is classified according to a World Health Organization (WHO) schema. WHO-1 is squamous cell carcinoma. WHO-2 is nonkeratinizing carcinoma. WHO-3 is undifferentiated carcinoma, including lymphoepithelioma.

E. Stage-directed approach to therapy

    1. Early-stage disease is rarely diagnosed because of lack of symptoms. EBV titers have been used in areas of high incidence to allow mass screenings. Radiation therapy (70 Gy) alone is the typical treatment for early disease. Surgical resection or repeated irradiation with chemotherapy may be considered for local recurrence.

    2. Advanced-stage disease had traditionally been treated with radiation, but the results of a randomized North American Intergroup trial have demonstrated a

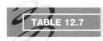

TABLE 12.7	**Staging of Nasopharynx Cancer**

Stage	Description
Primary tumor (T)	
TX	Primary tumor cannot be assessed
T0	No evidence of primary tumor
Tis	Carcinoma *in situ*
T1	Tumor confined to the nasopharynx
T2	Tumor extends to soft tissues of oropharynx and/or nasal fossa
T2a	Without parapharyngeal extension
T2b	With parapharyngeal extension
T3	Tumor invades bony structures and/or paranasal sinuses
T4	Tumor with intracranial extension and/or involvement of cranial nerves, infratemporal fossa, hypopharynx, or orbit
Regional lymph nodes (N)	
NX	Regional lymph nodes cannot be assessed
N0	No regional lymph node metastasis
N1	Unilateral metastasis in lymph node(s), ≤ 6 cm in greatest dimension, above the supraclavicular fossa
N2	Bilateral metastasis in lymph node(s), ≤ 6 cm in greatest dimension, above the supraclavicular fossa
N3	Metastasis in a lymph node(s)
N3a	>6 cm in dimension
N3b	Extension to the supraclavicular fossa
Distant metastasis (M)	
MX	Distant metastasis cannot be assessed
M0	No distant metastasis
M1	Distant metastasis

American Joint Committee on Cancer. *AJCC cancer staging manual,* 6th ed. New York: Springer-Verlag, 2002, with permission.

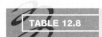

Stage	Tumor (T)	Node (N)	Metastasis (M)
Stage 0	Tis	N0	M0
Stage I	T1	N0	M0
Stage IIA	T2a	N0	M0
Stage IIB	T1	N1	M0
	T2	N1	M0
	T2a	N1	M0
	T2b	N0	M0
	T2b	N1	M0
Stage III	T1	N2	M0
	T2a	N2	M0
	T2b	N2	M0
	T3	N0	M0
	T3	N1	M0
	T3	N2	M0
Stage IVA	T4	N0	M0
	T4	N1	M0
	T4	N2	M0
Stage IVB	Any T	N3	M0
Stage IVC	Any T	Any N	M1

American Joint Committee on Cancer. *AJCC cancer staging manual,* 6th ed. New York: Springer-Verlag, 2002, with permission.

superior outcome with chemoradiation therapy. This study compared standard radiation therapy (70 Gy) alone with a schema of the same radiation therapy with concurrent cisplatin 100 mg/m^2 given every 21 days (total of three doses) during radiation therapy and three additional cycles of cisplatin and 5-FU given every 4 weeks after completion of radiation therapy. The 3-year progression-free survival was 24% versus 69% (p <0.001) and 3-year OS was 47% versus 78% ($p = 0.005$) for radiation versus chemoradiation, respectively. Both local control and distant metastasis were improved in the combined-modality arm (*J Clin Oncol* 1998;16:1310).

F. Natural history of disease. Nasopharyngeal carcinoma is a disease with unique features unlike other head and neck cancers. A younger age at presentation compared with that for other sites and a higher incidence in endemic areas are seen. Its greater radiation sensitivity leads to less need for neck dissection and a greater cure rate, despite advanced disease. Most patients are first seen with locally advanced disease, but the risk of distant metastasis is higher than with other sites. The role of genetic factors and EBV are well recognized but poorly understood. Viral titers, especially immunoglobulin (Ig) A (IgA) viral capsid antigen and early antigen, may be helpful, as titers that remain elevated may identify a group at risk for distant recurrence.

VIII. LESS COMMON TUMORS OF THE HEAD AND NECK

A. Salivary gland cancers most commonly arise in the parotid gland, but may arise in the submandibular or minor salivary glands that line the mucosa of the upper aerodigestive tract.

1. Pathology. The histology of salivary gland carcinoma is varied and affects prognosis and management. Perineural invasion and nodal metastases are adverse features.

a. Mucoepidermoid cancers are the most common type arising in the parotid glands and are classified as low, intermediate, or high grade. Low-grade tumors respond well to surgical resection, whereas higher-grade lesions are associated with more aggressive local invasion, and nodal and distant metastases.

   b. Adenoid cystic carcinoma has the most frequent histology in the submandibular and minor salivary glands. Perineural invasion may lead to facial nerve (CN VII) paralysis and involvement of the skull base. It is also classified by grade and has a significant incidence of distant metastatic disease.

   c. Malignant mixed tumors (carcinoma ex-pleomorphic adenoma) arise from a preexisting benign mixed tumor (pleomorphic adenoma).

   d. Adenocarcinomas commonly arise from the minor salivary glands but may also arise in the major salivary glands. They have aggressive behavior and significant risk of distant metastasis. Low-grade polymorphous adenocarcinomas arise in the oral cavity and have an excellent prognosis with complete resection.

   e. Acinic cell carcinomas usually arise in the parotid glands. They are typically low-grade, slow-growing tumors, but may invade adjacent structures. Late recurrences and distant metastases may occur.

   f. Squamous cell carcinomas arising from the excretory duct of the salivary glands have an aggressive course with a poor prognosis despite aggressive therapy.

   2. Treatment. Management of salivary gland cancers is complete surgical resection. In the parotid, this may consist of total or superficial parotidectomy, depending on the location of the tumor. When possible, the facial nerve may be preserved. High-grade tumors benefit from adjuvant radiation therapy. Recurrent or metastatic tumors may be treated with chemotherapy, including cisplatin, doxorubicin, 5-FU, and cyclophosphamide combinations.

B. Tumors of the nose and paranasal sinuses also include a variety of tumors. These are rare malignancies. Risk factors may include occupational exposures to wood dust, shoe manufacture, nickel refining, and Thorotrast contrast media.

   1. Squamous cell carcinoma is the most common type in the nose and paranasal sinuses, and the maxillary sinus is the most common primary site. Minor salivary gland histologies may also occur. Surgical resection and postoperative radiation therapy is the treatment.

   2. Esthesioneuroblastoma (olfactory neuroblastoma) arises from the olfactory neuroepithelium. Complete surgical resection with radiation therapy is the treatment. There may be a limited benefit to the addition of chemotherapy in a combined-modality approach.

   3. Sinonasal undifferentiated carcinomas (SNUCs) are high-grade epithelial malignancies that may occur with or without neuroendocrine differentiation. Treatment may include surgery, radiation, and chemotherapy.

IX. UNKNOWN PRIMARY AND MANAGEMENT OF THE NECK

A. The patient with a neck mass may not have a primary site identified on inspection of the oral cavity and pharynx, despite careful examination.

   1. Fine-needle aspiration for cytology of the neck mass should be pursued as the primary diagnostic procedure. Open biopsy should be pursued if a lymphoma is suggested. Evaluation of the thyroid, parotid, and any suggestive skin lesions should be performed. A mass in the supraclavicular fossa should prompt evaluation of possible primary sites below the clavicles.

   2. If squamous cell carcinoma is suggested by the cytology obtained, endoscopy with blind biopsy of potential primary sites should include the nasopharynx, tonsils, base of tongue, and pyriform sinuses.

   3. If no primary site is found, several approaches are considered. If the neck mass is unresectable, then primary radiation therapy with a nasopharyngeal port, which will include the likely potential primary sites, may be used. If a nasopharyngeal primary is suggested by the cytology, chemoradiation may be considered. Residual disease after radiation or neck masses larger than 6 cm should undergo subsequent neck dissection. If the neck mass is resectable, neck dissection may be pursued as primary therapy. If the pathology shows extracapsular extension or if multiple nodes are involved, postoperative radiation therapy with a nasopharyngeal port is given. If the neck mass is solitary and small, then radiation therapy may be held off and the patient closely observed, with radiation used at the time of relapse.

B. Management of the neck

1. **Control of disease in the neck** is a major challenge in patients with head and neck cancer. Much of the morbidity and mortality of this disease is related to disease in regional nodes, and effective control of nodal metastases is important in overall control and cure.

2. **Patients with clinically negative** neck nodes that are at significant risk for occult disease may be treated effectively with elective neck dissection (lymphadenectomy) or radiation therapy. Clinically involved nodes may require both modalities, especially if there is extracapsular extension, masses larger than 6 cm, or if multiple nodes are involved.

3. **Anatomy of the lymphatic drainage** of the neck is divided into various groups. Level I nodes include the submental and submandibular nodes. Level II includes the upper jugular or jugulodigastric nodes. Level III includes the midjugular nodes. Level IV includes the lower jugular nodes. Level V includes the posterior triangle of the neck.

4. **Radical neck dissection** consists of removing all five lymph node groups on one side of the neck, as well as the sternocleidomastoid muscle, the internal jugular vein, and the spinal accessory nerve (CN XI). Modified radical neck dissections remove all five lymph node groups but may spare one or more of the latter structures. In a selective neck dissection, only lymph node groups at the highest risk are excised, and the sternocleidomastoid, jugular vein, and CN XI are preserved.

X. CURRENT FOCUS OF RESEARCH. Areas of active investigation include the evaluation of induction chemotherapy before definitive chemoradiation; development of new targeted therapies; application of intensity-modulated radiation therapy (IMRT); and application of transoral CO_2 laser resection and reconstructive techniques.

Suggested Readings

Al-Sarraf M, LeBlanc M, Giri PG, et al. Chemoradiotherapy versus radiotherapy in patients with advanced nasopharyngeal cancer: phase III randomized Intergroup study 0099. *J Clin Oncol* 1998;16:1310.

Baselga J, Trigo JM, Bourhis J, et al. Phase II multicenter study of the antiepidermal growth factor receptor monoclonal antibody cetuximab in combination with platinum-based chemotherapy in patients with platinum-refractory metastatic and/or recurrent squamous cell carcinoma of the headneck. *J Clin Oncol* 2005;24:5568.

Bonner J, Harari PM, Giralt J, et al. Radiotherapy plus cetuximab for squamous-cell carcinoma of the head and neck. *N Eng J Med* 2006;354:567.

Choong N, Cohen EE. Epidermal growth factor directed therapy in head and neck cancer. *Crit Rev Hematol/Oncol* 2006;57:25.

Forastiere A, Goepfert H, Maor M, et al. Concurrent chemotherapy and radiotherapy for organ preservation in advanced laryngeal cancer. *N Engl J Med* 2003;349:2091.

Wolf G. Induction chemotherapy plus radiation compared with surgery plus radiation in patients with advanced laryngeal cancer: VA Laryngeal Cancer Study Group. *N Engl J Med* 1991;324:1685.

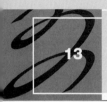

LUNG CANCER
Janakiraman Subramanian and Ramaswamy Govindan

I. NON–SMALL CELL LUNG CANCER
A. Presentation

1. **Subjective.** Although a few patients with non–small cell lung cancer (NSCLC) may be asymptomatic at presentation and detected only by "routine" radiographic examination, most patients present with symptoms related to local disease or distant metastasis. These symptoms may be secondary to a tumor in the lung, such as new or worsening cough, worsening or new dyspnea, chest wall pain, and fever, often secondary to postobstructive pneumonia. Hemoptysis, especially in the middle-aged or elderly smoker, should always raise the suspicion of lung cancer. Chest pain may signify chest-wall involvement; dyspnea and hoarseness of the voice may indicate involvement of recurrent laryngeal nerve. Because of its long intrathoracic course, the left recurrent laryngeal nerve is more commonly affected than the right. Superior sulcus tumors can cause Pancoast syndrome; a triad of shoulder pain, lower brachial plexus palsy, and Horner syndrome. Swelling and engorgement of the face, upper trunk, and arms signal superior vena cava (SVC) syndrome, which is associated more with right-sided tumors. Patients with pleural effusions may have dyspnea and cough. Occasionally dysphagia may be one of the dominant presenting symptoms secondary to mediastinal lymph node involvement. Symptoms suggesting distant metastasis are not specific and include weight loss, cachexia, and symptoms related to distant sites involved (e.g., bone pain or fractures from bone-involvement, right upper quadrant abdominal pain with liver metastases, and neurologic symptoms associated with central nervous system [CNS] involvement). Paraneoplastic syndromes associated with NSCLC include hypercalcemia (which can cause constipation, abdominal pain, and confusion) and hypertrophic pulmonary osteoarthropathy with marked clubbing, joint pains, and swelling.

2. **Objective.** Assessment of the performance status (PS) and signs of recent significant weight loss carry a significant prognostic importance. The superficial lymph nodes, particularly the supraclavicular nodes, should be carefully examined, as enlargement of these nodes raises the high likelihood of metastatic involvement. Signs on examination of the chest can detect not only those signs related to pleural effusion, atelectasis, and postobstructive pneumonia, but also can help assess the severity of any underlying lung disease (e.g., chronic obstructive pulmonary disease [COPD]) that may influence subsequent management options. Careful abdominal examination may detect hepatomegaly suggesting metastatic disease. New focal neurologic signs may signify brain or spinal cord involvement.

B. Workup and staging

1. **Imaging**

   a. **Chest radiograph (CXR).** A perfectly normal CXR does not necessarily exclude lung cancer, as conventional CXR may not always identify hilar or mediastinal lesions. Lung cancer can present as a mass, peripheral nodule, hilar or mediastinal changes suggestive of lymphadenopathy, or pleural effusions. CXR may reveal areas of atelectasis suggesting endobronchial lesion, and pneumonic infiltrates may be seen in association with obstructing lesions.

    b. Computed tomography (CT) scan of the chest is the most effective noninvasive study to evaluate suspected lung cancer. Although its sensitivity to detect mediastinal metastases is variable, it has a high negative predictive value. It can also help identify local invasion (e.g., chest wall, bones, pleura). The upper abdomen is usually included in this study, and the liver and adrenal glands should be carefully inspected for evidence of metastases.

    c. Magnetic resonance imaging (MRI) of the chest is not routinely used in the staging workup of patients with lung cancer. It is particularly helpful in the setting of suspected spinal cord, vascular, brachial plexus, or chest-wall involvement.

    d. Fluorodeoxyglucose (FDG) Positron emission tomography (PET) scan is a useful adjunct tool to complete the staging workup in patients with recently diagnosed NSCLC. The FDG PET scan has been demonstrated to be superior to CT scans in identifying mediastinal lymph node involvement and distant metastasis. FDG PET scan helps identify additional sites of disease in approximately 10% to 30% of patients that were not identified by the conventional workup.

  2. Pathological diagnosis. Flexible fiber optic bronchoscopy can help determine the extent of endobronchial lesions and to obtain tissue for diagnosis (washings, brushings, bronchoalveolar lavage, transbronchial biopsy). Cytologic examination of sputum is sometimes helpful in diagnosing centrally located squamous cell cancer in patients who are not candidates for CT-guided needle biopsy or bronchoscopy.

    Mediastinoscopy is very useful to determine status of mediastinal lymph nodes in patients who are considered to be candidates for surgical resection. Evaluation of mediastinal lymph nodes by mediastinoscopy is critical before surgical resection. Normal-appearing mediastinal lymph nodes may contain metastatic disease, and sometimes enlarged lymph nodes in the mediastinum may represent only hyperplastic lymph nodes from postobstructive pneumonia or may represent old granulomatous infection. Cervical mediastinoscopy is more accurate for staging superior mediastinal lymph nodes, whereas extended or anterior (Chamberlain) approach is better for anterior mediastinal lymph nodes. It is a safe procedure in experienced hands. Endoscopic and endobronchial ultrasonography are being increasingly utilized to biopsy the mediastinal lymph glands. Many thoracic surgeons do not perform preoperative mediastinoscopy if the CT chest and FDG PET reveal no abnormalities in the mediastinum.

    Video-assisted thoracoscopic surgery (VATS) can be used to access peripheral nodules, suspected pleural disease, and effusions.

  3. Pathology. Epithelial cancers are classified by the best-differentiated region but are graded by the most poorly differentiated region. There are two types: small cell lung cancer (SCLC) and NSCLC comprising of three subtypes, adenocarcinoma, squamous cell carcinoma, and large cell carcinoma. The distinction between NSCLC and SCLC is extremely important as they are treated very differently. The incidence of SCLC has been declining over the last decade and now accounts only for 13% of all primary lung cancers.

  4. Staging. The International Staging System (ISS) uses the TNM (tumor, node, metastasis) description system, which is shown in Table 13.1. Stage-specific survival is outlined in Table 13.2

C. Therapy and prognosis

  1. Overview of management of NSCLC.

    Stages I and II: surgical resection (or definitive radiotherapy (RT] if surgery is contraindicated) and adjuvant chemotherapy in IB (although a bit controversial) and II

      Stage IIIA: neoadjuvant therapy followed by surgery or definitive chemoradiation

      Stage IIIB (without pleural effusion): inoperable, chemoradiation

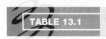

TABLE 13.1   **TNM Descriptions**

Primary tumor (T)
  TX: Primary tumor cannot be assessed, or tumor proved by the presence of malignant
    cells in sputum or bronchial washes but not visualized with imaging or bronchoscopy
  T0: No evidence of primary tumor
  Ti$_s$: Carcinoma *in situ*
  T1: Tumor ≤3 cm in greatest dimension, surrounded by lung or visceral pleura, without
    bronchoscopic evidence of invasion more proximal than the lobar bronchus a (i.e., not
    in the main bronchus)
  T2: Tumor with any of the following features of size or extent: > cm in greatest dimension;
    involves main bronchus, >2 cm distal to the carina; invades the visceral pleura;
    associated with atelectasis or obstructive pneumonitis that extends to the hilar region
    but does not involve the entire lung
  T3: Tumor of any size that directly invades any of the following: chest wall (including
    superior sulcus tumors), diaphragm, mediastinal pleura, parietal pericardium; or tumor
    in the main bronchus <2 cm distal to the carina, but without involvement of the carina;
    or associated atelectasis or obstructive pneumonitis of the entire lung
  T4: Tumor of any size that invades any of the following: mediastinum, heart, great vessels,
    trachea, esophagus, vertebral body, carina; or tumor with a malignant pleural or
    pericardial effusion, or with satellite tumor nodule(s) within the ipsilateral primary-tumor
    lobe of the lung

Regional lymph nodes (N)
  NX: Regional lymph nodes cannot be assessed
  N0: No regional lymph node metastasis N1: Metastasis to ipsilateral peribronchial and/or
    ipsilateral hilar lymph nodes, and
  Intrapulmonary nodes involved by direct extension of the primary tumor N2: Metastasis to
    ipsilateral mediastinal and/or subcarinal lymph node(s)
  N3: Metastasis to contralateral mediastinal, contralateral hilar, ipsilateral or contralateral
    scalene, or supraclavicular lymph node(s)

Distant metastasis (M)
  MX: Presence of distant metastasis cannot be assessed
  M0: No distant metastasis
  M1: Distant metastasis present including separate metastatic tumor nodule(s) in the
    ipsilateral nonprimary tumor lobe(s) of the lung

Stage Grouping: TNM subsets	
Stage	TNM subset
Stage 0	T$_{is}$: Carcinoma *in situ*
Stage IA	T1 N0 M0
Stage IB	T2 N0 M0
Stage IIA	T1 N1 M0
Stage IIB	T2 N1 M0
	T3 N0 M0
Stage IIIA	T3 N1 M0
	T1 N2 M0, T2 N2 M0, T3 N2 M0
Stage IIIB	T4 N0 M0, T4 N1 M0, T4 N2 M0
	T4 N3 M0
	T1 N3 M0, T2 N3 M0, T3 N3 M0
Stage IV	Any T, any N, M1

TABLE 13.2	Expected 5-Year Survival (with Treatment)	
Stage	**TNM subset**	**Average 5-year survival**
Stage IA	T1 N0 M0	82%
Stage IB	T2 N0 M0	68%
Stage IIA	T1 N1 M0	52%
Stage IIB	T2 N1 M0	40%
	T3 N0 M0	
Stage IIIA	T3 N1 M0	9%–15%, depending on subset
	T1–3 N2 M0	
Stage IIIB	T4 N0–2 M0	<5%
	T1–4 N3 M0	
Stage IV	Any T, any N, M1	NA

NA, not applicable.

Stage IIIB (with malignant pleural effusion) and stage IV: platinum-based doublet chemotherapy for those with good PS and single-agent chemotherapy or best supportive care (BSC) for those with poor PS. Patients with non squamous cell cancer with no brain metastasis, hemoptysis, or bleeding diathesis are appropriate candidates for chemotherapy with bevacizumab.

2. **Stages I and II.** Tl or T2 without extrapulmonary nodal disease (i.e., N2 or N3) is treated surgically whenever complete resection is possible. Preoperative assessment should determine stage (for potential resection), cardiopulmonary reserve (whether intended resection is possible), and perioperative risk of intended procedure. Suitable surgical candidates are those with estimated forced expiratory volume in 1 second (FEV_1) after pneumonectomy of more than 1.2 L, maximal O_2 consumption greater than 15 to 20 mL/kg/minute, no hypercarbia (more than 50 mm Hg), and no cor pulmonale. Patients are instructed to stop smoking at least 2 weeks before surgery. Stage of disease, age of patient, and extent of resection significantly affect mortality, which averages approximately 3% to 7%. Lobectomy is the most commonly used procedure and is equivalent to pneumonectomy when complete resection is achieved. Segmentectomy and wedge resection are associated with two- to threefold increased risk of local recurrence (*Ann Thorac Surg* 1995;60:615–623) and should be reserved for situations in which lobectomy cannot be done. Pneumonectomy is indicated if the tumor or lymph nodes involve the proximal bronchus or pulmonary artery or cross the major fissures. If chest wall is involved, then *en bloc* resection of tumor with the involved chest mass and a minimum of 2 cm of normal chest wall in all directions beyond the tumor are recommended.

Definitive RT is a good alternative for patients who are poor surgical candidates because of comorbid conditions. Selection of patients for RT is based largely on extent of the primary tumor and the prognostic factors. Survival after RT depends on PS (1 to 2), radiation dose (more than 60 Gy), tumor size, and complete response by 6 months after completion of RT.

Preoperative RT *is* not considered appropriate in early-stage lung cancer and postoperative radiotherapy (PORT) is not indicated in stage I disease. PORT meta-analysis revealed increased mortality (*Lancet* 1998;352:257–263). In patients with Nl or N2 disease, two studies by the Lung Cancer Study Group (LCSG) and British Medical Research Council (BMRC) concluded that PORT could improve local control but did not affect overall survival, possibly because of lack of effect on systemic disease (*N Engl J Med* 1986;315:1377–1381; *Br J Cancer* 1996;74:632–639). Patients with incompletely resected tumors or tumors with multiple nodal level involvement or bulky extracapsular extension, however, are generally treated with PORT.

Adjuvant chemotherapy is now considered standard treatment in the management of completely resected NSCLC tumors except stage IA. The International Adjuvant Lung Cancer Trial (IALT) reported a 4% improvement in the 5-year survival for patients receiving cisplatin-based adjuvant chemotherapy versus patients on observation alone after completely resected NSCLC (*N Engl J Med* 2004;350:351–360). Subsequently results from the (NCIC) National Cancer Institute of Canada JBR10 (stage IB and II) and Adjuvant Navelbine International Trialists Association (ANITA) (Stage IB, II, and IIIA) reported 8% to 15% improvement in survival with cisplatin-based chemotherapy. Interestingly, the Cancer and Leukemia Group B (CALGB) 9633 (included only Stage IB) initially reported improvement in overall survival with adjuvant paclitaxel and carboplatin, but a more recent follow-up failed to confirm these initial observations.

Results from a phase III trail by the Japanese Lung Cancer Research Group reported improved survival in resected adenocarcinoma stage IB patients receiving adjuvant chemotherapy with (uracil and tegafur) UFT (*N Engl J Med* 2004;350:1713–1721). Tegafur is administered orally and it is converted to 5-fluorouracil *in vivo*. It is currently not available in the United States.

We recommend cisplatin-based adjuvant chemotherapy in completely resected stage IB, II, and III NSCLC. There is no evidence that adjuvant chemotherapy improves survival in resected stage IA NSCLC.

3. **Stage III.** Stage IIIA includes T3 Nl or N2 nodal disease with a significant difference in prognosis, with the latter being worse. Patients with superior sulcus syndrome without mediastinal lymph gland involvement or disease involving the spine are candidates for surgery following induction chemoradiation.

Surgery is an option for patients with T3N1 disease followed by adjuvant chemotherapy. The role of surgery in patients with mediastinal lymph gland involvement was the subject of the intergroup study 0139. This study randomized patients with N2 disease to chemotherapy (cisplatin and etoposide [PE]) and radiation followed by surgery or chemotherapy and radiation alone. There was no improvement in overall survival with the addition of surgery following chemoradiation (*J Clin Oncol* 2005;23:624s). The study also reported higher treatment-related mortality in patients receiving pneumonectomy after preoperative radiation. The European Organization for Research and Treatment of Cancer (EORTC) 08941 randomized patients to surgery or RT after three cycles of platinum-based chemotherapy (*J Clin Oncol* 2006;24:18s). There was no significant difference in overall survival between the surgical and radiation arm. At present, it is a reasonable option to offer definitive chemoradiation for patients with locally advanced NSCLC. When mediastinal involvement is detected only at the time of resection, adjuvant chemotherapy should be considered as mentioned earlier. The role for PORT in this setting is uncertain. Patients with superior sulcus syndrome without mediastinal lymph gland involvement or disease involving the spine are candidates for surgery following induction chemoradiation.

The Radiation Therapy Oncology Group (RTOG) trial in 1987 established 60 Gy (in 30 daily fractions over a 6-week period) as the lowest optimal radiation dose for the treatment of lung cancer. Although a twice-daily fractionation regimen (total, 69.6 Gy) as well an accelerated fractionation regimen (54 Gy over a 2.5-week period) was found to have survival benefit at 2 years over the conventional regimen, the use is limited by increased esophagitis, pneumonitis, and logistic difficulties associated with twice-daily therapy. The use of three-dimensional or conformal RT may reduce the toxicity to the adjacent normal lung. RT alone is not an optimal therapy in patients with unresectable stage III NSCLC and good PS, as the 5-year survival rates are only 5%.

It has been proved now that addition of chemotherapy to RT improves survival in patients with stage III NSCLC over RT alone. Chemotherapy can be administered either before the initiation of RT (sequential) or in conjunction with RT (concurrent). Concurrent chemoradiation is superior to sequential chemotherapy followed by thoracic radiation (*J Clin Oncol* 1999;17:2692–2699; *Lung Cancer* 2000;29:93; *Proc Am Soc Clin Oncol* 2001;20:1246). The concurrent chemoradiation approach is associated with increased incidence of acute esophagitis and pneumonitis. The role of consolidation chemotherapy was evaluated in a phase II study. Concurrent administration of PE with RT, followed by three cycles of docetaxel, was associated with an impressive median survival of 26 months, and 3-year survival of 37% in patients with stage IIIB NSCLC (*J Clin Oncol* 2003;14:2004–2010). Preliminary results from a phase III study suggest a higher proportion of febrile neutropenia, pulmonary toxicity, and deaths in patients receiving docetaxel consolidation chemotherapy (*J Clin Oncol* 2006;24:7043).

Currently concurrent chemoradiation with cisplatin-based doublet is recommended in patients with good PS and unresected stage III disease. However, the role of consolidation chemotherapy and the optimal dosing of the regimen remain undefined. For patients with poor PS, radiation and chemotherapy are administered for symptom palliation and survival prolongation.

   a. Assessment of response. Although CT scans are commonly done approximately 2 months after the completion of RT, there is no clear correlation between the radiographic response (complete response, partial response, and stable disease) and survival, except for those who show evidence of progressive disease. There is no role for maintenance chemotherapy after the completion of chemoradiation in patients with stage III NSCLC.

4. Stage IV

   a. Initial therapy. Systemic chemotherapy improves survival in patients with previously untreated NSCLC over BSC. Some of the commonly used combination regimens in the treatment of NSCLC are listed in Table 13.3. It is important that both the patient and the physician realize that the goal of systemic chemotherapy is NOT to cure the disease but rather to achieve palliation of symptoms and prolongation of survival without unacceptable toxicity. It is now very clear that when administered at appropriate doses, platinum-based doublets that include a taxane, vinorelbine, or gemcitabine produce identical improvement in survival with slight differences in toxicity profile. An Eastern Cooperative Oncology Group (ECOG) trial that compared four of the commonly used platinum-based chemotherapeutic regimens found no significant difference in overall response rate (18.5%), median survival (7.5 months), 1-year survival (33%), or median time to progression (3.6 months) (*N Engl J Med* 2002;346:92–8). The treatment of stage IV disease should therefore be individualized and take into consideration the PS of the patient and the comorbid conditions. The addition of bevacizumab to carboplatin–paclitaxel regimen was associated with improved overall survival in patients with advanced nonsquamous NSCLC, with no brain metastases (*N Engl J Med* 2006;355:2542–50). There was a slightly increased incidence of treatment-related deaths (mainly from bleeding and myelosuppression) when patients were treated with chemotherapy and bevacizumab when compared with chemotherapy alone. Therefore, addition of bevacizumab would be indicated in patients with good PS, nonsquamous histology with no hemoptysis or brain metastasis. In patients with poor PS (PS2), single-agent chemotherapy (gemcitabine, vinorelbine, taxanes) is appropriate.

   Systemic chemotherapy should be given for approximately four to six cycles in the absence of progressive disease. There is no evidence to indicate that prolonged courses of chemotherapy result in improved survival. Patients

| TABLE 13.3 | Chemotherapy for Lung Cancer |

Drug	Dose	Route	Day	Cycle
Paclitaxel–carboplatin				
Paclitaxel	200 mg/m²	i.v. infused over 3-h period	d 1	Every 21 d
followed by				
Carboplatin	Dose calculated by the Calvert formula to an AUC of 6 mg/mL/min	i.v. infused over 1–2 h	d 1	
Premedications: Dexamethasone, 20 mg p.o., 12 and 6 h before paclitaxel; diphenhydramine, 50 mg i.v., and ranitidine, 50 mg i.v., both 30–60 min before paclitaxel.[a]				
Cisplatin–vinorelbine[b]				
Cisplatin	100 mg/m²	i.v.	d 1	Every 4 wk
Vinorelbine	25 mg/m²	i.v.	wkly	
Cisplatin–etoposide[c]				
Cisplatin	60 mg/m²	i.v.	d 1	Every 21–28 d
Etoposide	100 mg/m²/d	i.v.	d 1–3	
Cisplatin–gemcitabine[d]				
Cisplatin	100 mg/m²	i.v.	d 1, 2 or 15	Every 28 d
Gemcitabine	1,000 mg/m²	i.v.	d 1, 8, and 15	

NSCLC, non–small cell lung cancer; AUC, area under the time–concentration curve.

[a] Roa V, Connor A, Mitchell RB. *Proc Am Soc Clin Oncol* 1996;15:A1231, with permission.
[b] Wozniak, AJ, Crowley JJ, Balcerzak SP, et al. *J Clin Oncol* 1998;16:2459–2465, with permission.
[c] Longeval E, Klastersky J. *Cancer* 1982;50:2751–2756, with permission.
[d] Sandler A, Neumanitis C, Dehnam C, et al. *Proc Am Soc Clin Oncol* 1998;17:454a, and Ricci S, Antonuzzo A, Galli L, et al. *Proc Am Soc Clin Oncol* 1999;18:480a, with permission.

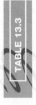

are closely monitored following completion of the initial chemotherapeutic regimen and should be considered for salvage chemotherapy if they are found to have progressive disease and have a good PS.

  b. **Second-line therapy.** Docetaxel has been shown to improve survival in patients who develop progressive disease following initial therapy with platinum-based doublet therapy over BSC. Moreover, docetaxel administered at a dose of 75 mg/m^2 every 3 weeks improved survival over vinorelbine or ifosfamide in a similar population of patients (*J Clin Oncol* 2000;18:2354–2362). More recent studies have shown weekly docetaxel to be as effective as an every 3-week regimen with lesser toxicity. Pemetrexed 500 mg/m^2 every 3 weeks in the second-line setting was reported to have response rate and overall survival similar to docetaxel (median survival of 8 months for both) and the toxicity profile was better than docetaxel. The epidermal growth factor receptor-tyrosine kinase (EGFR-TK) inhibitor erlotinib has been reported to improve survival compared to the best supportive in patients with advanced NSCLC following progressive disease (*N Engl J Med* 2005;353:123–132). In a phase I/II study, the combination of erlotinib and bevacizumab was shown to improve survival (median survival 13 months) in the second-line setting (*J Clin Oncol* 2005;23:2544–2555). A phase III study is under way to evaluate the efficacy of this combination. The future for NSCLC chemotherapy will depend on our better understanding the tumor signaling pathways and inhibition of these pathways with novel agents.

  c. **Role of surgery or RT in stage IV NSCLC.** An isolated metastatic lesion (e.g., brain) can be surgically resected before systemic therapy. Surgical intervention is also indicated in certain situations (e.g., metastatic lesion in weight-bearing bones, stabilization of spine). RT is indicated for palliation of the following:

    i. Atelectatic lobe, especially in COPD patients. Re-expansion is expected in 60% to 70% of patients if atelectasis has been present for less than 2 weeks.

    ii. Hemoptysis, intractable cough, and pain.

    iii. Metastatic disease. Bone: RT is used to alleviate pain and prevent impending fracture or compression syndrome. In case of pathologic fracture, RT is used in conjunction with orthopedic fixation to maintain function and activity. Brain: for solitary brain metastasis, better survival and function is seen when the lesion is resected before RT.

D. **Follow-up.** The recommendations with regard to follow-up imaging for patients who have been treated for NSCLC are somewhat arbitrary. We generally monitor patients with periodic physical examinations, CXR/CT imaging done at 6-month intervals for 3 to 5 years after they have had a curative resection.

  For patients who have completed chemoradiation for stage III NSCLC, we perform physical examinations, CXR/CT imaging every 6 months in the first 2 years and annually in the next 3 years.

E. **Background.** Lung cancer is the second most common cancer in both men and women in the United States. An estimated 213, 380 new cases will be diagnosed in 2007, accounting for 15% of all cancer diagnoses. On a global scale it is the most common cancer since 1985 and it is also the most common cause of cancer-related death (17.6%). Globally the age standardized incidence rates (ASR) are 35.5 per 100,000 in men and 12.1 per 100,000 in women. However, lung cancer incidence in men has declined by 3.3% and in women it has increased by 22%.

1. **Risk factors**

  a. **Tobacco use.** Cigarette smoking is responsible for at 90% of cases of lung cancer. The risk of dying of lung cancer is 22 times higher for male smokers and 12 times higher for female smokers compared with those who have never smoked. The risk of developing lung cancer is directly related to duration of smoking. This risk for developing lung cancer persists for a long time, even after stopping smoking.

b. **Asbestos.** Exposure increases the risk for the development of lung cancer, particularly in smokers.

c. **Age.** Both the incidence and the percentage of patients with advanced-stage disease increase with age.

d. **Genetic factors** (e.g., high metabolizers of debrisoquine, lack of class μ phenotype of glutathione transferase) probably contribute to the development of lung cancer in some patients.

e. **Exposure** to arsenic, beryllium, chromium, hydrocarbons, mustard gas, and uranium in mining workers and, less clearly, silicosis in smokers.

f. **Smoking status.** Approximately 90% of patients with lung cancer report a strong history of tobacco smoking. Lung cancer in "never smokers" (LCINS) is a distinct subset of lung cancer. Majority of patients with LCINS are women and the predominant histology is adenocarcinoma. EGFR-TK activating mutations are seen significantly more often in LCINS than tobacco-related lung cancer.

2. **Screening.** The regular use of the CXR as a method of screening for lung cancer has not been shown to affect long-term survival in three large prospective population studies. A large lung cancer screening study randomizing patients with a history of heavy tobacco use to conventional chest X-ray or CT screening is under way. Unless the study reports improved survival in the screened population with CT scans, the routine use of CT imaging for lung cancer screening is not recommended.

F. **Research initiatives.** Several molecularly targeted drugs are in development in advanced NSCLC. Some of these drugs include those that inhibit vascular endothelial growth factor (VEGF) pathway, epidermal growth factor (EGF) pathway and promote apoptosis

A large intergroup phase III study will compare conventional doses of thoracic radiation to higher doses of radiation (74 Gy) in patients with locally advanced NSCLC. On the basis of the promising results of bevacizumab in advanced NSCLC, a large intergroup study randomizing patients with resected NSCLC to cisplatin based doublet chemotherapy or chemotherapy with bevacizumab is currently underway.

1. **Prognostic factors.** The most important prognostic factors are stage, PS, and significant pretreatment weight loss (more than 5% to 10%). Women with lung cancer have a slightly better prognosis than men. Age and race have no prognostic significance per se. The role of other biologic factors (e.g., p53 mutations, *ras* oncogene activation) is less clear. The standardized uptake value (SUV) for fluorodeoxyglucose (FDG) in PET as a prognostic factor is being studied currently.

II. **SCLC**

A. **Presentation**

1. **Subjective.** Due to the primarily central endobronchial location of this tumor, presenting symptoms often include shortness of breath, wheezing, cough, hemoptysis, chest pain, and postobstructive phenomena such as pneumonitis. As the mediastinal lymph nodes are involved very commonly, patients can demonstrate SVC syndrome (10% of patients at time of diagnosis), hoarseness from recurrent laryngeal nerve involvement, and dysphagia. Thirty percent of patients at some point in their disease course will have brain metastases; 90% of such patients will be symptomatic from brain metastases. However, bone metastasis only rarely results in pain or pathologic fractures.

2. **Objective.** The importance of a good physical examination in these patients cannot be emphasized enough because more than two thirds of patients have obvious distant metastases, some of which can be recognized in the physical examination. This may include hepatomegaly, subcutaneous nodules, focal neurologic signs, palpable adenopathy, and bony tenderness. The most common sites of extrathoracic disease include bone (19% to 38% of all presenting patients), liver (17% to 34%), bone marrow (17% to 23%), and CNS (0% to 14%).

3. **Laboratory.** Approximately 50% to 60% of patients with liver metastasis will have mildly abnormal liver function on hepatic enzyme laboratory tests; most of these patients will not have severely compromised liver function, however. When bone marrow is involved, it takes extensive involvement to lead to myelosuppression evident in the complete blood count. Seventy percent of patients will have mediastinal lymph node involvement. Paraneoplastic syndromes are also much more common in small cell than NSCLC, and in one large series, 11% of patients had syndrome of inappropriate secretion of antidiuretic hormone (SIADH; see later).

On radiographic examination, these tumors are found to cavitate very infrequently. In comparison to those with non–small cell tumors, CXRs of small cell patients more often demonstrate hilar and mediastinal adenopathy, pneumonitis, and atelectasis and do not as often exhibit pleural effusions or involvement of the chest wall.

B. Workup and staging

1. **Workup.** The physician should aim for a cost effective workup that adequately stages the tumor for necessary therapeutic decisions. The key question is whether the patient has limited- or extensive-stage disease (defined later), because the therapy for patients with limited-stage disease includes thoracic radiation in addition to chemotherapy, whereas patients with extensive-stage disease would be treated with chemotherapy alone. Therefore once metastasis has been documented with extensive-stage disease, there is no need to document any other metastatic locations unless they are symptomatic, requiring palliative therapy.

Patients who do not have any evidence of overt metastatic disease should undergo CT of the chest and abdomen with contrast, a bone scan, and CT of the head with contrast to establish that disease is confined to one hemithorax (limited-stage disease). The role of a PET scan in staging workup of patients with SCLC remains investigational. Given the low yield associated with bone marrow biopsies, we do not advocate bone marrow biopsy in patients with SCLC for the purpose of staging.

2. **Staging.** The Veterans Administration Lung Group staging system currently in use in North America categorizes patients into limited-stage and extensive-stage disease. Limited stage is defined as tumor confined to one hemithorax and regional lymph nodes and is often subjectively defined by what can fit into one RT portal. Extensive stage is defined as any disease outside limited stage. Generally, 30% to 40% of patients will have limited-stage, and 60% to 70%, extensive-stage disease.

C. Therapy and prognosis

1. **Limited stage**

   a. **Therapy.** The current standard of care is combined-modality therapy with chemotherapy and RT.

      i. **Chemotherapy.** Although patients with SCLC respond to chemotherapy initially, almost all will relapse and die from the disease. Combination chemotherapy results in higher response rates and longer survival than does single-agent chemotherapy. The overall response rate for limited stage is estimated to be 80% to 90%. The combination of PE has been repeatedly demonstrated to yield similar or improved results as compared with any other studied combination and is easily one of the most commonly used chemotherapeutic regimens for patients with SCLC. In addition, this combination is tolerated well when administered in conjunction with thoracic radiation. We typically administer PE for four to six cycles for those patients who have no evidence of progressive disease.

      ii. **RT.** Administration of thoracic RT in conjunction with systemic chemotherapy has been shown to improve survival. A meta-analysis of 13 trials including 2,140 patients with limited disease demonstrated a higher survival rate for combined-modality approach with the combination of chemotherapy and thoracic RT as compared with combination chemotherapy alone (3-year survival increased from 8.9% to 14.3%; *N Engl J Med* 1992;327:1618–1624). Another meta-analysis of 11 randomized trials confirmed this improvement in survival and demonstrated improved local tumor control with this regimen as well; however, this analysis also demonstrated a mild increase in therapy-related mortality when combined modality was used instead of chemotherapy alone (*J Clin Oncol* 1992;10:890–895). The schedule of RT and temporal coordination with chemotherapy may be of some importance. It is possible but not proved that radiation early in the treatment course may be advantageous because of its ability to eradicate tumor cells before they have a chance of acquiring chemotherapy drug resistance. Additionally, it has been shown that radiation administered twice a day concurrent with chemotherapy results in an increased 5-year survival rate and decreased local failure rate compared with the same chemotherapeutic regimen administered concurrent with daily radiation (*N Engl J Med* 1999;340:265–271).

iii. **Prophylactic cranial irradiation (PCI).** For those limited-stage patients who demonstrate a complete response to induction chemotherapy , PCI should be considered to reduce the incidence of brain metastasis and improve survival. The role of PCI in patients with SCLC has been debated for a while, because of initial randomized studies demonstrating no definite improvement in survival and because of concerns about effects on brain function. A meta-analysis of 987 patients demonstrated a 16% decrease in mortality, 5.4% increase in 3-year survival, decreased incidence of brain metastasis, and prolonged disease-free survival in limited-stage patients who received PCI after complete response to induction chemotherapy (*N Engl J Med* 1999;341:476–484). In addition, studies have failed to consistently demonstrate cognitive deterioration after PCI. Administering PCI after chemoradiation and in low doses per fractions could further reduce the risk of neurologic sequelae.

iv. **Surgery.** Addition of surgical resection after chemoradiation has not been shown to improve survival in patients with SCLC (*Chest* 1994;106: 320S–323S). If patients are found to have SCLC after resection and have no evidence of distant disease, they should be treated with chemotherapy with or without radiation.

2. **Extensive stage**
   a. **Therapy.** The current standard of care is combination chemotherapy. There is no role for thoracic irradiation in this stage except for palliation of symptoms. Chemotherapy improves survival in patients with extensive-stage disease; the overall response rate is 60% to 80%. Regimens used in this stage are similar to those used for limited-stage therapy. The combination PE is a commonly used regimen in patients with extensive-stage SCLC. It has demonstrated that the combination of carboplatin and etoposide (CE) is as efficacious as PE in offering improved survival in patients with SCLC (*Semin Oncol* 1994;21:23–30). Higher doses of PE, when compared with standard doses of CE, resulted only in increased toxicity without any increase in survival. *In vitro* drug-sensitivity testing on pathologic samples of patients has been evaluated in a prospective trial to determine if patient-specific chemotherapy is a possibility, because this could eliminate the problem of tumor resistance to therapy; however, the results of this trial revealed that this is of limited clinical utility, partly because of the time the testing takes (*J Natl Cancer Inst* 1990;82:117–124). Maintenance chemotherapy has not been shown to improve overall survival (*J Clin Oncol.* 2001;19(8):2114–22).

   Initial reports indicated addition of paclitaxel to PE improved response rates. However, two phase III randomized trials failed to detect significant improvement in survival with the addition of paclitaxel. In addition, treatment-related mortality was higher in the paclitaxel arm. In a phase II study from Japan the combination of cisplatin and irinotecan was reported to be superior to PE (median survival 12.8 vs. 9.4 months) in patients with extensive-stage SCLC (*N Engl J Med* 2002;346:85–91). A multicenter study in the United States did not detect any significant difference in survival between the treatment arms (*J Clin Oncol* 2006;24(13):2038–43). Similar results have been reported with cisplatin–topotecan combination (*J Clin Oncol* 2006;24:2044–2051). The combination of platinum etoposide continues to be the standard treatment of small cell lung cancer. Administration of PCI following chemotherapy improves survival in patients with extensive stage SCLC (*J Clin Oncol* (Meeting Abstracts) 200725:4).

- **i. Relapsed SCLC.** In spite of a high response rate, most patients with SCLC eventually have relapse of the disease and die of progressive disease. There are two categories of relapsed SCLC: sensitive relapse, those who relapse 3 months after the completion of therapy, and resistant relapse, those who have progressive disease during initial chemotherapy or those who have relapse within 3 months of completion of therapy. Although the response rates for the subgroup of patients with sensitive relapse is approximately 25%, fewer than 10% of patients with resistant relapse respond to salvage therapy. A number of single agents have been reported to be active in this setting. They include topotecan, paclitaxel, gemcitabine, and vinorelbine. Topotecan is the recommended single agent for salvage chemotherapy in sensitive relapse patients. A phase III trial comparing topotecan to cyclophosphamide, adriamycin, and vincristine (CAV) reported similar survival and response rates, but lesser toxicity with topotecan (*J Clin Oncol* 1999;17:658–667). In addition, topotecan achieved better symptom (dyspnea, anorexia, hoarseness, fatigue) control than CAV. When possible, patients with relapsed SCLC should be enrolled in clinical trials.

D. Prognosis. Unfavorable prognostic factors include extensive stage, poor PS, older age, hyponatremia, male gender, and elevated serum lactate dehydrogenase (LDH) and alkaline phosphatase. Of these, stage and PS are most powerfully associated with prognosis. The most important risk factor for treatment-related mortality, which can approach 5% in aggressive limited-stage therapy, is PS. Additionally, amplification of the *c-myc* oncogene is linked with shorter survival.

The natural history of the progression of this disease is that of rapid growth and early dissemination. The median survival of patients with limited-stage SCLC is 10 to 16 months. The reported 5-year survival varies from 14% to 28%. One third of limited-stage patients who remain disease-free for 2 years will still develop recurrent cancer. Median survival in extensive stage is 7 to 11 months, but only 2 to 4 months if untreated. From 50% to 80% of patients who survive longer than 2 years will have metastases to the brain. Only 10% to 15% of patients with extensive disease will survive to 2 years. An extremely small number of 5-year survivors (fewer than 1%) have been documented.

E. Complications
1. **Therapy related.** Therapy-related mortality overall is from none to 8%, greater in extensive-stage patients. The most common therapeutic complication is that of myelosuppression and associated neutropenia and thrombocytopenia.
   a. **Chemotherapy.** The chemotherapeutic regimens used in the treatment of this disease are very toxic. Oral etoposide has been associated with alopecia, nausea, and myelosuppression in a significant number of patients. CE has been demonstrated to produce less nausea, vomiting, neurotoxicity, and nephrotoxicity than PE (i.e., 18% of CE patients experienced neurotoxicity as compared with 53% of PE patients). Most of these side effects in PE therapy are attributed to the cisplatin component, which is well known to cause nephrotoxicity and neurotoxicity. Irinotecan is associated with GI (gastrointestinal) toxicity, nausea, and vomiting. Topotecan is associated

with hematologic toxicity, including anemia and thrombocytopenia. Furthermore, cyclophosphamide is associated with hemorrhagic cystitis, and rarely patients will experience secondary acute myelocytic leukemia (AML), especially those who received prolonged therapy with nitrosoureas and procarbazine. Although chemotherapy initiation is associated with acute tumor lysis syndrome for many cancers, SCLC is not often associated with this syndrome, and therefore routine use of allopurinol is not necessary. Finally, patients with ectopic Cushing's syndrome are more prone to experience chemotherapeutic complications.

b. RT. Twice-daily RT has been associated with more severe esophagitis than once-daily therapy. Esophagitis can lead to dehydration from decreased oral intake, which often requires administration of intravenous fluids. Combined-modality pneumonitis, seen as cough, dyspnea, and/or infiltrates on CXR, can be treated with corticosteroids. Chemotherapy combined with radiation, especially in cases of concurrent administration, leads to significantly greater myelosuppression than does either modality alone. In one trial, 26% of patients required hospitalization for severe pulmonary toxicity related to combined-modality therapy.

c. Infection. While undergoing chemotherapy, one third of patients will have a fever, but infection can be documented in only 5%. Anorectal infections, seen often as only perirectal pain or tenderness, are documented in 6% to 32% of patients; the major risk factor for anorectal infections is chemotherapy-induced neutropenia. Additionally, herpes zoster can be problematic in these patients; one study reported an incidence of 12% in patients undergoing the initial course of chemotherapy, whereas previous studies had reported a much lower incidence. Adrenocorticotropic hormone (ACTH)-producing tumors are associated with higher rates of infection. Granulocyte colony-stimulating factor (G-CSF) administration during chemotherapy can decrease the incidence of culture-documented infections and neutropenic fever (decreased from 77% to 40% in one prospective trial). In randomized trials, irinotecan with cisplatin combinations have demonstrated less hematologic toxicity including neutropenia than the PE regimen.

2. Disease related

a. SVC syndrome. This neoplasm is often associated with SVC syndrome. Chemotherapy is adequate treatment for this if patients are not otherwise going to receive thoracic radiation; however, radiation is acceptable therapy for SVC syndrome in patients for whom thoracic radiation is already indicated.

b. Brain metastasis. Of patients with SCLC, 30% will have metastasis to the CNS, and 90% of these patients will be symptomatic from this at some point. Symptoms can often be palliated with RT (using a higher dose than that used for PCI), but chemotherapy alone has also been shown to induce regression of these metastatic tumors. Some radiation oncologists also use steroids with radiation to help with symptom palliation. Unfortunately, symptom response duration is often short after palliative therapy for CNS metastasis.

c. Carcinomatous leptomeningitis. Approximately 2.5% of patients at some point in their disease course will have carcinomatous leptomeningitis. Median survival after this diagnosis is made in less than 2 months. Treatment is often intrathecal methotrexate with or without irradiation. This will sterilize the cerebrospinal fluid (CSF) malignant cells in some cases, but such sterilization is not always associated with amelioration of neurologic derangements.

F. Follow-up

1. Secondary malignancies. These patients are at high risk of developing other malignancies related to smoking. The cumulative risk for a second malignancy 15 years after diagnosis of SCLC is 70%. Overall, in 20% of long-term survivors in one large analysis, secondary malignancies developed. The risk of having a second primary lung cancer increases with time (14.4% after 10 years). If a new lung mass develops in a long-term survivor, the physician must obtain a biopsy to rule out a new primary malignancy that may not be SCLC. Additionally, these patients are at increased risk for other tobacco-related malignancies such as cancer of the upper aerodigestive tract (12.6% after 10 years).

2. Smoking. These patients should be strongly encouraged to stop smoking. Once a smoker quits, the risk of any type of lung cancer begins to decline, but it takes at least a decade for such patients to approach a risk equivalent to that of a nonsmoker.

G. Background

1. Epidemiology. The incidence of SCLC has been declining over the last few decades, accounting for only 14% of all newly diagnosed lung cancer. It is a disease of the elderly, with age peaks at 70 to 74 years in men and 60 to 69 years in women. The incidence of SCLC in the United States has decreased in the recent years (*J Clin Oncol* 2006;24:4539–4544). The proportion of SCLC among all primary lung cancer subtypes has decreased from 17.3% in 1986 to 12.9% in 2002. In addition, there has been a dramatic increase in the incidence among women from 28% in 1973 to 50% in 2002.

2. Risk factors. Almost all patients with this cancer have a history of tobacco abuse: only 2% of 500 patients treated at the National Cancer Institute in one series denied ever smoking. Exposure to radioactive radon in mining also may be a risk factor.

3. Pathogenesis. SCLC is thought to arise from peptide hormone-secreting basal neuroendocrine cells, which are much more common in fetal than in adult lung tissue. Often, but not always, these cells will stain positive with silver staining. Electron microscopy can demonstrate neurosecretory granules in these cells. Most small cell lines have upregulated expression of L-Dopa decarboxylase, gastrin-releasing peptide (GRP), and enolase, all of which point to the neuroendocrine origin of the cells. GRP is an autocrine growth factor. Antibodies to bombesin, a molecule analogous to GRP, can inhibit small cell line growth *in vitro*. Unfortunately, this has not been found to be clinically effective as an antitumor agent.

4. Pathology. The classic "oat cell" type of small cell is represented by small round cells characterized by dark-staining nuclei, scant cytoplasm, and few to no nucleoli. The 1988 International Association for Study of Lung Cancer (IASLC) classified SCLC into three subtypes. They are pure small cell, mixed small cell/large cell and a mixed tumor with predominant SCLC and some areas of NSCLC. All subtypes demonstrate the classic "salt and pepper" chromatin distribution, cell size two to three times that of a mature lymphocyte, nuclear molding, and numerous atypical mitoses. Additionally, these mixed tumors and large cell/small cell mixed tumors have not been found to demonstrate any significant difference in disease progression or response to treatment. Histologically, the distinction between SCLC and NSCLC can be difficult, and often a tumor is classified as combined, meaning it contains elements of both SCLC and NSCLC but should be clinically addressed as a small cell tumor.

5. Paraneoplastic syndromes. SCLC has a strong association with certain paraneoplastic syndromes that result from peptide hormone secretion from tumor cells. Syndromes that are specifically associated with SCLC include ectopic ACTH secretion (leading to Cushing's syndrome), SIADH, and Lambert-Eaton syndrome. The endocrinologic paraneoplastic syndromes can be relieved by chemotherapy; however, often the neurologic syndromes are not affected by antitumor therapy.

H. Current focus

1. New chemotherapeutic regimens. Despite some promising results with molecularly targeted therapy in NSCLC, several molecularly targeted agents (imatinib, gefitinib, matrix metalloproteinase inhibitors) have had disappointing results in the treatment of SCLC. Drugs inhibiting VEGF pathway are being actively studied in SCLC.

Suggested Readings

American Society of Clinical Oncology. Clinical practice guidelines for the treatment of unresectable non–small-cell lung cancer. Adopted on May 16, 1997 by the American Society of Clinical Oncology. *J Clin Oncol* 1997;15:2996–3018.

Ettinger D, Johnson B. Update: NCCN small cell and non–small cell lung cancer clinical practice guidelines. *J Natl Compr Canc Netw* 2005;3(Suppl 1):S17–S21.

Faivre-Finn C, Lee LW, Lorigan P, et al. Thoracic radiotherapy for limited stage small cell cancer: controversies and Future developments. *Clin Oncol* 2005;17:591–598.

Osterland K. Chemotherapy in small cell lung cancer. *Eur Respir* 2001;18:1026–1043.

Penland SK, Socinski MA. Management of unresectable stage III non–small cell lung cancer: the role of combined chemoradiation. *Semin Radiat Oncol* 2004;14:326–334.

Pfister DG, Johnson DH, Azzoli CG, et al. American Society of Clinical Oncology treatment of unresectable non–small cell lung cancer guideline: update 2003. *J Clin Oncol* 2004;22:330–353.

Schrump AN, Altorki NK, Henschke CL. Non–small cell lung cancer. In: DeVita VT, Hellman S, Rosenberg SA, eds. *Cancer: principles and practice of oncology*, 7th ed. Philadelphia: Lippincott Williams & Wilkins, 2005.

Spira A, Ettinger DS. Multidisciplinary management of lung cancer. *N Engl of Med* 2004;350:379–392.

Turrisi AT, Kim K, Blum R, et al. Twice-daily compared with once-daily thoracic radiotherapy in limited small-cell lung cancer treated concurrently with cisplatin and etoposide. *N Engl J Med* 1999;340:265–271.

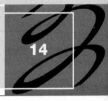

BREAST CANCER

14

Rama Suresh and Mathew J. Ellis

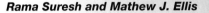

I. BACKGROUND

A. Epidemiology. In developed countries, breast cancer is the most commonly diagnosed malignancy in women and is the second leading cause of cancer death. In 2006, estimated new breast cancers in the United States were 212,920 and deaths, 40,600. Analysis of the Surveillance, Epidemiology, and End Results (SEER) data showed that breast cancer incidence rates were stable between 1973 and 1980. In the early 1980s, the incidence rates increased steeply because of increased detection by screening mammography. More recently, total incidence of breast cancer has marginally declined (by 4.8% between 2001 and 2003—SEER data). The overall mortality from breast cancer has also seen recent declines due to better screening and adjuvant treatment.

B. Identifiable risk factors. Many women with breast cancer do not have any of the known risk factors, and the relative risks associated with each known factor are often quite modest. However, these factors have been formulated into several models to predict overall risk, of which the Gail model is the one most often used in the United States (http://www.cancer.gov/bcrisktool/). Other, perhaps better, models may also be used (e.g., Tyler-Cuzick) and the question of which model is best remains controversial.

1. Demographic factors. Women are 100 times more likely to have breast cancer as compared to men. SEER data analysis indicates that the incidence of breast cancer increases sharply between the ages 35 and 75, starts to plateau between 75 and 80, and then decreases. In the United States, breast cancer incidence is the highest in whites and the lowest in the Native American population (Fig. 14.1).

2. Hereditary factors. Only approximately 10% of patients with breast cancer have first-degree relatives with the disease. The risk of true hereditary breast cancer, where the inheritance pattern suggests the presence of a dominant cancer gene, is determined by the number of first- or second-degree maternal or paternal relatives with breast cancer and their age at diagnosis. When a genetic anomaly can be detected it is usually in either the *BRCA1* or the *BRCA2* gene. Women with a loss-of-function mutation in a *BRCA1* and *BRCA2* allele have a 65% and 45% cumulative risk of developing breast cancer respectively (*Am J Hum Genet* 2003;72(5):1117–1130). BRCA1 and BRCA2 mutations are more common in Ashkenazi Jews, where 2% of the population are carriers. Importantly, ovarian cancer has also been strongly linked to BRCA1 mutations (44% by age 70) and to a less extent BRCA2 mutations (11% by age 70) and all patients with BRCA1 or BRCA2 mutations should consider a prophylactic bilateral oophorectomy after child bearing has been completed. Although an occasional case of primary peritoneal adenocarcinoma despite bilateral oophorectomy is described, the incidence is low, particularly if the surgeon was careful to remove all ovarian and fallopian tube tissue. A hysterectomy is not medically necessary since there is no increased risk of endometrial cancer. Both *BRCA1* and *BRCA2* are also general cancer predisposition genes with an increase in carriers of male breast, prostate, stomach, and pancreatic cancers. Other less common familial syndromes associated with inherited breast cancer risk include Li-Fraumeni and Li-Fraumeni-like syndrome (TP53 and CHK2), Cowden syndrome (PTEN), Peutz-Jaegers syndrome (LKB1), and homozygotes with ataxia telangiectasia (ATM).

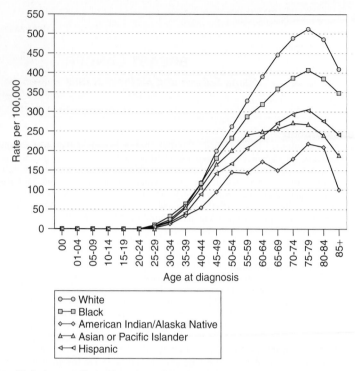

Figure 14.1. Age specific incidence rate of female breast cancer by race from SEER registries 1992 to 2002.

3. **History of breast cancer.** Women with a previous invasive breast cancer are at risk of developing second breast cancer at an annual rate of 0.5% to 0.7%. Women with history of ductal carcinoma *in situ* (DCIS) are at an increased risk of developing ipsilateral and contralateral breast cancers (cumulative incidence of 4.1% after 5 years).

4. **Benign breast disease.** Nonproliferative breast lesions such as cysts and ductal ectasia do not increase the risk for cancer. Proliferative breast lesions with atypia such as atypical ductal hyperplasia carry a 4- to 6-fold increase in the risk of developing cancer. Proliferative lesions without atypia such as fibroadenoma, intraductal papilloma, sclerosing adenosis, and radial scar carry a 1.5- to 2-fold risk of cancer. LCIS is associated with a 1% annual risk of developing cancer in either breast.

5. **Endocrine factors.** Higher endogenous estrogen levels are associated with an increased risk of breast cancer (Multiple Outcomes for Raloxifene Evaluation (MORE) trial and the Nurses Health Study). Early menarche, late menopause, nulliparity, and later age at first pregnancy increase the risk of breast cancer presumably by elevating endogenous estrogen levels. Oral contraceptives (OCP) were initially thought to increase breast cancer risk slightly but subsequent studies have not confirmed this association (*N Engl J Med* 2002;346:2025–2032). Randomized studies of hormone replacement therapy (HRT) in postmenopausal women show that HRT increases incidence of breast cancer, particularly when a combined estrogen-progestin formulation is used. In the Women's Health Initiative trial, there was a 1.24-fold increased risk with combined estrogen and progesterone but no increased risk with estrogen-alone preparations (*JAMA*

2003;289:3243–3253, *JAMA* 2006;295:1647–1657). The Million Women Study, however, showed that both estrogen-alone and combined estrogen and progesterone preparations increase the risk. The risk is higher with estrogen and progesterone combination (hazard ratio of 2.0) as compared to estrogen alone (hazard ratio of 1.3) (*Lancet* 2003;362:419–427).

6. **Dietary Factors.** Postmenopausal obesity is associated with an increased incidence and mortality from breast cancer—perhaps through increased levels of circulating estrogen as a result of aromatization of adrenal androgens in adipose tissue. There have been mixed results regarding associations with dietary fat intake, vitamins E, C, and A, selenium, alcohol, and caffeine.

7. **Environmental factors.** Women exposed to chest wall radiation, especially as children, adolescents, and young adults have been shown to be at substantially increased risk for developing breast cancer throughout their lives. This a particularly severe problem in young women who received mantle radiation for Hodgkin's disease, where the lifetime risk for breast cancer is at least 19% by age 50 (average population risk at that age is approximately 4%) and one suspects that the lifetime incidence may be even higher. Other environmental factors such as organochlorines, silicone breast implants, electromagnetic field, cigarette smoking, antibiotic use, and hair dyes have not been shown conclusively to be associated with an increased risk of breast cancer.

C. **Histopathology of breast cancer.** The *in situ* carcinomas of the breast are classified as ductal (DCIS), lobular (LCIS), or Paget's disease of the nipple (which may have an associated component of DCIS or invasive carcinoma). Most invasive breast cancers are adenocarcinomas, with invasive ductal carcinoma being the commonest (80%) and invasive lobular carcinoma occurring approximately 10% of the time. Less common histopathologic types represent the remaining 10% and include the medullary, tubular, mucinous, papillary, squamous cell, adenoid cystic, metaplastic, secretory, cribriform, and undifferentiated types. Paget's disease of the nipple is a specialized form of ductal carcinoma that arises from the main excretory ducts in the breasts and extends to involve the skin of the nipple and areola. The pathologic hallmark is the presence of malignant intraepithelial adenocarcinoma cells (Paget's cells) occurring singly or in small groups within the epidermis of the nipple. It can just involve the nipple/areolar complex or be associated with either DCIS or invasive carcinoma. Inflammatory carcinomas infiltrate widely throughout the breast tissue and involve the lymphatic structures in the dermis, producing swelling, erythema, and tenderness in the involved breast. The diagnosis is clinical and requires redness or erythema to be present. Peau d'orange can be present without erythema and should not be considered inflammatory breast cancer (IBC). Traditionally the prognosis for IBC has been considered to be poor; however, *HER2* gene amplification is present in approximately 50% of cases and with trastuzumab therapy prognosis, is likely to be considerably better than in the past.

D. **Screening.** American Cancer Society has the following recommendations for breast cancer screening.

1. Starting at age 40, yearly mammograms should be done and continued for as long as a woman is in good health.

2. Clinical breast examination by a physician approximately every 3 years for women in their 20s and 30s and annually for women aged 40 and above.

3. Breast self-examination monthly starting with women in their 20s.

4. Women at increased risk for breast cancer such as those with genetic mutation or significant family history of breast cancer should have more frequent examinations, and probably have earlier mammograms (starting at age 25 or 5 years earlier than when the youngest relative was diagnosed with breast cancer), ultrasonography (US) or magnetic resonance imaging (MRI).

Full-field digital mammography is a technique similar to film mammography but the images are captured electronically and stored in a computer. Digital mammography is more expensive but has the advantage of easy storage and ability to manipulate the image for clearer definition. Studies have shown that the diagnostic accuracy is superior to that with film mammography in women with dense breasts, women under the age of 50, and premenopausal and peri-menopausal women (N *Engl J Med* 2005;353:1773–1783). US of the breast may help in women with dense breasts as an adjunct to screening mammography (*Ann Oncol* 2004;15(Suppl 1):15–16). MRI of the breast as a screening technique is recommended only for women who are at an increased familial risk (more than 20% lifetime risk) of breast cancer with or without BRCA1 or BRCA2 mutation. In those patients, MRI is recommended in addition to yearly mammography. In other patients, MRI of the breast is not recommended for routine screening (N *Engl J Med* 2004;351:427–437; *J Clin Oncol* 2005;23:8469–8476). Ductal lavage is considered investigational and has, to date, not proved to be useful for screening or diagnosis.

II. PRESENTATION

A. History. The most common symptom is a painless breast mass. Some patients may have pain associated with the mass, unilateral nipple discharge, skin changes over the breast mass and nipple retraction. Patients who have had the breast mass for a longer time may present with an ulcerating mass and patients with inflammatory disease will complain of a "warm or hot" breast and have obvious erythema.

B. Physical examination. A careful examination of the area should be performed after the patient has disrobed to the waist. Inspection of the area should include nipple and areolar complex for ulceration, thickening, and nonmilky nipple discharge; the breast for size, symmetry, and visible masses, skin for color and thickening called the *peau d'orange* or *orange skin* appearance; and the axilla and supraclavicular area for visible enlarged lymph nodes. The inspection should be done with the patient sitting in four views; with the arm against the side, the arm above the head, the arm on the hip position, and leaning forward. For palpation of the patient's breast, the patient should be supine with her arms raised above head. The entire breast including the tail of the breast should be palpated using the palmar aspect of the fingers in concentric circles. If a mass is felt then its size, shape, location, tenderness, consistency, and mobility should be noted. If nipple discharge is elicited by pressing the areolar area, the color, consistency, and quantity of any discharge should be recorded. The axilla, infraclavicular, and supraclavicular area should be palpated for lymph nodes in the sitting posture with the arm muscles relaxed.

III. WORKUP AND STAGING OF BREAST CANCER

A. Evaluation of a breast mass. Though the physical characteristics on examination can make a physician suspect breast cancer, a biopsy provides definitive pathologic diagnosis. Mammogram helps evaluate the mass as well the rest of the ipsilateral breast and the contralateral breast. DCIS is usually an incidental finding on mammography as a cluster of microcalcifications. Suspicious lesions on mammogram should be biopsied by a core needle technique. Palpable masses may be biopsied by core needle, and although fine needle aspiration can also be used, a core has the advantage of distinguishing between invasive disease (requiring a lymph node evaluation) and DCIS (where nodal exploration can often be avoided). Incisional/excision biopsy for diagnosis is rarely necessary and should be discouraged because once the diagnosis has been established by core biopsy many patients can have their definitive breast surgery in a single procedure. If the mass is not palpable, biopsy can be conducted using the needle localization technique under mammographic guidance, US-guided core needle biopsy, or a stereotactic core biopsy using a special mammographic machine and table to localize the lesion. When the lesion is visible only by MRI, it may be used to guide the biopsy in some centers. If the biopsy result is benign and the lesion is considered to be of relatively low risk for cancer radiologically, then close follow-up (6 months) may be recommended. If the biopsy result is benign and the lesion is suggestive of cancer, a wire-localized surgical biopsy should be considered. If there are atypical epithelial changes in the biopsy, a surgical biopsy is often conducted because a more advanced lesion is ultimately present in a significant number of cases. A US can help differentiate solid from cystic lesions. A simple cyst should resolve with aspiration and the aspirate should not be hemorrhagic. A cystic lesion should be biopsied if the aspirate produces hemorrhagic fluid, the lesion does not resolve, or recurs after aspiration. If there is a palpable mass, it needs to be core-biopsied to rule out malignancy, regardless of radiologic studies. MRI has 88% sensitivity, 67% specificity, and a 72% positive predictive value (superior to mammography) in breast cancer detection. It does not obviate the need for subsequent biopsy of a mass as it is not specific enough to exclude a malignancy (*JAMA* 2004;292:2735–2742). MRI is particularly useful in detecting the extent of tumors that are mammographically subtle or occult (e.g., lobular carcinomas). It is useful in the setting of adenocarcinoma of unknown primary site involving the axillary lymph node, where the detection of breast cancer by MRI can help direct further treatment. It is also useful to evaluate ipsilateral multifocal cancer in patients who are considering breast conservation therapy and contralateral breast cancer when clinically suspected (*Cancer* 2003;98:468–473). MRI of the breast can also differentiate scar tissue from cancer and can be used to detect local recurrence and residual cancer in patients with positive margin. MRI can also help assess response to neoadjuvant chemotherapy (*Radiol Clin North Am* 2002;40:443–466).

Pathologic evaluation should include standard tumor, node, metastasis (TNM) staging according to the latest American Joint Committee on Cancer (AJCC) criteria, estrogen receptor (ER), progesterone receptor (PgR), and HER2 measurements, tumor grade by Scarff-Bloom-Richardson (SBR) or Nottingham score, and the margin status. ER is expressed in 60% of all breast cancers and indicates responsiveness to endocrine therapies. Twenty-five percent of all breast cancers overexpress HER2 (a transmembrane tyrosine kinase receptor), a poor prognostic factor that is associated with high-grade, ER negativity and a response to trastuzumab and other HER2-targeting agents. HER2 status can be measured by immunohistochemistry (IHC), but the fluorescent *in situ* hybridization (FISH) test for gene amplification is increasingly considered the gold standard.

B. Staging of breast cancer. The AJCC staging system uses the TNM classification (Table 14.1). The stage of the tumor has a strong influence on prognosis (Table 14.2) and treatment.

C. Staging workup of breast cancer

1. **Clinical examination.** A good clinical examination is required with careful inspection and palpation of the local lymph nodes, including supraclavicular nodes, skin, both breasts, abdomen, and spine.

2. **Laboratory tests.** Laboratory tests help physicians focus their workup for metastasis. An abnormal complete blood count (CBC) should prompt evaluation of the bone marrow for metastatic disease. Elevated levels of liver enzymes may suggest liver metastasis, and an elevated calcium/alkaline phosphatase level suggests bone metastasis. Levels of tumor markers CA 15-3, CA 27-29, and carcinoembryonic antigen (CEA) can be elevated in breast cancer. CA 15-3 and CA 27.29 have been evaluated for their ability to help in diagnosis, determine prognosis, predict recurrence of breast cancer after curative therapy, and monitor treatment response. The American Society of Clinical Oncology (ASCO) recommended in 2000 that there is not enough evidence to routinely use tumor markers. There is some evidence suggesting their use in the metastatic setting to monitor tumor response in select patients (*J Clin Oncol* 2001;19:1865–1878).

3. **Radiologic tests.** Radiologic studies complete the clinical staging for breast cancer by detecting metastatic disease. A chest radiograph is fairly routine for almost all patients with invasive breast cancer and a computed tomographic (CT) scan is recommended in patients who have stage III disease, localizing symptoms, or abnormal laboratory values suggesting liver disease. In stage II breast cancer, the use of CT is more controversial but it is often ordered when the lymph nodes are positive. A bone scan should be obtained in patients with stage III disease, or localizing symptoms, or abnormal alkaline phosphatase. The role of fluorodeoxyglucose-positron emission tomography (FDG-PET) scan in staging breast cancer is evolving. It may be useful to detect occult systemic

TABLE 14.1   AJCC TNM Staging for Breast Cancer

Primary tumor (T)

Classification	Definition
TX	Primary tumor cannot be assessed
T0	No evidence of primary tumor
Tis	Carcinoma *in situ*
Tis (DCIS)	Ductal carcinoma *in situ*
Tis (LCIS)	Lobular carcinoma *in situ*
Tis (Paget)	Paget's disease of the nipple with no tumor (*Note:* Paget's disease associated with a tumor is classified according to the size of the tumor.)
T1	Tumor $\leq$2 cm in greatest dimension
T1mic	Microinvasion $\leq$0.1 cm in greatest dimension
T1a	Tumor >0.1 cm but not more than 0.5 cm in greatest dimension
T1b	Tumor >0.5 cm but not more than 1 cm in greatest dimension
T1c	Tumor >1 cm but not more than 2 cm in greatest dimension
T2	Tumor >2 cm but not more than 5 cm in greatest dimension
T3	Tumor >5 cm in greatest dimension
T4	Tumor of any size with direct extension to (a) chest wall or (b) skin, only as described in subsequent text
T4a	Extension to chest wall, not including pectoralis muscle
T4b	Edema (including peau d'orange) or ulceration of the skin of the breast, or satellite skin nodules confined to the same breast
T4c	Both T4a and T4b
T4d	Inflammatory carcinoma

Regional lymph nodes (N) — Clinical

NX	Regional lymph nodes cannot be assessed (e.g., previously removed)
N0	No regional lymph node metastasis
N1	Metastasis in movable ipsilateral axillary lymph node(s)
N2	Metastases in ipsilateral axillary lymph nodes fixed or matted, or in clinically apparent[a] ipsilateral internal mammary nodes in the absence of clinically evident axillary lymph node metastasis
N2a	Metastasis in ipsilateral axillary lymph nodes fixed to one another (matted) or to other structures
N2b	Metastasis only in clinically apparent[a] ipsilateral internal mammary nodes and in the absence of clinically evident axillary lymph node metastasis
N3	Metastasis in ipsilateral infraclavicular lymph node(s) with or without axillary lymph node involvement, or in clinically apparent[a] ipsilateral internal mammary lymph node(s) and in the presence of clinically evident axillary lymph node metastasis; or metastasis in ipsilateral supraclavicular lymph node(s) with or without axillary or internal mammary lymph node involvement
N3a	Metastasis in ipsilateral infraclavicular lymph node(s)
N3b	Metastasis in ipsilateral internal mammary lymph node(s) and axillary lymph node(s)
N3c	Metastasis in ipsilateral supraclavicular lymph node(s)

Regional lymph nodes (pN) — Pathologic

pNX	Regional lymph nodes cannot be assessed (e.g., previously removed or not removed for pathologic study)

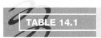

TABLE 14.1 *(Continued)*

Classification	Definition
pN0	No regional lymph node metastasis histologically, no additional examination for isolated tumor cells (ITC) *Note*: ITC are defined as single tumor cells or small cell clusters not greater than 0.2 mm, usually detected only by immunohistochemical (IHC) or molecular methods but which may be verified on H&E stains. ITCs do not usually show evidence of malignant activity, e.g., proliferation or stromal reaction
pN0(i−)	No regional lymph node metastasis histologically, negative IHC
pN0(i+)	No regional lymph node metastasis histologically, positive IHC, no IHC cluster >0.2 mm
pN0(mol−)	No regional lymph node metastasis histologically, negative molecular findings (RT-PCR)[c]
pN0(mol+)	No regional lymph node metastasis histologically, positive molecular findings (RT-PCR)[c]
pN1	Metastasis in one to three axillary lymph nodes, and/or in internal mammary nodes with microscopic disease detected by sentinel lymph node dissection but not clinically apparent[b]
pN1mi	Micrometastasis (>0.2 mm, none greater than 2.0 mm)
pN1a	Metastasis in one to three axillary lymph nodes
pN1b	Metastasis in internal mammary nodes with microscopic disease detected by sentinel lymph node dissection but not clinically apparent[b]
pN1c	Metastasis in one to three axillary lymph nodes and in internal mammary lymph nodes with microscopic disease detected by sentinel lymph node dissection but not clinically apparent[b] (If associated with more than three positive axillary lymph nodes, the internal mammary nodes are classified as pN3b to reflect increased tumor burden)
pN2	Metastasis in four to nine axillary lymph nodes, or in clinically apparent[a] internal mammary lymph nodes in the absence of axillary lymph node metastasis
pN2a	Metastasis in four to nine axillary lymph nodes (at least one tumor deposit >2.0 mm)
pN2b	Metastasis in clinically apparent[a] internal mammary lymph nodes in the absence of axillary lymph node metastasis
pN3	Metastasis in 10 or more axillary lymph nodes, or in infraclavicular lymph nodes, or in clinically apparent[a] ipsilateral internal mammary lymph nodes in the presence of one or more positive axillary lymph nodes; or in more than three axillary lymph nodes with clinically negative microscopic metastasis in internal mammary lymph nodes; or in ipsilateral supraclavicular lymph nodes
pN3a	Metastasis in 10 or more axillary lymph nodes (at least one tumor deposit >2.0 mm), or metastasis to the infraclavicular lymph nodes
pN3b	Metastasis in clinically apparent[a] ipsilateral internal mammary lymph nodes in the presence of one or more positive axillary lymph nodes; or in more than three axillary lymph nodes and in internal mammary lymph nodes with microscopic disease detected by sentinel lymph node dissection but not clinically apparent[b]
pN3c	Metastasis in ipsilateral supraclavicular lymph nodes

(Continued)

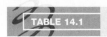

TABLE 14.1	*(Continued)*

Classification	Definition
Distant metastasis (M)	
MX	Distant metastasis cannot be assessed
M0	No distant metastasis
M1	Distant metastasis

[a]Clinically apparent is defined as *detected by imaging studies* (excluding lymphoscintigraphy) or by clinical examination.
[b]Not clinically apparent is defined as *not detected by imaging studies* (excluding lymphoscintigraphy) or by clinical examination.
[c] RT-PCR: Reverse transcriptase/polymerase chain reaction.

Stage Grouping

Stage 0	Tis N0 M0
Stage I	T1[a] N0 M0
Stage II A	T0 N1 M0 T1[a] N1 M0 T2 N0 M0
Stage II B	T2 N1 M0 T3 N0 M0
Stage III A	T0 N2 M0 T1[a] N2 M0 T2 N2 M0 T3 N1 M0 T3 N2 M0
Stage III B	T4 N0 M0 T4 N1 M0 T4 N2 M0
Stage III C	Any T N3 M0
Stage IV	Any T Any N M1

[a]T1 includes T1mic.
Reprinted with permission of the American Joint Committee on Cancer (AJCC). *The original source for this material is the AJCC cancer staging manual*, 6th ed. Chicago: Springer-Verlag New York, 2002.

metastasis but care should be taken to never consider a patient to have advanced disease on the basis of PET alone without other corroboration, preferably by biopsy, because the false-positive rate associated with inflammatory conditions is high. Cardiac systolic function should be evaluated (multiple gated acquisition (MUGA) scan/echocardiogram) before and during treatment with trastuzumab or anthracycline-based chemotherapy.

IV. THERAPY AND PROGNOSIS

A. Ductal carcinoma *in situ*. DCIS is a direct precursor of invasive breast cancer. The incidence of DCIS has increased with screening mammography where it is often diagnosed through the presence of a cluster of microcalcifications (more

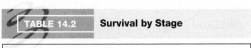

| TABLE 14.2 | Survival by Stage |

Stage	5-yr survival (%)	10-yr survival (%)
0	99	95
I	97	88
II	83	66
III	54	36
IV	16	7

Reprinted with permission Bland KI. The national cancer data base 10-year survey of breast carcinoma treatment at hospitals in the United States. *Cancer* 1998;83:1262.

TABLE 14.3	Modified Van Nuys Prognostic Index		
Score	1	2	3
Size (mm)	≤15	16–40	≤41
Margins (mm)	≤10	1–9	≤1
Pathology	Non-high grade without necrosis	Non-high grade with necrosis	High grade with or without necrosis
Age (yr)	≤61	40–60	≤39

5-year disease-free survival for VNPI 4 to 6 = 100%, VNPI 7 to 9 = 100%, VNPI 10 to 12 = 97.6%
10-year disease-free survival for VNPI 4 to 6 = 100%, VNPI 7 to 9 = 97.7%, VNPI 10 to 12 = 97.6%
Adapted with permission from Silverstein MJ. Ductal carcinoma *in situ*: USC/Van Nuys prognostic index and the impact of margin status. *Breast* 2003;12:457–471.

than 90% of the cases). Uncommonly patients may have a mass, nodule, or other soft tissue changes. Although MRI may pick up some foci that are not visible by mammography, it may also miss some mammographically visible foci. The pathologic subtypes of DCIS are the comedo, cribriform, micropapillary, papillary, and solid subtypes. Prognostically they can be divided into comedo and noncomedo subtypes where the former is more often associated with subsequent recurrence. The modified Van Nuys prognostic index system (VNPI, Table 14.3), which takes into account several factors to predict the likelihood of recurrence after local excision, maybe useful in clinical decision making.

1. **Local Treatment**
   a. **Surgery.** Options include local excision and mastectomy. The cure rate with mastectomy is high at 98% but may be considered unnecessarily aggressive surgery for a preinvasive condition when the amount of breast tissue involvement is low. As an alternative, patients may undergo breast-conserving therapy (BCT) should consider adjuvant radiation therapy. A wide margin (>10 mm) is necessary to achieve the lowest chance of local recurrence (*J Clin Oncol* 2001;19:2263–2271). Axillary lymph node involvement is rare (only 3.6%) and so is not routinely biopsied.
   b. **Radiation Therapy.** The NSABP (National Surgical Adjuvant Breast Project) B17, EORTC (**European Organisation for Research and Treatment of Cancer**) 10853 and the UK trials showed that adjuvant radiation therapy after BCT for DCIS reduces the relative risk of local recurrence by 50% without improving overall survival (OS) and is usually recommended. In patients with a small, low VNPI DCIS, omitting adjuvant radiation therapy is controversial but can be considered in motivated patients, particularly in the setting of older patients with small, low-grade ER-positive lesions.
   c. **Systemic therapy.** In patients undergoing BCT and radiation therapy, the NSABP B24 study showed that tamoxifen reduces the relative risk of ipsilateral invasive breast cancer by 44% and noninvasive cancer by 18%, but the benefit was limited to ER-positive DCIS. In contrast the UK/ANZ trial did not show a clear benefit for adjuvant tamoxifen. The NSABP B35 trial is looking at tamoxifen versus anastrozole in postmenopausal women with DCIS undergoing BCT and adjuvant radiation therapy. There is no role for chemotherapy in this disease.

B. **Lobular carcinoma *in situ*.** LCIS is a histologic biomarker that identifies women at increased risk for subsequent development of an invasive cancer in either breast (approximately 1% per year to a maximum risk of approximately 17.6% by year 25). It is usually not detected clinically and is an incidental finding in patients undergoing breast biopsy. The increased risk of breast cancer persists beyond 20 years and so lifelong follow-up is suggested. Most of the subsequent cancers are infiltrating ductal (rather than lobular) carcinomas.

1. **Local treatment.** LCIS can be managed by close follow-up with clinical breast examination every 6 to 12 months and annual mammogram. It is usually multicentric and bilateral and there is no evidence that re-excision to obtain histologically negative surgical margins is beneficial. Bilateral prophylactic mastectomy can be considered in select patients who are unwilling to accept the risk of bilateral breast cancers, unable to follow up closely, or take prophylactic endocrine therapy. There is no role for radiation therapy.

2. **Systemic therapy.** The NSABP tamoxifen prevention trial (NSABP P1) showed that the use of tamoxifen at 20 mg daily for 5 years is associated with a decrease in the risk of developing breast cancer by 56% in women with LCIS (*J Natl Cancer Inst* 1998;90:1371). The NSABP P2 trial showed equivalent benefit with raloxifene 60 mg daily for 5 years when compared with tamoxifen. There was decreased risk of thrombotic events and uterine cancer with raloxifene. There is no role for chemotherapy.

C. **Treatment of early-stage invasive breast cancer (stages I and II).** A multi-disciplinary approach which includes surgery, radiation therapy, chemotherapy, hormone therapy, and immunotherapy with trastuzumab is used to treat these patients.

1. **Local treatment**

   a. **Surgery**

   i. **Primary tumor surgical approaches.** Lumpectomy/BCT with adjuvant radiation therapy and modified radical mastectomy (with or without reconstructive surgery) shows similar survival and local control (*N Engl J Med* 1995;332:907–911). Radical mastectomy is no longer performed after the NSABP B04 trial showed that the procedure is not superior and has more morbidity than total mastectomy without muscle resection. The selection of a surgical approach depends on the size of the tumor in relation to the size of the breast, patient preference, and the presence or absence of contraindication to BCT. The absolute contraindications are multicentric disease (two or more primary tumors in separate quadrants), extensive malignant-appearing microcalcifications, persistent positive margins despite repeat re-excision surgery after BCT, and previous breast or mantle irradiation. The relative contraindications include pregnancy, history of collagen vascular disease, and large pendulous breasts because of the risk of marked fibrosis and osteonecrosis after adjuvant radiation in these patients. Tumors more than 5 cm and focally positive margins are also relative contraindications to BCT, although for unifocal large T2 and T3 breast masses, neoadjuvant systemic therapy to improve the chance of breast-conserving surgery (BCS) can be considered. The age of the patient is not a criterion for selection of the type of local surgery. Family history of breast cancer is not a contraindication to BCT. In patients who are positive for BRCA1 or BRCA2 mutation, bilateral mastectomy is often recommended because of the very high risk for second breast cancer. If the patient still chooses to undergo BCT, then very close follow-up with MRI and mammography is recommended.

   ii. **Axillary lymph node surgical approaches.** Axillary lymph node status is the most important prognostic factor in breast cancer and so axillary lymph node dissection (ALND) is important diagnostically and thera-peutically. The sentinel lymph node (SLN) is the first lymph node that drains the tumor. In an effort to decrease the chances of arm lymphedema with ALND, SLN biopsy was evaluated in patients with a clinically neg-ative axilla. ASCO has endorsed SLN biopsy as an alternative to full ALND in this setting (*J Clin Oncol* 2005;23:7703). SLN biopsy has been evaluated in women with T1 and T2 disease, without multifo-cal involvement and without clinically positive axillary lymph nodes (*N Engl J Med* 1998;337:941). Vital blue dye and/or technetium-labeled sulfur is injected in and around the tumor or biopsy site. The ipsilateral axilla is explored and the first lymph node that has taken up the dye or radioactive material is excised and examined pathologically. The negative predictive value of this procedure in experienced hands is 93% to 97%. If the SLN is negative, further exploration of the axilla is not required. When the SLN is positive, ALND should be performed. When disease is detected by keratin IHC, management remains controversial.

iii. **Breast-reconstruction techniques.** If a patient undergoes mastectomy, her options for breast reconstruction are a saline implant under the pectoralis muscle and myocutaneous flaps such as a transverse rectus abdominis myocutaneous (TRAM) flap or a latissimus dorsi flap. To improve cosmesis, the patient may elect to undergo another surgery to reconstruct the nipple/areolar complex. The only contraindication to reconstructive surgery is comorbid conditions that would make it difficult to do a longer surgery or reduce the vascular viability of a tissue flap (small vessel disease). Surgery to the contralateral breast may be needed to achieve a symmetrical appearance.

iv. **The role of neoadjuvant chemotherapy.** Neoadjuvant chemotherapy is considered in patients with early-stage breast cancer who meet the criteria for BCT except for tumor size. The chemotherapy regimens used are similar to those used in the adjuvant setting for node-positive disease. Tumor regression increases the opportunities for BCT. There is no difference in survival if the chemotherapy is given before or after the surgery. See Section IV.D.1 for more details on neoadjuvant chemotherapy administration.

b. **Adjuvant radiation therapy.** Adjuvant radiation therapy in patients undergoing BCT for early-stage breast cancer decreases the chances of local recurrence from 39% to 14% (NSABP B-06 trial [*N Engl J Med* 2002;347:1233–1241]). Radiation is effective and necessary in both node-positive and node-negative patients undergoing BCT (*Lancet* 2005;366:2087–2106). There is no clear improvement in survival with this treatment. A dose of 4,500 to 5,000 cGy is given to the breast over 5 to 6 weeks. A radiation boost of 1,000 to 1,500 cGy to the tumor bed is often administered. For patients found to have negative axillary nodes by sentinel lymph node biopsy (SLNB) or ALND, regional nodal irradiation is not recommended. Patients with positive axillary nodes may benefit from regional nodal irradiation in addition to irradiation of the intact breast. In patients with 4 or more positive axillary nodes, the radiation field should include the supraclavicular nodes and the upper internal mammary nodes should also be considered. In patients with one to three positive nodes, radiation to the supraclavicular area and internal mammary is optional, but is often performed because subset analyses of chest wall radiation studies have suggested there may be a survival benefit for nodal radiation in this subgroup. The internal mammary nodes must be irradiated if they are clinically or pathologically positive. Partial breast radiation with interstitial implants have been studied in early-stage breast cancer patients after BCT as an alternative to whole breast irradiation. Although the early results are promising, long-term results are still awaited. The risk of local recurrence in postmastectomy patients is high when the tumor is more than 5 cm, there are positive margins, more than four positive nodes, lymphovascular invasion, and the patient is young, and premenopausal with ER-negative tumor. In these patients chest wall, axillary, and supraclavicular radiation should be administered to reduce locoregional recurrence. In patients with less number of positive nodes, the axilla and supraclavicular area should be evaluated. The internal mammary nodes should be evaluated in all the patients receiving postmastectomy radiation therapy and should be treated if the nodes are clinically or pathologically positive. Adjuvant radiation therapy is given after completing all adjuvant chemotherapy as concurrent therapy increases the side effects of radiation therapy.

2. **Systemic therapy.** Adjuvant systemic therapy addresses the possibility of occult micrometastasis, which can, with time, grow into overt metastatic

disease. Over the last three to four decades, stepwise improvements in adjuvant systemic therapy regimens have improved OS in early-stage breast cancer. Adjuvantonline.com is a web site that enables the treating oncologist to give an approximate average estimate of the benefit from adjuvant chemotherapy (of various types) and endocrine therapy. More recently the Oncotype DX test has been developed to examine the likelihood of distant recurrence in patients with node-negative, ER-positive breast cancers despite the administration of adjuvant tamoxifen. It is a reverse transcriptase-polymerase chain reaction (RT-PCR) assay of 21 selected genes (16 "cancer" genes and 5 reference genes) in paraffin-embedded tumor tissue. The use of chemotherapy may be guided by the Oncotype risk; however, this approach needs to be validated in the setting of an ongoing clinical trial called *TAILORx*.

a. **Adjuvant endocrine therapy.** ER and PgR status of the tumor is routinely identified by immunohistochemical staining of breast cancer tissue. Estrogen binds to the receptor and stimulates cell proliferation, survival, and angiogenesis. The goal of adjuvant endocrine therapy is to suppress these tumor-promoting effects. ER and PgR are both prognostic factors as positivity indicates better prognosis. However, these biomarkers are much stronger predictive factors since the outcome of endocrine therapy is dependent on the level of ER expression. The value of PgR expression remains to be debated and does not provide useful clinical information independent of the ER status. ER-negative, PgR-positive breast cancer should be treated as if it were ER positive.

In premenopausal women, ovaries are the main source of estrogen production. Before the menopause, estrogen can be targeted either by tamoxifen, or by suppression of estrogen levels, or using both approaches in combination. Estrogen suppression can be achieved with luteinizing hormone-releasing hormone (LHRH) agonists (goserelin and leuprolide), oophorectomy, or ovarian radiation, although this latter approach is obsolete as radiation exposure is not justified, given the less toxic alternatives. In postmenopausal women, the predominant source of estrogen is peripheral conversion of adrenal androgens to estrogen by the enzyme aromatase. The action of estrogen can therefore be blocked by tamoxifen, or estrogen synthesis can be inhibited with a third-generation aromatase inhibitor (letrozole, anastrozole and exemestane).

The Early Breast Cancer Trialists Collaborative Group (EBCTCG) meta-analysis of trials in women with early-stage breast cancer, showed that after a median of 15 years of follow-up, tamoxifen reduced annual breast cancer mortality in women with ER-positive breast cancer by 31%, and the annual breast cancer recurrence rate by 41%. This effect was irrespective of age, chemotherapy use, menopausal status, PgR status, involvement of axillary lymph nodes, tumor size, or other tumor characteristics (*Lancet* 2005;365:1687–1717). It also showed that tamoxifen given for 5 years is better than tamoxifen given for 1 to 2 years. The benefits of tamoxifen persisted long after the course of therapy was finished. In fact, the rate of benefit at 15 years is the same as at 5 years. There was a trend toward a detrimental effect after treatment for more than 5 years. The incidence of contralateral breast cancer was not further reduced with prolonged administration of tamoxifen.

The NSABP B-14 trial that looked only at patients with node-negative, ER-positive breast cancer in the 15-year follow-up report, showed that tamoxifen reduced breast cancer recurrence in the ipsilateral breast, contralateral breast, and distant sites by 42% and also reduced mortality by 20% (*Lancet* 2004;364:858–868).

In patients receiving adjuvant chemotherapy, tamoxifen should be administered after the completion of chemotherapy. (Intergroup trial 0100 (SWOG-8814) San Antonio Breast Cancer Symposium;2004:abstract#37). The meta-analysis shows that chemotherapy and endocrine therapy are complementary adjuvant treatments in ER-positive patients with independent and additive benefits but the question of which patients with ER-positive disease require chemotherapy remains controversial, particularly in the setting of low risk ER-positive HER2-negative disease in older patients.

For ER-positive premenopausal patients, the EBCTCG meta-analysis also showed that ovarian ablation/suppression reduced breast cancer mortality but appears to do so only in the absence of other systemic treatments (*Lancet* 2005;365:1687–1717). Oophorectomy may be considered in women with hereditary breast cancer syndromes who are at an increased risk of development of ovarian malignancies and desire oophorectomy. The potential additive role of ovarian ablation to chemotherapy and/or endocrine therapy is presently being explored in the TEXT and SOFT clinical trials.

The use of aromatase inhibitors (AIs) as adjuvant hormonal therapy either instead of tamoxifen or in sequence with tamoxifen has been recommended in postmenopausal women on the basis of ATAC, MA17, IES, and BIG 1-98 trials. ASCO recommended in 2004 that an AI be considered as part of adjuvant hormone therapy for all postmenopausal women with ER-positive breast cancer. The ATAC (5 years of anastrozole vs. 5 years of tamoxifen) and BIG 1-98 (5 years of letrozole vs. 5 years of tamoxifen) trials have shown that AI improved disease-free survival (DFS) in comparison to tamoxifen. The MA17 trial (5 years of letrozole after 5 years of tamoxifen vs. 5 years of tamoxifen alone) showed improved DFS and improved OS in the node-positive subset with adding letrozole to 5 years of tamoxifen. The IES trial (2 to 3 years of exemestane following 2 to 3 years of tamoxifen for a total of 5 years of hormone therapy vs. 5 years of tamoxifen) has demonstrated improvement in both DFS and OS with exemestane. The optimal timing or duration of AI has yet to be established. In general, for all hormone receptor-positive postmenopausal women, 5 years of AI or sequential therapy of 2, 3, or 5 years of tamoxifen followed by 2, 3, or 5 years of AI, up to a total period of 10 years is recommended. There is no data on use of tamoxifen after AI. AIs as single agents are contraindicated in premenopausal women as inhibition of the aromatase enzyme can lead, by a feedback mechanism, to stimulation of the ovaries to produce more estrogen (*J Clin Oncol* 2005;23:619–629). These agents should only be combined with LHRH agonists in the adjuvant setting in clinical studies. The main side effects of AI include hot flashes, myalgias, arthralgias, and osteoporosis whereas the main side effects of tamoxifen include thromboembolic events, uterine cancer, weight gain, hot flashes, and rarely, visual changes.

b. **Adjuvant chemotherapy.** The EBCTCG meta-analysis published the following conclusions on adjuvant chemotherapy after 15 years of follow-up (*Lancet* 2005;365:1687–1717). Adjuvant chemotherapy benefits early-stage breast cancer patients irrespective of their menopausal status, ER status, and nodal status. Longer chemotherapeutic regimens (longer than 6 months) were not superior to shorter chemotherapeutic regimens. Anthracycline-based chemotherapeutic regimens were better than nonanthracycline-based chemotherapy regimens reducing the breast cancer death rate by 38% for women younger than 50, by 20% for women aged 50 to 69. Few women older than 70 entered these trials. Patients in the EBCTCG meta-analysis did not receive a taxane, trastuzumab, or AI and conclusions regarding these agents must currently be drawn from the individual trials, although meta-analyses are planned to examine the value of all these therapies. The findings from the meta-analysis have been incorporated into a web-based algorithm that provides a calculation of benefit of treatment called *adjuvantonline.com* (*J Clin Oncol* 2001;19:980–991). A key issue to understand is that although the reduction in annual odds of recurrence may be impressive, in low-risk groups the absolute benefit can be very small and not worth the cost of the intervention to the patient. For example, a patient with a 90%

chance of being free of disease at 10 years without systemic treatment can expect only a very small absolute benefit, even from an agent that reduces the risk of recurrence by 50%.

In general, for patients with node-negative and ER-positive disease, chemotherapy can be offered in addition to endocrine therapy when the tumor has "high-risk features," for example, high-grade, HER2 gene amplification, size greater than 2 cm, or young age (which is a strong adverse risk factor for ER+ disease). More recently, the Oncotype Dx risk score has been introduced and is currently the focus of the TAILORx trial. For patients whose tumors have a high recurrence risk score by Oncotype Dx, chemotherapy should also be offered. Patients whose tumors have a low recurrence risk score can be potentially treated with adjuvant hormone therapy alone. In patients whose tumors are at intermediate risk, a careful discussion of the benefit and risk of adjuvant chemotherapy should be undertaken by the treating medical oncologist with the patient (*N Engl J Med* 2004;351:2817–2826). In the TAILORx trial, intermediate risk patients are offered a treatment randomization to endocrine therapy versus endocrine therapy plus chemotherapy. The Oncotype Dx assay is not of value in patients with ER-negative disease as all tumors are typed to be high risk (*N Engl J Med* 2006;355:560–569).

Chemotherapy can be considered when the tumor is more than 1 cm, or when it is less than 1 cm and is ER negative, HER2 positive, high grade, or has lymphovascular invasion. The common regimens used in node-negative breast cancer are shown in Table 14.4 and include AC × four cycles, EC × four cycles, FAC/CAF × six cycles, FEC × six cycles, oral CMF (Bonadonna regimen), and i.v. CMF × six to eight cycles. Taxanes have not been well studied in node-negative breast cancer. The ongoing Cancer and Leukemia Group B (CALGB) 40101 trial is comparing AC four versus six cycles or paclitaxel four versus six cycles.

For patients with node-positive disease (both ER-positive and -negative), chemotherapy should be given if there are no contraindications. The addition of taxanes to anthracycline-based regimens has been studied extensively. Although the 2000 National Institutes of Health (NIH) consensus conference concluded that the use of taxane in this setting is inconclusive, since this meeting the benefit of taxane has become more apparent. The CALGB 9344 trial showed an OS benefit in favor of paclitaxel (Taxol) and the NSABP B28 trial showed a DFS benefit with Taxol. The Breast Cancer International Research Group (BCIRG) 001 (TAX 316) trial and the PACS 01 trial showed an OS benefit with docetaxel (Taxotere). The Eastern Cooperative Oncology Group (ECOG) 1199 trial showed that there was no difference in DFS when comparing taxanes (Taxol to Taxotere) or schedule of the taxanes. There was a trend toward improved DFS with weekly Taxol as compared to the standard treatment arm.

The CALGB 9741 study showed an improvement in OS and DFS with dose-dense (every 2-week administration with granulocyte colony–stimulating growth factor (GCSF) support) doxorubicin (Adriamycin), cyclophosphamide (Cytoxan, AC) and paclitaxel (T). There was no difference between concurrent (AC then T) and sequential administration of these drugs (A then T then C).

The best taxane-containing regimen is unclear but reasonable choices include dose-dense AC × four followed by paclitaxel × four, FEC × three followed by docetaxel 100 mg/m2 × three, or TAC × six.

c. **Adjuvant trastuzumab therapy.** In patients whose tumors overexpress HER2 as assessed by FISH or are designated 3+ by IHC, trastuzumab, a humanized monoclonal antibody to HER2 improves DFS by approximately 50%. This has been shown by the combined analysis of the North Central Cancer Treatment Group (NCCTG) N 9831 and NSABP B31 trials (AC × four cycles, weekly paclitaxel × 12 cycles, and trastuzumab for 1 year

TABLE 14.4   **Common Adjuvant Chemotherapy Regimens**

Regimen	Dosage
CMF every 28 days × 6 cycles (Bonadonna regimen)	Cyclophosphamide 100 mg/m^2 PO days 1 to 14 Methotrexate 40 mg/m^2 IV on days 1 and 8 5FU 600 mg/m^2 IV on days 1 and 8
CMF every 21 days × 6 cycles (IV regimen)	Cyclophosphamide 600 mg/m^2 IV on day 1 Methotrexate 40 mg/m^2 IV on day 1 5FU 600 mg/m^2 IV on day 1
FAC every 28 days × 6 cycles	5FU 400 mg/m^2 IV on days 1 and 8 Doxorubicin 40 mg/m^2 IV on day 1 Cyclophosphamide 400 mg/m^2 IV on day 1
CAF every 21 days × 6 cycles	Cyclophosphamide 500 mg/m^2 IV on day 1 Doxorubicin 50 mg/m^2 IV on day 1 5FU 500 mg/m^2 IV on day 1
FEC 100 every 21 days × 6 cycles	5FU 500 mg/m^2 IV on day 1 Epirubicin 100 mg/m^2 on day 1 Cyclophosphamide 500 mg/m^2 on day 1
AC every 21 days × 4 cycles	Doxorubicin 60 mg/m^2 on day 1 Cyclophosphamide 600 mg/m^2 on day 1
TAC every 21 days × 6 cycles	Docetaxel 75 mg/m^2 IV on day 1 Doxorubicin 50 mg/m^2 IV on day 1 Cyclophosphamide 500 mg/m^2 IV on day 1
FEC 100 every 21 days × 3 cycles and then Docetaxel 100 every 21 days × 3 cycles	5FU 500 mg/m^2 IV on day 1 Epirubicin 100 mg/m^2 IV on day 1 Cyclophosphamide 500 mg/m^2 IV on day 1 Docetaxel 100 mg/m^2 IV on day 1
AC every 2 weeks × 4 cycles followed by single-agent paclitaxel every 2 weeks × 4 cycles (dose dense AC + T)	Doxorubicin 60 mg/m^2 IV on day 1 Cyclophosphamide 600 mg/m^2 IV on day 1 Paclitaxel 175 mg/m^2 IV on day 1
AC every 3 weeks × 4 cycles and then weekly Paclitaxel + trastuzumab × 12 cycles	Doxorubicin 60 mg/m^2 IV on day 1 Cyclophosphamide 600 mg/m^2 IV on day 1 Paclitaxel 80 mg/m^2 IV every week Trastuzumab 4 mg/kg IV loading dose and then 2 mg/kg IV weekly
AC every 3 weeks × 4 cycles followed by docetaxel every 3 weeks × 4 cycles with trastuzumab given for 1 year	Doxorubicin 60 mg/m^2 IV on day 1 Cyclophosphamide 600 mg/m^2 IV on day 1 Docetaxel 100 mg/m^2 IV on day 1 Trastuzumab 4 mg/kg IV loading dose and then 2 mg/kg IV weekly
TCH every 3 weeks × 6 cycles then trastuzumab given for 1 year	Docetaxel 75 mg/m^2 IV on day 1 Carboplatin AUC 6 IV on day 1 Trastuzumab 8 mg/kg IV loading dose and then 6 mg/kg IV on day 1 every 3 weeks

IV, intravenous; PO, orally; BID, twice a day.
This is a list of some of the common regimens used. There are other regimens reported that have not been included in this list.

either concurrently with Taxol or sequentially after paclitaxel), HERA trial (chemotherapy of choice followed by trastuzumab for 1 year or 2 years), and the BCIRG 006 trial (AC × four cycles followed by docetaxel × four cycles and trastuzumab for 1 year starting weekly during docetaxel and then every 3 weeks) as well as docetaxel, carboplatin, and trastuzumab [TCH] × six cycles followed by trastuzumab for 1 year). The NCCTG 9831/NSABP B31 trial also showed an improvement in OS by 33% (*N Engl J Med* 2005:353;1673–1684).

In the NCCTG 9831/NSABP B31 study, concurrent paclitaxel + trastuzumab treatment had a better DFS but a higher congestive heart failure incidence (4.1%) as compared to sequential therapy with Taxol followed by trastuzumab (1.2%). Close follow-up of the cardiac function (echocardiogram or MUGA scan) is recommended while the patient is receiving adjuvant trastuzumab. In the study, all patients with cardiac dysfunction recovered their cardiac function after discontinuing trastuzumab.

The results of the 2-year adjuvant trastuzumab arm of the HERA trial are awaited. There are other trials also exploring shorter durations of adjuvant trastuzumab.

See Table 14.4 for adjuvant chemotherapy doses.

d. Sequence of adjuvant chemotherapy and radiation therapy. The administration of radiation therapy concurrently with chemotherapy increases the side effects of radiation therapy and it not recommended. In terms of optimal sequencing, a randomized clinical trial addressing this question showed that giving chemotherapy first followed by radiation therapy reduced recurrence rate for all sites from 38% to 31% and improved OS from 73% to 81%. There was a slight increase in local recurrence rate in the chemotherapy-first arm, but it was not statistically significant (*N Engl J Med* 1996;334:1356). Radiation therapy can be delayed up to 6 months postsurgery to allow completion of adjuvant chemotherapy. After completing chemotherapy, radiation therapy can be given concurrently with adjuvant trastuzumab with no increase in side effects including cardiac toxicity, although pneumonitis is a concern with patients receiving chest wall radiation.

D. Treatment of locally advanced breast cancer and inflammatory breast cancer (stage III A, stage III B, stage IIIC). More advanced stages of primary breast cancer are associated with a poorer prognosis and a higher rate of local and distant recurrences as compared to earlier stages of the disease. With aggressive multimodality treatment, 5-year OS is approximately 75% in patients who have a pathologic complete response (CR) with neoadjuvant chemotherapy. Patients with disease at surgery (i.e., those with invasive cancer) have a significantly worse outcome.

1. Systemic therapy. Neoadjuvant chemotherapy will facilitate tumor regression to allow surgical resection with clear margins and is an *in vivo* test of the cancer cell sensitivity to the regimen used. Several studies have shown that patients with pathologic complete response (pCR) in the breast and axilla (more so axillary pCR) are associated with better DFS and OS. Whether increasing the pCR rate will increase the DFS and OS rate is currently being investigated. Fewer than 5% of breast cancers progress while receiving neoadjuvant chemotherapy.

The following recommendations have been made on neoadjuvant chemotherapy by the 2003 NIH consensus conference (*Cancer* 2004;100:2512).

a. Anthracycline-based regimen or a taxane for four cycles followed by evaluation of the response.

b. When there is complete or almost complete clinical response to induction therapy, definitive local treatment is advised.

c. In cases where the clinical response is not complete, four additional cycles of chemotherapy with a non-cross-resistant drug may be used. (Anthracycline may be used if taxane was used initially and vice versa.)

d. As in the case of adjuvant therapy, eight cycles of chemotherapy is recommended either preoperatively or split before and after surgery.

e. Two to four cycles of chemotherapy are necessary before labelling the tumor as a nonresponder (in the absence of progressive disease).

In the Aberdeen trial, adding four cycles of docetaxel after four cycles of CAVP resulted in a 31% pCR rate as compared to only 15% with CAVP (*Breast Cancer Res Treat* 2003;82(Suppl 1):S9, Abstr# 11). In the NSABP B27 trial giving docetaxel four cycles of AC preoperatively was associated with a pCR rate of 26.1% (*J Clin Oncol* 2003;21:4165–4174, San Antonio Breast Cancer Symposium 2004, Abstr# 26). Whether a taxane should be given sequentially after or concurrently with anthracycline is still controversial but hematologic toxicity is definitely less with sequential therapy. In patients whose tumors overexpress HER2, trastuzumab can be used initially with a taxane neoadjuvantly and subsequently adjuvantly for 1 year. Neoadjuvant endocrine therapy with an aromatase inhibitor is an alternative for postmenopausal women with ER-positive HER2-negative disease and offers similar benefits to chemotherapy with an improvement in breast conservation rates. The AI is generally offered for 4 to 6 months preoperatively. In carefully selected patients (ER-rich tumors), a 60% response rate and a 50% rate of conversion to breast conservation can be expected (*J Clin Oncol* 2001;19:3808–3816).

In ER-positive locally advanced breast cancer (LABC) patients, an AI is often offered as therapy in preference to tamoxifen because high-risk tumors are more prone to relapse early on in follow-up justifying agents that show improved relapse-free survival over tamoxifen.

Several studies have looked at high-dose chemotherapy and stem cell transplantation in patients with breast cancer. Improvements in OS have not been observed so it is not recommended as a standard of care.

2. Locoregional therapy

a. Surgery of primary tumor. The surgical options are mastectomy and BCT. The selection of the type of surgery is based on response to neoadjuvant treatment, the involvement of nipple/areolar complex, extent of skin involvement/chest wall involvement, and the size of the breast in relation to the size of the residual tumor. Preoperative breast MRI can be helpful in determining if the residual tumor is of limited extent and amenable to wide excision. In patients with multicentric tumors, extensive microcalcifications associated with an extensive intraductal component persisting postchemotherapy, mastectomy should be performed. In patients with connective tissue diseases (systemic lupus erythematosus, scleroderma, or active dermatomyositis), a relative contraindication to adjuvant radiation therapy, mastectomy should be considered. Where BCT is an option following neoadjuvant chemotherapy, a radiopaque clip should be placed in the central portion of the tumor under US guidance before starting neoadjuvant chemotherapy, so that the tumor can be located if complete clinical response is achieved with neoadjuvant treatment. In patients with IBC, mastectomy should be performed even in those with complete clinical response as the incidence of local recurrence is higher with BCT.

b. Axillary staging. Most patients with LABC and IBC have clinically palpable nodal disease. For the minority of patients whose axilla is clinically negative, some physicians consider SLN biopsy before neoadjuvant therapy although most studies have restricted SLNB testing to early-stage breast cancer. This topic is still being debated.

c. Radiation therapy. Radiation therapy to the breast should be given in patients undergoing BCT. In patients undergoing mastectomy, the chest wall should be irradiated in patients whose tumor size was more than 5 cm before neoadjuvant therapy, and who had positive margins, more than four positive axillary nodes, lymphovascular invasion, ER-negative and high-grade tumors. The ECOG study showed that adjuvant radiation therapy helps lower the local recurrence rate even in patients undergoing mastectomy

(*Cancer* 1997;79:1138), and an MD Anderson retrospective study showed improvement in local recurrence and OS with postmastectomy adjuvant radiation therapy (*J Clin Oncol* 2004;22:4691).

In patients who had SLNB, the axilla should be included in the radiation field if it was positive. In patients undergoing ALND, the axilla should be irradiated if the nodes are persistently positive after neoadjuvant chemotherapy. The supraclavicular nodes should be included in patients receiving radiation therapy to the axilla. The internal mammary nodes, if clinically or pathologically positive, should also be included in the radiation field.

V. FOLLOW-UP. There is data to recommend monthly self-breast examination, annual mammography to the preserved and contralateral breast, careful history and physical examination every 3 to 6 months for 3 years and then every 6 to 12 months for years 4 and 5 and then annually. Data is not sufficient to recommend routine bone scans, chest x-rays, blood counts, tumor markers, liver ultrasounds, or CT scans. CT and bone scans should only be done for suggestive symptoms (*J Clin Oncol* 1999;17:1080).

In patients taking tamoxifen, yearly pelvic examination by a gynecologist is recommended. There is no evidence for endometrial cancer screening on a regular basis. In women with irregular or excessive bleeding or pelvic pain, a careful pelvic examination, US, and endometrial biopsy should be performed. While on tamoxifen, yearly ophthalmologic evaluation is recommended to identify corneal, macular, and retinal changes.

In patients taking AI, an initial bone density scan is recommended. Patients with normal bone mineral density (BMD) can be followed up clinically with only sparing use of repeat scans. Osteopenic patients should be offered calcium and vitamin D supplements and yearly BMD and lifestyle advice (exercise). Osteoporotic patients should be offered a bisphosphonate as well and followed up closely. Fasting lipids levels should also be followed up because AIs do not protect from heart disease and in low-risk breast cancer patients cardiovascular disease is the most common cause of death.

Physicians should also monitor their patients for long-term side effects from treatment including sexual dysfunction, premature ovarian failure, infertility in younger patients, cognitive dysfunction, lymphedema, decreased arm mobility, postmastectomy pain syndrome, cardiac dysfunction, psychological stress, and second cancers (soft tissue sarcoma from RT, acute leukemia/myelodysplasia (MDS) from chemotherapy).

VI. LOCOREGIONAL RECURRENT BREAST CANCER. Locoregional recurrence can present as a breast lump or nipple discharge following BCT, chest wall rash, or nodules following mastectomy or enlargement of axillary, supraclavicular, or internal mammary lymph nodes.

Breast cancer can recur locally after BCT and mastectomy. In patients who undergo mastectomy, recurrence is usually within the first 3 years of surgery, but in patients who undergo BCT, tumor can recur even at 20 years postsurgery (*Cancer* 1989;63:1912–1917). In patients who undergo BCT, the locoregional recurrence rate is higher in women who do not undergo adjuvant RT, and have positive margins, high-grade tumor and lymphovascular invasion.

When a patient has cancer in the ipsilateral breast after BCT, it could either be a locally recurrent tumor or a second primary. Mastectomy is recommended for these patients. Radiation therapy is limited by earlier whole breast radiation therapy and other contraindications to RT. Systemic therapy is based on the size, nodal status, hormone receptor status, HER2/neu status and other tumor characteristics and follows treatment principles similar to a first diagnosis of early-stage breast cancer.

When cancer recurs in the chest wall after mastectomy, 20% to 30% of patients have metastatic disease at the time. In patients with isolated chest wall recurrence, full-thickness chest wall resection can palliate symptoms, improve survival, and even result in cure (*Am Surg* 2005;71:711–715). Node-negative patients at the first presentation and those patients with a DFS of more than 24 months before chest wall recurrence had a better prognosis with outcomes improved by chest wall radiation therapy and systemic chemotherapy (*Ann Surg Oncol* 2003;10:628–634). Endocrine therapy or a change in endocrine therapy should also be considered for ER-positive chest wall recurrences.

VII. **METASTATIC BREAST CANCER.** The common sites for breast cancer to metastasize are the lung, liver, and bones. Metastatic breast cancer (MBC) is incurable except perhaps in a very small percentage of patients, who are chemotherapy naïve, receive multiagent chemotherapy, and may remain in durable remission for unexpectedly long periods of time. On an average, patients live with MBC for 2 to 3 years, although with the advent of newer therapies, 5-year survival has become more common. Patients with bone or lymph node metastasis survive longer than patients with visceral metastasis. Treatment aims to control the cancer, palliate symptoms, improve quality of life, and prolong survival. The choice of treatment in these patients is dependent on the hormone receptor status, HER2 status, site and extent of disease as well as the patient's performance status and comorbidities.

A. **Local treatment**

1. **Surgery.** In patients with solitary/limited metastasis of the lung, liver, brain, and sternum, case reports and retrospective studies have suggested improved survival with surgical resection; however, these are uncontrolled patient series and there are no definitive data. Patients should be chosen carefully on the basis of operative morbidity, disease-free interval since their primary tumor, the possibility of achieving negative margins, extent of metastasis, performance status, and comorbidities.

   In patients who present with metastatic disease at the time of diagnosis, most oncologists do not routinely recommend primary breast tumor surgery. Surgery is done to palliate any symptoms related to the primary tumor. Retrospective studies have suggested improved survival with removal of the primary tumor in patients with metastatic disease but this remains controversial.

   Spinal cord compression from metastasis is a medical emergency and has improved outcomes with neurosurgical decompression of the spinal cord followed by radiation therapy as compared to radiation therapy and steroids alone (*Lancet* 2005;366:643–648).

   Prophylactic pinning/rod placement of long bones that have cancer destroying more than 50% of the cortical bone is done to prevent fractures, which can lead to a poor quality of life and decrease in survival.

2. **Radiation therapy.** Radiation therapy is used to palliate symptoms and can help with pain in patients with bone metastasis and chest wall metastasis. Some patients can have significant mediastinal/hilar adenopathy or lung metastasis causing obstruction of the bronchus leading to collapse of a lung lobe or postobstructive pneumonia. Palliative radiation therapy can be used to open up the bronchus in these situations. In patients with spinal cord compression, who are not candidates for neurosurgery, radiation therapy is used to relieve the cord compression.

   In patients with unresectable brain metastasis, whole-brain radiation therapy (WBRT) is shown to help improve symptoms and improve median survival from 4 to 6 months. Stereotactic radiosurgery (gamma knife) is used in patients with limited brain metastasis that is in an inaccessible place, as a boost to WBRT, and in patients with recurrences after WBRT. In patients with HER2-positive brain metastasis, lapatinib, a HER2 kinase inhibitor, holds some promise.

   Radioactive isotopes such as strontium-89 and samarium-153 can be used to palliate bone pain from multifocal osteoblastic bone metastasis.

B. **Systemic therapy.** Endocrine therapy is recommended as first-line therapy in patients with hormone receptor–positive tumor, if they have bone, lymph node, soft tissue, or asymptomatic visceral metastasis. Chemotherapy is recommended in patients with hormone receptor–negative tumor or symptomatic visceral metastasis. Trastuzumab is added to chemotherapy if the tumor overexpresses HER2.

1. **Hormone therapy.** In premenopausal patients, options include tamoxifen (±LHRH agonists) and oophorectomy (±AIs). In postmenopausal patients, options include AI, tamoxifen, fulvestrant, and megestrol acetate. High-dose estrogen (for example estradiol 10 mg TID) is an option in patients with tamoxifen and AI-resistant disease, although the mechanism of action of high-dose estrogen is not clear. The onset of action for hormonal therapy is slow, in the order of months, and is most effective in slowly progressive disease. Compared to megestrol acetate or tamoxifen, AIs have a superior response rate and better time to disease progression and may improve OS. One of these agents is therefore considered appropriate first-line endocrine therapy in postmenopausal patients.

   When the tumor progresses through one endocrine agent, further endocrine therapy is recommended as long as the patient does not have symptomatic visceral disease or rapidly progressing disease. Second- and third-line endocrine therapy agents are chosen from a different drug class. With each subsequent endocrine therapy, the response rate and time to progression (TTP) decrease. Chemotherapy should be started when the disease eventually becomes resistant to hormone therapy, while considering the patient's performance status and comorbidities.

2. **Chemotherapy.** Whether the chemotherapeutic drugs should be given in combination or sequentially is uncertain. Combination chemotherapy is associated with better response rate, better TTP, and, at best, marginally improved OS, but is associated with more side effects. Combination chemotherapy should be used when the patient has visceral disease and organ function is threatened, otherwise single-agent approaches offer the best chance at palliation.

   Anthracyclines (doxorubicin, liposomal doxorubicin, epirubicin, mitoxantrone) and taxanes (paclitaxel, docetaxel, nab-paclitaxel) are the two most active drug classes against breast cancer. Many patients have often received these agents in the adjuvant setting, but they may be reused at relapse, particularly if there has been an interval of more than a year. Capecitabine is used when the disease has recurred or progressed after anthracyclines and taxanes. The other active drugs include cytoxan, methotrexate, vinorelbine, gemcitabine, oral etoposide, and irinotecan.

   MBC that does not overexpress HER2 can be treated with chemotherapeutic regimens listed in Table 14.5. Approximately 25% of MBC overexpress HER2 and can be treated with a single-agent trastuzumab with response rates of 35%. If the primary tumor had initially been treated with trastuzumab, the response rate decreases to approximately 10% (Table 14.6). The combination of chemotherapy with trastuzumab was associated with higher response rates, a longer TTP, and a statistically significant improvement in OS.

   Trastuzumab is well tolerated as compared to standard chemotherapy. The use of trastuzumab in combination with anthracyclines has been associated with severe cardiac toxicity in up to 27% of patients (*N Engl J Med* 2001;349:783).

   Whether trastuzumab should be continued upon tumor progression has not been answered by randomized phase III clinical trials. On the basis of the extension study of the pivotal trastuzumab trial and retrospective studies, it appears safe to do so.

   Bevacizumab is a monoclonal antibody against vascular endothelial growth factor (VEGF). The ECOG 2100 trial showed benefit to adding this drug to paclitaxel. There was higher response rate (28% vs. 14%) and longer progression-free survival (11 vs. 6 months) for the combination. The main side effects of bevacizumab include high blood pressure, bleeding risk, and proteinuria. This treatment is considered in patients who have no brain metastasis or hemostatic problems. At the time of writing, bevacizumab is not approved for the treatment of breast cancer.

   Lapatinib (Tykerb) is a dual tyrosine kinase inhibtor drug that blocks both HER1 and HER2. It is FDA approved in combination with capecitabine for the treatment of patients with advanced or metastatic breast cancer whose

| TABLE 14.5 | Metastatic Breast Cancer Chemotherapy Regimens |

Regimen	Dosage
Doxorubicin every 3 weeks	40 to 75 mg/m^2 IV on day 1
Pegylated liposomal doxorubicin every 3 to 4 weeks	45 to 60 mg/m^2 IV on day 1
Epirubicin every 3 weeks	60 to 90 mg/m^2 IV on day 1
Paclitaxel every 3 weeks	175 to 200 mg/m^2 IV on day 1
Paclitaxel every week	80 to 100 mg/m^2 IV on day 1
Docetaxel every 3 weeks	80 to 100 mg/m^2 IV on day 1
Docetaxel every week	30 to 35 mg/m^2 IV on day 1
Abraxane every 3 weeks	260 mg/m^2 IV on day 1
Abraxane weekly on 3 weeks off 1 week q 28 days	125 mg/m^2 IV on days 1, 8, and 15 IV
Capecitabine on 2 weeks off 1 week every 3 weeks	850 to 1,250 mg/m^2 PO BID on days 1 to 14
Gemcitabine weekly on 3 weeks off 1 week every 28 days	725 mg/m^2 IV on days 1, 8, and 15
Vinorelbine weekly	30 mg/m^2 IV on day 1
Etoposide on 2 weeks off 1 week every 3 weeks	50 mg PO every day
Gemcitabine and paclitaxel every 21 days	Gemcitabine 1,250 mg/m^2 IV days 1 and 8 Paclitaxel 175 m/m^2 IV day 1
Capecitabine and docetaxel every 21 days	Capecitabine 1,250 mg/m^2 PO BID on days 1 to 14 Docetaxel 75 mg/m^2 IV on day 1
Capecitabine and paclitaxel every 21 days	Capecitabine 850 mg/m^2 PO BID on days 1 to 14 Paclitaxel 175 mg/m^2 IV on day 1
Capecitabine and Navelbine every 21 days	Capecitabine 1,000 mg/m^2 PO BID on days 1 to 14 Navelbine 25 mg/m^2 IV on days 1 and 8
CMF every 28 days (PO regimen)	Cyclophosphamide 100 mg/m^2 PO days 1 to 14 Methotrexate 40 mg/m^2 IV on days 1 and 8 5FU 600 mg/m^2 IV on days 1 and 8
CMF every 21 days (IV regimen)	Cyclophosphamide 600 mg/m^2 IV on day 1 Methotrexate 40 mg/m^2 IV on day 1 5FU 600 mg/m^2 IV on day 1
FAC every 28 days	5FU 400 mg/m^2 IV on days 1 and 8 Doxorubicin 40 mg/m^2 IV on day 1 Cyclophosphamide 400 mg/m^2 IV on day 1
CAF every 21 days	Cyclophosphamide 500 mg/m^2 IV on day 1 Doxorubicin 50 mg/m^2 IV on day 1 5FU 500 mg/m^2 IV on day 1
FEC 100 every 21 days	5FU 500 mg/m^2 IV on day 1 Epirubicin 100 mg/m^2 IV on day 1 Cyclophosphamide 500 mg/m^2 on day 1
AT every 21 days	Doxorubicin 60 mg/m^2 IV on day 1 Paclitaxel 200 mg/m^2 IV on day 1
Docetaxel and doxorubicin every 21 days	Docetaxel 75 mg/m^2 IV on day 1 Doxorubicin 50 mg/m^2 IV on day 1

IV, intravenous; PO, orally; BID, twice a day.
This is a list of some of the common regimens used. There are other regimens reported that have not been included in this list.

| TABLE 14.6 | Metastatic Breast Cancer Overexpressing HER2 |

Regimen	Response rate (%)
Trastuzumab	10–35
Paclitaxel + trastuzumab	38–63
Docetaxel + trastuzumab	41–70
Vinorelbine + trastuzumab	68–78
Gemcitabine + trastuzumab	37
Capecitabine + trastuzumab	53
Liposomal doxorubicin + trastuzumab	58
Cisplatin + trastuzumab	24
Cisplatin + docetaxel + trastuzumab	76–79
Carboplatin + docetaxel + trastuzumab	54–64
Carboplatin + paclitaxel + trastuzumab	52–57
Cisplatin + gemcitabine + trastuzumab	40
Paclitaxel + gemcitabine + trastuzumab	62
Epirubicin + cyclophosphamide + trastuzumab	62–71

This is a list of some of the common regimens used. There are other regimens reported that have not been included in this list.

tumors overexpress HER2 and who have received prior therapy including an anthracycline, a taxane, and trastuzumab. The median time to progression was 8.4 months for lapatinib and capecitabine compared to 4.4 months for capecitabine alone. (*N Engl J Med* 2006;355:2733).

High-dose chemotherapy and stem cell transplantation trials have not shown an improvement in OS despite the cost and toxicity.

C. Follow-up while on treatment. Monitoring treatment can be done by physical examination if there is palpable adenopathy or chest wall/soft tissue nodules. Significant cancer-related symptoms such as pain can also be monitored. Monitoring of tumor markers is useful only if elevated (*J Clin Oncol* 1999;17:1080). Tumor marker levels may not correlate with tumor burden (by imaging). The tumor marker may be spuriously elevated due to cytolysis. The tumor marker level may be lower with clearly progressive disease because the tumor has changed and is secreting lower levels of the marker. The physical examination and radiologic findings should then determine treatment decisions. Imaging (CT, MR, and bone scans) should be done periodically to assess response to treatment. Little data is available regarding the use of PET scans to monitor treatment. Recently, studies looking at circulating tumor cell (CTC) levels have been published. High levels of CTC before starting treatment have been associated with poorer DFS and OS (*N Engl J Med* 2004;351(8):781). When the CTC level has not declined after 3 to 6 weeks of starting a new regimen, those patients are unlikely to benefit from chemotherapy.

D. Duration of chemotherapy treatment. Randomized studies have shown that OS is not significantly different whether chemotherapy is continued until disease progression or withheld after an optimum number of cycles (approximately six cycles). Patients who tolerate chemotherapy well may accept continued treatment, and randomized trials suggest that this may be the best option in terms of progression-free survival and quality of life (*N Engl J Med* 1987:317:1490–1495). However, when toxicity is a problem, chemotherapy "holidays" may improve the quality of life, after which treatment can be resumed even if disease progression has not yet occurred.

E. Bone metastasis. Local therapy for bone metastasis has been outlined above. Pamidronate (90 mg i.v. q 3 to 4 weeks) and zoledronic acid (4 mg i.v. q 3 to 4 weeks) are U.S. Food and Drug Administration (FDA)-approved drugs for use in patients with bone metastasis to palliate pain and prevent skeletal complications. These drugs have not shown an improvement in OS. Zoledronic acid is preferred, as it can be given over a shorter time. While administering these drugs, the serum creatinine, electrolytes, calcium, and magnesium levels should be monitored. The drugs should be continued as long as the patient receives treatment for MBC. These drugs are being studied in clinical trials to see if they prevent bone metastasis.

VIII. FUTURE DIRECTIONS. Major advances have been made in the diagnosis and treatment of breast cancer, resulting in a decrease in mortality from breast cancer over the last four decades. However, there is still a subset of patients dying from breast cancer and we need to understand the biology of these cancers to be able to treat these patients better. Every effort should be made to enroll patients in clinical trials to enable us to achieve this goal. There are a lot of ongoing exciting clinical trials with targeted therapies that act on various receptors and cellular pathways.

Patients differ in their ability to tolerate treatment and tumors differ in how they proliferate, metastasize, and respond to treatment. New technologies such as gene microarray, gene polymorphism studies, and proteomics are being used to help us understand these important differences at a molecular level.

While we are making an effort to better understand and treat breast cancer, efforts are also being made to improve the quality of life of patients undergoing treatment for breast cancer. Research is ongoing in the field of antiemetics, memory loss, fatigue, postmenopausal symptoms, and other symptoms related to the treatment of this disease.

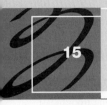

THYMOMA AND MESOTHELIOMA
Daniel Morgensztern

15

I. THYMOMA
- **A. Subjective complaints.** The clinical presentation for patients with thymic neoplasms can be quite variable. Up to 50% of patients present with an asymptomatic anterior mediastinal mass on the chest radiograph. Symptoms may occur due to local compression or as paraneoplastic syndromes. The most common local complaints include cough, chest pain, and dyspnea. Other symptoms include hemoptysis, hoarseness, and dysphagia. Systemic complaints such as weight loss, fatigue, fever, and night sweats are less common, and more typically associated with lymphoma. The most common paraneoplastic syndrome is myastenia gravis (MG), occurring in approximately, one third of the patients. Among patients with MG, 10% to 15% are found to have thymoma during further investigation. Pure red cell aplasia (PRCA) occurs in approximately, 5% to 10% of the patients with thymoma but half of the patients with this disorder have thymoma. This syndrome is suspected in patients with isolated anemia and low reticulocyte count. Hypogammaglobulinemia is present in up to 10% of the patients. The association of thymoma, and combined B and T cell immunodeficiency is commonly termed Good's syndrome and the patients are characterized by an increased susceptibility to infections by encapsulated bacteria, and opportunistic viruses and fungi (*J Clin Pathol* 2003;56:12–16). Several other paraneoplastic syndromes have been described in association with thymoma (Table 15.1).
- **B. Objective findings.** At an early stage, patients often have a completely normal physical examination. The thoracic expansion of the tumor with invasion or compression of the superior vena cava may cause the characteristic findings of facial and upper extremity swelling, whereas invasion of the innominate vein will cause a predominantly left arm swelling. Phrenic nerve invasion may cause decreased breath sounds on the affected side. Most patients develop ocular findings such as ptosis or diplopia and some may have involvement of the respiratory muscles.

II. WORKUP AND STAGING
- **A. Imaging studies.** Most cases of thymoma are detected initially by standard chest radiographs. On the posteroanterior view, there is usually a round or oval lesion, with smooth or lobulated border, near the junction of the heart and great vessels. Although the tumor may be located in the midline, it usually protrudes more predominantly into one of the hemithoraces. The trachea is rarely displaced and the presence of an elevated hemidiaphragm may suggest the invasion of a phrenic nerve. A small percentage of tumors have calcification in the periphery or within the tumor. On the lateral view, the mass causes opacification of the anterior cardiac window. Further evaluation is obtained with a computed tomography (CT) scan of the chest, which may detect the unusual cases not visualized in the chest radiographs and help to evaluate the extent of the mass. Although CT scan is unreliable for the detection of mediastinal invasion, highly suggestive findings include complete obliteration of fat planes, encasement of mediastinal vessels, pericardial or pleural thickening. The tendency to metastasize to the posterior basilar pleural space is unique of thymomas. Magnetic resonance imaging (MRI) is useful in the investigation of vascular invasion. Thymic tumors often express somatostatin receptors and may be detected by an indium-labeled octreotide scan. The use of positron emission tomography (PET) in the evaluation of patients with thymoma remains investigational.

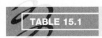

TABLE 15.1	Paraneoplastic Syndromes Associate With Thymoma
Endocrine	Addison's disease, Cushing's syndrome, panhypopituitarism, thyroiditis
Cardiovascular	Myocarditis, pericarditis
Hematologic	Agranulocytosis, hypogammaglobulinemia, pernicious anemia, red cell aplasia
Neuromuscular	Myastenia gravis, limbic encephalopathy, polymyositis, radiculopathy
Rheumatologic	Rheumatoid arthritis, scleroderma, sistemic lupus erithematosus, Sjogren's
Miscellaneous	Alopecia areata, sarcoidosis, ulcerative colitis

B. Biopsy. The diagnosis of thymoma is usually made clinically, particularly in patients with paraneoplastic syndrome. When the tumor is small and confined to the thymus, the surgical excision may provide both diagnosis and treatment. Furthermore, it allows the staging required for the decision whether the patient will need adjuvant therapy. Biopsy has an important role in patients with large and invasive tumors that may require a nonsurgical approach or neoadjuvant treatment, as well as in cases where lymphoma remains a strong possibility, because this malignancy is not primarily treated with surgery. The histopatologic diagnosis may be obtained through a fine-needle aspiration (FNA) or surgical biopsy with success rates of approximately, 60% and 90% respectively. The sensitivity and specificity of FNA is limited due to the cytologically benign appearance of many thymomas. There is limited data to support the concerns over seeding thymic tumors to the pleural space during the biopsy procedure. There are no reports of tumor seeding through the needle tract or biopsy site and the pattern of spreading to the pleural space appears to be inherent of this malignancy, regardless of previous biopsy.

C. Pathology. The term thymoma should be restricted to neoplasms of thymic epithelial cells. Therefore, other tumors that may also involve the thymus such as seminomas and lymphomas should not be considered variants of thymoma. Most of the thymomas arise in the upper portion of the anterior mediastinum, corresponding to the location of the normal thymus gland. Rare locations include the posterior mediastinum, lower neck, perihilar tissues, lung parenchima, and pleura. Grossly, the thymomas are largely or entirely solid, separated in lobules by connective tissue septa, and usually well-encapsulated. Microscopically, the thymomas are composed of a mixture of neoplastic epithelial cells and a lymphocyte infiltrate. After many years of debate and several proposed schemes, the **World Health Organization** (WHO) developed a standard and unified classification for thymic epithelial neoplasms in 1999 (Table 15.2). In this report, two major types of

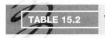

TABLE 15.2	WHO Classification Of Thymomas

WHO scheme	Other histologic classifications
Type A	Medullary, spindle cell
Type AB	Mixed
Type B1	Lymphocyte-rich, predominantly cortical, organoid
Type B2	Cortical
Type B3	Epithelial, atypical thymoma, well-differentiated thymic carcinoma
Type C	Thymic carcinoma

WHO, World Health Organization.

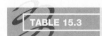

TABLE 15.3	Masaoka Staging System For Thymoma

Stage	Description
I	Completely encapsulated tumor
IIa	Microscopic invasion into surrounding fatty tissue or mediastinal pleura
IIb	Macroscopic invasion into the capsule
III	Macroscopic invasion into neighboring organs (pericardium, great vessels, lung)
IVa	Pleural or pericardial metastases
IVb	Lymphatic or hematogenous metastases

thymoma were identified based on the characteristics of the malignant epithelial cells, which could have a spindle or oval shape in type A or epithelioid appearance in type B. Tumors with both characteristics were designated as AB. Type B tumors were further subdivided in three groups, B1 to B3, depending on the progressive increase of the epithelial-to-lymphocyte ratio and degree of atypia. An additional category, type C, was reserved for patients with thymic carcinoma, where there are overt characteristics of malignancy. There is a significant correlation between the WHO subtype and paraneoplastic syndromes, with MG occurring most commonly in subtype B and PRCA in subtype A.

D. Staging. The most commonly used staging system is the one proposed by Masaoka et al. in 1981 (Table 15.3). In this system, four clinical stages are created based on the degree of invasion through the capsule into the surrounding structures.

III. THERAPY AND PROGNOSIS
A. Resectable disease
   1. Surgery. Surgery is a treatment of choice for thymoma and should be offered to all patients except those with clinically grossly unresectable disease or where it is spread beyond the thorax. In patients with grossly encapsulated lesions, the procedure of choice is a complete excision with total thymectomy. Patients with gross fixation of the tumor to nonvital adjacent structures such as lung, pleura or pericardium, should undergo the resection of the adjacent involved tissues. The presence of intrapulmonary metastasis does not constitute a contraindication for the surgery if accomplished by lobectomy. The role for pneumonectomy in this setting is questionable. Patients with unilateral phrenic nerve involvement should undergo surgery with curative intent, provided that they can tolerate the loss of function in that hemidiaphragm, which can be particularly problematic in patients with MG. The operative mortality is approximately, 2.5% and overall survival for patients with resected thymoma is usually very good (Table 15.4). Patients with stage III or IV are considered unresectable when there is extensive involvement of the trachea, great arteries or heart, extensive bilateral pleural metastases, or distant metastases. The role of debulking or subtotal resection in

TABLE 15.4	Overall Survival For Resected Thymomas

Masaoka stage	5-year survival (%)	10-year survival (%)
I	92	88
II	82	70
III	68	57
IVa	61	38

advanced stages remains controversial. Patients with relapsed disease following a complete resection should be considered for a second operation.

2. **Adjuvant radiation therapy.** The use of adjuvant radiation therapy remains controversial, although this therapeutic modality is frequently recommended for patients with stages II and III as well as in incomplete resections. Adjuvant radiation is probably not justified in patients with encapsulated disease due to the very low risk of relapse. Adjuvant radiation however, may decrease the recurrence rate after complete resection in patients with invasive disease and particularly, in Masaoka stage III patients, has been recommended by several authors.

B. **Locally advanced disease**

1. **Neoadjuvant therapy.** Although the use of preoperative single modality radiation therapy has not been associated with survival benefit, several studies suggested improvement in both resectability and survival with the use of multimodality treatment in patients with Masaoka stage III and IV patients. Small studies using three cyces of neoadjuvant cisplatin-based chemotherapy and adjuvant radiation with or without chemotherapy, have shown response rates between 77% and 100%, complete resection in 57% to 80%, pathologic complete remission in 4% t 31%, and 5-year survival between 57% and 95%. Although the outcomes compare favorably with historic controls, further prospective trials are required to better define the role of trimodality therapy.

C. **Advanced disease.** Thymomas are sensitive to chemotherapy and several chemotherapeutic agents, either as a single agent or in combination regimens have been shown to be active. In a phase II study, 2 out of 21 patients with metastatic or recurrent thymomas treated with single agent cisplatin (50 mg/m^2 every 3 weeks) achieved partial response (*Am J Clin Oncol* 1993;16:342–345). Single agent ifosfamide (1.5 g/m^2 on days 1 to 5 every 3 weeks with mesna) was evaluated in 17 patients with advanced thymoma or thymic carcinoma and resulted in a 46% partial remission with a 5-year survival of 57% (*J Clin Oncol* 1999;17:2737–2744). The intergroup phase II trial evaluated the PAC regimen (cisplatin 50 mg/m^2, doxorubicin 50 mg/m^2, and cyclophosphamide 500 mg/m^2 every 3 weeks) in 30 patients with metastatic or recurrent thymoma and thymic carcinoma (*J Clin Oncol* 1994;12:1164–1168). The overall response rate was 50% with median survival of 38 months and a 5-year estimated survival of 32%. The combination of cisplatin (60 mg/m^2 on day 1) and etoposide (120 mg/m^2 on days 1 to 3) resulted in a 56% response rate and median survival of 4.3 years (*J Clin Oncol* 1996;14:814–820). The triplet therapy VIP (cisplatin 20 mg/m^2, etoposide 75 mg/m^2, and ifosfamide 1.2 g/m^2 all for 4 days every 3 weeks) led to a 32% partial response with median survival of 31 months (*Cancer* 2001;91:2010–2015). For patients with thymoma and positive indium-labeled octreotide scan, octreotide 0.5 mg subcutaneously three times daily for upto one year resulted in a 12.5% response rate. When combined with prednisone (0.6 mg/kg/day), octreotide showed a 31% response rate with median survival of 15 months (*Cancer* 2002;94:1414–1420).

D. **Prognosis.** Most of the thymomas are slow-growing encapsulated tumors which can be cured by surgical resection. Prognosis is usually related to the stage at presentation, presence or absence of complete resection, and the histologic type. Staging, regardless of the system used, remains the single most important prognostic determinant and the outcomes are significantly better in patients undergoing complete resection. There is a linear progression of malignancy among the WHO histologic subtypes, with A and AB thymomas behaving as benign tumors, B1 and B2 as low-grade tumors, and B3 as an aggressive tumor similar to thymic carcinoma. This correlation is reflected in both the likelihood of invasion and the overall survival.

IV. **THYMIC CARCINOMA.** Thymic carcinoma are rare tumors characterized by overt traditional histologic and cytologic features of malignancy such as nuclear atypia, increased mitotic activity, and necrosis. Tumors are usually located in the anterosuperior mediastinum and patients usually present with symptoms of local invasion such as dyspnea, cough, and chest pain. Most of the patients present with advanced disease with invasion of contiguous mediastinal structures and lymphadenopathy seen in approximately, 80% and 40% of patients respectively. Paraneoplastic syndromes are rarely seen. Due to the paucity of cases, the optimal treatment remains undefined. Surgical resection is the mainstay of treatment but complete resection is possible in a few patients due to the advanced stage. Most patients receive sequential radiation therapy and there may be a role for chemotherapy as well.

V. BACKGROUND. Thymomas are the most common primary tumors of the anterior mediastinum in adults. Most of the patients are between the ages of 40 and 60 at the time of diagnosis and there is no sex predilection. The overall incidence is 0.15 cases per 100,000 person-years.

VI. MESOTHELIOMA

A. Presentation

1. **Subjective.** Mesothelioma symptoms are usually insidious and nonspecific, commonly leading to a delay in the diagnosis. The median time between the onset of symptoms and the diagnosis is two to three months. The most commonly presenting complaints are dyspnea and nonpleuritic chest wall pain. Constitutional symptoms such as weight loss and fatigue are more common in the later stages of the disease but may occur in approximately, one third of the patients at presentation. Some patients may be asymptomatic and their disease is first noticed incidentally on a routine chest radiograph.

2. **Objective.** Common findings on physical examination include signs of unilateral pleural effusion including dullness to percussion and decreased air entry at one lung base. Fixed hemothorax, characterized by the lack of expansion in one side of the chest, is present in large tumors and usually represents a late finding. Occasionally, patients with advanced disease may have palpable supraclavicular lymph nodes or a palpable chest wall mass. Clubbing is rare. Some patients may have no physical signs due to the presence of a localized pleural mass without effusion.

B. Workup and staging

1. **Imaging studies.** Radiographic evaluation begins with a posteroanterior (PA) and lateral chest radiograph, which usually demonstrates a unilateral pleural effusion and occasionally, a pleural-based mass. Approximately, 20% of the patients have radiologic evidence of asbestos exposure on chest radiograph such as pleural plaques. CT scan often shows the effusion with or without pleural mass and allows the evaluation of tumor extent. In some patients, mesothelioma produces a localized lobular thickening whereas in others, it causes a rind of tumor encasing the lung. MRI may help to further define the local extension of pleural mesothelioma to the chest wall and diaphragm. PET scan can be used to differentiate between benign and malignant pleural masses. It may also allow the detection of lymph node or extrathoracic involvement.

2. **Diagnosis.** Despite the presence of typical, clinical or radiographic findings, the definitive diagnosis of mesothelioma should be made by pathologic evaluation. The initial diagnostic procedure is usually a thoracentesis. Cytology however, not always provides a definitive diagnosis because the yield can be low and when abnormal cells are present, it is often difficult to differentiate mesothelioma cells from reactive mesothelial cells and other malignancies, particularly adenocarcinomas. The diagnostic value of cytology may improve with the use of immunohistochemical (IHC) stains. When the cytology is inconclusive, patients should undergo a pleural biopsy. Histology samples may be obtained either by a CT-guided biopsy or through direct thoracoscopy.

3. **Pathology.** Mesothelioma is classified into three histologic subtypes: epithelial, sarcomatoid, and mixed. The epithelial type is the most common, comprising 50% to 60% of all cases. The sarcomatoid type is present in approximately 15% of cases and is characterized by spindle cells that are similar to fibrosarcomas. The mixed or biphasic subtype contains features of both epithelioid and sarcomatoid elements. Because the diagnosis of mesothelioma may not be easily accomplished from the pathologic specimen, IHC studies are commonly used to differentiate between mesothelioma and metastatic or primary lung adenocarcinomas. Stains, typically positive in mesothelioma include epithelial membrane antigen (EMA), Wilms tumor antigen-1 (WT1), cytokeratins 5 and 6, calretinin, and mesothelin. Negative stains include carcinoembryonic antigen (CEA), thyroid transcription

factor-1 (TTF-1), B72.3, CD15, MOC-31, Ber-P4, and Bg8. Electron microscopy should be reserved for difficult cases with equivocal IHC results. The epithelial form is composed of polygonal cells with long microvilli, prominent desmosomes, and abundant tonofilaments. The electron microscopy on the sarcomatoid variant reveals elongated nuclei and abundant rough endoplasmatic reticulum.

4. **Serum markers.** Serum mesothelin-related protein (SMRP) is a soluble form of mesothelin, which is elevated in most of the patients with mesothelioma. SMRP levels correlate with disease progression or response to therapy, and may be useful in in the early detection for patients at risk.

5. **Staging.** Although several staging systems have been proposed for mesothelioma, none achieved universal acceptance. The International Mesothelioma Interest Group (IMIG) proposed a new staging system for mesothelioma (Table 15.5). This tumor (T), lymph node (N), and metastases (M) staging system includes T descriptors that are much more detailed than those in previous systems. In addition, the descriptors for nodal involvement are the same as those used in the staging of non-small cell lung cancer. This new system allowed a more a accurate staging of mesothelioma patients according to prognosis. Median survival by stage was 35 months, 16 months, 11.5 months, and 5.9 months for stages I through IV, respectively. The difference in survival by tumor stage remained statistically significant when assessed with multivariate analysis. Based on these data, adoption of the IMIG staging system may allow a more accurate comparison of results between different therapies in patients with mesothelioma.

C. **Treatment.** Mesothelioma is an essentially incurable disease and the primary goal of therapy is to improve the quality of life and prolong survival. The tumor spreads along the serosal surface and infiltrates the underlying vital thoracic organs preventing a complete surgical resection. Furthermore, mesothelioma often arises from multiple sites in the parietal pleura. Patients are commonly elderly with significant comorbidities, and the insidious symptoms frequently delay the diagnosis. The choice of treatment is determined by the stage of the disease and the patients' comorbidities.

1. **Surgery.** There are three main surgical procedures used in the management of patients with mesothelioma: pleurodesis, pleurectomy with decortication (PD), and extrapleural pneumonectomy (EPP). Pleurodesis is commonly used in the treatment of persistent dyspnea caused by large pleura effusions. This procedure is effective in preventing fluid reaccumulation and should be performed earlier during the treatment. As the disease progresses, the tumor grows along the visceral pleura and encases the lung preventing the re-expansion. The resulting trapped lung is usually refractory to pleurodesis. PD refers to the surgical removal of the visceral, parietal, and pericardial pleura from the lung apex to the diaphragm, without the removal of the lung. This procedure has not been associated with survival benefit. A complete resection is only possible in very early stages of the disease, and most of the patients develop a disease recurrence. EPP is the most aggressive procedure and involves the *en bloc* resection of the visceral and parietal pleura, lung, pericardium, and ipsilateral diaphragm. EPP achieves the greatest degree of cytoreduction and allows higher doses of adjuvant radiation to be delivered to the ipsilateral hemithorax because the lung has already been removed. Although both PD and EPP are performed with curative intent, neither appear to provide a significant improvement in survival when used as a single modality therapy. Therefore, more recent studies have focused on the role of adjuvant therapy.

2. **Radiation therapy.** Mesothelioma cells are relatively sensitive to radiation therapy. However, due to the diffuse nature of the cancer, the dose of radiation for mesothelioma is limited by the need to irradiate the entire hemithorax, which includes vital organs such as lung, heart, esophagus, and spinal cord. Radiation therapy has minimal effects on increasing survival. There are three main indications for the use of radiation therapy: palliation of pain, prophylaxis against needle tract metastases, and adjuvant therapy. Most of the patients treated with radiation therapy achieve a short-lived pain control. Because mesothelioma is characterized by direct local invasion, it often invades tracts after local

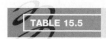

TABLE 15.5 The International Mesothelioma Interest Group Staging System

T: Tumor

T1	T1a, tumor limited to the ipsilateral parietal pleura, including mediastinal, and diaphragmatic pleura No involvement of the visceral pleura T1b, tumor involving the ipsilateral parietal pleura, including mediastinal, and diaphragmatic pleura Scattered foci of tumor also involving the visceral pleura
T2	Tumor involving each of the ipsilateral pleural surfaces (parietal, mediastinal, diaphragmatic, and visceral pleura) with at least one of the following features: ■ Involvement of the diaphragmatic muscle ■ Confluent visceral pleural tumor (including the fissures) or extension of tumor from visceral pleura into the underlying pulmonary parenchyma
T3	Describes locally advanced but potentially resectable tumor Tumor involving all the ipsilateral pleural surfaces (parietal, mediastinal, diaphragmatic, and visceral pleura) with at least one of the following features: ■ Involvement of the endothoracic fascia ■ Extension into the mediastinal fat ■ Solitary, completely resectable focus of tumor extending into the soft tissues of the chest wall ■ Nontransmural involvement of the pericardium
T4	Describes locally advanced technically unresectable tumor Tumor involving all of the ipsilateral pleural surfaces (parietal, mediastinal, diaphragmatic, and visceral) with at least one of the following features: ■ Diffuse extension or multifocal masses of tumor in the chest wall, with or without associated rib destruction ■ Direct transdiaphragmatic extension of tumor to the peritoneum ■ Direct extension of tumor to the contralateral pleura ■ Direct extension of tumor to one or more mediastinal organs ■ Direct extension of tumor into the spine ■ Tumor extending through to the internal surface of the pericardium with or without a pericardial effusion; or tumor involving the myocardium

N: Lymph nodes

NX	Regional lymph nodes cannot be assessed
N0	No regional lymph node metastases
N1	Metastases in the ipsilateral bronchopulmonary or hilar lymph nodes
N2	Metastases in the subcarinal or the ipsilateral mediastinal lymph nodes, including the ipsilateral internal mammary nodes
N3	Metastases in the contralateral mediastinal, contralateral internal mammary, ipsilateral, or contralateral supraclavicular lymph nodes

M: Metastases

MX	Presence of distant metastases cannot be assessed
M0	No distant metastasis
M1	Distant metastases present

Stage groupings:

Stage	Ia	T1a	N0	M0
	Ib	T1b	N0	M0
Stage	II	T2	N0	M0
Stage	III	Any T3	N0–2	M0
		T1–3	N1–2	M0
Stage	IV	Any T	N3	M0
		Ty	Any N	M0
		Any T	Any N	M1

procedures. In these cases, prophylactic radiation may be used as a prophylactic measure. Due to the high rates of local relapse after surgery, radiation therapy has been used in the adjuvant setting in an attempt to eradicate residual tumor. Studies in patients undergoing EPP have shown decreased local relapse with disease palliation, but no definitive survival improvement.

3. **Chemotherapy.** Chemotherapy has been used in the neoadjuvant or adjuvant setting in patients treated with multimodality treatment or as single modality in advanced cases. The role of chemotherapy remains palliative because even trimodality therapy does not appear to achieve cure or prolong survival. Several chemotherapeutic agents have been tested in mesothelioma, either alone or in combination therapy. Among several regimens, the combination of pemetrexed and cisplatin emerged as the standard of care after a phase III study showing improved survival compared with single agent cisplatin (*J Clin Oncol* 2003;21:2636–2644). In this study, 456 patients were assigned to cisplatin alone (75 mg/m^2 day 1 every 3 weeks) or in combination with pemetrexed (500 mg/m^2 day 1 every 3 weeks). The combination arm resulted in significant benefit including improved response rate (41% vs. 16%, p <0.0001), median time to progression (5.7 months vs. 3.9 months, p = 0.001), and median survival (12.1 months vs. 9.3 months, p = 0.02). Several novel approaches for the systemic treatment of mesothelioma have been recently developed. The Cancer and Leukemia Group B conducted a phase II study evaluating the role of gefitinib, an oral epidermal growth factor receptor (EGFR) tyrosine kinase in previously untreated patients with mesothelioma (*Clin Cancer Res* 2005;11:2300–2304). Among the 43 enrolled patients, the response rate was 4% and median survival 6.8 months. EGFR expression was not correlated with response or survival. The ribonuclease ranpirnase was evaluated in a large phase II study involving 105 patients with mesothelioma (*J Clin Oncol* 2002;20:274–281). Among the 81 patients evaluated for response, 4 had partial response, 2 had minor response, and 35 patients had stabilization of a previously progressive disease. Although the median survival for the entire group was 6 months, the treatment was very well tolerated and patients with tumor response or stable disease had a markedly prolonged survival. Other therapeutic strategies include immunotherapy, gene therapy, proteasome inhibitors, and angiogenesis inhibitors such as bevacizumab and thalidomide.

D. **Prognosis.** The prognosis for patients with mesothelioma is poor, with median survival of approximately 12 months from diagnosis. Factors associated with poor prognosis include advanced stage, poor performance status, male sex, chest pain, weight loss, thrombocytosis, leukocytosis, anemia, older age, and sarcomatoid histology. Two prognostic systems have been developed based on data collection from patients enrolled into large cooperative group trials. In the European Organization for Research and Treatment of Cancer (EORTC) study, the risk factors identified were Eastern Cooperative Oncology Group (ECOG) performance status 1 or 2, white blood cells more than 8,300/μL, hemoglobin decrease equal to or greater than 1 g/dL, probable or possible diagnosis, and sarcomatoid histology (*J Clin Oncol* 1998;16:145–152). Patients were subdivided into two prognostic groups: good prognosis with upto two risk factors and poor prognosis with three or more risk factors. Outcomes were significantly better for patients in the good prognosis category, with improved median survival (10.8 months vs. 5.5 months), 1-year overall survival (40% vs. 12%), and 2-year survival (14% vs. 0%). In the Cancer and Leukemia Group B (CALGB) study, the significant risk factors included poor performance status, chest pain, dyspnea, platelet count greater than 400,000/μL, weight loss, serum lactate dehydrogenase (LDH) greater than 500 IU/L, pleural involvement, anemia, leukocytosis, and age above 75 (*Chest* 1998;113:723–731). There were six identified prognostic subgroups with median survival times ranging from 1.4 to 13.9 months.

E. **Background.** Malignant mesothelioma is an aggressive tumor of the serosal surfaces. The incidence is increasing worldwide as a result of widespread exposure to asbestos. There are approximately, 2,500 new cases per year in the United States. The main risk for the development of mesothelioma is exposure to asbestos. Although approximately, 80% of patients with mesothelioma have a history of asbestos exposure, only approximately 10% of those will develop mesothelioma. The role of Simian virus 40 (SV40), a double-stranded DNA polyoma virus, remains unclear. SV40 is a potent oncogenic virus in human and rodent cells, and may have contaminated humans through injectable Salk poliomyelitis vaccines 35 to 40 years ago.

Suggested Readings

Thymoma

Detterbeck FC, Parsons AM. Thymic tumors. *Ann Thorac Surg* 2004;77:1860–1869.

Duwe BV, Sterman DH, Musani AI. Tumors of the mediastinum. *Chest* 2005;128:2893–2909.

Eng TY, Fuller CD, Jagirdar J, et al. Thymic carcinoma: state of the art and review. *Int J Radiat Oncol Biol Phys* 2004;59:654–664.

Giaccone G. Treatment of malignant thymoma. *Curr Opin Oncol* 2005;17:140–146.

Giaccone G, Wilmink H, Paul MA, et al. Systemic treatment of malignant thymoma. A decade of experience at a single institution. *Am J Clin Oncol* 2006;29:336–344.

Johnson SB, Eng TY, Giaccone G. Thymoma: update for the new millennium. *Oncologist* 2001;6:239–246.

Suster S, Moran CA. Thymoma classification. Current status and future trends. *Am J Clin Pathol* 2006;125:542–554.

Thomas CR, Wright CD, Loehrer PJ. Thymoma: state of the art. *J Clin Oncol* 1999;17:2280–2289.

Mesothelioma

Curran D, Sahmoud T, Therasse P, et al. Prognostic factors in patients with pleural mesothelioma: the European Organization for Research and Treatment of Cancer experience. *J Clin Oncol* 1998;16:145–152.

Herndon JE, Green MR, Chahinian AP, et al. Factors predictive of survival among 337 patients with mesothelioma treated between 1984 and 1994 by the Cancer and Leukemia Group B. *Chest* 1998;113:723–731.

Krug LM. An overview of chemotherapy for mesothelioma. *Hematol Oncol Clin North Am* 2005;19:1117–1136.

Masaoka A, Monden Y, Nakahara K, et al. Follow-up study of thymomas with special reference to their clinical stages. *Cancer* 1981;48:2485–2492.

Pistolesi M, Rusthoven J. Malignant pleural mesothelioma. Update, current management, and newer therapeutic strategies. *Chest* 2004;126:1318–1329.

Robinson BWS, Lake RA. Advances in malignant mesothelioma. *N Engl J Med* 2005;353:1591–1603.

Robinson BWS, Musk AW, Lake RA. Malignant mesothelioma. *Lancet* 2005;366:397–408.

Scaglioti GV, Novello S. State of the art in mesothelioma. *Ann Oncol* 2005;16:240s–245s.

Volgelzang NJ, Porta C, Mutti L. New agents in the management of advanced mesothelioma. *Semin Oncol* 2005;32:336–350.

Volgelzang NJ, Rusthoven JJ, Symanowsky J, et al. Phase III study of pemetrexed in combination with cisplatin versus cisplatin alone in patients with malignant pleural mesothelioma. *J Clin Oncol* 2003;21:2636–2644.

West SD, Lee YCG. Management of malignant pleural mesothelioma. *Clin Chest Med* 2006;27:335–354.

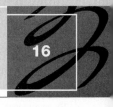

I. ESOPHAGEAL CANCER

A. Subjective. Patients with esophageal cancer often do not have symptoms until the esophageal lumen is greatly narrowed. The most common symptom for patients with esophageal cancer is dysphagia. Ninety-five percent of symptomatic patients will report dysphagia. It typically begins with solid food only but often progresses to occurring with liquids as the esophageal lumen becomes blocked by the cancer. Other common symptoms include weight loss (50%), regurgitation (40%), pain on swallowing (20%), and cough (20%).

B. Objective. Physical examination findings are varied. It may be normal, suggest cachexia only, or there may be evidence of metastases such as supraclavicular lymphadenopathy, hoarseness from recurrent laryngeal nerve involvement, pleural effusion, hepatomegaly, or bony tenderness.

C. Workup. Symptoms or signs suggesting esophageal cancer should prompt further evaluation. The most important test is an esophagogastroduodenoscopy (EGD). This test allows the visualization and biopsy of an esophageal lesion. If an esophageal cancer is found, a complete blood count (CBC), comprehensive metabolic panel (CMP), and a computed tomogram (CT) of the chest and abdomen need to be performed.

CT is an excellent initial staging tool but further specialized testing may be necessary. If the patient does not have evidence of metastasis, an endoscopic ultrasound should be performed. This procedure, involving insertion of an ultrasound probe into the esophagus and stomach, allows the most precise assessment of depth of tumor involvement, length of esophagus affected, and magnitude of lymph node metastases, particularly paraesophageal and celiac nodes. A biopsy of suspicious lymph nodes can be done during the study.

Positron emission tomographic (PET) scans are an important part of the staging evaluation of patients without clear evidence of metastasis on CT. FDG (2-fluoro-2-deoxy-D-glucose)-avid lymph nodes should be biopsied to confirm metastasis.

A primary tumor located above the carina is a risk for a tracheoesophageal fistula so a bronchoscopy should be preformed.

D. Staging. Esophageal cancer staging depends on the tumor, node, metastases (TNM) system established by the American Joint Commission for Cancer (AJCC) and the International Union Against Cancer (UICC) (Table 16.1).

E. Therapy

1. Therapy for localized esophageal cancer

   a. General considerations. The treatment of esophageal cancer requires a multidisciplinary approach. It frequently involves the combination of surgery, radiation, chemotherapy, and supportive treatments. The functional status of the patient and location of the tumor play a key role in determining the management of the patient. Patient comorbidities may preclude potentially curative therapies.

   b. Surgery. Surgery is considered the standard therapy for stage I, II, and III esophageal cancers located outside the cervical esophagus. If an early-stage cancer is located in the cervical esophagus, however, the preferred treatment is a combination of chemotherapy and radiation.

   The best chance for surgical cure involves removal of the entire tumor and draining lymph nodes with adequate proximal and distal margins. The three

181

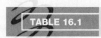

TABLE 16.1	Staging Classification of Esophageal Cancer		
Primary tumor (T)	**Regional lymph nodes (N)**	**Distant metastasis (M)**	**Stage**
TX: primary tumor cannot be assessed	NX: regional lymph node involvement cannot be assessed	MX: presence of metastasis cannot be assessed	Stage 0: TisN0M0
T0: no evidence of primary tumor	N0: no regional lymph nodes metastasis	M0: no distant metastasis	Stage 1: T1a/bN0M0
Tis: carcinoma *in situ*	N1: regional lymph node metastasis	M1: distant metastasis	Stage IIA: T2N0M0; T3N0M0
T1: tumor invades lamina propria or submucosa	N1a: one to three nodes involved	Tumors of the lower thoracic esophagus:	Stage IIB: T1a/bN1M0; T2N1M0
		M1a: metastasis to celiac lymph nodes M1b: other distant metastasis	
T1a: tumor invades mucosa or lamina propria	N1b: four to seven nodes involved	Tumors of the midthoracic esophagus:	Stage III: T3N1M0; T4 any N M0
		M1a: n/a M1b: non-regional lymph nodes and/or other distant metastasis	
T1b: tumor invades submucosa	N1c: >7 nodes involved	Tumors of the upper thoracic esophagus: M1a: metastasis to cervical lymph nodes M1b: other distant metastasis	Stage IVA: any T any N M1a
T2: tumor invades muscularis propria			Stage IVB: any T any N M1b
T3: tumor invades adventitia			
T4: tumor invades adjacent structures			

most frequently used approaches for resection are (a) the Ivor-Lewis approach, in which a laparotomy and right thoracotomy are performed for esophageal resection and gastric mobilization with an anastomosis in the upper thorax; (b) a transhiatal esophagectomy, through a cervical and abdominal approach with cervical anastomosis; and (c) a left thoracoabdominal approach, with an anastomosis below the aortic arch. After an esophagectomy, most patients are reconstructed with a primary esophagogastric anastomosis in the neck or chest.

Esophageal resection is a major surgery with a mortality rate of approximately 4% in experienced hands. Other complications of the surgery may include anastomotic leak, chylothorax, damage to the left recurrent laryngeal nerve, severe hemorrhage, and pulmonary embolus.

The ability of surgery to cure is dependent on the stage of the cancer. Thirty percent to fifty percent of patients with stage I esophageal cancer will be cured by surgery alone. For patients with stage IIA and IIB disease, the 5-year survival following surgery is 15% to 30% and 5% to 15%, respectively. Locoregional relapse after surgical resection ranges from 15% to 25%.

c. **Neoadjuvant and adjuvant therapy.** In order to improve outcomes with surgery, neoadjuvant and adjuvant treatment with chemoradiotherapy, radiation, and combined chemotherapy have been attempted. This is one of the most controversial areas in oncology. Randomized phase III trials have been performed often with mixed results.

Neoadjuvant and adjuvant chemotherapy has been examined. The two most prominent trials are Intergroup 0113 and MRC. In Intergroup 0113, more than 400 patients with resectable esophageal cancers of both histologic subtypes (squamous and adenocarcinoma) were randomly assigned to immediate surgery or neoadjuvant cisplatin/5-fluorouracil (5-FU) for three cycles. The patients in the chemotherapy arm also received adjuvant cisplatin/5-FU for two cycles. The 2-year survival (approximately 35%) was the same in both arms (*N Engl J Med* 1998;339:1979). In the MRC trial, 800 patients were randomized to immediate surgery or two cycles of neoadjuvant cisplatin/5-FU. Neoadjuvant chemotherapy increased the 2-year survival from 34% to 43% (*Lancet* 2002;359:1727). There are, however, some methodologic concerns with the MRC trial. Approximately 10% of patients received radiation therapy (RT) to the esophagus. Given the lack of convincing data and other treatment options, neoadjuvant and adjuvant chemotherapy are not currently recommended by the National Comprehensive Cancer Network (NCCN).

Neoadjuvant and adjuvant RT has also been tried. At least five trials have tested neoadjuvant radiation versus surgery alone, and none of them have shown a survival advantage. Few randomized trials of postoperative radiation have been performed, and it has been largely replaced by postoperative chemoradiotherapy.

Postoperative chemoradiotherapy clearly has a role in the treatment of esophageal cancer. Patients with gross or microscopic residual disease following surgery are felt to benefit from combined modality chemotherapy/RT. Adjuvant chemoradiotherapy in patients without residual disease is less defined. In the current NCCN guidelines, observation is recommended for those with squamous cell carcinoma. For patients with adenocarcinoma, those with lymph node–positive disease and large tumors (T3 or greater) should receive chemoradiotherapy. Chemoradiotherapy is a consideration in patients with T2N0 adenocarcinoma. Adjuvant chemoradiation in esophageal cancer is most commonly cisplatin 75 mg/m^2 on day 1 and 5-FU 1,000 mg/m^2/day c.i.v.i. on days 1 to 4 in weeks 1, 5, 8, and 11, along with daily radiation.

The role of preoperative chemoradiotherapy is less defined. Since 1982, there have been at least 46 trials performed involving approximately 2,700 patients. The most prominent trials were performed by Walsh et al. and Bosset et al. Walsh et al. randomized 113 resectable patients to either immediate surgery or cisplatin/5-FU combined with radiation before surgery. There was a significant downstaging with chemoradiotherapy with a 25% pathologic complete response (CR) rate at the time of surgery. Median survival was significantly lengthened with chemoradiation from 11 months to 16 months and 3-year survival was 6% versus 32% (*N Engl J Med* 1996;335:462). Bosset et al. randomized 282 resectable patients to cisplatin plus radiation or immediate surgery. There was no difference in median survival but there was an increased perioperative death rate (3.6% vs. 12.3%) (*N Engl J Med* 1997;337:161). This increase in perioperative death rate was not found in the other trials performed. A recent meta-analysis has shown a significant survival advantage and decreased local failure with neoadjuvant chemoradiotherapy. Neoadjuvant chemoradiation remains investigational, but it is a reasonable option for patients with a good performance status and locally advanced disease.

d. **Therapy for unresectable locally advanced esophageal cancer.** The standard of care for unresectable locally advanced esophageal cancer is concurrent chemoradiotherapy. Herscovic et al. randomized 120 patients to radiation alone (64 Gy) or cisplatin 75 mg/m^2 on day 1 and 5-FU 1,000 mg/m^2/day c.i.v.i. on days 1 to 4 to be repeated in weeks 1, 5, 8, and 11 along with 50 Gy of radiation over 5 weeks. The median survival for the chemoradiotherapy arm was 14.1 months versus 9.3 months in the radiation-alone arm. The 5-year survival for chemoradiotherapy was 27%, as compared to 0% in the radiation-alone group (*N Engl J Med* 1992;326:1593).

2. **Therapy for metastatic esophageal cancer**
   a. **General considerations.** Metastatic esophageal cancer is incurable and the toxicity of therapy must be weighed against its potential benefit. Palliative therapy for swallowing and nutritional support is especially important. There are a number of options for palliation of swallowing. These include esophageal dilatation, stent placement, brachytherapy, external-beam radiation, and laser therapy. In regard to nutritional support, patients with metastatic esophageal cancer frequently require a gastrostomy tube.
   b. **Chemotherapy.** Several chemotherapeutic agents have activity in esophageal cancer. Unfortunately, no large phase III trials comparing chemotherapeutic regimens have been performed in recent years. The agents that have the most activity in esophageal cancer are cisplatin, carboplatin, 5-FU, paclitaxel, docetaxel, vinorelbine, oxaliplatin, and irinotecan. In general, platinum-based doublets have the highest response rate and are typically used as first-line therapy. One could also consider treating adenocarcinoma of the lower esophagus like a gastric carcinoma. NCCN currently lists cisplatin-based and 5-FU–based chemotherapeutic regimens as category 1 recommendations (strongest recommendation). The other agents are category 3 (disagreement among committee members regarding the usefulness of therapy).

F. **Course of the disease.** Metastatic esophageal cancer has a poor prognosis with a median survival of approximately 9 months despite systemic chemotherapy. Three fourths the number of patients present with mediastinal node involvement or distant spread at the time of diagnosis. Death often occurs from progression of their metastatic disease or aspiration pneumonia from local disease.

G. **Complications.** Complications of the esophageal cancer include hemorrhage, obstruction, tracheoesophageal fistula, and aspiration pneumonia.

H. **Epidemiology.** Esophageal cancer is a commonly found neoplasm and is the seventh in the most common causes of cancer death in the world. There is vast geographic variation in the incidence of this cancer. The incidence in the United States is about 5 per 100,000, although in African-American men, it may be as high as 18 per 100,000, whereas China and Iran have an incidence of 20 per 100,000. In parts of Africa, Central America, and Western Asia, the incidence is only 1.5 per 100,000.

The two most common pathologic subtypes of esophageal cancer are squamous cell carcinoma and adenocarcinoma. Other histologic types such as sarcomas, small cell carcinomas, and lymphomas are extremely rare. Of the two most common histologies, squamous cell tumors make up 98% of malignancies in the upper and middle one third of the esophagus, whereas adenocarcinoma is found predominantly in the lower third. Previously, squamous cell carcinoma was the most frequent subtype, but over the past 20 years, the incidence of adenocarcinoma has been increasing rapidly in the Western world. The reason for this shift is unknown.

The incidence of esophageal cancer increases with age and is rarely found among patients younger than 40 years. Squamous cell carcinoma affects African-American men six times more than it affects white men, whereas adenocarcinoma affects whites four times as much. All subtypes of esophageal cancers afflict men three times as often as they do women.

Several factors can increase the risk of developing esophageal cancer. The long-term use of tobacco and alcohol are predisposing factors for development of squamous cell carcinoma of the esophagus. Dietary factors such as inadequate vegetable and fruit intake may also increase the risk of the development of this cancer. Nitrosamines and their precursors (found in pickled vegetables, moldy or fermented foods, and smoked fish) are known to promote cancerous changes in the esophagus. Tylosis, a rare genetic syndrome, carries the highest risk of developing squamous cell carcinoma from chronic inflammation and stasis (1,000-fold risk). It is an autosomal dominant trait that is characterized by hyperkeratosis of the palms and soles and may produce defective vitamin A metabolism. Other conditions associated with esophageal cancer are head and neck malignancies, celiac disease, and gastroesophageal reflux disease.

Barrett's esophagus (BE) predisposes to the development of adenocarcinoma of the esophagus. BE increases the risk of adenocarcinoma by 30 to 125 times that of the healthy patient population. In BE, the normal squamous epithelium of the esophagus is destroyed by chronic gastroesophageal reflux of acid, pepsin, and bile, and is ultimately replaced by a specialized intestinal columnar epithelium.

I. **Research initiatives.** The role of epidermal growth factor receptor (EGFR) targeted therapies is currently being studied. Defining the role of neoadjuvant chemoradiation is also an important area of research.

II. GASTRIC CANCER

A. **Subjective.** Gastric cancer usually presents with nonspecific constitutional symptoms. The most common is weight loss that occurs in approximately 80% of patients. Other common symptoms include anorexia, fatigue, vague stomach pain, dysphagia (from gastroesophageal [GE] junction tumors), and vomiting (from gastric outlet obstruction).

B. **Objective.** The physical findings in gastric cancer are typically manifestations of metastatic disease. Several eponymic terms have been created to describe specific sites of metastatic gastric cancer. *Virchow's node* describes metastasis to the left supraclavicular node. *Sister Mary Joseph's node* is a periumbilical lymph node metastasis. A *Krukenberg tumor* is a gastric cancer metastatic to the ovaries. *Blumer's shelf* describes a "drop metastasis" into the perirectal pouch. Other common physical findings in patients with metastatic gastric cancer include cachexia, palpable abdominal masses, and malignant ascites.

C. **Workup.** EGD is useful for the evaluation of suspected gastric cancer. This technique allows visualization of lesions and easy biopsy. EGD is used in the Japanese screening program for gastric cancer, which is credited with the increased proportion of early gastric cancers diagnosed in that country.

Once a diagnosis of gastric carcinoma is made, further staging is necessary. As in esophageal cancer, endoscopic ultrasound may be used to gauge tumor depth and involvement of local lymph nodes. CT scans and PET/CT are used to evaluate for metastatic disease. Unfortunately, metastatic peritoneal deposits may not be seen on routine imaging and a diagnostic laparotomy is necessary to rule this out before definitive resection.

Gastric cancer is staged with the AJCC TNM criteria (Table 16.2).

D. **Therapy**

1. **Localized gastric adenocarcinoma**

a. **Surgery.** Surgery is the most effective curative therapy for gastric cancer. In the United States, patients with resected stage I cancer have a 5-year survival of 58% to 78%. For stage II, survival ranges from 20% to 34%, and for stage III from 8% to 20%.

A controversy exists over the extent of surgery required. There is general agreement that patients with cancers localized to the distal stomach may be cured with subtotal gastrectomy. Other sites are usually treated with total gastrectomy. In Japan, the standard of care is a total gastrectomy including a D2 lymph node dissection that removes the perigastric nodes along the greater and lesser curvature (the N1 group of nodes) as well as the nodes along the left gastric artery, the common hepatic artery, the celiac artery, and the splenic artery (the N2 group of nodes). The tail of the pancreas and the spleen are sometimes removed additionally in a D2 dissection but this has been noted to increase morbidity and mortality. Japanese investigators credit the D2 dissection for the superior outcomes in Japanese patients stage for stage, and survival is double or triple that of North American patients.

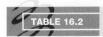

| TABLE 16.2 | Staging Classification of Gastric Cancer |

Primary tumor (T)	Regional lymph nodes (N)	Distant metastasis (M)	Stage
TX: primary tumor cannot be assessed	NX: regional lymph node involvement cannot be assessed	MX: presence of metastasis cannot be assessed	Stage 0: TisN0M0
T0: no evidence of primary tumor	N0: no regional lymph node metastasis	M0: no distant metastasis	Stage IA: T1N0M0
Tis: intraepithelial tumors without invasion of lamina propria	N1: regional lymph node metastasis in 1–6 nodes	M1: distant metastasis	Stage IB: T1N1M0; T2a/bN0M0
T1: tumor invades lamina propria or submucosa	N2: regional lymph node metastasis in 7–15 nodes		Stage II: T1N2M0; T2a/bN1M0; T3N0M0
T2: tumor invades lamina propria/submucosa	N3: regional lymph node metastasis in >15 nodes		Stage IIIA: T2a/bN2M0; T3N1M0; T4N0M0
T2a: tumor invades muscularis propria			Stage IIIB: T3N2M0
T2b: tumor invades submucosa			Stage IV: T4 any N M0; any T N3 M0; any T any N M1
T3: tumor penetrates serosa (visceral peritoneum)			
T4: tumor invades adjacent structures			

Outside of Japan, D2 dissection is associated with greater morbidity. Controlled, randomized studies have not shown D2 dissection to be better than the more limited D1 dissection in which only the N1 group of nodes is removed. In a more recent trial, D1 dissection is the generally accepted standard in the United States, although it is likely that many patients receive even less than this. Currently, NCCN recommends that at least a D1 resection be performed.
   b. Neoadjuvant and adjuvant therapy. Adjuvant therapies have been tried in an attempt to improve survival following resection. Adjuvant radiotherapy alone has not shown benefit. Adjuvant chemotherapy has also not clearly shown a benefit but meta-analysis has suggested that there may be some. Adjuvant combination chemoradiotherapy, however, clearly has benefit for some patients. This is based on the Intergroup 116 (INT-116) study. In this study, 556 patients with at least stage IB gastric carcinoma, who had undergone definitive resection to negative margins, were randomized to observation or 5 months of therapy. The adjuvant therapy consisted of one cycle consisting of 5-FU (425 mg/m^2) plus leucovorin (20 mg/m^2) daily for 5 days. One month of rest followed this cycle of chemotherapy. Combination chemoradiotherapy was then started. Radiation dose of 4,500 cGy was given over 5 weeks with

5-FU (400 mg/m^2) and leucovorin (20 mg/m^2) on days 1 to 4 and for the last 3 days of radiation. A 1-month rest then followed. Then 5-FU (425 mg/m^2) plus leucovorin (20 mg/m^2) on days 1 to 5 was repeated monthly for two cycles. Adjuvant therapy increased overall survival from 27 months to 36 months (*p* less than 0.005) (*N Engl J Med* 2001;345:725). Therefore, adjuvant chemoradiotherapy is considered standard of care for patients who have had completely resected stage IB or more advanced gastric adenocarcinoma. For patients who had positive margins at resection, combination chemoradiation is also considered standard of care.

Neoadjuvant/perioperative chemotherapy has been tested in order to make unresectable cancers operable and to improve overall survival. The most prominent trial is the MAGIC trial published by Cunningham in 2006. In this trial, 503 patients with at least stage II adenocarcinoma of the stomach, gastroesophageal junction, and distal esophagus were randomized to surgery alone or chemotherapy in addition to surgery. The chemotherapeutic regimen was ECF (epirubicin 50 mg/m^2 on day 1, cisplatin 60 mg/m^2 on day 1, and 5-FU 200 mg/m^2 by c.i.v.i. on days 1 to 21) every 3 weeks for three cycles before surgery and then three cycles after surgery. The chemotherapy arm showed a statistically significant downsizing of the tumor as well as significant improvement in survival. The 5-year survival was 36% in the chemotherapy arm versus 23% in the surgery-only arm. Interestingly, only 42% of the chemotherapy patients were able to complete the three cycles of postoperative chemotherapy (*N Engl J Med* 2006:355:11).

On the basis of the results of Intergroup 116 and the MAGIC trials, it is clear that surgery alone is not sufficient therapy for gastric cancer. What is not clear is whether adjuvant or neoadjuvant/perioperative therapy is best and what the role of RT is. Currently, NCCN recommends the adjuvant chemoradiotherapy approach until more information on the neoadjuvant/perioperative chemotherapy is collected.

c. **Therapy for medically unresectable patients.** Combination chemoradiation is considered the standard of care for medically unresectable localized gastric adenocarcinoma. It typically combines 5-FU with 4,500 to 5,000 cGy of radiation. Notably, only a very small percentage of patients can be cured with chemoradiotherapy alone.

2. **Metastatic gastric adenocarcinoma**
a. **Chemotherapy.** Chemotherapy has been shown to improve survival and quality of life in patients with metastatic gastric carcinoma. Several chemotherapeutic agents have activity in gastric cancer. These include 5-FU, cisplatin, oxaliplatin, irinotecan, capecitabine, anthracyclines, and taxanes. In a recent retrospective Cochrane meta-analysis, combination chemotherapy appears to offer a small survival benefit over single-agent chemotherapy. Commonly used combination chemotherapeutic regimens include CF (cisplatin 100 mg/m^2 on day 1 every 4 weeks, and infusional 5-FU 1,000 mg/m^2/day on days 1 to 5 every 4 weeks), DCF (docetaxel 75 mg/m^2 on day 1 every 3 weeks, cisplatin 75 mg/m^2 on day 1 every 3 weeks, and infusional 5-FU 750 mg/m^2/day on days 1 to 5 every 3 weeks), ECF (epirubicin 50 mg/m^2 on day 1 every 3 weeks, cisplatin 60 mg/m^2 on day 1 every 3 weeks, and infusional 5-FU 200 mg/m^2/day continuously), EOF (epirubicin 50 mg/m^2 on day 1 every 3 weeks, oxaliplatin 130 mg/m^2 on day 1 every 3 weeks, and infusional 5-FU 200 mg/m^2/day continuously), EOX (epirubicin 50 mg/m^2 on day 1 every 3 weeks, oxaliplatin 130 mg/m^2 on day 1 every 3 weeks, and capecitabine 625 mg/m^2 p.o. b.i.d. continuously), and FOLFIRI (irinotecan 180 mg/m^2 on days 1 and 15 every 4 weeks, leucovorin 400 mg/m^2 on days 1 and 15 every 4 weeks, 5-FU 1200 mg/m^2/day on days 1,2,15, and 16 every 4 weeks). Although there are some interesting phase III trials comparing combination chemotherapies such as the TAX 325 (that showed an increased TTP for DCF vs. CF) and the REAL-2 trial (that showed at least equivalence of EOX, ECF, EOF, and ECX), there is no clear standard of care first-line combination chemotherapy (*Proc*

Am Soc Clin Oncol 2005;23:4002; *Proc Am Soc Clin Oncol* 2006;24:4017). Also, there is no clear standard of care second-line chemotherapy.

   b. Other palliative procedures. Debulking/diverting surgery may improve quality of life in selected patients with discrete obstructing tumors. Radiotherapy may palliate bleeding or painful metastases. Other procedures are similar to those discussed earlier for esophageal cancer.

E. Course of the disease. Like esophageal cancer, gastric cancer is aggressive. The median survival of patients with metastatic gastric cancer is approximately 9 months. Common sites of metastasis include the liver, peritoneum, and lymph nodes.

F. Complications. Gastric cancer can lead to hemorrhage, gastric obstruction, and malignant ascites. Anastomotic leaks are the most common complication of gastrectomy. Development of B12 deficiency following gastric surgery is also a concern.

G. Pathology. Ninety percent of gastric carcinomas are adenocarcinomas. The remainder are non-Hodgkin's lymphomas (NHLs) and leiomyosarcomas (gastrointestinal [GI] stromal tumors). NHL and GI stromal tumors are discussed in depth in other chapters 26, Hematologic Malignancies: Lymphoma and 31, Sarcoma.

   Two classification systems for gastric adenocarcinoma are used. The Lauren classification divides gastric adenocarcinomas into the intestinal and diffuse types. The intestinal type arises from a background of intestinal metaplasia and shows differentiation resembling that of a colonic adenocarcinoma. Intestinal type is predominant in epidemic areas, affects older patients, and often metastasizes first to the liver. The diffuse type is poorly differentiated, affects younger patients, and has a tendency to metastasize to the peritoneum, resulting in implants and malignant ascites. Patients with the intestinal type appear to have better outcomes overall.

   The Borrmann classification divides adenocarcinomas by their growth pattern. Types I and II are polypoid and heaped-up ulcers, respectively, and are associated with the intestinal type. Type III is an ulcerated, infiltrating tumor, and type IV, diffusely infiltrating. This last type is also referred to as *linitis plastica* or leather bottle stomach. These are associated with the diffuse type of adenocarcinoma. GE-junction tumors are usually the diffuse type. The boundaries between these groupings are not sharp, and some tumors are not easily categorized.

H. Epidemiology. Gastric cancer was once the most common malignancy in the United States, but its incidence has decreased since the 1930s. Worldwide, gastric cancer is surpassed only by lung cancer in frequency. It is the most frequent visceral cancer in Japan, where the incidence reaches 93.3 per 100,000. The high incidence in Japan has resulted in the creation of an endoscopic screening program, which is credited for the high frequency of early-stage cancers (50%) in Japanese patients. In contrast, more than 80% of Western patients have advanced cancers at diagnosis.

   The intestinal and diffuse types of gastric cancer differ in regard to epidemiology and risk factors. The intestinal type is associated with consumption of large amounts of salt and preserved foods, and possibly with *Helicobacter pylori* infection. These irritants lead to intestinal metaplasia of the stomach, which can then transform into frank malignancy. Other predisposing factors include achlorhydria associated with pernicious anemia and previous partial gastrectomy for peptic ulcer. It is thought that the lack of stomach acid in these conditions predisposes to intestinal metaplasia. Despite this, long-term use of H_2 blockers does not appear to be a risk factor.

   The intestinal type of gastric cancer is more prevalent in Japan, where preserved and salty foods are widely consumed. The decrease in the incidence of gastric cancer in the United States may relate to the availability of refrigeration and a dietary shift toward fresh foods. Asian patients may have genetic predispositions increasing cancer risk as well, as the rate decreases in Japanese immigrants in the United States who adopt local diets, but remains elevated as compared with the U.S. populace as a whole. The diffuse type is more sporadic and is not associated with diet. It is the most common form found in the United States. Diffuse types have a tendency to be more aggressive.

I. Research areas. A comparison of adjuvant versus neoadjuvant therapy for gastric cancer is currently under way. Novel chemotherapeutic agents such as S-1 are currently in Phase III trials.

Suggested Readings

Bosset J, Gignoux M, Triboulet JP, et al. Chemoradiotherapy followed by surgery compared with surgery alone in squamous-cell cancer of the esophagus. *N Engl J Med* 1997;337:161.

Cunningham D, Allum WH, Stenning SP, et al. Perioperative chemotherapy versus surgery alone for gastric cancer. *N Engl J Med* 2006;355:11.

Herskovic A, Martz K, al-Sarraf M, et al. Combined chemotherapy and radiotherapy compared with radiotherapy alone in patients with cancer of the esophagus. *N Engl J Med* 1992;326:1593.

Kelson D, Ginsberg R, Pajak TF, et al. Chemotherapy followed by surgery compared with surgery alone for localized esophageal cancer. *N Engl J Med* 1998;339:1979.

Macdonald J, Smalley SR, Benedetti J, et al. Chemoradiotherapy after surgery compared with surgery alone for adenocarcinoma of the stomach or gastroesophageal junction. *N Engl J Med* 2001;345:725.

MRC Oesphogeal Working Party. Surgical resection with or without preoperative chemotherapy in oesophageal cancer: a randomised controlled trial. *Lancet* 2002;359:1727.

Walsh T, Noonan N, Hollywood D, et al. A comparison of multimodal therapy and surgery for esophageal adenocarcinoma. *N Engl J Med* 1996;335:462.

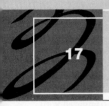

17

GASTROINTESTINAL CANCER: COLORECTAL AND ANAL

Benjamin R. Tan

I. PRESENTATION

A. Subjective. Colorectal cancer (CRC) is usually diagnosed after a positive screening test or workup of a symptomatic patient. Symptoms associated with CRC include rectal bleeding, abdominal pain, changes in bowel habits, weight loss, fatigue, anorexia and abdominal distension. Patients could also present with bowel obstruction, perforation, peritonitis, or fever. A thorough family history and past medical/oncologic history should be done to exclude any familial CRC syndromes.

B. Objective. Physical examination should always include a thorough abdominal and rectal examination and may reveal abdominal tenderness, hepatomegaly, ascites, a palpable mass, palpable adenopathy, and gross blood- or heme-positive rectal examination. Extracolonic manifestations in patients with hereditary CRC syndromes should also be noted (discussed in subsequent text).

II. WORKUP AND STAGING

A. Initial evaluation. Patients found to have a pedunculated or sessile polyp or mass in the colon or rectum require careful pathologic review of the excised specimen and precise marking of the polyp site. If invasive cancer is detected, additional workup should include a CBC (complete blood count), chemistry panel with liver function tests, carcinoembryonic antigen (CEA), computed tomography (CT) of the abdomen and pelvis and a chest x-ray. Although routine positron emission tomography (PET) scans are not standard, it may be valuable in assessing the extent of metastatic disease in a patient considered for potentially curative resection. If the specimen is fragmented, or has unfavorable histology, or if margins cannot be assessed, further resection should be planned.

III. TREATMENT

A. Colon cancer

1. Surgical principles. Surgery remains the primary modality for cure in patients with CRC. Select patients with synchronous or metachronous solitary or limited hepatic/pulmonary metastatic disease should still be considered for potentially curative resection of both the primary and metastatic sites. The extent, type, and timing of resection are dependent on the location of the tumor and presence of bleeding, obstruction, or perforation and the presence and extent of polyposis. The number of lymph nodes harvested and examined (13 or more recommended) impacts staging accuracy and prognosis.

Laparoscopic colectomy has been associated with higher cancer-related survival, reduced relapse rates, decreased morbidity, blood loss, and hospital stays as compared to open colectomy (Lacy, *Lancet* 2002;359:2224).

2. Pathology and staging. Five-year survival rates for colon cancer patients using the sixth edition of the new American Joint Committee on Cancer (AJCC)-based on surveillance, epidemiology, and end results (SEER) data from 1991 to 2000 (O'Connell, *J Natl Cancer Inst* 2004;96:1420) are summarized in the table on the following page.

Earlier studies on stage III patients revealed lower 5-year survival rates— 60% for IIIa, 42% for IIIb, and 27% for IIIc (Greene, *Am Surg* 2002;236:416). Unfortunately, information about chemotherapy is not available in the SEER data, which may contribute to the differences observed between the two studies.

3. Prognostic factors

a. Tumor grade. Low-grade tumors are significantly associated with better survival in stages II, III and IV, but not in stage I colon cancer.

	T	N	M	5-yr overall survival (%)
I	T1 or T2	N0	M0	93
IIa	T3	N0	M0	84
IIb	T4	N0	M0	72
IIIa	T1 or T2	N1	M0	83
IIIb	T3 or T4	N1	M0	64
IIIc	Any T	N2	M0	44
IV	Any T	Any N	M1	8

T1, tumor invades submucosa; T2, tumor invades muscularis propria; T3, tumor invades through the muscularis propria into the subserosa or into nonperitonealized pericolic tissues; T4, tumor directly invades other organs or structures and/or perforates visceral peritoneum; N0, no regional lymph node metastasis; N1, metastasis to one to three regional lymph nodes; N2, metastasis to four or more regional lymph nodes; M0, no distant metastasis; M1, distant metastasis.

b. Histologic subtype. Adenocarcinoma comprises more than 85% of colorectal cancer, whereas mucinous and signet-ring types occur in 12% and 1%, respectively. Patients with signet ring cell carcinomas had the worse prognosis as compared to adenocarcinomas and mucinous types (5-year overall survival [OS] 36%, 66%, and 62%, respectively).

c. Tumor location. Sigmoid colon cancers confer the best 5-year survival (70%) as compared to tumors in the right colon (64%), transverse colon (65%), and the left colon (65%).

d. Number of positive lymph nodes. Worse survival rates are seen in patients with more lymph nodes involved with cancer, as seen in the above table. Further subcategorizing lymph node involvement to N2 (4 to 5 LN+), N3 (6 to 8 LN+), and N4 (more than 9 LN+) could provide a more accurate prognosis among stage III CRC patients with 5-year OS of 52%, 43% and 27%, respectively.

e. Lymphovascular involvement is associated with poorer prognosis.

f. Molecular markers including microsatellite instability, 18q LOH, thymidylate synthase (TS) and dihydropyrimidine dehydrogenase (DPD) levels also carry predictive and prognostic information.

4. Treatment by stage

a. Stage I colon cancer (T1–T2, N0 M0). Since surgical resection confers a high cure rate for patients with stage I cancer, no adjuvant therapy is recommended.

b. Stage II colon cancer (T3–T4, N0 M0). Although the American Society of Clinical Oncology does not recommend the routine use of adjuvant therapy for stage II CRC patients, "high-risk" patients including those with **inadequately sampled nodes, T4 lesions, perforation, or poorly differentiated histology** should be considered for chemotherapy (Benson, *J Clin Oncol* 2004;22:3408).

- The **IMPACT B2 Study** reported a 2% to 3% absolute difference in 5-year disease-free survival (DFS) (76% vs. 73%) and OS (82% vs. 80%) in patients treated with adjuvant 5-FU–leucovorin chemotherapy versus observation (IMPACT B2 *J Clin Oncol* 1999;17:1356).

- The **QUASAR study** showed a significant improvement in recurrence rates (22.2% vs. 26.2%) and 5-year survival (80.3 vs. 77.4%, HR 0.83) with 5-FU versus observation (Gray, *PASCO* 2004:A3501].

- A systematic review of published literature included 37 randomized studies and 11 meta-analysis with 20,317 patients demonstrated a 5% to 10% absolute improvement in DFS associated with adjuvant therapy, although this was not statistically significant (Figueredo, *Cancer Prev Control* 1997;1:379).

- With more aggressive oxaliplatin-based adjuvant chemotherapy, patients with stage II colon cancer treated on the **MOSAIC study** had an absolute 5-year DFS benefit of 3.8% (83.7% vs. 79.9%) as compared to those treated with 5-FU/leucovorin alone. In high-risk stage II patients, the benefit is higher at 7.2% (PASCO 2007, A4007). OS was similar (86.9% vs. 86.8%) in both arms. (De Gramont, *N Engl J Med* 2004;350:2343 and *PASCO* 2005:A3501).

  Therefore, a careful assessment of risk of recurrence based on tumor and patient characteristics, and a thorough discussion with the patient regarding the absolute and relative benefits and toxicities are necessary in considering adjuvant therapy in a patient with stage II CRC.

c. **Stage III colon cancer (Tany, N1–N2, M0).** Adjuvant oxaliplatin-based chemotherapy is standard for patients with stage III CRC.

- Stage III CRC patients treated with FOLFOX4 on the **MOSAIC** study had an 7.5% absolute benefit in 5-year DFS (66.4% vs. 58.9%) and 4-year DFS (69.7% vs. 61%) as compared to 5-FU/leucovorin (LV). OS at 5-years was superior to SFU alone with a 4.4% absolute benefit (7.3% vs. 68.6%) [De gramont, *PASCO* 2005:A3501).

- The NSABP C-07 confirmed the efficacy of oxaliplatin with bolus 5-FU showing a significant improvement in 3-year DFS (76.5% vs. 71.5%) as compared to bolus 5-FU/LV (Wolamrk, *PASCO* 2004:A3500).

- For patients unsuitable for oxaliplatin-based therapy, capecitabine or 5-FU with LV are alternative therapies. In the X-ACT study, adjuvant capecitabine resulted in a trend toward improved 3-year relapse-free survival (64.2% vs. 60.6%) but OS (77.6% vs. 81.3%) did not differ significantly as compared to Mayo Clinic schedule of 5-FU/LV (Twelves, *N Engl J Med* 2005;353:2696).

- Irinotecan-based therapies cannot be considered for the adjuvant treatment of stage III CRC on the basis of three large randomized trials (ACCORD, PETACC-3 and CALGB 89803) showing no benefit over 5-FU alone.

d. **Metastatic CRC–first-line therapy.** The goal of therapy is potential cure versus palliation, and may help determine the choice of whether regimen used for initial therapy for patients with metastatic CRC. More aggressive regimens associated with the best response rates (RR) may be favored for patients with limited metastatic sites potentially amenable for resection or patients with rapidly growing symptomatic visceral metastases whereas, the toxicity profiles of equally effective regimens may determine the choice of palliative therapy for patients with widely metastatic CRC (Table 17.1).

- Oxaliplatin-based (FOLFOX) or irinotecan-based 5-FU regimens (FOLFIRI) are appropriate first-line treatment for metastatic CRC. The N9741 study demonstrated superiority of FOLFOX over irinotecan with bolus 5-FU (IFL) in terms of RR (45% vs. 31%) and OS (19.5 months vs. 14.8 months) (Goldberg, *Clin Oncol* 2004;22:23). Two studies have shown equal efficacy between FOLFOX and FOLFIRI regimens. Substitution of infusional 5-FU with capecitabine in oxaliplatin-based regimen resulted in similar outcomes (Tournigand, *J Clin Oncol* 2004;22:229; Colucci, *J Clin Oncol* 2005;22:4866).

- Bevacizumab is the first antiangiogenic drug approved for cancer treatment. This anti-vascular endothelial growth factor (VEGF) antibody, when added to chemotherapy, significantly improved outcomes. Hurwitz demonstrated a 4.7-month survival advantage with bevacizumab and IFL, as compared to IFL alone (20.3 months vs. 15.6 months). Furthermore, RR (45% vs. 35%) and duration of response (10.4 months vs 7.1 months) are superior in the bevacizumab arm. Moreover, when bevacizumab is combined with 5-FU/LV alone, median survival of 18.3 months was achieved with RR of 40% (Hurwitz, *J Clin Oncol* 2005;23:3502).

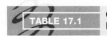

| TABLE 17.1 | Colorectal Chemotherapeutic Regimens |

Oxaliplatin-based
FOLFOX4: q 2 weeks
Oxaliplatin 85 mg/m^2 day 1
Leucovorin 200 mg/m^2 days 1,2
5-FU 400 mg/m^2 i.v. bolus days 1,2
5-FU 600 mg/m^2 c.i.v.i. days 1,2
Modified FOLFOX: q 2 weeks (TREE)
Oxaliplatin 85 mg/m^2 day 1
Leucovorin 350 mg/m^2 day 1
5-FU 400 mg/m^2 i.v. bolus
5-FU 2400 mg/m^2 c.i.v.i. over 46H day 1
Oxaliplatin + Capecitabine: q 3 weeks
Oxaliplatin 130 mg/m^2 day 1
Capecitabine 850 mg/m^2 p.o. b.i.d. x 14 days
Irinotecan-based
FOLFIRI: q 2 weeks
Irinotecan 180 mg/m^2 day 1
Leucovorin 200 mg/m^2 day 1
5-FU 400 mg/m^2 i.v. bolus day 1
5-FU 2400 mg/m^2 c.i.v.i. over 46 H day 1
Bevacizumab: 5–10 mg/kg i.v. q 2 weeks with chemotherapy
Cetuximab: 400 mg/m^2 i.v. day 1, then 250 mg/m^2 weekly

Bevacizumab with FOLFOX or FOLFIRI also resulted in high RR and relatively long survival (Hochster, *PASCO* 2006:A3510; Fuchs, *PASCO* 2006:A3506).

■ Cetuximab, an antiepidermal growth factor receptor has also been combined with oxaliplatin and irinotecan-based chemotherapy in the first-line CRC setting with encouraging results (Venook, *PASCO* 2006:A3509).

e. **Metastatic Colorectal Cancer — second-line and subsequent therapy**

■ For patients who received oxaliplatin-based therapy, irinotecan-based therapy can be considered after progression, and vice versa. Tournigand demonstrated survival rates of 21 months with this strategy (Tournigand, *J Clin Oncol* 2004;22:229).

■ Bevacizumab is approved for second-line therapy when combined with FOLFOX. This regimen improved OS (12.5 months vs. 10.7 months) as compared to FOLFOX alone in patients who progressed after irinotecan first-line therapy (Giantonio, *PASCO* 2005:A2).

■ Cetuximab alone or with irinotecan conferred RR of 10.8% and 23%, respectively. Bevacizumab added to cetuximab also resulted in a 23% RR and when all three drugs are given, RR is 38%. The EPIC study reported superior PFS & RR for cetuximab + irinotecan compound to irinotecan alone in the second-line setting (Saltz, *PASCO* 2005:A3508).

B. **Rectal cancer.** A multimodality approach, including colorectal surgery, radiation oncology, and medical oncology is necessary for the optimal treatment of patients with rectal cancer. Initial workup should include a transrectal ultrasound to assess depth of invasion and lymph node involvement, CT or magnetic resonance imaging (MRI) to assess distant metastases, and biopsy to rule out other rectal tumors (i.e., squamous cell carcinoma, melanoma, sarcoma or lymphoma). Low anterior resection (LAR) is suitable for tumors located in the middle and upper third of the rectum whereas an abdominoperineal resection (APR) may be necessary for low-lying rectal cancer. Tumor stage and grade, lymphovascular involvement, lymph node metastases, and achievement of a negative radial margin are important prognosticators and are predictive of local and distant recurrences. Total mesorectal excision (TME) in conjunction with LAR or APR has been advocated as the optimal surgical procedure for rectal cancer. A sharp (rather than blunt or avulsive) dissection is performed to remove the entire rectum. This technique has been shown to achieve a higher negative radial margin rate than blunt dissection (93% vs 80%). Laparoscopic procedures are safe in the hands of experienced surgeons.

1. **T1–T2 N0 Rectal cancer.** Transrectal ultrasound staged rectal lesions confined to the submucosa may be treated with full thickness local resection. Regional lymph node involvement occurs in 10% to 15% of these patients. T1 tumors invading the deepest part of the submucosa (SM3) carry a significantly higher risk of lymph node involvement than more superficial lesions (SM1 or SM2). Lesions invading the muscularis propia (T2) have a higher incidence of lymph node involvement (12% to 22%). If pathologically confirmed, patients require additional chemoradiotherapy. Preoperative radiation may be indicated for low-lying rectal lesions in an attempt to convert an APR to a potential sphincter-preserving LAR.

2. **Locally advanced T3–T4 or N1 rectal cancer.** Neoadjuvant chemoradiation is a standard treatment for locally advanced rectal cancer. 5-FU-based infusional chemoradiation is associated with lower local recurrence rate (6% vs. 13%), reduced acute and long-term toxicities, improved compliance, and higher sphincter preservation, but achieved similar 5-year OS as compared to postoperative therapy (Sauer, *N Engl J Med* 2004;351:1731). The degree of downstaging achieved with neoadjuvant therapy also provides prognostic information. Resection generally is done 6 to 10 weeks after chemoradiation and the decision to administer adjuvant chemotherapy is based on the initial clinical staging.

IV. **COMPLICATIONS**
   A. **Cancer-related.** Bowel obstruction, hemorrhage, abdominal pain, perforation, fistula formation, peritonitis, anemia, and malnutrition. Extensive liver metastases hepatomegaly, liver failure, or jaundice.
   B. **Treatment-related**
      1. Surgical and radiation complications: Common bowel dysfunction after surgery includes stool frequency, episodic frequency, pressure sensation, urgency, nocturnal movements, and soilage. Anastomotic stricture, leak, ulceration, bleeding obstruction, infection, and bladder and sexual dysfunction may occur.
      2. Chemotherapy and targeted therapy
         a. Fluoropyrimidines. 5-FU or capecitabine—myelosuppression, mucositis, diarrhea, excessive lacrimation, skin discoloration, dehydration, palmar-plantar erythrodysesthesia (PPE), and rare cardiotoxicity. In patients with DPD deficiency—severe myelosuppression, ataxia, and diarrhea.
         b. Oxaliplatin. Cold-induced peripheral neuropathy, laryngodysesthesias, myelosuppression, nausea, and fatigue.
         c. Irinotecan. Acute and delayed diarrhea, nausea, vomiting, myelosuppression, and alopecia. Patients with the UGT1A1 7/7 polymorphism may require irinotecan dose reductions due to increased risk for grade 4 to 5 neutropenia.
         d. Bevacizumab. Epistaxis, hypertension, and proteinuria are common. Rarer side effects include arterial thrombotic events (ATEs) such as myocardial infarction or stroke, perforation, wound dehiscence, and reversible leukoencephalopathy among others.
         e. Cetuximab. Acneform rash, diarrhea, fatigue, hypomagnesemia and rare pulmonary toxicities.

V. **FOLLOW-UP.** After curative resection and completion of therapy, a history, physical examination, and CEA determination are recommended every 3 months for the first 2 years and then every 4 to 6 months until the fifth year. Colonoscopy is recommended 1 year after diagnosis, and repeated in 1 year if abnormal, otherwise repeated in 2 to 3 years. For patients without an earlier full colonoscopy (i.e., due to obstructing lesion or emergent surgery), colonoscopy in 6 months is recommended.

VI. EPIDEMIOLOGY AND SCREENING. CRC ranks third in frequency among men and women with approximately 150,000 new cases/year. As regards mortality rates, it ranks second in men and third in women.

Patients with average risk (age 50 or less, no previous history of adenoma, no IBD) should have a colonoscopy done. If no polyps are seen, colonoscopy should be repeated in 10 years. If polyps are seen, polypectomy should be done. Alternatively, fecal occult blood tests (FOBT) annually with flexible sigmoidoscopy every 5 years or double-contrast barium enema every 5 years could be performed.

VII. RISK FACTORS. The lifetime risk for developing CRC are as follows:

A. General population, 6%

B. Personal history, 15% to 20%

C. Inflammatory bowel disease, 15% to 40%

D. Hereditary nonpolyposis colorectal cancer (HNPCC) or Lynch syndrome—70% to 80%—is characterized by early onset of colon cancer and adenomas but not polyposis. HNPCC is autosomal dominant with 80% penetrance and is due to a mutation in mismatch repair genes MLH1, MSH2, MSH6, PMS1, PMS2, and MSH3. Extracolonic manifestations include endometrial, ovarian, gastric, urogenital, bile duct, and sebaceous gland (Muir-Torre) cancer.

E. Familial adenomatous polyposis (FAP)—more than 95%—is characterized by the presence of thousands of polyps with an autosomal dominant inheritance with high penetrance and a prevalence of 1 in 8,000. The APC suppressor gene is located on chromosome 5q21, which is important in cell adhesion, signal transduction, and transcriptional activation in its interaction with β catenin and the Wnt pathway. Cyclin D1 and c-myc are downstream targets. Cancer occurs at a median age of 39 and more than 90% will develop adenomas by age 30. Extracolonic manifestations include cholangiocarcinoma, duodenal carcinoma, gastric cancer, desmoid tumors, osteomas, thyroid cancer, and brain tumors.

F. Other risk factors include age above 50, high red meat intake and low fiber diets, Peutz-Jeghers syndrome, juvenile polyposis, and others.

VIII. PATHOGENESIS. There are two major pathways to CRC:

A. Chromosomal instability or suppressor pathway accounts for 85% of sporadic CRC with an adenoma as the precursor lesion. FAP coli is the prototype for this model characterized by the loss of APC gene. A potential subtype of this model is characterized by the silencing of methylation of the DNA repair enzyme methylguanine DNA methyltransferase with serrated polyps as a precursor lesions.

B. Microsatellite instability or mutator pathway, accounts for 15% of sporadic CRC. HNPCC is the prototype for this model characterized by a loss of mismatch repair genes (MLH1, MSH2, MSH6 etc).

IX. ANAL CANCER

A. Presentation. Bleeding, pain, constipation, tenesmus, diarrhea, discharge and pruritus. Often the symptoms are ascribed to other benign conditions such as hemorrhoids, fistula in ano, fissure, or anal condylomata. A careful history on risk factors also need to be obtained.

Physical examination findings include a firm, indurated or exophytic anal mass or inguinal lymphadenopathy. A careful digital examination and anoscope is necessary to evaluate the extent of the tumor. Women with anal cancer should also have a thorough gynecologic examination. Diagnosis is made with incisional biopsy of the mass and any inguinal lymphadenopathy.

Pathology usually reveals squamous cell carcinoma or cloacogenic carcinoma. Adenocarcinomas involving the anus should be treated similar to rectal cancer. Rare cases of melanomas or neuroendocrine cancers may occur. Workup should include chest x-ray and CT or MRI of the abdomen and pelvis. Human immunodeficiency virus (HIV) testing should be considered in high-risk individuals in addition to baseline laboratory tests.

B. Staging. Staging is based on the tumor, node, metastasis (TNM) system.

Tis, carcinoma *in situ*

T1, tumor 2 cm or smaller

T2, tumor between 2 cm and 5 cm

T3, tumor larger than 5 cm

T4, tumor of any size that invades adjacent organs such as the vagina, urethra, or bladder

N0, no regional lymph nodes involved

N1, metastases in unilateral internal iliac or inguinal lymph node

N3, metastases in perirectal and one inguinal lymph node and/or bilateral internal iliac or inguinal lymph nodes

M0/1, no or (+) distant metastases present

Stage I, T1, N0, M0

Stage II, T2, 3, N0, M0

Stage IIIA, T1–3, N1, M0 or T4, N0, M0

Stage IIIB, T4, N1, M0 or any T, N2–3, M0

Stage IV, any T, any N, M1

- **C. Prognosis.** Prognosis is based on staging. T1 and T2 tumors have a more than 80% 5-year survival, whereas T3 and T4 tumors have 5-year survival of less than 50%. Inguinal lymphadenopathy and male sex are also related to a poorer prognosis. Tumors in the anal margin have a more favorable prognosis than do those in the canal.
- **D. Treatment.** Standard therapy includes the Nigro protocol chemoradiation with mitomycin C and 5-FU. Higher DFS (73% vs. 51%) and lower colostomy rates (9% vs. 22%) are associated with chemoradiation as compared to radiation alone (Flam, *J Clin Oncol* 1996;14:2527). Five-year survival varied between 64% and 83% with combined-modality therapy. Patients with HIV/AIDS and anal cancer may be treated with the same Nigro protocol, but caution should be applied as they may not tolerate full doses of chemotherapy. Patients with T1 lesions may be considered for local excision alone or with chemoradiation.
- **E. Epidemiology and risk factors**
  - **1. Epidemiology.** Anal cancer accounts for approximately 1.6% of all digestive system cancers in the United States. It is more common in men than in women. Its incidence generally increases with age, with the peak incidence in the sixth and seventh decades of life. The incidence is increasing in men younger than 40 years.
  - **2. Risk factors.** Human papillomavirus (HPV) infection—HPV 16 and 18, women with HPV-related cervical cancer, smoking, HIV infection, and anal receptive sex.

Suggested Readings

Andre T, Boni C, Mounedji-Boudiaf L, et al. Oxaliplatin, fluorouracil, and leucovorin as adjuvant therapy for colon cancer. *N Engl J Med* 2004;350:2343–2351.

Benson AB III, Schrag D, Somerfield MR, et al. American Society of Clinical Oncology recommendations on adjuvant chemotherapy for stage II colon cancer. *J Clin Oncol* 2004;22:3408–3419.

Desch CE, Benson AB III, Somerfield MR, et al. Colorectal cancer surveillance. *J Clin Oncol* 2005;23:8512–8519.

Ryan DP, Compton CC, Mayer RJ. Medical progress: carcinoma of the anal canal. *N Engl J Med* 2000;342:792–800.

Sauer R, Becker H, Hohenberger W, et al. Preoperative versus postoperative chemoradiation for rectal cancer. *N Engl J Med* 2004;351:1731–1740.

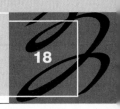

HEPATOBILIARY AND PANCREATIC CANCER

18

Steven Sorscher

HEPATOCELLULAR CARCINOMA

I. PRESENTATION

A. Subjective. Common symptoms of hepatocellular carcinoma (HCC) include anorexia, weight loss, abdominal pain, increasing abdominal girth, and jaundice. Up to 25% of patients will be asymptomatic at presentation. Paraneoplastic syndromes include hypoglycemia, erythrocytosis, hypercalcemia, and dysfibrinogenemia and these or progressive signs of liver failure may be the presenting symptoms.

B. Objective. Hepatomegaly, ascites, fever, bleeding, and splenomegaly can be seen.

II. WORKUP AND STAGING.
High-risk patients should have periodic screening with ultrasonography (USN) of liver, α-fetoprotein (AFP), albumin, and alkaline phosphatase levels (*Cancer* 1996;78:977–985), although there is no clear evidence that screening results in more patients being cured. There may be a role for retenoids in HCC prevention. A rising AFP with negative liver imaging should result in frequent radiographic follow-up. Magnetic resonance imaging (MRI) or computed tomography (CT) should be used to better define tumor extent and helical CT or MRI with arterial phase enhancement may still better define disease extent (*Br J Radiol* 2004;77:663–640).

A variety of histologic subtypes are described, with the fibrolamellar histology noteworthy for its higher likelihood of resectability and the lack of association with cirrhosis. Current American Joint Committee on Cancer/*Union Internationale Contre Cancer* (AICC/UICC) staging includes noting the presence or absence of cirrhosis/fibrosis, which are histologic features which predict prognosis after surgery.

A tissue diagnosis can be obtained by fine needle aspiration (FNA) (*Am J Clin Pathol* 1995;104:583), core biopsy, or laparoscopic biopsy. The potential for tumor "spillage" appears to be very small. Although occasionally patients may be treated for HCC based on the clinical, radiologic, and biochemical features, generally an attempt should be made to obtain a tissue diagnosis.

III. MANAGEMENT.
Surgical resection represents the only known curative therapy. In cirrhotic patients, resection is controversial (*Cancer J* 2004;10:74–87). Child-Pugh classification and other scoring systems, which help predict liver function and reserves with surgery, have been used to help identify patients eligible for resection (*J Hepatolbiliary Pancreat Surg* 2002;9:469–477). The hepatic venous pressure gradient (HVPG) may measure potential hepatic decompensation after resection (*Gastroenterology* 1996;111:1018–1022).

According to the United Network for Organ Sharing (UNOS), transplantation is considered in patients who are not eligible for resection and have small tumors (equal to or less than 5 cm or two to three tumors equal to or less than 3 cm each), and without macrovascular invasion or extrahepatic spread. Survival after transplant may be as high as 75%, with vascular invasion predicting lower survival. Patients with unresectable but small tumors may be considered for tumor ablation and later liver transplantation (*Hepatology* 2005;41:1130–1137; *Ann Surg* 2003;238:508–518).

Other "local" therapies such as radiofrequency ablation (RFA), alcohol injection, cryotherapy, and chemoembolization may improve symptoms and control local disease in selected patients. The likelihood of success with these approaches may involve the expertise of the clinician, the number, size, and location of the tumors, as well as whether there is vascular involvement by the tumors. Systemic therapy with single-agent or combination chemotherapy has been studied. However, cytotoxic chemotherapy has traditionally been associated with low response rates and questionable disease control. The results of an international Phase III placebo controlled trial in which 602 patients with hepatocellular carcinoma were randomly assigned to receive sorafenib or placebo, demonstrated an overall survival (OS) benefit for those receiving sorafenib (10.7 vs. 7.9 months) which represented a 44% improvement in OS (HR = 0.69; p = 0.0006). Supportive care is often the most reasonable option. Enrollment on clinical trials utilizing novel agents and approaches should be considered.

IV. **EPIDEMIOLOGY.** HCC is among the most frequent causes of cancer death worldwide, more commonly affecting men than women. In the United States, HCC is relatively less common, but is increasing in frequency , in part due to hepatitis C infection (*Am Intern Med* 2003;139:817–823). Of those with hepatitis C–induced cirrhosis, 1% to 2% per year develop HCC. Cirrhosis due to other causes such as alcohol use, hepatitis B, aflatoxin B1 (produced by Aspergillus), and exposure to certain carcinogens as well as exogenous steroid use are also risk factors.

Suggested Readings

Goudolesi GE, Roayaie S, Munoz L, et al. Adult living donor liver transplantation for patients with hepatocellular carcinoma: extending UNOS priority criteria. *Ann Surg* 2004;239:142–149.

Greten TF, Papendorf F, Bleck JS, et al. Survival rate in patients with hepatocellular carcinoma: a retrospective analysis of 389 patients. *Br J Cancer* 2005;92:1862–1868.

Groupe d'Etude et de Traitement du Carcinome Hepatocllulaire. A comparison of lipidol chemoembolization and conservative treatment for unresectable hepatocellular carcinoma. *N Engl J Med* 1995;332:1256–1261.

Llovet JM, Real MI, Montana X, et al. Arterial embolization or chemoembolization versus symptomatic treatment in patients with unresectable hepatocellular carcinoma: a randomized controlled trial. *Lancet* 2002;359:1734–1739.

Lo CM, Ngan H, Tso WK, et al. Randomized controlled trial of transarterial lipiodol, chemoembolization for unresectable hepatocellular carcinoma. *Hepatology* 2002;35: 1164–1171.

Mazzaferro V, Regalia E, Doci R, et al. Liver transplantation for the treatment of small hepatocellular carcinomas in patients with cirrhosis. *N Eng J Med* 1996;334:693–699.

 CANCER OF THE GALLBLADDER

I. **PRESENTATION**
   A. **Subjective.** Patients typically present with symptoms referable to the biliary tract and often cholecystitis or biliary colic are suspected. Suspicion of malignancy should particularly be raised in older patients with weight loss and more continuous pain.
   B. **Objective.** Physical examination may reveal icterus, scratch marks from pruritis, and hepatomegaly.
II. **WORKUP AND STAGING.** A carbohydrate antigen 19-9 (CA19-9) greater than 20 u/dL has a reported 79% sensitivity and 79% specificity. Approximately 93% of patients with gallbladder cancer where surgery is planned for benign disease will have carcinoembryonic antigen (CEA) greater than 4mg/mL (*Int J Cancer* 1990; 45:821).

   An abnormality on USN may imply the need for CT or MRI or MRI/magnetic resonance cholangiopancreatography (MRCP) as these tests can better characterize the extent of disease. However, CT is not very sensitive for distinguishing involved from involved lymph nodes (*Am J Surg* 1992;163:239). Endoscopic retrograde cholangiopancreaticography (ERCP) with endoscopic USN may identify patients with unresectable disease, or allow for a tissue diagnosis. There is no clear risk of dissemination in obtaining cytology using ERCP and endoscopic USN.

   Diagnosis is often made at the time of surgery, and definitive resection rather than cholecystectomy should be planned in suspicious, yet resectable cases. In addition to cytology specimens obtained with ERCP, percutaneous needle biopsy and core biopsy are used, although core biopsy, in particular, may carry significant "tracking" risk and should be reserved for unresectable cases (*Acta Cytol* 1995;39:494). Gallbladder cancer is typically adenocarcinoma, although other histologies occur infrequently. Higher-grade tumors are associated with a worse prognosis whereas the rare papillary tumors are associated with a better prognosis (*Cancer* 1992;70:1493).

Dysplasia, *in situ* carcinoma, and invasive carcinoma are often seen together in pathologic specimens, and mutation in the *p53* tumor suppressor gene may be an early event in tumorigenesis (*J Clin Pathol* 1994;47:453).

If no distant metastases are identified radiographically, laparoscopy should be considered to complete preoperative staging.

III. MANAGEMENT. Patients with incidentally found gallbladder tumors who are identified as having resectable disease should be considered for cholecytectomy, *en bloc* hepatic resection, lymphadenectomy, and possible bile duct resection. A similar approach is warranted for patients with preoperative radiographic staging, which reveals the possibility of resection of all radiographically evident tumors. If jaundice is present, the evaluation should include ERCP/percutaneous transhepatic cholangiography/MR cholangiography. If, at choleycystectomy, the gallbladder is removed intact, and a T1a tumor with negative margins is identified, no additional surgery is recommended. Lymph node involvement is very rare for T1.For T1b or greater disease, more extensive surgery (e.g., extended cholecystectomy for T2 disease) including the possibility of removing the port site from previous laparoscopy has been recommended.

In combining retrospective reviews, 5-year survival for patients with T1 tumors generally approaches 100%; whereas for T2, 70% to 90% survival may be expected (*Ann Surg* 1992;215:326; *Eur J Surg* 1997;163:419; *Surgery* 1994;115:751), but again, may be as high as 100%.Surgery remains the only curative therapy with 5-year survivals of 45% to 63% for patients with N1 disease (*World J Surg* 1995;19:758; *Ann Surg* 1996;224:639; *Ann Surg* 1992;216:565).

In a small trial, adjuvant 5-fluorouracil (FU) and radiation demonstrated an improved 5-year survival compared to surgery alone (64% vs 33%) (*Int J radiat Oncol Biol Phys* 2002;52:167–175) and, as a result, has been recommended for those with greater than T1 disease. Also, another small trial showed a 5-year survival benefit to 5-FU/mitomycin after surgery compared to observation after surgery (26% vs. 4%) (*Cancer* 2002;95:1685–1695).

Patients with unresectable, but not metastatic disease may benefit from chemotherapy/radiation therapy (RT), although this approach has not been extensively studied. Gemcitabine or capecitabine alone or in combination have been used in patients with metastatic disease (*Cancer* 2004;101:578–586). The overall prognosis from metastatic gallbladder cancer remains poor, with average survival of approximately 6 months and only approximately 5% of patients surviving 5 years. Biliary decompression may be necessary before initiation of chemotherapy and may also relieve obstructive symptoms. Given the lack of a clear survival benefit from the currently used agents, patients should be considered for clinical trials or supportive care only.

IV. EPIDEMIOLOGY. Marked regional and ethnic differences are seen in the incidence of gallbladder cancer. For example, gallbladder cancer has been reported as the leading cause of cancer death in Chilean women. High rates are seen in other South Americans countries as well as in central Europe, Israel, and in Native Americans, Japanese men, and others. In the United States, gallbladder cancer is the most common biliary tract cancer, and is more common in women than in men. There are approximately 2,800 deaths per year from gallbladder cancer.

Chronic inflammation, often due to gallstones, is associated with gallbladder cancer. In fact, 75% to 98% of gallbladder cancer patients will have had gallstones (*Cancer Treat Res* 1994;69:97). The so-called "porcelain gallbladder" will be associated with cancer in up to 25% of patients (*Radiology* 1973;106:29). Gallbladder polyps, particularly those greater than 1 cm and in older patients warrant special attention (*Br J Surg* 1992;79:227). There are associations between gallbladder cancers and anomalous biliary ductal malformations as well as with typhoid (*Am Surg* 1993;59:430; *Lancet* 1979;311:1791).

Suggested Readings

de Aretexaba XA, Roa IS, Burgos LA, et al. Curative resection in potentially resectable tumors of the gallbladder. *Eur J Surg* 1997;163:419.

Daines WP, Rajagopalan V, Groosbard ML, et al. Gallbladder and biliary tract carcinoma: A comprehensive update, part 2. *Oncology (Huntington)* 2004;18:1049.

Lazcano-Ponce EC, Miquel JF, Munoz N, et al. Epidemiology and molecular pathology of gallbladder cancer. *CA Cancer J Clin* 2001;51:349.

Matsumoto Y, Fujii H, Aoyama H, et al. Surgical treatment of primary carcinoma of the gallbladder based on histologic analysis of 48 surgical specimens. *Am J Surg* 1992;162:239.

Shirai Y, Yoshida K, Tsukada K, et al. Inapparent carcinoma of the gallbladder: an appraisal of a radical second operation after simple cholecystectomy. *Ann Surg* 1992; 215:326.

Tsukada K, Kurosaki I, Uchida K, et al. Lymph node spread from carcinoma of the gallbladder. *Cancer* 1997;80:661.

Wistuba II, Sugio K, Hung J, et al. Allele-specific mutations involved in the pathogenesis of endemic, gallbladder carcinoma in Chile. *Cancer Res* 1995;55:2511–2515.

 CHOLANGIOCARCINOMA

I. PRESENTATION
   A. Subjective. Patients typically present with weight loss or symptoms related to biliary obstruction such as jaundice, pruritis, or fever from infection.
   B. Objective. Physical examination may reveal icterus, a palpable gallbladder (Courvoisier's sign), and enlarged liver.
II. WORKUP AND STAGING. Laboratory findings often reveal elevated liver function tests, CEA, and CA19-9. A variety of radiographic studies, such as USN and delayed contrast CT scanning, are used to define disease extent. Retrograde cholangiopancreatography with ERCP is used for stent placement and to obtain cytology for diagnosis. Cytology sampling has demonstrated 62% sensitivity (Blumgart L, Fong Y eds. *Surgery of the Liver and Biliary Tract*. United Kingdom: WB Saunders, 2001:419). For hilar tumors, percutaneous transhepatic cholangiography is used to define proximal bile ducts involvement. MRI cholangiography, angiography, and endoscopic USN (may define a mass for biopsy) have potential roles in defining disease extent and vascular involvement.
   Adeoncarcinoma is the most common histology. Subtypes include sclerosing, nodular, and papillary variants. In addition to AJCC staging, a preoperative staging system which predicts survival, likelihood of metastatic disease, and resectability has been proposed.
III. MANAGEMENT. Surgery offers the best chances of cure for those with disease confined to a localized portion of the liver. Involvement of both liver lobes indicates generally unresectable disease. Nodal involvement or more distant metastases are usually considered contraindications to curative surgery. In summarizing multiple series, 5-year survival rates of 13% to 42% are expected, with an average survival of 15 to 59 months after surgery. Papillary variants have improved prognosis (*Histol Histopathol* 2002;17:851). With positive margins after surgery, additional surgery, ablation, and/or RT with or without chemotherapy (5-FU or gemcitabine based) should be considered. Transplant is considered in some select patients (*Liver Transpl* 2004;10:S65–S68).
   Patients with disease involving the proximal third of the ducts should undergo hilar resection and lymphadenectomy with or without *en bloc* liver resection. A 5-year survival rate of 20% to 25% is anticipated. For more distal disease (typically with tumor involving the common hepatic duct or intrapancreatic portion of the duct), pancreaticoduodenectomy, and lymphadenectomy is usually recommended. The more distal cholangiocarcinomas appear to have a 20- to 33-month median survival. Patients with tumors of the mid third of the duct are candidates for major bile duct excision and lymphadenectomy.

Before or after surgery, patients should be considered for additional therapy such as chemotherapy with RT (external beam, brachytherapy, or both),although large randomized studies demonstrating a clear benefit are not available. One study showed a statistically significant improved outcome for patients with locally advanced disease involving the main hepatic duct with radiation (intraoperative radiation therapy (IORT) and external beam) versus no therapy (*Am J Surg* 1997;174:605–608; *Int J Radiant Oncol Biol Phys* 2000:46:581). Adjuvant RT has been used, particularly for tumors resected with positive margins (including *in situ* carcinoma) or positive lymph nodes, and has been recommended for patients with tumors involving the muscularis layer.

Either stents or surgery can be used to improve biliary drainage and reduce symptoms and potentially delay hepatic function deterioration (*Lancet* 1992;340:1488–1492; *Gastrointest Endosc* 1998;47:1–7). Preoperative stenting is somewhat controversial. Silastic stents are changed regularly to reduce infectious risk whereas metal stents do not require changing, but cannot be removed once obstructed (*Gastrointest Endosc* 1998;47–51).

For metastatic disease and unresectable disease, chemotherapy with radiation or chemotherapy alone (typically gemcitabine or 5-FU–based) is the usual consideration along with supportive care only (*Hepatogastroenterology* 2001;39:783–789). Photodynamic therapy and combination chemotherapy for metastatic disease are being explored, including regimens such as gemcitabine in combination with capecitabine (*Gastrointest Endosc* 2004;60:68–75; *Am J of Oncol Rev* 2005;4:634–644).

IV. EPIDEMIOLOGY. Cholangiocarcinomas arise in the biliary tree and are classified as intrahepatic or extrahepatic tumors. Extrahepatic cholangiocarcinomas account for more than 90% ofcholangiocarcinomas and include hilar cholangiocarcinomas, which are commonly called Klatskin's tumors (*Ann Surg* 1996;224:463). These tumors are associated with conditions causing chronic inflammation such as primary sclerosing cholangitis, choledocal cysts, and liver flukes. Cholangiocarcinomas are more common in Southeast Asia and China and the incidence and mortality from cholangiocarcinomas is rising (*J Gastroenterol Hepatol* 2002;17:1049).

Suggested Readings

Heimbach JK, Haddock MG, Alberts SR, et al. Transplantation for hilar chlangiocarcinoma: 5-year follow-up of a prospective phase II study. *Gastrointest Endosc* 2004;60:68–75.

Jarnagin WR, Fong Y, DeMatteo RP, et al. Staging, resectability and outcome in 225 patients with hilar cholangiocarcinoma. *Ann Surg* 2001;234:507–517; discussion 517–519.

Klatskin G. Adenocarcinoma of the hepatic duct at its bifurcation within the porta hepatic. An unusual tumor with distinctive clinical and pathologic features. *Am J Med* 1965;38:241.

Lee CC, Wy CY, Chen JT, et al. Comparing combined hepatocellular-cholangiocarcinoma and cholangiocarcinoma: a clinicopathologic study. *Hepatogastroenterology* 2002;49:1487.

Rajagopalan V, Daines WP, Grossbard ML, et al. Gallbladder and biliary tract carcinoma: a comprehensive update, Part 1. *Oncology* 2004;18:889–896.

Sudan D, DeRoober A, Chinnakotla S, et al. Radiochemotherapy and transplantation allow long-term survival for nonresectable hilar cholangiocarcinoma. *Am J Transplant* 2002;2:774–779.

 # CANCER OF THE PANCREAS

I. PRESENTATION

A. Subjective. Typical presenting symptoms include weight loss, abdominal pain, nausea and vomiting, jaundice, or pruritis. Pancreatitis without an obvious cause might occasionally be the first sign of pancreatic cancer. Occasionally, new-onset diabetes will be due to pancreatic cancer.

B. Objective. Physical examination findings may include jaundice, hepatomegaly, ascites, left supraclavicular adenopathy (Virchow's node), periumbilical adenopathy (Sister Mary Joseph's node) or perirectal drop metastases (Blummer's shelf).

II. **WORKUP AND STAGING.** Although the tumor, node, metastasis (TNM) system is used to stage pancreatic cancer, for the purpose of choosing appropriate therapy, pancreatic cancer is typically divided into resectable, locally advanced/unresectable, and metastatic stages. CT scan (including high-speed helical scanning) with contrast enhancement and thin sectioning will often delineate the extent of the disease and identify potential sites for FNA in order to establish the diagnosis. Endoscopic USN provides high resolution of the pancreas and nearby vasculature and also allows for FNA. If done in conjunction with ERCP, therapeutic common bile duct stenting can be done as well. Laparoscopy may demonstrate intraperitoneal metastasis. In fact, up to 37% of cases with apparent locally advanced disease have intraperitoneal metastases seen at laparoscopy (*Gastrointest Surg* 2004;8:1068–1071). Histology is nearly always adenocarcinoma with cells harboring a *ras* mutation in nearly all cases. However, other histologies, such as neuroendocrine tumors, occur in small but significant numbers and prognosis and treatment differs compared to that for patients with adenocarcinoma.

III. **MANAGEMENT**

A. **Localized disease.** Surgery remains the only modality clearly established to cure pancreatic adenocarcinoma. Less than 10% to 20% of patients present with apparently resectable disease and of these, only approximately 20% are apparently cured with surgery. There is lack of complete agreement regarding the features which identify patients ineligible for curative surgery. Features which seem to identify patients as poor candidates for curative resection include peripancreatic lymph node involvement, occlusion or encasement of the superior mesenteric vein or the superior mesenteric vein/portal vein confluence, or involvement of the superior mesenteric artery, inferior vena cava, celiac access or aorta. Some surgeons will consider surgery in select patients with superior mesenteric vein or lymph node involvement. Surgery can also be used as a palliative procedure for locally advanced pancreatic cancer.

Preoperative chemotherapy/RT has been used in nonrandomized series for patients with resectable tumors or for patients with tumors potentially resectable with successful downstaging. The rationale for exploring neoadjuvant approaches include the potential to identify patients with rapidly progressive disease (in order to avoid unsuccessful surgery), improve the effectiveness of RT (because surgery may interfere with the effectiveness of postoperative RT as a result of vascular damage from surgery), and downstage tumors such that unresectable or marginally resectable tumors may become resectable. Studies have explored this approach although the role of preoperative therapy remains unclear at this time.

The gastrointestinal treatment study group (GITSG, 1987) demonstrated a median survival of 21 months for patients receiving RT and concurrent 5-FU (followed by prolonged treatment with 5-FU) compared to 10.9 months' median survival with observation alone after surgery ($p = 0.03$) (*Arch Surg* 1985;120:899–903). This study remains the primary basis for adjuvant 5-FU/RT as a standard adjuvant treatment after surgery for pancreatic adenocarcinoma.

More recently, the European Study of Pancreatic Cancer (ESPAC) 1, the largest randomized adjuvant study reported to date for pancreatic cancer, showed a median survival advantage favoring the chemotherapy alone (20.1 months) ($p = 0.009$) and 2- and 5-year survival better than with no chemotherapy (40% and 12% vs. 30% and 8% respectively). The no-chemotherapy arm showed an average survival of 15.5 months. Chemotherapy was also compared to chemoradiation therapy and there appeared to be a small median survival disadvantage with the chemo/RT (15.9 vs. 17.9 months) (*N Engl J Med* 2004;350:1200–1210).

Each of these studies has been criticized. The GITSG study involved a small number of patients ($n = 43$) and a long accrual time (8 years) whereas ESPAC 1 included a large number of patients who did not complete the full planned protocol and the radiation given was not centrally controlled for quality. Therefore, in spite of the ESPAC 1 results and a meta-analysis also showing no clear benefit for RT/chemotherapy, chemoradiotherapy has remained a standard approach for adjuvant therapy for pancreatic adenocarcinoma.

With more recent studies suggesting a benefit for continuous 5-FU versus bolus 5-FU when combined with RT and split-course RT no longer considered optimal in this setting, continuous 5-FU is also chosen frequently as the chemotherapy of choice in the adjuvant setting. The current ESPAC 3 trial is randomly assigning patients to chemotherapy with bolus 5-FU versus gemcitabine therapy whereas the Radiation Therapy Oncology Group (RTOG) study (R9704) is comparing infusional 5-FU with RT and either gemcitabine or 5-FU for 2 months before and 2 months after the chemoradiation therapy phase.

B. Locally advanced pancreatic cancer. Patients with unresectable disease, but without distant metastases, are considered to have locally advanced pancreatic cancer. On the basis of limited studies, chemoradiation therapy has become an established standard of care. External beam RT with concurrent 5-FU chemotherapy has been compared to external beam RT alone and shown to have an improved 1-year and overall survival (10.4 vs. 6.3 months) (*Cancer* 1981;48:1705–1710). Chemoradiation therapy has also shown improved 1-year survival compared to chemotherapy alone. Several studies demonstrate RT with continuous 5-FU (with maximum tolerated dose of 250 mg/m^2 per day) appears to be preferred compared to bolus 5-FU with the dose limiting toxicity being mucositis (*J Clin Oncol* 1995;13:227–232; *Int J Radiat Oncol Biol Phys* 2001;51:736–740; *Tumori* 2001;87:398–401). Capecitabine in combination with RT has also been studied (*Int J Radiat Oncol Biol Phys* 2001;51:736–740; *Int J Radiat Oncol Biol Phys* 2002;53:675–679).

Although the toxicity of gemcitabine chemotherapy is greatly enhanced when given concurrently with RT, multiple trials have now evaluated gemcitabine with concurrent RT and RT has been studied with concurrent paclitaxel as well, and limited results appear promising (*J Clin Oncol* 1999;17:2208–2212; *Int J Gastrointest Cancer* 2003;34:107–116; *J Clin Oncol* 2001;19:4202–4208; *ASCO Gastrointestinal Cancer Symposium* 2004, abstract 96; *Am J Clin Oncol* 2004;27:51–66).

C. Metastatic Pancreatic Cancer. Patients with metastatic pancreatic cancer may present with pain, weight loss, anorexia, or fatigue. Average survival is very poor. Gemcitabine was compared to 5-FU chemotherapy in patients with metastatic disease and the median survival favored gemcitabine (5.7 vs. 4.4 months, $p = 0.0025$). Clinical benefit was defined as improvement for equal to or greater than 4 weeks in either pain, analgesic use, weight loss, or performance status without worsening of a second of these symptoms. The likelihood of clinical benefit favored gemcitabine (24% vs. 5%). As a consequence of this study, gemcitabine was soon established as standard therapy (*J Clin Oncol* 2003;21:3402–3408; *Ann Oncol* 1998;9:1003–1008). Although gemcitabine has been studied in a randomized manner alone compared to combinations with 5-FU, premetrexed, irinotecan, cisplatin, and oxaliplatin, none of these combinations have shown clear median survival benefit compared to gemcitabine alone (*Proc Am Soc Clin Oncol Ann Meeting* 2004;22:4007; *J Clin Oncol* 2004;22:3776–3783; *Cancer* 2002;94:902–910; *Proc Am Soc Clin Oncol* 2004;22:4008; *ASCO Gastrointestinal Cancer Symposium*, 2004, abstract 96).

In a large study (n = 569), gemcitabine in combination with erlotinib was compared to gemcitabine alone and a small, but statistically significant survival advantage was seen in the combination therapy group (6.37% vs. 5.9 months, $p = 0.001$) as well as an improved estimated 1-year survival (23.8% vs. 16.8%). Rash and diarrhea were increased in the erlotinib arm (*ASCO Gastrointestinal Cancer Symposium*, 2005, abstract 77). The National Cancer Research Network (NCRN) has preliminarily reported that in a large randomized trial (*n* = 533) patients receiving gemcitabine/capecitabine compared to gemcitabine alone, had superior median survival (17.4 vs. 6.0 months HR 0.8, $p = 0.014$). A randomized trial comparing standard dose gemcitabine to fixed dose gemcitabine or gemcitabine/oxaliplatin appears not to favor the experimental arms.

IV. EPIDEMIOLOGY. Pancreas cancer is the fourth most common cause of cancer death in United States. Approximately 31,000 patients are diagnosed with pancreatic cancer and about the same number die each year, underscoring the extremely poor prognosis associated with this disease. Less than 10% of cases appear to have a hereditary basis. Cigarette smoking has been shown to increase risk (*Arch Intern Med* 1996;156:2255–2260).

V. FUTURE DIRECTIONS. Phase II studies involving gemcitabine and bevicizumab and gemcitabine and cetuximab have shown promising results (*Proc Am Soc Clin Oncol* 2004;22:4009; *J Clin Oncol* 2004;22:2610–2616). However, a phase III study randomizing patients to gemcitabine or gemcitabine and bevicizumab did not improve survival (Cancer and Leukemia Group B (CALGB) 80303). Other targeted agents are being investigated as well.

Suggested Readings

American Cancer Society. *Cancer facts and figures 2004.* 2004.

Burris HA III, Moore MJ, Andersen J, et al. Improvements in survival and clinic benefit with gemcitabine as first – line therapy for patients with advanced pancreas cancer a randomized trial (see comment). *J Clin Oncol* 1997;15:2403–2413.

Gastrointestinal Tumor Study Group. Further evidence of effective adjuvant combined radiation and chemotherapy following curative resection of pancreatic cancer. *Cancer* 1987;59:2006–2010.

Gastrointestinal Tumor Study Group. Treatment of locally unresectable carcinoma of the pancreas: comparison of combined-modality therapy (chemotherapy plus radiotherapy to chemotherapy alone). *J Natl Cancer Inst* 1988;80:751–755.

Lynch HT, Smyrk T, Kern SE, et al. Familial pancreatic cancer: a review. *Semin Oncol* 1996;23:251–275.

Moertel CG, Childs DS, Reitmeier RJ, et al. Combined 5-fluorouracil and supervoltage radiation therapy of locally unresectable gastrointestinal cancer. *Lancet* 1969;2:865–861.

Poplin E, Levy DE, Berlin J, et al. Phase III trial of gemcitabine (30-minute infusion) versus gemcitabine (fixed-dose-reate infusion [FDR]) versus gemcitabine + oxaliplatin (GEMOX) in patients with advanced pancreatic cancer (E6201). *Proceedings of the American Society of Clinical Oncology Annual Meeting.* 2006:24; abstract LBA4004.

Silverman DT, Schiffman M, Everhart J, et al. Diabetes mellitus, other medical conditions and familial history of cancer as risk factors for pancreatic cancer. *Br J Cancer* 1999;80:1830–1837.

Stocken DD, Buchler MW, Dervenis C, et al. Meta-analysis of randomized adjuvant therapy trials for pancreatic cancer. *Br J Cancer* 2005;92:1372–1381.

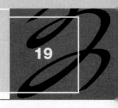

I. PRESENTATION

A. Subjective. Renal cell carcinoma (RCC) has been referred to as the *internists' tumor* because of its protean clinical manifestations. Despite a number of interesting clinical syndromes and paraneoplastic syndromes associated with this disease, many of these cancers remain asymptomatic until bulky metastatic disease produces symptoms, leading to diagnosis. The diagnosis of small asymptomatic tumors has increased rapidly in the past several decades, likely because of an increase in utilization of imaging procedures, such as computed tomography (CT) scans.

The most common presenting symptoms of RCC are anemia (20% to 40%), cachexia, fatigue, weight loss (33% each), and fever (30%). Less commonly, patients may be seen first with erythrocytosis, related to increased erythropoietin production, or elevated liver-function test (LFT) values in the absence of metastatic disease (Stauffer syndrome). The classic triad of symptoms (flank pain, hematuria, and a flank mass) is seen in fewer than 10% of patients and usually heralds the presence of metastatic disease. Almost 50% of patients will have gross hematuria at some time in the disease course.

B. Objective. Hematuria is the most common objective finding in RCC. The presence of a flank mass is not uncommon, being present in up to 45% of patients in some series. A variety of laboratory abnormalities can be seen, including anemia, erythrocytosis, hypercalcemia, and elevated LFT values. An uncommon but interesting physical finding associated with kidney cancer is a varicocele that does not subside in the supine position.

II. EVALUATION AND STAGING.
As described in Section I, a large number of RCCs are diagnosed serendipitously when seen on imaging studies obtained for another indication, or because of symptoms related to metastatic disease. A smaller number of patients have symptoms related to local disease, such as hematuria or flank pain related to the stretching of the renal capsule. In this section, we focus on the evaluation of a renal mass and the appropriate staging evaluation after an RCC has been diagnosed.

III. EVALUATION OF A RENAL MASS

A. Radiology. The evaluation of a renal mass, noted either incidentally or during evaluation of related symptoms, should proceed according to a rational algorithm. It should be noted that there is great reluctance to perform a biopsy of a renal mass. There is good reason for this reluctance. Several authors have reported the seeding of needle tracts, and although the risk of such occurrence appears to be low, even a small chance of making a curable lesion incurable is unacceptable. In addition, the risk of a false-negative biopsy results due to sampling error limits the utility of percutaneous biopsies.

The first step in evaluating a renal mass is determining whether it is solid or cystic. The best imaging modality to answer this question is ultrasonography. If the lesion is cystic, no further evaluation is necessary. If the lesion is solid, or cystic with solid components, a CT scan should be performed. A CT scan should help differentiate benign solid renal masses, such as angiomyolipomas and oncocytomas, from RCC. If a solid renal mass cannot be confirmed to be benign on the basis of CT appearance, excision is indicated.

Newer imaging modalities, such as magnetic resonance imaging (MRI) and positron emission tomography (PET) have not yet proved to be of sufficient sensitivity and specificity to alter this algorithm. Despite the high resolution and ability to detect vascular enhancement achieved by MRI, no difference was seen in the ability to detect RCCs by MRI in comparison to contrast-enhanced CT. The role of MRI in the evaluation of renal masses is probably limited to patients who cannot tolerate contrast-enhanced CT because of contrast allergy or impaired renal function. Although PET scans are a promising adjunctive imaging modality, there is as yet insufficient experience with this modality to define a role in the diagnosis of renal masses.

B. Pathology. Cancers of the kidney can generally be broken down into cancers of the renal parenchyma (80%) and cancers of the renal pelvis. Cancers of the renal parenchyma are generally adenocarcinomas (RCCs), and those of the renal pelvis are generally transitional cell tumors. This chapter focuses on cancers of the renal parenchyma. Histologically, RCC is classified into clear cell type (75% to 85%), chromophilic type (12% to 14%), chromophobic type (5%), and collecting duct type (1%).

C. Staging. Once an RCC is diagnosed, treatment planning must be based on preoperative or clinical staging. The keys to staging RCC, such as those for most other malignancies, are to define the local extent of disease and to determine whether there is distant spread of disease. The approach to staging RCC outlined here is depicted in Fig. 19.1.

The principal tool for determining the local extent of disease is the abdominal CT scan. The size of the lesion, the degree of invasion, the presence of lymphadenopathy, and the presence of vascular invasion are the essential pieces of information for determining T and N stage (Table 19.1). CT scan is currently the most effective tool for correctly assessing these issues. In a comparison of CT scans with pathologic stage in 100 patients with RCC, Johnson et al. found that CT scans had 46% sensitivity for perinephric invasion, 78% for venous invasion, 83% for adenopathy, and 60% for adjacent organ invasion. Overall, 91% of patients were correctly staged by CT scan. There are certain limitations of CT scans for staging. Lymph node status is generally determined by size criteria, with lymph nodes larger than 1 cm being considered to be involved, and those smaller than 1 cm being considered not to be involved by tumor. CT scans are notoriously poor for determining tumor extension to the liver. This determination is based on obliteration of fat planes between the two organs, and intraoperative findings frequently do not correlate with CT findings in this regard.

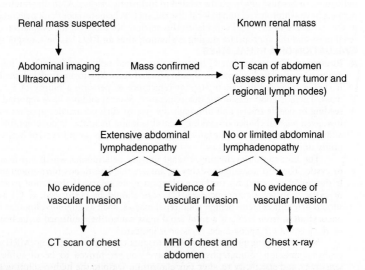

Figure 19.1.   Approach to staging evaluation of renal cell carcinoma.

TABLE 19.1	AJCC Staging of Renal Cell Carcinoma (from the AJCC Cancer Staging Manual, Fifth Edition)	

Primary tumor		
Tx	Primary tumor cannot be assessed	
T0	No evidence of primary tumor	
T1	Tumor ≤7 cm in greatest dimension limited to the kidney	
T2	Tumor >7 cm in greatest dimension limited to the kidney	
T3	Tumor extends into major veins or invades the adrenal gland or perinephric tissues, but not beyond Gerota's fascia	
T3a	Tumor invades the adrenal gland or perinephric tissues but not beyond Gerota's fascia	
T3b	Tumor grossly extends into the renal vein(s) or vena cava below the diaphragm	
T3c	Tumor grossly extends into the renal vein(s) or vena cava above the diaphragm	
T4	Tumor invades beyond Gerota's fascia	
Regional lymph nodes		
Nx	Regional lymph nodes cannot be assessed	
N0	No regional lymph node metastases	
N1	Metastases in a single regional lymph node	
N2	Metastases in more than one regional lymph node	
Distant metastases		
Mx	Distant metastases cannot be assessed	
M0	No distant metastases	
M1	Distant metastases	
Stage grouping		
Stage I	T1	N0	M0
Stage II	T2	N0	M0
Stage III	T1	N1	M0
	T2	N1	M0
	T3a	N0	M0
	T3a	N1	M0
	T3b	N0	M0
	T3b	N1	M0
	T3c	N0	M0
	T3c	N1	M0
Stage IV	T4	N0	M0
	T4	N1	M0
	Any T	N2	M0
	Any T	Any N	M1

AJCC, American Joint Commission on Cancer.

CT scans are of limited value in identifying tumor thrombus. The presence or absence of tumor thrombus significantly affects surgical planning. The presence of thrombus is not a contraindication to surgery, but will affect the surgical approach. Modern CT scanning techniques have improved the sensitivity and specificity for detection of tumor thrombus, but MRI scans with gadolinium enhancement do appear to provide superior assessment of the extent of thrombus, as well as in discriminating bland thrombus from tumor thrombus. Obtaining a preoperative MRI is probably not necessary in all patients, but in patients with evidence of venous extension on CT scan, it is an important part of the preoperative evaluation.

In addition to determining the T and N stages, metastatic disease must be ruled out before proceeding with surgery. The most common sites of metastatic spread of RCC are the adrenal glands, liver, lung, and bone. An abdominal CT scan obtained to evaluate the primary tumor is usually sufficient to evaluate the adrenal glands and liver. In the case of elevated LFT values without liver metastases on CT scan, it may be worthwhile obtaining an MRI of the abdomen before attempting surgical resection. As mentioned earlier, abnormal LFT values may be a manifestation of Stauffer syndrome, but basing this diagnosis on CT findings alone may lead to attempted resection in the presence of liver metastases.

A chest radiograph is generally considered sufficient to rule out pulmonary metastases. A chest CT scan should be obtained if a complex surgical resection, such as extensive thrombectomy, is being considered. The presence of enlarged retroperitoneal lymph nodes on abdominal imaging also warrants a staging chest CT.

A bone scan is indicated if there is bone pain or laboratory evidence suggestive of possible bony metastases (elevated calcium or alkaline phosphatase).

IV. TREATMENT

A. Early disease (T1 or T2, N0). The treatment for localized, that is, nonmetastatic RCC is primarily surgery. In general, a radical nephrectomy is performed. Partial nephrectomy, or nephron-sparing surgery, is performed in certain situations, such as bilateral RCC, RCC in a solitary kidney, and in patients at risk for future insults to the nondiseased kidney. The nephron-sparing approach seems to offer satisfactory outcomes with respect to disease recurrence, especially for low-stage tumors.

Radical nephrectomy includes *en bloc* resection of the kidney and the perinephric fat outside Gerota capsule. Ipsilateral adrenalectomy is performed for large, upper-pole tumors. Removing a clinically uninvolved adrenal gland with small tumors, or mid- or lower-pole primaries, is more controversial. Resection of the regional lymph nodes at the time of radical nephrectomy is also controversial. Lymph node resection certainly provides more accurate staging than does clinical staging alone. It may also be that removing involved lymph nodes improves the outcome in node-positive disease, but no clear data support this belief.

Radical nephrectomy can be performed from a number of approaches. Incisions can be midline upper abdominal, flank, subcostal, or thoracoabdominal. The selection of incision depends on which approach is likely to provide adequate exposure.

Partial nephrectomy is indicated if a radical nephrectomy would lead to the immediate need for dialysis. Partial nephrectomy is also considered in patients with small (smaller than 4 cm) tumors that are clearly localized. A number of operative techniques are used to perform partial nephrectomies, including segmental polar nephrectomy, wedge resection, and major transverse resection.

Laparoscopic radical nephrectomy is also gaining popularity because of diminished operative morbidity and shortened hospital stays. The first laparoscopic nephrectomy was performed in 1990 for benign disease. Since then, this technique has been applied to both benign and malignant diseases. Early reports indicate that laparoscopic nephrectomy is safe, and at least for short-term follow-up, provides outcomes similar to those of radical nephrectomy. Laparoscopic nephrectomy is associated with less postoperative pain, shorter hospital stays, and shorter convalescence time. This approach is a reasonable option for patients at centers with expertise with this procedure. As with most operative techniques, complications associated with this procedure decline dramatically as operators gain experience with the technique.

B. Locally advanced disease (T3 or T4, N1 or N2). In approximately half the number of patients, RCC is first seen as locally advanced disease (T3 to T4), presenting a number of therapeutic challenges. Involvement of the inferior vena cava (IVC) by direct extension of tumor down the renal vein (T3) is not an uncommon scenario. Resection of these tumors involves specialized surgical approaches determined by the superior extension of the tumor thrombus. Tumors involving the IVC, even up to the right atrium, are technically resectable, and these tumors may still be cured with surgery alone. Ten-year survival rates of up to 40% have been reported for patients undergoing tumor thrombectomy.

Renal artery embolization has been used in a variety of circumstances. In locally advanced disease, embolization of the renal artery may be used to attempt to shrink large tumors, or to diminish the extent of IVC thrombus. The efficacy of embolization in these settings is unclear. Embolization may also be used to diminish perioperative blood loss, or as a palliative intervention for hematuria. Embolization can be complicated by a postinfarction syndrome. This syndrome is characterized by pain, fever, nausea, and vomiting. The syndrome may last several days after embolization.

Locally invasive disease, that is, direct extension of primary tumors into adjacent organs such as the liver, pancreas, or colon, sometimes occurs in the absence of metastatic disease (T4). The mainstay of treatment in this setting is again surgery. Few patients with extension to adjacent organs are cured with surgery. Their quality of life may be improved if a complete resection can be performed, allowing local control of the tumor and tumor-related symptoms. Resection may be considered in patients with a good performance status, with few competing morbidities, and tumors that can be completely resected. Survival at 1 year is unusual in this group of patients.

C. Adjuvant therapy. At this time, there is no proven role for adjuvant therapy in the treatment of RCC, even though a proportion of patients will develop recurrence. Postoperative radiation was evaluated in a randomized trial and was not found to be effective. Interferon-α has been evaluated in this setting and was not found to be effective. The use of high- and intermediate-dose interleukin 2 (IL-2) is still being evaluated.

D. Metastatic disease. Approximately 33% of patients with RCC are first seen with metastatic disease, and in up to 50% of patients treated with surgery for local disease, metastatic disease eventually develops. Metastatic disease is generally treated with systemic therapy, although surgery and radiation do have roles in the treatment of metastatic RCC.

1. Solitary metastasis. RCCs first seen with a solitary metastasis represent a relatively unique situation. Patients whose solitary site of metastatic disease can be completely resected have between 35% and 60% chance of surviving 5 years. Radiation therapy (XRT) is often delivered after surgery. Despite this favorable outcome, it is unclear whether the improved survival is a result of surgical intervention or of the indolent nature of the tumor.

A number of patient and disease characteristics help predict survival after resection of metastatic disease in RCC. Features favoring long-term survival include a disease-free interval of longer than 12 months (55% vs. 9% overall survival), solitary versus multiple sites of metastases (54% vs. 29% 5-year survival), and age younger than 60 (49% vs. 35% 5-year survival). Survival is longer after resection of lung metastases than of brain metastases. Anecdotal evidence suggests that patients may derive benefit from resection for a second or third recurrence. For patients with a solitary metastatic site that cannot be resected, XRT can be considered. Radiation is also effective in relieving symptoms from metastatic lesions, with approximately 66% of patients receiving symptomatic benefit, especially those with bony pain, and 50% achieving objective tumor regressions.

2. Multiple metastases. RCCs frequently have multiple metastatic lesions, with lung and bone being the most frequently affected sites. The treatment of metastatic RCC is systemic therapy, with local modalities used for palliative purposes. A recent increase in the understanding of RCC molecular biology has altered our treatment modalities greatly. Immunotherapy has long been the basis of most of the systemic treatment regimens of RCC, whereas more conventional chemotherapeutic agents have demonstrated little activity in this disease.

Insights gained from study of patients with von Hippel Lindau disease (VHL) have shown that RCC overexpresses vascular endothelial growth factor (VEGF) through a variety of biochemical pathways. This has led to the development and use of small-molecule receptor inhibitors in RCC.

E. The role of systemic therapy

1. Molecular-targeted therapy. Some of the greatest recent advances is cancer therapeutics involve an increased understanding of the pathogenesis of various diseases at the molecular level, with new therapies specifically designed to inhibit pathways crucial to pathogenesis. Initial insights into the pathogenesis of RCC have come from studies of patients with VHL, with the discovery that loss of heterozygosity of the VHL locus results in overexpression of multiple pathways, including that of VEGF. Further gene expression profiling studies have demonstrated that approximately 90% of sporadic cases of RCC also demonstrate these abnormalities. A new agent, temsorolimus, has just been approved for the treatment of metastatic RCC. This drug is an mtor inhibitor. It is given weekly by intravenous infusion, and has generally been well tolerated. This offers an additional option in the treatment of metastatic RCC.

Sorafenib, a small-molecule, multiple tyrosine kinase inhibitor, was one of the first demonstrated VEGF receptor inhibitors. It was evaluated in a phase III study of patients with advanced RCC who had previously failed immunotherapy. Those patients receiving sorafenib had significantly increased progression-free survival (24 weeks as compared to 12 weeks in the placebo arm), although an actual partial response was seen in very few patients.

Sunitinib, another small-molecule multiple tyrosine kinase inhibitor, has been evaluated in the treatment of RCC as well. Several studies are currently ongoing to elucidate its full potential. However, a phase II study of sunitinib demonstrated a 40% objective partial response rate in patients treated with the medication.

On the basis of these results, sorafenib and sunitinib have gained U.S. Food and Drug Administration (FDA) approval for the treatment of advanced and metastatic RCC. They are generally very well tolerated with similar side effect profiles; hand-foot syndome, worsening hypertension, and mild gastrointestinal (GI) side effects are most common.

2. Immunotherapy. Standard cytotoxic chemotherapeutic agents have been uniformly disappointing in the treatment of RCC. Immunotherapy, which refers to treatment with agents that stimulate the patient's own immune system to combat the cancer, has shown some limited success in the treatment of RCC. The primary agents studied are IL-2 and interferon α (IFN-α). IL-2 works through the activation of cytotoxic T-cell subgroups and stimulation of cytokine release. A number of clinical trials have documented modest but reproducible response rates to IFN-α and IL-2 in RCC.

a. Interleukin 2 in renal cell carcinoma. IL-2 was initially studied as a high-dose, intravenous regimen (600,000 IU/kg i.v. bolus every 8 hours for a total of 14 doses over 5 days, then repeated 2 weeks later. This regimen resulted in an overall response rate of 14%, with 5% complete responses. Complete responders had a significant chance of long-term survival. Since this finding, a number of studies have looked at doses, schedules, and routes of administration of IL-2. The response rates in these studies vary from none to 40%. The dose-limiting toxicities of IL-2 are generally hypotension and a vascular leak syndrome. In general, during high-dose therapy with IL-2, doses are skipped rather than reduced for toxicity. A significant proporrtion of patients treated with this regimen will require hemodynamic support with vasopressors. In the initial National Cancer Institute (NCI) study, a 4% mortality rate was observed. This mortality rate has been significantly reduced as experience with the regimen and supportive care improved, but this regimen should be delivered in a monitored setting by physicians well versed in the regimen.

Several studies have reported the use of lower-dose subcutaneous IL-2 given on an outpatient basis. These studies have demonstrated overall survival rates comparable to that of traditional high-dose therapy, but response rates for subcutaneous regimens have been significantly less, with a trend toward more durable responses with the conventional therapy.

b. **Interferon α in renal cell carcinoma.** IFN-α has been widely studied in phase II studies, using different preparations and dosing schemes. Published response rates have been in the 15% to 20% range. The optimal dosing and schedule of IFN-α has not been determined, but 5 to 10 million IU/m^2 given s.c. 3 to 5 days per week is the generally accepted dosage.

c. **The combination of interleukin 2 and interferon α.** The combination of IL-2 and IFN-α has been evaluated in a number of studies with inconclusive results. At least one randomized study showed improved response rates and survival with the combination of the two cytokines as compared with either used alone. Negrier et al. reported the results of a three-arm randomized study comparing IL-2, IFN-α, or the combination (*N Engl J Med* 1998;338:1272–1278). Response rates were significantly higher (18.6% vs. 6.5% and 7.5%) for the combination as compared with IL-2 and IFN-α, respectively. Event-free survival at 1 year was 20% in the combination arm, as compared with 15% and 12% in the single-agent arms ($p = 0.01$). Overall survival was not different between treatment groups. Toxicity was most pronounced in the combination arm. The relatively small improvement in event-free survival is generally not thought to justify the toxicity of this regimen. The very low response rates in the single-agent arms were also disappointing.

3. **Immunochemotherapy.** Another randomized study recently compared the combination of IL-2 and IFN-α with the same combination given with continuous-infusion 5-fluorouracil (*J Clin Oncol* 2000;24:4009–4015). In this study, the response rate to IL-2 and IFN-α was 1.4%, and in the group that received IL-2 and IFN-α and 5-fluorouracil, the response rate was 8.2%. This difference was not statistically significant, and the survival at 1 year was not different between the groups. This result was disappointing, not only because it failed to show any improvement with the addition of 5-fluorouracil, but also because the response in the "standard arm" was so low.

F. **Current standard of systemic therapy for advanced renal cell carcinoma.** There is no current accepted standard for the treatment of advanced or metastatic RCC. On the basis of the recent institution of molecular-targeted therapies, much more progress needs to be made in elucidating optimum treatment strategies, combination therapies, and roles for new medications. Therefore, patients with advanced or metastatic RCC should be evaluated for potential incorporation into clinical trials, if available.

Otherwise, use of high-dose IL-2 should be reserved for patients with good performance status who have access to centers with experience with this regimen. Patients with poor performance status, widespread disease, and those who are unlikely to tolerate the side effects of high-dose IL-2 should be offered a trial of either sorafenib or sunitinib.

G. **Radical nephrectomy in metastatic renal cell carcinoma.** There remains interest in removing the primary tumor in patients with metastatic RCC. This is derived from reports of regression of metastatic disease after removal of the primary tumor. In theory, removing the primary tumor may provide an immunologic impetus that leads to response in the metastatic disease. The Southwest Oncology Group reported a large randomized trial in which nephrectomy plus systemic interferon immunotherapy was compared with immunotherapy alone (interferon) for patients with advanced RCC. A statistically significant survival benefit was seen in favor of the nephrectomy arm (12 months vs. 8.5 months). It seems reasonable for the moment to view a combination of nephrectomy and immunotherapy as a new standard of care, although it is possible that even newer cytokines will improve results. Patients with a good performance status who are being considered for systemic therapy should therefore be considered for nephrectomy as well.

V. **COMPLICATIONS**

A. **Of the disease.** The complications of RCC may be related to local progression of disease or metastatic spread. Local progression of disease often leads to pain and hematuria. RCC frequently metastasizes to lung and bone. Bone pain and pathologic fractures are relatively common. Shortness of breath, cough, hemoptysis, and malignant pleural effusions all occur relatively frequently.

B. Of therapy. Serious complications occur in approximately 20% of patients undergoing radical nephrectomy, and the mortality rate associated with this procedure is approximately 2%. Common complications include perioperative myocardial infarction, cerebrovascular accident, pulmonary embolism, and pneumonia. Early mobilization and incentive spirometry may help reduce the incidence of some of these complications.

Intraoperative injuries to the liver, spleen, pancreas, and bowel may occur. These should be recognized and repaired in the operating room. A pancreatic fistula can develop as a result of an unrecognized injury to the pancreas.

Pneumothorax, retroperitoneal bleeding, and wound infection can also occur.

As described earlier, laparoscopic nephrectomy is associated with less postoperative pain, shorter hospital stays, and shorter overall convalescence.

The complications of systemic therapy are related to agents and doses used. IL-2 regimens are generally more toxic than IFN-α regimens. Combinations regimens are more toxic than single-agent regimens. The common toxicities of high-dose IL-2 include hypotension requiring vasopressors, fever, and decreased performance status.

VI. NATURAL HISTORY. RCC is well known for its unpredictable behavior. Spontaneous regressions of metastatic disease have been reported more often than for any other solid tumor. Late recurrences are also seen. These cases represent extremes, however, and most RCCs follow relatively predictable patterns.

Pathologic stage is the most important determinant of prognosis. Five-year survival rates are approximately 75% for stage I, 60% for stage II, 40% for stage III, and 10% for stage IV. The median survival of patients with metastatic disease is in the range of 14 months.

VII. BACKGROUND

A. Epidemiology. Approximately 30,000 cases of RCC occur in the United States each year, resulting in 12,000 deaths. There is a slight (1.5:1) male predominance, and RCC is more common among urban than among rural populations. The incidence increases with increasing age, although cases have been reported at essentially all ages.

The incidence of RCC has increased gradually over the past two decades. It is unclear whether this represents a true increase in the incidence of disease or increased diagnosis related to the use of CT scans and MRI of the abdomen on a more routine basis.

B. Identifiable risk factors. Several risk factors have been identified for kidney cancer. Cigarette smoking has been associated with kidney cancer in case–control studies, and cohort studies have demonstrated a clear association with a dose–response relation. Obesity is associated with RCC, with the risk increasing with increasing body mass index. Hypertension and the use of antihypertensive agents are considered risk factors for RCC. Renal cell cancers have no clear relation to occupational exposures.

By far most RCCs are sporadic, but three distinct family syndromes have been described.

VHL carries a high risk of clear cell RCC. This disorder is caused by germline mutations of the tumor suppressor VHL gene located on chromosome 3p. Familial occurrence of clear cell carcinomas in the absence of VHL has been associated with balanced translocations of 3p. Hereditary papillary RCC is related to mutations of the proto-oncogene met on chromosome 7q.

C. Molecular pathology. Studies of the molecular pathology of RCC have focused on genetic alterations. Mutations of the VHL gene (3p) are closely associated with clear cell RCC, whereas mutations of met (7q) are associated with papillary RCC (*J Urol* 1999;162:1246–1258).

D. Pathogenesis. The VHL gene has been found to be mutated in a high percentage of patients with clear cell RCC, and have also been noted in patients with granular and sarcomatoid RCC. Such mutations are not seen in patients with papillary RCC. It is thought that acquired mutations of the gene may contribute to the development of nonpapillary RCC.

VIII. **FUTURE DIRECTIONS.** Much of the ongoing research in RCC is focusing on immunotherapy and molecularly targeted approaches to this disease.

An approach to immunotherapy is allogeneic stem cell transplantation. The theory is to achieve a graft-versus-tumor effect, as seen in leukemia. In general, a nonmyeloablative induction regimen is used, followed by infusion of donor stem cells from a human leukocyte antigen (HLA)–matched sibling. One small study from the National Heart, Lung, and Blood Institute reported 10 responses in 19 patients treated in this manner. Two patients died of treatment complications. Regression from metastases occurred late, often after discontinuation of cyclosporins used to suppress graft-versus-host reaction, being consistent with graft-versus-tumor effect. In the three complete responders, responses lasted 27, 25, and 16 months (*N Engl J Med* 2000;343:750–758). It is not clear whether case selection and nature of metastases influenced results. This approach also remains experimental, but offers promise for the future of the treatment of metastatic RCC.

Further evaluation of small molecule–targeted therapies is underway. Dosing schedules and combinations of the VEGF receptor inhibitors are being evaluated. Bevacizumab, a monoclonal antibody to circulating VEGF, is currently being evaluated for use in RCC. An initial phase II study of bevacizumab demonstrated significantly prolonged median time to progression in patients receiving the drug as compared to those receiving placebo (4.8 months as compared to 2.5 months).

Other targeted therapies, including inhibition of mTOR (mammalian target of rapamycin) and inhibition of epidermal growth factor are being evaluated, although early studies with endothelial growth factor receptor (EGFR) inhibitors have not demonstrated significant activity.

Suggested Readings

Childs R, Chernoff A, Contentin N, et al. Regression of metastatic renal-cell carcinoma after nonmyeloablative peripheral-blood stem-cell transplantation. *N Engl J Med* 2000;343:750–758.

Coughlin SS, Neaton JD, Randall B, et al. Predictors of mortality from kidney cancer in 332,547 men screened for the multiple risk factor intervention trial. *Cancer* 1997;79:2171–2177.

Goldberg MA, Mayo-Smith WW, Papanicolaou N, et al. FDG-PET characterization of renal masses: preliminary experience. *Clin Radiol* 1997;52:510–515.

Jayson M, Sanders H. Increased incidence of serendipitously discovered renal cell carcinoma. *Urology* 1998;51:203–205.

Johnson CD, Dunnick NR, Cohan RH, et al. Renal adenocarcinoma: CT staging of 100 tumors. *AJR Am J Roentgenol* 1987;148:59–63.

Maclure M, Willett W. A case-control study of diet and risk of renal adenocarcinoma. *Epidemiology* 1990;1:430–440.

McLaughlin JK, Hrubec Z, Blot WJ, et al. Smoking and cancer mortality among U.S. veterans: a 26-year follow-up. *Int J Cancer* 1995;60:190–193.

Motzer RJ, Michaelson MD, Redman BG, et al. Activity of SU11248, a multitargeted inhibitor of vascular endothelial growth factor receptor, and platelet-derived growth factor receptor, in patients with metastatic renal cell carcinoma. *J Clin Oncol* 2006;1:16–24.

Negrier S, Caty A, Lesimple T, et al. Treatment of patients with metastatic renal carcinoma with a combination of subcutaneous interleukin-2 and interferon alpha with or without fluorouracil. *J Clin Oncol* 2000;24:4009–4015.

Negrier S, Escudier B, Lasser C, et al. Recombinant human interleukin-2, recombinant alfa-2a, or both in metastatic renal cell carcinoma. *N Engl J Med* 1998;338:1272–1278.

Oto A, Herts BR, Remer EM, et al. Inferior vena cava tumor thrombus in renal cell carcinoma: staging by MR imaging and impact on surgical treatment. *AJR Am J Roentgenol* 1998;171:1619–1624.

Rosenberg SA, Lotze MT, Yang JC, et al. Experience with the use of high dose interleukin-2 in the treatment of 652 cancer patients. *Ann Surg* 1989;210:474.

Semelka RC, Shoenut JP, Kroeker MA, et al. Renal lesions: controlled comparison between CT and 1.5-T MR imaging with non-enhanced fat-suppressed spin-echo and breath-hold FLASH techniques. *Radiology* 1992;182:425–430.

Waters WB, Richie JP. Aggressive surgical approach to renal cell carcinoma: review of 130 cases. *J Urol* 1979;122:306–309.

Wynder EL, Mabuchi K, Whitmore WF Jr. Epidemiology of adenocarcinoma of the kidney. *J Natl Cancer Inst* 1974;53:1619–1634.

Yuan JM, Castelao JE, Gago-Dominguez M, et al. Hypertension, obesity and their medications in relation to renal cell carcinoma. *Br J Cancer* 1998;77:1508–1513.

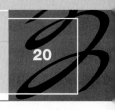

I. PRESENTATION

A. Subjective. The most common presenting symptom of bladder cancer is hematuria in 80% to 90% of patients. Gross hematuria obviously warrants a thorough evaluation of the genitourinary system. When gross hematuria is painless and total (present during the entirety of the urinary stream), it especially causes concern for bleeding from the bladder or upper tracts. In a study of 1,000 patients with total, gross, painless hematuria, 15% were found to have bladder cancer (*JAMA* 1957;153:783). Irritative urinary symptoms are relatively common at presentation, including frequency, urgency, and dysuria. The combination of these symptoms with hematuria is very suggestive and warrants full urologic evaluation. Depending on the location of their tumors, patients may have symptoms of bladder-outlet obstruction or ureteral obstruction. A small subset of 5% to 10% of patients, have symptoms related to metastatic disease.

B. Objective. Physical findings may be conspicuously absent in early bladder cancer. With more advanced disease, a pelvic mass may become palpable. Lower extremity edema may also develop with advanced disease. Either microscopic or gross hematuria will usually be present. It may, however, be intermittent.

II. WORKUP AND STAGING

A. Workup. Evaluation of gross hematuria should include a urine culture, cytologic evaluation of the urine, imaging of the kidneys and upper urinary tracts, and cystoscopy. Microscopic hematuria potentially presents a more difficult diagnostic decision making. Microscopic hematuria is an extremely common finding, and most cases of microscopic hematuria are nonneoplastic in origin. The question becomes how to evaluate the finding adequately without putting most of the patients through unnecessary diagnostic tests. The initial evaluation of urine that tests positive for blood on a dipstick is microscopic evaluation to confirm the presence of red cells. Again, culture and cytology should be performed. Bladder cancer is generally diagnosed with cystoscopy. At cystoscopy, the gross appearance of the cancer can be assessed (focal vs. multiple, flat vs. papillary or nodular), and biopsies can be obtained. If a bladder tumor was anticipated before cystoscopy, and appropriate anesthesia arranged, the evaluation can proceed to transurethral resection (TUR) of the bladder tumor and examination under anesthesia (EUA). If anesthesia was not arranged before cystoscopy, then this takes place in two stages, cystoscopy with biopsy followed by TUR and EUA. EUA allows bimanual palpation of the bladder wall. Induration of the bladder wall without a palpable mass likely portends a better-prognosis tumor, whereas the presence of a palpable mass likely indicates gross extravesical tumor. TUR provides a more sensitive method for defining the depth of invasion. Ideally, a full-thickness bladder wall specimen would be obtained to allow for definitive staging. Specimens should be obtained with clear indications of the superficial and deep aspects of the biopsy. Small papillary tumors that appear to be superficial may be resected completely, without resecting deep into the detrusor muscle. Larger tumors, especially nodular or solid masses, require deeper resection done in layers. Resection to the depth of the perivesical fat can be performed in attempts to resect completely, the muscle-invasive tumors.

B. Pathology

1. Staging. In the 1940s, Jewett and Strong noted a relation between the depth of invasion into the muscle wall of bladder tumors and survival. This observation

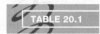

TABLE 20.1	AJCC Staging of Bladder Cancer (2002)

Primary tumor

(T)

Tx	Primary tumor cannot be assessed
T0	No evidence of primary tumor
Ta	Noninvasive papillary carcinoma
Tis	Carcinoma *in situ*
T1	Tumor invades subepithelial connective tissue
T2	Tumor invades muscle
T2a	Tumor invades superficial muscle (inner half)
T2b	Tumor invades deep muscle (outer half)
T3	Tumor invades perivesical tissue
T3a	Microscopically
T3b	Macroscopically
T4	Tumor invades prostate, uterus, vagina, pelvic wall, abdominal wall
T4a	Tumor invades prostate, uterus, vagina
T4b	Tumor invades pelvic wall, abdominal wall
Nx	Regional lymph nodes cannot be assessed
N0	No regional lymph node metastasis
N1	Metastasis in a single lymph node, ≤ 2 cm in greatest dimension
N2	Metastasis in a single lymph >2 cm but ≤ 5 cm in greatest dimension, or multiple lymph nodes, none >5 cm in greatest dimension
N3	Metastasis to a single lymph node >5 cm
M0	No distant metastasis
M1	Distant metastasis

Stage grouping

Stage 0a	Ta	N0	M0
Stage 0is	Tis	N0	M0
Stage I	T1	N0	M0
Stage II	T2a	N0	M0
	T2b	N0	M0
Stage III	T3a	N0	M0
	T3b	N0	M0
	T4a	N0	M0
Stage IV	T4b	N0	M0
	Any T	N1, 2, or 3	M0
	Any T	Any N	M1

led to the first staging system for bladder cancer, the Jewett system. The staging of bladder cancer has since been modified to correlate with the tumor, node, metastasis (TNM) system used by the American Joint Committee on Cancer (AJCC). The TNM system (Table 20.1) is still largely based on the depth of tumor invasion into the muscular wall of the bladder, and the most important information regarding clinical stage comes from results of transurethral biopsies or resection specimens. Treatment and prognosis are to a large extent defined by T stage. Patients with Ta or T1 disease are generally treated with TUR, whereas patients with muscle-invasive or T2 disease generally require cystectomy or radical radiation. Bladder cancers are initially staged clinically; if cystectomy is performed, they are staged pathologically.

There are two main prognostic groups. Superficial tumors occur at the level of the bladder mucosa and include carcinoma *in situ* (CIS; Tis), papillary lesions (Ta), and those that invade (but not through) the lamina propria

(T1). T2, T3, and T4 tumors that penetrate the muscularis propria are more aggressive and have a strong tendency to metastasize.

Determining the T stage of bladder tumors by TUR has its limitations. The correlation between TUR and cystectomy staging is in the range of 60%. The single most important determination made by TUR is whether muscle invasion is present. Superficial, that is non–muscle-invasive tumors, are treated much differently than muscle-invasive tumors. Even this determination can be challenging. The **muscularis mucosae,** a muscular layer that is sometimes seen in the lamina propria, can be confused with the **muscularis propria** or detrusor muscle.

In addition to the depth of invasion, information regarding gross appearance, grade, and the presence of **CIS** can be determined at cystoscopy. Papillary tumors are more likely to be superficial and may be completely resected without deep muscle resection. Solid or nodular tumors are more likely to be muscle invasive, and will likely require deeper resection. High-grade tumors are more likely to be muscle invasive, and cystectomy studies have documented a 95% rate of muscle invasion for high-grade tumors. The presence of CIS is generally thought to portend a worse prognosis, and CIS is generally characterized as high grade. The risk of invasion increases when tumors are found to be multifocal. Lymphatic or vascular invasion is also associated with increased risk for metastasis.

For patients without invasion into the **muscularis propria,** the risk of nodal or systemic metastases is quite low, and further staging studies are generally not indicated. For patients with muscle-invasive disease, more complete staging is indicated before determination of the treatment plan. In general, a computed tomography (CT) scan or magnetic resonance imaging (MRI) of the abdomen is obtained to help define the local extension of the tumor, the presence or absence of nodal metastases, and the presence or absence of other abdominal metastases. Both CT and MRI have relatively high specificity (greater than 90%) for the presence of nodal metastases when size criteria are used, but also relatively poor sensitivity ($\sim$50%). A chest radiograph is generally sufficient to exclude pulmonary metastases, and a bone scan should be obtained to rule out bone metastases.

III. THERAPY AND PROGNOSIS. The therapy and prognosis of bladder cancer is dependent on the stage of disease at presentation. Treatment options and prognosis can best be described according to the clinical presentation: superficial, muscle invasive, or metastatic.

IV. SUPERFICIAL BLADDER CANCER. Most of the bladder cancers, in the neighborhood of 75%, are superficial at presentation. Treatment of superficial bladder tumors consists of resection (TUR), intravesical chemotherapy or immunotherapy, and in very selected cases, cystectomy. Most superficial tumors can be completely resected by TUR. The most important determinations to be made in regard to these tumors are the risk for recurrence and the risk for progression to muscle-invasive disease. Most patients with superficial bladder tumors will experience recurrence within 5 years of diagnosis. Approximately 30% of these patients will progress to muscle-invasive disease. For patients at high risk of recurrence or progression, intravesical therapy may be added to TUR to reduce these risks. For patients with refractory superficial disease or extremely high risk for progression, cystectomy may be considered.

The risk of progression is related to the initial tumor stage. Most patients with Ta disease will recur with superficial disease. Patients with T1 disease and Tis, especially multifocal Tis, are at much greater risk for progression to muscle-invasive disease. Grade also affects the likelihood of progression. Ta disease that is grade 2 or 3 has a significant (20%) risk of progression, whereas Ta grade 1 disease has a negligible risk of progression (Table 20.2).

Determining the risk of progression plays a role in defining treatment. As stated earlier and depicted in Table 20.2, most patients with superficial bladder cancer will experience recurrence. Therefore, it is recommended that patients undergo repeated cystoscopy 3 months after their initial resection. Recurrent tumors are resected and evaluated for evidence of progression, in terms of both invasiveness and grade. For

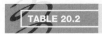

TABLE 20.2	Approximate Risk of Recurrence and Progression of Superficial Bladder Cancer by Stage			
	Recurrence at			**Rate of progression to muscle invasion**
Stage	**1 yr**	**3 yr**	**5 yr**	
Ta G1	25%	50%	65%	Rare
Ta G2,3	35%	65%	85%	20%
Tis, focal	25%	50%	65%	20%
Tis, multicentric	50%	75%	100%	50–80%
T1	50%	80%	90%	50%

patients at high risk for recurrence and/or progression, consideration must be given to intravesical therapy.

The indications for intravesical therapy have not been clearly defined. Some general guidelines have been proposed. At Memorial Sloan-Kettering Cancer Center, the indications for prophylaxis have included four or more recurrences in 1 year, tumor involvement of more than 40% of the bladder surface, diffuse Tis, and T1 disease. Intravesical therapy has been shown to reduce the likelihood of recurrence and the rate of progression to muscle-invasive disease.

A number of agents have been used for intravesical therapy, including chemotherapeutic and immunologic agents. Chemotherapeutic agents used have included mitomycin-c, doxorubicin, epirubicin, and thiotepa. All have been found to reduce recurrence rates by 15% to 20%. None has been shown to prevent progression to muscle-invasive disease or alter overall survival.

Immunotherapies used for this purpose have primarily included Bacille Calmette-Guérin (BCG) and Interferon-α (IFN-α). BCG is thought to be the most active agent for preventing recurrence and progression of superficial bladder cancer. Randomized studies have shown BCG to be superior to thiotepa, doxorubicin, and epirubicin. Mitomycin-c has shown results, equivalent and inferior to BCG in randomized studies. A number of treatment regimens with BCG have been used. The most standard is probably a regimen evaluated by the Southwest Oncology Group (SWOG). They found a regimen of 6 weekly instillations followed by instillations for 3 consecutive weeks every 3 months for 3 years to be superior to a 6-week induction regimen. The mechanism of action of BCG is not well understood, but there is evidence that the bacillus attaches to the bladder cells and evokes an immune response, or perhaps nonspecific immune stimulation or an alteration of suppressor/helper T-cell ratios in the bladder. BCG has been shown to reduce the rate of recurrence and prolong the disease-free state, but it may not affect the ultimate rate of progression to invasive cancer. Patients may experience flulike symptoms. A granulomatous infection can occur at various sites including the liver, lung, prostate, and kidney. BCG sepsis can be life threatening. If dissemination is documented, 6 months of antituberculous therapy is needed.

A small number of patients with superficial bladder cancer will require cystectomy for effective management. Patients with recurrent high-grade papillary tumors or CIS, tumors that have progressed to muscle invasion, and tumors involving the prostatic stroma or ducts should be considered for cystectomy. Cystectomy results in high rates of cure for patients with superficial cancer who require this aggressive treatment.

V. MUSCLE-INVASIVE DISEASE. The standard treatment for muscle-invasive bladder cancer is radical cystectomy. Over the recent years, interest in bladder-sparing approaches for muscle-invasive disease has grown. Such approaches include aggressive TUR, with or without intravesical therapy, radiation, and/or chemotherapy. These approaches are still considered investigational.

    A. Radical cystectomy. Early series using radical cystectomy for the treatment of bladder cancer reported disappointing results. This was due to very high rates of operative mortality. As the care of operative patients has improved over the last several decades, the mortality rate associated with this procedure has been reduced to less than 5%, and radical cystectomy with pelvic lymph node dissection (PLND) is considered the standard of care for muscle-invasive bladder cancer. Modern series report 5-year survival rates in the ranges of 60% to 80% for stage II disease, and 30% to 60% for stage III disease.

In male patients, radical cystectomy involves the *en bloc* removal of the bladder, prostate, seminal vesicles, proximal vas deferens, proximal urethra, and a margin of adipose tissue, and peritoneum. In female patients, the procedure involves the *en bloc* removal of the bladder, urethra, uterus, fallopian tubes, ovaries, anterior vaginal wall, and surrounding fascia.

After removal of the bladder, a route for elimination of urine must be created. This is accomplished either with a noncontinent urinary diversion, usually an ileal conduit, or with a continent urinary diversion. An ileal conduit is created by connecting the ureters to a segment of ileum, and the segment of ileum to the abdominal wall. A number of surgical approaches have been designed for the creation of continent diversions. These include approaches that use the abdominal wall, orthotopic bladders, and the rectum as sites of drainage. All forms of urinary diversion entail a number of potential complications including metabolic and electrolyte disturbances, pyelonephritis, urinary calculi, and altered drug metabolism. The continent diversions generally entail longer operations and increase the risk of complications. They should be considered for patients with a reasonable life expectancy and the ability to catheterize themselves.

B. Radiation therapy. In many countries, external-beam radiation is considered standard therapy for muscle-invasive bladder cancer. This is not the case in the United States. The ability to perform radical cystectomy and PLND with greatly reduced morbidity and mortality has made this a procedure with an acceptable risk profile for most patients with muscle-invasive bladder cancer. For patients who are not thought to be candidates for radical surgery, radiation therapy (RT) would be an alternative.

Radiation has been evaluated in both pre- and postoperative settings. Several randomized trials of preoperative RT have failed to demonstrate significant improvement in outcomes and have shown significant increases in gastrointestinal (GI) toxicity. Postoperative radiation has also been evaluated and not found to improve survival over surgery alone. Pre- and postoperative radiation are generally not indicated, unless they are incorporated into a multimodality bladder-sparing approach, as described later.

C. Chemotherapy. Chemotherapy has been evaluated in the neoadjuvant and adjuvant settings. The commonly used chemotherapeutic regimens in the treatment of transitional cell carcinoma (TCCA) of the bladder are discussed in more detail in the section on metastatic disease. In general, regimens containing cisplatin have been found to be most efficacious in this disease, and most of the regimens evaluated in these settings have included cisplatin.

There is a reasonable consensus that perioperative chemotherapy improves outcomes in stage III bladder cancer. Chemotherapy in the neoadjuvant setting has shown the clearest benefit. The Nordic 1 Trial randomized patients with muscle-invasive disease or high-grade T1 tumors to two cycles of cisplatin (70 mg/m^2) and doxorubicin (30 mg/m^2) or no chemotherapy before radiation and cystectomy. This trial included 304 patients and demonstrated a significantly improved 5-year survival for the chemotherapy group for patients with muscle-invasive disease (*Scand J Urol Nephrol* 1993;27:355). A larger randomized trial compared three cycles of cisplatin, methotrexate, and vinblastine (CMV) before radiation or surgery, versus no chemotherapy. This trial enrolled 976 patients and demonstrated a small (5.5%) but not statistically significant difference in a 3-year survival (*Lancet* 1999;354:1650). The SWOG reported a survival benefit in a trial of neoadjuvant MVAC (methotrexate, vinblastine, doxorubicin, cisplatinum) plus radical cystectomy versus radical cystectomy alone in patients with locally advanced bladder cancer (T2–T4a). Of patients treated with chemotherapy, 38% had no disease at surgery. Median survival was 6.2 years for the chemotherapy group versus 3.8 years for cystectomy alone (*Proc ASCO* 2001;20:3).

Adjuvant chemotherapy has also been evaluated in a number of trials, but this issue also remains controversial. Three completed randomized studies have suggested a survival benefit to adjuvant chemotherapy. One trial, from the University of Southern California, compared four cycles of cyclophosphamide, doxorubicin, and cisplatin (CISCA) with surgery alone. A difference in median survival of 51 versus 29 months, favoring the chemotherapy group, was seen, but this was not statistically significant ($p = 0.062$), and only 91 patients were randomized in this trial. A second trial using methotrexate, vinblastine, epirubicin, and cisplatin (M-VEC) was terminated early because of a higher rate of relapse in the no-treatment group at an interim analysis. This study eventually reported a survival difference, but this was difficult to interpret, because relapsing patients in the no-treatment arm did not receive chemotherapy at the time of relapse. A third trial randomized 50 patients to CMV or no chemotherapy, and showed no significant survival difference.

Overall, it appears that perioperative chemotherapy improves outcomes in the treatment of stage III bladder cancer. The benefit has been most clearly demonstrated in the neoadjuvant setting. The data in the adjuvant setting has trended towards showing a benefit, but the trials have not had the statistical power to be definitive. It does appear that the most effective regimens include cisplatin.

VI. BLADDER-SPARING/COMBINED-MODALITY APPROACHES. Radical cystectomy is associated with an operative mortality rate of approximately 3%, and results in significant lifestyle changes. A number of approaches have been evaluated in muscle-invasive TCCA to find alternatives that would allow patients to be successfully treated for their cancer and maintain normal urinary function. For instance, patients who are found to have muscle-invasive disease on TUR, and are found to have no residual disease at repeated TUR, may not require further treatment. Patients with papillary tumors and those with minimal muscle invasion may be successfully treated with TUR alone. This does require regular follow-up, and patients must understand that they may require cystectomy, should their disease recur.

Given the relatively high response rates to chemotherapy and RT, and the morbidity and quality-of-life issues associated with radical cystectomy, a number of centers have actively evaluated bladder-sparing approaches for the treatment of muscle-invasive bladder cancer. Trials of neoadjuvant chemotherapy have documented pathologic complete responses to the neoadjuvant therapy in a subset of patients. RT can also result in pathologic complete responses. Using one or both of these modalities, followed by a more limited surgical procedure such as partial cystectomy or aggressive TUR, may result in equivalent outcomes to radical cystectomy.

A number of single-arm studies have demonstrated 5-year survival rates similar to those achieved with conventional treatment (~50%), and a significant portion (~40%) of patients surviving with an intact bladder. These-single arm studies do not necessarily demonstrate equivalence to radical cystectomy. Patients are often highly selected, and patients who do not achieve significant responses to chemotherapy may be removed from the bladder-sparing approach and undergo radical cystectomy. They do demonstrate that selected patients may be able to survive with their bladders intact, despite muscle-invasive bladder cancer.

One approach reported from Massachusetts General Hospital involves CMV chemotherapy, radiation with concurrent cisplatin, and TUR. Patients undergo aggressive TUR followed by two cycles of CMV. They then undergo repeated cystoscopy and assessment of response. Then they receive radiation to a maximum of 40 Gy with concurrent cisplatin. A third cystoscopy is performed after completion of the RT, and patients without a complete response are referred for cystectomy. Other groups have reported on similar approaches, with acceptable survival, and bladder preservation in the range of 40%.

Some patients with muscle-invasive bladder cancer may be managed without a cystectomy. Patients with small, papillary tumors and with the ability to maintain regular follow-up are reasonable candidates for bladder-sparing approaches. We hope

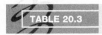

TABLE 20.3 | **Common Chemotherapeutic Regimens for the Treatment of Transitional Cell Carcinoma**

Regimen	Drug	Dose	Schedule	Response rate
MVAC, every 28 d	Methotrexate	30 mg/m^2	d 1, 15, 22	46% (12% CR)
Vinblastine	3 mg/m^2	d 2, 15, 22		
Doxorubicin (Adriamycin)	30 mg/m^2	d 2		
Cisplatin	70 mg/m^2	d 2		
CMV, every 21 d	Cisplatin	100 mg/m^2	d 2	56% (28% CR)
Methotrexate	30 mg/m^2	d 1 and 8		
Vinblastine	3 mg/m^2	d 1 and 8		
GC, every 28 d	Gemcitabine	1,000 mg/m^2	d 1, 8, and 15	49% (12% CR)
Cisplatin	70 mg/m^2	d 2		
ITP	Ifosfamide	1,200 mg/m^2	d 1,2,3	79% (20% CR)
Paclitaxel	200 mg/m^2	d 1		
Cisplatin	70 mg/m^2	d 1		

CR, complete response.

that ongoing trials will help define the optimal combination of therapies to obtain tumor control while minimizing toxicity.

VII. METASTATIC DISEASE. Patients with locally advanced, usually thought to include T4b and N2 or N3 disease, and metastatic bladder cancer die of their disease unless they receive effective chemotherapy. These patients generally receive limited benefit from local-treatment modalities and are considered for systemic therapy.

A number of single agents have been found to produce a significant number of partial remissions. Unfortunately, these remissions tend to be brief, in the range of a few months. These findings led investigators to pursue combinations of active single agents, and these efforts have led to a number of active combinations in the treatment of bladder cancer (Table 20.3).

Several combination regimens have been evaluated and found to produce high response rates, with some durable responses in advanced TCCA of the bladder. The most commonly used regimens are the combination MVAC and the combination CMV. Another highly active regimen is ifosfamide, paclitaxel, and cisplatin. Both MVAC and CMV have been found to be superior to single-agent cisplatin. In a study comparing MVAC with cisplatin, the response rate of MVAC was 39% with a median survival of 12.5 months, statistically significant compared to the 12% response rate and 8.2-month median survival with cisplatin alone. MVAC has been demonstrated to be superior to CISCA. MVAC and CMV have not been directly compared.

In general, MVAC has been thought to be the standard regimen for metastatic TCCA. Some clinicians prefer CMV, and as stated earlier, the regimens have not been directly compared. MVAC has been associated with significant toxicity, including treatment-related mortality in the range of 5%. Newer agents are being studied, and paclitaxel, docetaxel, ifosfamide, and gemcitabine have all been shown to have significant activity. Combinations have resulted in response rates between 50% and 80%. The ITP regimen of ifosfamide, paclitaxel, and cisplatin was reported to have a median survival of 18 months. Recently the combination of gemcitabine and cisplatin (GC) has been found to have similar clinical activity to MVAC with significantly fewer side effects in the treatment of advanced TCCA of the bladder.

Unfortunately, despite high response rates, nearly all patients with advanced TCCA of the bladder die of their disease. Median survival in most series using an effective combination regimen is in the range of 12 months. Up to 20% to 30% of patients with nodal and up to 10% of patients with metastatic disease may obtain long-term remission. Most authors currently recommend six cycles of therapy for responding patients, with consideration of surgical resection of residual disease after four cycles, followed by two additional cycles.

Patients with poor performance status, or extensive bony or visceral metastases, are unlikely to achieve a complete response or long-term survival. The median survival for these patients is in the range of 6 months. For these patients, consideration could be given to using one of the many active single agents (cisplatin, gemcitabine, or paclitaxel) or no chemotherapy, as opposed to the aggressive combination regimens.

VIII. COMPLICATIONS OF THERAPY

A. **Surgery.** The major surgical treatments for TCCA of the bladder are TUR and radical cystectomy. Each is associated with its own potential complications.

TUR is generally accomplished with a resectoscope inserted into the bladder through the urethra. A resecting loop is passed beyond the tumor, and then pulled back toward the scope with application of electric current. The tumor is generally resected until healthy muscle can be seen at the base of the resection site. The most common complication of this procedure is perforation of the bladder. Often the perforations are minor and of limited clinical consequence. A cystogram can confirm the diagnosis, and patients are generally treated with a drainage catheter and prophylactic antibiotics.

Other complications of TUR include clot retention due to bleeding, obturator nerve injuries, and injury to the urethra or ureteral orifice. Late complications include bladder contracture.

Radical cystectomy with PLND is a major operative procedure. As described earlier, advances in operative and perioperative care have greatly reduced the mortality rate associated with this procedure. Reported mortality rates in recent series are generally less than 3%. The incidence of significant early postoperative complications is in the range of 10%, and this includes hemorrhage requiring transfusion, partial small bowel obstruction, and urine leakage. Early ambulation and the use of pneumatic compression stockings have greatly reduced the incidence of deep venous thrombosis and pulmonary embolism.

The long-term complications of this procedure are to a great extent related to the type of urinary diversion used. The most common type of diversion used at this time is the ileal conduit. In addition to common postoperative complications such as wound infections or dehiscence, urine leakage, and bowel obstruction, these patients are at risk for a number of complications specifically related to the urinary diversion. These include stomal stenosis, parastomal hernia, pyelonephritis, urinary calculi, and metabolic problems. The metabolic problems encountered depend on the type and length of bowel used in creating an anastomosis. Hypochloremic, hyponatremic, hyperkalemic, metabolic acidosis occurs in up to 40% of patients with a small bowel conduit. Drugs that are urine and can be reabsorbed in the intestine may build up toxic levels. This phenomenon has been described for phenytoin, among others. B_{12} and fat malabsorption may occur. Chronic acidosis may lead to osteomalacia.

B. **RT.** As with surgery, radiation techniques have advanced over recent years, and this has resulted in a significant decrement in the toxicities associated with this form of treatment. Three-dimensional treatment planning has been a major advance. This has allowed higher doses of radiation to be delivered to tumors, with less radiation delivered to surrounding normal tissues. The most common complications of radiation to the bladder include irritative bowel or bladder symptoms, chronic proctitis, and reduced bladder capacity. Occasionally severe bowel obstruction or severe bladder dysfunction requiring surgical diversion will occur.

C. **Chemotherapy.** As would be expected, the toxicities of chemotherapy are predicated by the agents and doses used. The most commonly used regimens in bladder cancer are multiagent regimens including cisplatin (MVAC, CMV, or GC). Common toxicities of these regimens include neutropenia and fever (10% to 30%) and mucositis (10% to 20%). Peripheral neuropathy, hearing loss, and renal impairment occur less frequently. Anticipated treatment-related mortality is in the range of 3% for MVAC and 1% for GC.

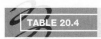

TABLE 20.4	Follow-up of Patients with Superficial Bladder Cancer	

Presentation	3-month cystoscopy	Follow-up
Single tumor	No recurrence	Annual follow-up
	Recurrence	Cystoscopy every 3 mo
Multiple tumors	No recurrence	Cystoscopy every 3 mo
	Recurrence	Intravesical therapy

Modified from Parmer MKB, Freedman CS, Hargreave TB, et al. Prognostic factors for recurrence and follow-up policies in the treatment of superficial bladder cancer: report from the BMRC subgroup on superficial bladder cancer (Urological Working Group Party). *J Urol* 1989;142:284–288, with permission.

D. **Follow-up.** Specific follow-up recommendations depend on the clinical presentation of disease. The most specific recommendations address the care of patients with superficial bladder cancer. Given the high rate of recurrence of superficial bladder cancer, most authors recommend regular follow-up, usually with cystoscopy and urine cytology 3 months after initial diagnosis. Subsequent follow-up is determined by the findings at the 3-month evaluation (Table 20.4). Patients with a single tumor at diagnosis and no recurrence at 3 months may be followed up with annual cystoscopy. Patients with a single tumor at diagnosis and a recurrence at 3 months, or multiple tumors at diagnosis and no recurrence at 3 months should undergo cystoscopy every 3 months. Patients with multiple tumors at diagnosis and recurrence at 3 months should receive intravesical therapy. These guidelines have been validated only retrospectively. The duration of follow-up has not been defined, but given the propensity of this disease for late recurrences, many authors recommend indefinite follow-up.

The follow-up of patients with muscle-invasive disease is less clearly defined. Certainly, patients undergoing bladder-sparing treatment require frequent cystoscopy to document response to treatment, and they will require regular follow-up after completion of treatment. Even patients treated with radical cystectomy warrant follow-up. They remain at risk for local recurrence, metastatic disease, and new tumors occurring anywhere in the remaining urothelium. Unfortunately, the follow-up evaluations are even less clearly defined in these patients.

Patients with metastatic disease are generally monitored with radiographic tests to document their response to therapy. If a complete response is obtained, regular radiographic evaluation of the areas previously involved with disease will likely be undertaken. The value of such follow-up is not proved.

IX. **BACKGROUND**

A. **Epidemiology.** Bladder cancer is relatively common, with approximately 60,000 cases diagnosed in the United States in 2005. The median age at diagnosis is 65 years, and this disease is uncommon in patients younger than 40. It is more common in men than in women (3:1), in urban than in rural settings, and in African Americans than in whites. Superficial tumors account for 75% of disease at diagnosis, whereas muscle-invasive disease accounts for 20% to 25%. This helps to explain why 50,000 cases were diagnosed in 1995 and 10,000 deaths occurred.

B. **Identifiable risk factors.** The most well-defined risk factor for bladder cancer in the United States is cigarette smoking. Exposure to polycyclic aromatic hydrocarbons, including 2-naphthylamine and benzene, result in increased risk. Several occupations pose increased risk, including chimney sweeping, dry cleaning, and manufacturing preservatives. Infection with *Schistosoma haematobium,* a parasite found in many third world countries, increases the risk of bladder cancer, and greatly increases the risk of squamous cell bladder cancer. In the United

States, 90% to 95% of bladder cancers are TCCAs. In countries with endemic *S. haematobium,* squamous cell tumors compose a larger portion.

C. **Molecular biology.** Alterations in a number of oncogenes and tumor-suppressor genes have been associated with bladder cancer. Oncogenes associated with bladder cancer include *p21 ras, c-myc,* and *c-jun.* The tumor-suppressor genes most commonly associated with bladder cancer are *p53* (17p) and the retinoblastoma gene *(RB)* (13q). Overexpression of *erb*-b2 has also been associated with higher grade tumors and higher risk of recurrence *(Urol Res* 1993;21:39).

D. **Pathogenesis.** Bladder cancer is thought to arise because of a field defect of the urothelium, resulting in a genetically unstable urothelium. This helps explain why bladder tumors tend to recur either locally or at anatomically distinct sites. Smokers have been found to have atypia in the urothelium when examined at autopsy. There appears to be a progression of genetic changes from low-grade, noninvasive tumors to higher grade, invasive tumors. Deletions of 17p *(TP53* gene locus), 18q *(DCC* gene locus), and 13q *(RB* gene locus) are associated with invasive tumors.

E. **Current focus.** Bladder cancer has offered a unique opportunity for cancer researchers. These tumors are relatively accessible for obtaining tissue. In addition, the natural history of this disease, with recurrences and progression from relatively innocuous to more malignant behavior has allowed evaluation of molecular changes as tumors advance through this course.

A number of important molecular associations of bladder cancer have been described. Mutations of the *p53* gene have been found to be present in up to 80% of CIS and invasive tumors at diagnosis. The p53 protein is an important transcription factor, regulating genes involved in cell-cycle control. Mutations of the *p53* gene lead to aberrant cell-cycle regulation and appear to play a role in malignant transformation. Other prognostic factors include the absence of blood group antigens on the tumor cell surface, DNA ploidy, and expression of epidermal growth factor receptor. As the molecular abnormalities underlying bladder cancer are more clearly elucidated, it is likely that clinical interventions based on these findings will be developed. One area of investigation is gene transfer to correct existing gene abnormalities in the urothelium and prevent progression to invasive cancer. These strategies are in very early development.

Another major area of ongoing interest is the development of bladder-sparing approaches for muscle-invasive disease. As described earlier, a number of these strategies have been piloted. Ongoing studies should help define the optimal approach in this setting and will help more clearly to define which of the patients are appropriate for this strategy.

Strategies for screening and prevention in high-risk groups are also under evaluation. As molecular abnormalities are identified and their significance determined, they may be incorporated into screening strategies. Specifically, precancerous abnormalities that can be identified in shed cells of the urothelium may help with early detection and even prevention of TCCA of the bladder.

Suggested Readings

Brosman SA. Experience with bacillus Calmette-Guerin in patients with superficial bladder carcinoma. *J Urol* 1982;128:27–30.

Cote RJ, Chatterjee SJ. Molecular determinants of outcome in bladder cancer. *Cancer J Sci Am* 1999;5:2–15.

Dreicer R. Chemotherapy for muscle-invasive bladder cancer in the perioperative setting: current Standards. *Urol Oncol* 2007;25:72.

Esrig D, Elmajian D, Groshen S, et al. Accumulation of nuclear p53 and tumor progression on bladder cancer. *N Engl J Med* 1994;331:1259–1264.

Grossman H, Natale R, Tangen C, et al. Neoadjuvant chemotherapy plus cystectomy compared with cystectomy alone for locally advanced bladder cancer. *N Engl J Med* 2003;349:859.

Harker WG, Meyers FJ, Freiha FS, et al. Cisplatin, methotrexate, and vinblastine (CMV): an effective chemotherapy regimen for metastatic transitional cell carcinoma of the urinary tract: a Northern California Oncology Group study. *J Clin Oncol* 1985;3:1463–1470.

Kim HL, Steinberg GD. The current status of bladder preservation in the treatment of muscle invasive bladder cancer. *J Urol* 2000;164:627–632.

Lancet. Neoadjuvant cisplatin, methotrexate, and vinblastine chemotherapy for muscle-invasive bladder cancer: a randomized controlled trial: international collaboration of trialists. 1999;354:1650.

Lee LW, Davis E Jr. Gross urinary hemorrhage: a symptom, not a disease. *JAMA* 1953;153:783.

Rintala E, Hannisdal E, Fossa SD, et al. Neoadjuvant chemotherapy in bladder cancer: a randomized study: nordic cystectomy trial I. *Scand J Urol Nephrol* 1993;27:355.

Skinner DG, Daniels JR, Russell CA, et al. The role of adjuvant chemotherapy following systemic chemotherapy for invasive bladder cancer: a prospective comparative trial. *J Urol* 1991;145:459.

Smith J, Labasky RF, Cockett ATK, et al. Bladder cancer clinical guidelines panel: summary report on the management of nonmuscle invasive bladder cancer (stages Ta, T1, and TIS). *J Urol* 1997;xx:162.

Sternberg CN, Yagoda A, Sher HI, et al. Preliminary results of methotrexate, vinblastine, adriamycin, and cisplatin (M-VAC) in advanced urothelial tumors. *J Urol* 1985;133:403.

Von der Maase H, Hansen SW, Roberts JT, et al. Gemcitabine and cisplatin versus methotrexate, vinblastine, doxorubicin, and cisplatin in advanced or metastatic bladder cancer: results of a large, randomized, multinational, multicenter, phase III study. *J Clin Oncol* 2000;17:3068–3077.

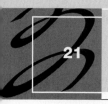

21 GENITOURINARY CANCER: PROSTATE
Ramakrishna Venkatesh and Donald P. Lombardi

I. PRESENTATION
A. Subjective.
Prostate cancer rarely causes symptoms early in the course of the disease as most of the adenocarcinomas arise in the periphery of the gland away from the urethra.

In the prostate-specific antigen (PSA) era, the most common finding is the *absence* of symptoms. The presence of symptoms due to prostate cancer often suggests locally advanced or metastatic disease. Growth of prostate cancer around or into the urethra, or involvement of bladder neck can result in decreased urinary force of stream, frequency, urgency, nocturia, or hematuria. However, many of these symptoms are not specific and may occur with benign prostatic hyperplasia and aging. Involvement of ejaculatory ducts can cause hemospermia, and extraprostatic disease involving the branches of pelvic plexus can cause erectile dysfunction (ED).

Metastatic disease can cause a wide variety of symptoms related to the sites of metastases. Bone is the favored site of metastasis, with pain being a common, and at times, debilitating symptom. Men with spinal metastases may live for years; therefore, careful and thoughtful, serial histories and examinations are mandatory. The most devastating consequences of bone involvement are pain, fractures, and spinal cord or nerve root compression. Spinal cord compression is usually accompanied by back pain that is often made worse by coughing, sneezing, or straining (and other activities that increase intradural pressure). Unlike nonmalignant causes of back pain, the back pain of metastatic prostate cancer is usually worse at night. If a peripheral nerve is pinched by tumor, the back pain may radiate around to the front of the patient in the thorax or abdomen or down the legs. Patients with early spinal cord compression will have weakness, with progression to paralysis occurring, on the one hand, over a period of weeks to even months. On the other hand, late spinal cord compromise leads to loss of sensation distal to the level of metastasis, urinary retention and incontinence in a matter of minutes to hours. The classic symptoms of cauda equina syndrome are low back pain, bilateral sciatica, sensory and motor deficits, including sacral and perianal anesthesia, and loss of sphincter control of bladder and anus. Delays in management result in permanent loss of sensation, motor function, and continence.

Fatigue is a prominent complaint of patients, but it may occur for very different reasons depending on the state of the tumor and the patient. If due to advanced or metastatic disease, it may be an indicator of bone marrow infiltration by tumor with associated anemia. Liver involvement occurs in only 15%, usually at the end of life. Hepatic metastases are usually due to poorly differentiated adenocarcinomas or to tumors with small cell (neuroendocrine) differentiation.

Androgen deprivation therapy (ADT) and/or chemotherapy can cause anemia, but the former is usually mild, whereas the latter may be moderate or severe. Lower limb edema can result from pelvic lymph node involvement, compression of iliac veins, and/or deep vein thrombosis (DVT).

Shortness of breath may be due to chemotherapy treatment, anemia, pulmonary embolism, and/or lung metastases, but the latter occurs late in only 15% of patients. Later in the course of the disease, older men complain of fatigue and gradually fail to thrive at home, with debilitating bone pain, weakened legs, decreased activity, poor appetite, weight loss, and other symptoms of advanced metastatic disease.

B. **Objective.** With the widespread use of PSA screening and early detection programs, the most common finding on examination of the prostate is, or will soon
become, the *absence* of findings. Despite the lead-time bias that PSA screening intro-
duces, physicians must be able to perform an excellent digital rectal examination
(DRE) to diagnose and clinically stage localized prostate cancer. Attention should
be directed to defining the presence or absence of a nodule and its location with
respect to the right or left lobe and median raphe. Clearly, the absence of a nodule
does not preclude the diagnosis of prostate cancer, and simply hardness of the
prostate may indicate the presence of tumor. As patients become more obese, the
DRE becomes more difficult to perform, but one should try to define extracapsular
extension and/or involvement of the seminal vesicles. The sensitivity and specificity
of the DRE is modest to poor, depending on the examiner, which can lead to both
over- and underdiagnosis.

   As with all cancer patients, the oncologist must do a careful, comprehensive
physical examination, with special attention to signs of anemia, lymphadenopathy,
bone tenderness, neuropathy, and lower extremity edema. For men treated with
ADT, the testicular examination ought to show atrophy, whereas its absence should
alert the physician that the patient does not have castrate levels of testosterone.
Because of the potential for extended periods of good quality of life (QOL) and
survival, even with metastatic disease, prostate cancer remains one of several
neoplasms that physicians must rule out in the evaluation of carcinoma of unknown
primary tumor (see Chapter 22, Genitourinary Cancer: Penile).

II. **WORKUP AND STAGING.** Autopsy studies have shown localized prostate cancer in
approximately 30% of men older than 50 years and 70% of men older than 80
years. However, with the availability of serum PSA and transrectal ultrasonogram-
guided needle biopsy of the prostate, clinically organ-confined prostate cancer is
increasingly diagnosed, with continuing uncertainty regarding the clinical significance
of some tumors. Defining the grade of the tumor and anatomic stage are critical in
understanding the prognosis and formulation of a treatment plan. Various predictive
models (e.g., Partin table, Kattan nomograms) have been developed and available for
use in clinical practice for counseling patients and for planning a rational management
plan. Most of these validated models include prognostic variables such as PSA, Gleason
score, and clinical stage of the cancer.

A. **Laboratory testing**

   1. **PSA.** PSA is a serum marker that is central to the diagnosis and management of
      prostate cancer. The use of PSA testing has helped to identify cases of prostate
      cancer that are or will become clinically significant, rather than simply identifying
      cases of cancer that are unlikely to be detected until autopsy. PSA is directly
      associated with tumor volume and clinical stage. Normal PSA ranges depend on
      factors such as age and race, and PSA level is affected by prostatic biopsy but
      not significantly by DREs.

      Absolute PSA levels and the rate of change of those levels with respect to
      time can predict the likelihood of organ-confined disease and influence opinions
      on the likelihood of a cure. PSA levels greater than 10 μg/L are associated
      with increased risk for extracapsular extension. The positive predictive value for
      a PSA between 4 and 10 ng/mL in a patient with normal DRE is only 30%
      approximately. To improve the performance of the PSA test, modifications, such
      as PSA velocity, PSA density, and free-to-total PSA ratio have been used. Some
      physicians advocate the use of free PSA versus bound PSA to quantify further
      the risk of cancer and need for biopsy; higher percentage free PSA levels are
      associated with more favorable histopathologic features in prostate tumors. A
      cutoff of 25% free PSA detects 95% of cancer while avoiding 20% of unnecessary
      biopsies.

      More recently PSA kinetics has been explored. A study showed men whose
      PSA level increased by more than 2.0 ng/mL during the year before diagnosis
      of prostate cancer were at high risk for cancer-specific death even if they had
      "favorable" clinical parameters (such as a PSA level less than 10 ng/mL and
      Gleason score less than 6 at diagnosis) and that they should undergo radical

prostatectomy (RP). For these men, watchful waiting may not be an appropriate option. Their increased risk also makes them candidates for enrollment in clinical trials examining various combination treatment strategies. Physicians must use caution when using such measures because men with tumors with Gleason scores of 8, 9, and 10 may be so poorly differentiated that they do not synthesize and secrete large amounts of PSA.

2. **Complete blood count and chemistries.** The laboratory workup should include a complete blood count and comprehensive metabolic panel. Widely metastatic disease may cause anemia or thrombocytopenia because of marrow infiltration, but most patients will have normal peripheral counts and normal chemistries at the time of diagnosis. Abnormal tests should prompt investigation, especially in patients thought to have only localized disease. For example, an elevated alkaline phosphatase may be due to bone metastases and, therefore, a bone scan should be done to rule out this possibility.

B. **Imaging.** Computed tomography **(CT)**, magnetic resonance imaging (MRI), and bone scans are important in the assessment of advanced disease, but they are not often indicated in the standard workup of low-risk prostate cancer because of their low sensitivity and high cost. Physicians should adopt a symptom-directed approach to the use of imaging of low-risk disease. Patients with high-risk disease are more likely to have benefit from routine imaging, and many physicians use CT of the abdomen and bone scan as adjuncts to clinical staging in this group. Imaging in these patients may help to identify those with lymph node involvement, but sensitivity is poor even in this risk group. It has been suggested that endorectal coil MRI can be used to categorize risk further in intermediate-risk tumors by identifying seminal vesicle involvement and extraprostatic extension before surgery, but favorable results found with its use have not yet been reproduced. Current imaging studies (CT, MRI, or positron emission tomography [PET] scan) do not adequately stage prostate cancer, and they do not provide data on risk stratification as readily as that provided by clinical tumor stage, serum PSA, or Gleason grade.

C. **Pelvic lymphadenectomy.** In patients with intermediate or high-risk disease, such as with PSA greater than 10 ng/mL, high Gleason score 7 to 10, and clinical stage T3, laparoscopic pelvic lymphadenectomy should be considered to rule out metastatic disease before definitive therapy. These patients are at higher risk for lymphatic involvement, and positive findings will affect future therapy decisions.

D. **Staging.** The first purpose of a staging system is to provide a well-accepted classification where health care workers from around the world may interpret the extent of disease of the patient. However, in addition, the clinical and/or pathologic stage of the prostate cancer patient may guide discussions about the optimal modality for treatment. The clinical or pathologic stage of the patient is the stage that is defined at the time of initial diagnosis. One does not "re-stage" the patient because it confuses the discussions about prognosis. If the patient relapses, one may refer to the patient as one who has "recurrent" or "relapsed, metastatic" disease. The first stage that is assigned is the clinical tumor (T) stage, where the physician performs a prostate examination and assigns a score (Table 21.1).

To answer queries from patients about prognosis and treatment options, one must weigh the clinical and/or pathologic tumor, node, metastasis (TNM) staging, Gleason grade, and serum PSA level in the context of the general health of the patient. The oncologist should give estimates of both prostate cancer-specific survival and overall survival. The median age at diagnosis for U.S. men is declining, but is still approximately 68, and the average man lives to 75 years at this time. In the future, men will get diagnosed earlier and will live longer, leading to more treatment, more "cures," more PSA relapses, and longer times with side effects from therapies for recurrent disease.

1. **TNM** tumor staging is more commonly used than the older Whitmore–Jewett system (Table 21.1).

2. **Histologic grade** is best determined with the Gleason scoring system. The Gleason grade is a classification of gland formation from a relatively low power view. It is not a histologic classification in the basic sense, such as a comment

	Primary tumor (T)
	Clinical
TX	Primary tumor cannot be assessed
T0	No evidence of primary tumor
T1	Clinically inapparent tumor neither palpable nor visible by imaging
T1a	Tumor incidental histologic finding in ≤5% of tissue resected
T1b	Tumor incidental histologic finding in >5% of tissue resected
T1c	Tumor identified by needle biopsy (e.g., because of elevated PSA)
T2	Tumor confined within the prostate[a]
T2a	Tumor involves ≤$\frac{1}{2}$ of one lobe
T2b	Tumor involves >$\frac{1}{2}$ of one lobe but not both lobes
T2c	Tumor involves both lobes
T3	Tumor extends through the prostatic capsule[b]
T3a	Extracapsular extension (bilateral)
T3b	Extracapsular extension (unilateral)
T3c	Tumor invades the seminal vesicle(s)
T4	Tumor is fixed or invades adjacent structures other than seminal vesicles; bladder neck, external sphincter, rectum, levator muscles, and/or pelvic wall

[a]Note: Tumor found in one or both lobes by needle biopsy, but not palpable or reliably visible by imaging, is classified as T1c.
[b]Note: Invasion into the prostatic apex or into (but not beyond) the prostatic capsule is not classified as T3, but as T2.

	Regional lymph nodes (N)
	Clinical
NX	Regional lymph nodes were not assessed
N0	No regional lymph node metastasis
N1	Metastasis in regional
Pathologic	
pNX	Regional nodes not sampled
pN0	No positive regional nodes
pN1	Metastases in regional node(s)
Distant Metastasis (M)[a]	
MX	Distant metastasis cannot be assessed (not evaluated by any modality)
M0	No distant metastasis
M1	Distant metastasis
M1a	Non-regional lymph node(s)
M1b	Bone(s)
M1c	Other site(s) with or without bone disease

[a]Note: When more than one site of metastasis is present, the most advanced category is used. pM1c is most advanced.

Pathologic (pT)

pT2[a]	Organ confined
pT2a	Unilateral, involving $\frac{1}{2}$ of the lobe or less
pT2b	Unilateral, involving more than $\frac{1}{2}$ of one lobe but not both lobes
pT2c	Bilateral disease
pT3	Extraprostatic extension
pT3a	Extraprostatic extension[b]
pT3b	Seminal vesicle invasion
pT4	Invasion of bladder, rectum

[a] Note: There is no pathologic T1 classification.
[b] Note: Positive surgical margin should be indicated by an R1 descriptor (residual microscopic disease).

Stage Grouping

Stage I	T1a	N0	M0	G1
Stage II	T1a	N0	M0	G2, 3,4
	T1b	N0	M0	Any G
	T1c	N0	M0	Any G
	T1	N0	M0	Any G
	T2	N0	M0	Any G
Stage III	T3	N0	M0	Any G
Stage IV	T4	N0	M0	Any G
	Any T	N1	M0	Any G
	Any T	Any N	M1	Any G

on nucleoli, nuclear to cytoplasmic ratio and so on. The tumor pattern is graded from 1 for well differentiated to grade 5 for poorly differentiated pattern. **Gleason score** is the sum of the scores for the primary and secondary Gleason patterns seen on the biopsy or prostatectomy specimen. Because the prognosis varies according to the primary and secondary Gleason grades, each should be assessed along with the sum score. Most men have intermediate-range Gleason scores (Gleason 6 or 7), and it is important to recognize that Gleason scores from transrectal ultrasonogram-guided biopsies may underscore a tumor. Pathologic review from subsequent prostatectomy may increase Gleason scores; for example, a "Gleason 3 + 3 = 6" may be upgraded to a "Gleason 3 + 4 = 7."

3. **The combination of clinical stage, Gleason score, and PSA level** allows physicians to prognosticate most accurately. Patients at highest risk for progression/relapse have PSA greater than 20, Gleason sum score greater than 7, extraprostatic disease and presence of tumor at the surgical margin. Intermediate-risk disease is T2b, PSA 10 to 20, Gleason 7; and high-risk disease is greater than T2c, PSA more than 20, and Gleason 8. Histologic grade is a good predictor of the outcome, but is not as good as the Gleason sum score. Patients with well-differentiated, moderately differentiated, and poorly differentiated tumors had 15-year death rates for untreated disease of 9%, 28%, and 51%, respectively.

III. TREATMENT

A. **Localized disease (T1 to T3 N0 M0).** The discussion of treatment options for localized disease should encompass risks and benefits of surgery or radiation (either external beam or brachytherapy). The 5-year disease-free survival for both RP and radiation therapy (XRT) is approximately 60% to 70%.

1. **RP.** For most men, the treatment of choice for early-stage prostate cancer remains surgical resection. The optimal post-RP outcome for the patient is to be cancer free (with undetectable serum PSA) and to recover preoperative urinary and erectile function. Anatomic RP, also known as *radical retropubic prostatectomy*, is the most common technique for resection currently and allows for the possibility of nerve-sparing techniques that increase the likelihood of preserving potency as well as total continence. The procedure is performed through a midline lower-abdominal incision and may involve pelvic (hypogastric and obturator) lymph node dissection. External iliac nodes are not generally removed to reduce the risk of future lower-extremity edema. Nerve-sparing techniques allow preservation of neurovascular bundles if uninvolved by tumor. Indications for removal of the neurovascular bundle and surrounding tissues are induration along the posterolateral margin of the prostate, palpable induration of the lateral pelvic fascia, and fixation of the neurovascular bundle to the prostate. RP is likely curative for organ-confined prostate cancer, somewhat less likely to be so in more locally advanced tumors with capsular penetration or high Gleason score, and rarely curative in lymph node-positive/metastatic disease. In a study looking at 1,745 patients undergoing RP with curative intent, surgical excision controlled prostate cancer effectively in 1,441 (83%) of the patients. At 5, 10, and 15 years, 82%, 77%, and 75% of patients, respectively, remained free from disease progression (i.e., from biochemical or clinical recurrence).

a. **Laparoscopic radical prostatectomy (LRP) with or without robotic assistance.** Surgeons have demonstrated that LRP with or without robotic assistance can be performed with excellent results. LRP is technically demanding, requiring a significant learning curve. The average intraoperative blood loss is less with robotic or laparoscopic approach. The perceived advantages that laparoscopic or robotic prostatectomy with a magnified surgical image would markedly improve patient outcomes has not been realized. However, the short-term outcomes of robotic RP are no worse than open prostatectomy. Robotic prostatectomy is more expensive than RP. To date, no prospective randomized trials have compared the two approaches, and it is unlikely that such a study will be performed. As with open surgical procedures, laparoscopic outcomes, including surgical margin status, continence, and potency, reflect technique more than approach. Current data suggest that a skilled surgeon is the most important factor for improving outcomes, whether open RP or LRP is performed.

2. **Pelvic lymphadenectomy** does not provide additional curative benefit, but may provide prognostic information. It can be especially useful in patients with high-risk or locally advanced disease in which future hormonal therapy will be an important consideration, and, likewise, it may not be indicated in low-risk patients. Most urologists perform pelvic lymphadenectomy by using laparoscopic techniques. The finding of malignant involvement of pelvic nodes should lead to medical rather than surgical therapy. However, more recently some authors have recommended extended pelvic lymph node dissection for high-risk disease patients to adequately stage the disease with potential therapeutic benefit.

3. **XRT.** XRT for the prostate is a continually evolving field as new and better technologies make it possible to deliver higher doses of targeted local radiation, sparing normal tissues, with less local toxicity. **External-beam radiation**. At least two prospective studies have shown that a dose of 78 to 79 Gy is better than 70 Gy. Advanced computer modeling has led to the development of **intensely modulated radiation therapy (IMRT)**, which is currently available only in highly specialized centers. This technique uses complicated tools that precisely control both the dose of radiation and the tissue targeted. Also, with IMRT doses more than 81 Gy can be administered, although the outcome is no better than 79 Gy. Outcomes for T1/T2 disease are similar to those seen with surgery, with 87% of patients free of local recurrence at 10 years. Pelvic lymph node analysis before definitive XRT may be useful in patients at high risk for advanced disease.

An alternative to external-beam therapy is **interstitial XRT with seed implants (brachytherapy)** which is popular. **High-dose-rate (HDR) brachytherapy** has been reported to be associated with lesser incidence of dysuria, frequency, and rectal pain compared to the low-dose-rate brachytherapy.

4. **Active surveillance (AS).** AS may be a safe alternative to immediate treatment in compliant men with a low risk of cancer progression. The goal of AS is to avoid overtreatment for most patients while administering curative therapy to those in need of more aggressive treatment. A complete baseline reevaluation, including DRE, measurement of free and total PSA levels, imaging study of the prostate (preferably endorectal MRI with spectroscopy), and ultrasonogram-guided systematic needle biopsy is required. If these studies confirm a low-risk cancer, and the patient chooses AS, checkups with DRE and PSA every 6 months indefinitely are recommended, with repeat imaging and biopsy 12 to 18 months after the baseline evaluation and then every 2 to 3 years.

5. **Cryotherapy.** With better ultrasonographic imaging along with real-time monitoring of freezing and improvements in the cryotherapy technology with smaller cryoprobes, interest in cryotherapy has been rekindled. With the "third generation" cryotherapy technology, the reported morbidity is significantly less compared to the older generation cryotechnology. Cryotherapy is currently limited to patients who are poor candidates for RP or XRT and who have poor sexual function. It can also be used as salvage therapy for locally recurrent prostate cancer following RP or failed brachytherapy or external-beam XRT. However, currently the role of cryotherapy as a primary treatment of prostate cancer continues to be controversial. Focal-targeted therapy seems attractive, if we can identify significant cancer focus or foci. The University of Colorado, in partnership with other institutions, is conducting a phaseII trial to study the feasibility of focal-targeted cryoablation. Their protocol uses three-dimensional topographic prostatic reconstruction to aid in the identification of significant cancer foci.

B. **Locally advanced disease (T3 N0)**

1. **Surgery or radiation** remains first-line therapy for locally advanced disease. Neoadjuvant therapy with hormonal blockade has been shown to decrease the rate of positive margins at surgery in these patients, but it did not affect overall survival. When extraprostatic cancer within the pelvis is detected, there is benefit to the use of hormonal blockade after surgery or radiation. However, physicians

must weigh the toxicities of hormonal therapy versus the possible benefits. There is substantial debate regarding the efficacy of **immediate hormonal blockade versus delayed hormonal blockade** (waiting until there is evidence of disease progression) in the management of locally advanced prostate cancer after RP. A number of studies with conflicting results have been performed. A small percentage of these studies have demonstrated survival benefit to the immediate-treatment group, but most of the studies have found no survival difference. In a randomized prospective study, patients with node-positive (microscopic) disease discovered at the time of RP were assigned to immediate surgical or hormonal castration or to observation and castration only when metastatic disease was found. The group of patients who had immediate castration had significant survival benefit. It should be noted that this study had a small sample size. In addition, patients were considered to have progressive disease only when they had measurable disease by imaging. Patients with increasing PSA were not treated until they had measurable disease, and perhaps because of this additional delay, the study found a survival difference between groups.

The Medical Research Council (MRC) study also compared immediate versus delayed therapy in locally advanced disease after surgery, and although survival differences were not impressive, early treatment had QOL **benefits** with decreased incidence of cord compression, ureteral obstruction, and pathologic fractures versus delayed treatment.

2. **The combination of hormone therapy with radiation alone** in locally advanced disease has also been evaluated. The benefit of adding hormone therapy in this setting continues to be a matter of debate and the subject of several ongoing clinical studies. The combination of XRT and hormonal therapy in locally advanced disease has been shown to result in superior survival when compared with XRT alone in this setting. (It is unclear whether these data can be extrapolated to use of higher-dose conformational XRT now commonly given. A similar study, in contrast, did not show survival benefit to combined hormonal and XRT. However, there was improved duration of disease-free survival and decreased local failure with combined therapy. The combination of hormonal therapy with brachytherapy in locally advanced disease has not yet shown convincing evidence of survival benefit.

3. **Increasing PSA after prostatectomy or radiation.** Asymptomatic progressive increase in PSA is a common problem in patients with prostate cancer after XRT or surgery. Prognostic factors to consider in this setting are doubling time of PSA, time from definitive therapy to increase in PSA, age of the patient, and comorbidities. Many methods have been used to predict failure, and most physicians consider higher risk patients to be those with seminal vesicle involvement, aggressive histology (Gleason greater than 6), and PSA greater than 10. D'Amico et al. reported that PSA doubling time of less than 6 months is highly predictive of disease progression compared to doubling time of more than 10 months.

Local control after initial failure can be attempted. XRT may provide additional local control after RP, but it has not shown survival benefit and may be associated with higher rates of radiation-related complications. Salvage prostatectomy after XRT is rarely an option because of higher surgical complication rates. Other surgical options in this setting include cryotherapy and brachytherapy, but current studies show only negative results.

Most men who have increasing PSA levels after initial management are given medical therapy (see section C). Ongoing trials will attempt to determine whether combined hormonal and XRT is beneficial in patients with increasing PSA after definitive surgery.

C. **Metastatic disease**
1. **Initial therapy (hormone-sensitive disease).** Medical or surgical castration remains the first-line therapy for metastatic disease, as it is associated with a response rate greater than 80% and can often reduce PSA levels to undetectable levels. In the recent past, metastatic prostate cancers have remained sensitive to

the effects of hormonal blockade for an average of 12 to 18 months. Currently, with lead-time bias of diagnosis, more widespread use of PSA as a serum marker, improved imaging, and early hormonal intervention, men can respond to androgen deprivation for 2 or more years, with some living up to a decade.

Given the psychological impact of surgical castration, most men in the United States prefer medical androgen blockade to **bilateral orchiectomy.** However, surgery is certainly the most cost-effective treatment. **Gonadotropin-releasing hormone (GnRH) agonists** are the most commonly employed first line agents. Because these agents are agonists, they will initially **increase** serum testosterone levels and could result in progression of pain, disease, and even spinal cord compression. Therefore, before GnRH injection, treatment with an androgen receptor antagonist (bicalutimide 50 mg daily; nilutimide 150 mg daily, or flutamide 250 mg three times a day) is warranted. Routinely, these drugs are started 2 weeks before injections and are prescribed for 1 month. Then, leuprolide acetate (Lupron) may be given as 4-month (30 mg), 3month (22.5 mg) or 1-month (7.5 mg) intramuscular injections. Another GnRH agonist, goserelin (Zoladex), is introduced as a depot injection into the anterior abdominal wall, subcutaneously, every 3 months (10.6 mg) or every month (3.6 mg). The most common side effects are hot flashes and ED. However, over the first year of ADT, (), many men will become anemic and fatigued, lose muscle mass and gain fat tissue, and lose bone density. Combined androgen blockade (CAB), with both a GnRH agonist and an androgen-receptor blockade (ARB), is not substantially better than GnRH agonist alone.

Failure of first line ADT is often marked by an asymptomatic rise in PSA, although symptoms of urinary track outlet obstruction, bone pain and so on may be observed as well. This transition may be referred to as *castrate-independent* disease, but the androgen receptor is still present and can still respond to androgens. Therefore, it is important to maintain patients on ADT with GnRH agonists. If the patient was treated with a GnRH agonist alone, then one may add an ARB (preferred: Casodex). If the patient was managed with CAB, then it is wise to stop treatment with the ARB, to rule out "flutamide withdrawal syndrome." Only approximately 10% of these patients will respond, but sometimes it may take 6 weeks to observe a decrease in PSA levels. Some data suggest that in tumors of a subset of patients, mutations of the androgen receptor result in flutamide acting as an agonist, instead of an antagonist of the androgen receptor.

Eventually, second-line hormonal therapy will no longer work and this stage may be treated with inhibitors of adrenal androgen synthesis (ketoconazole, hydrocortisone, or the combination), estrogens, progestins and so on. However, the patient should have mild to moderate symptoms and no impending visceral crisis. Randomized trials have not shown a clear benefit to the use of third-line hormonal therapy, but clearly a subset of patients respond.

2. **Hormone refractory disease.** Once the patient has progressed through ADT plus antiandrogen therapy, we consider his tumor to be "castrate-refractory." Again, the tumor can still respond to androgens, so it is important to maintain castrate levels of testosterone. Chemotherapy was tried in metastatic prostate cancer for 4 decades and was considered a failure. However, the improvement with antiemetics, supportive care, pain control, and hematopoietic growth factors finally allowed for adequate trials in this elderly men. In a randomized trial, the anthracycline, mitoxantrone, plus prednisone proved to be superior to prednisone alone in terms of QOL, but not in survival. Nevertheless, this regimen became the control group for future chemotherapy trials. Finally, the taxanes and other microtubule inhibitors showed activity in prostate cancer in the late 1990s. Then, two randomized, controlled, prospective, multicenter studies were performed testing docetaxel-based chemotherapy versus mitoxantrone plus prednisone in castrate-independent, metastatic prostate cancer. For the first time, docetaxel-based therapy resulted in superior median and overall survival rates. Docetaxel plus prednisone was approved by the U.S. Food and Drug Administration (FDA)

and is considered the standard of care in the United States. Current studies are designed to ask whether the addition of antiangiogenesis agents will improve outcome. The prominent side effects of docetaxel include fatigue, aches and pain in muscles and joints, nail changes, diarrhea, and sequelae of bone marrow suppression.

IV. COMPLICATIONS

A. Complications of therapy

1. **Complications of surgery.** The complications of RP are predominantly urinary incontinence and impotence, but the nerve-sparing and retropubic approach has decreased complication rates. In the best series, an estimated 8% of men will have stress incontinence after surgery, with only 1% to 2% requiring more than one pad daily. Larger, population-based studies, unfortunately, have shown higher complication rates. Patients are less likely to complain about urinary incontinence to their surgeons, and in some reports, 11% of men after prostatectomy were using two or more pads per day.

    Impotence is still a major problem, and the rate of total impotence increases with advanced disease, advanced age, and poor surgical technique. An estimated 20% to 80% of men who are fully potent before surgery will retain potency after the procedure, but the erections may not be of the same quality. In men younger than 50 years, some degree of potency is preserved in an estimated 91%, even if one neurovascular bundle is excised. However, in men older than 70 years, potency rates decrease to approximately 25% with excision of the neurovascular bundles. It is important to make men aware of available therapies designed to restore potency, both pharmacologic and nonpharmacologic. Sensation to the penis is preserved after RP (through the pudendal nerve), although the autonomic innervation of the corporal bodies are damaged. Medications such as sildenafil, verdanafil, and tadalafil may help men regain erectile function and improved sexual activity and QOL.

    The reported blood transfusion rate for robotic or laparoscopic prostatectomy is 1% to 2% compared to 5% to 10% for open RP. Other rare complications include DVT (1% to 3%), rectal injury (less than 1%). The risk of postoperative mortality after RP is relatively low (less than 0.5%) for otherwise healthy older men up to age 79. In one large study, 61,039 patients with prostate cancer had undergone RP as the principal procedure at 1,552 U.S. hospitals. The post-RP mortality rate was 0.11% (66 deaths). Procedure-specific volumes predominantly affected the odds of in-hospital mortality from RP.

2. **Complications of XRT.** Toxicities of XRT most commonly involve the rectum and the bladder. An estimated 60% of patients will have moderate rectal symptoms including pain, tenesmus, or diarrhea. Others will have symptoms of cystitis, hematuria, impotence, incontinence, or difficulty with urination around the period of XRT. Most of these symptoms resolve on completion of the therapy. Less than 1% of conventional XRT patients require hospitalization for local toxicities including rectal pain, rectal/urinary bleeding, or other urinary complaints.

3. **Complications of hormone deprivation therapy and antiandrogens.** Men who are contemplating treatment with ADT should be made aware of the potential side effects of therapy. Decreased total and free serum testosterone levels lead to hypogonadism, impotence, and decreased libido. In addition, over the first year or so, the patient will notice decreased muscle mass and increased adipose tissue, especially centripetally. A decrease in bone mineral density may lead to osteoporosis. An increase in estrogen to testosterone ratio may result in hot flashes, sweats, and gynecomastia. Endocrine changes may result in an increase in components of the metabolic syndrome, such as hyperglycemia, hyperinsulinemia and insulin resistance, dyslipidemia (hypertriglyceridemia and low high density lipoprotein (HDL) cholesterol levels). These metabolic changes may lead to an increased risk of cardiovascular disease. As we detect more men with prostate cancer at younger ages and these men live longer, the metabolic consequences of ADT will work against the very benefits of treatment.

4. **Complications of chemotherapy.** Docetaxel has a complicated structure that is poorly soluble in water. Therefore, it is formulated in polysorbate-60, and the side effects of treatment may be due to both the chemotherapy agent and its solvent. Allergic reactions such as shortness of breath, facial flushing, fever, chest pain, dizziness, lightheadedness, or skin rash may occur, but are rare with premedication with dexamethasone. Musculoskeletal and bone and joint symptoms of pain and stiffness are among the most common reported by patients. Other common symptoms include fatigue (50%), diarrhea (33%), and alopecia (40%). Docetaxel is only mildly emetogenic, but 40% of patients report nausea, vomiting or both. Patients should expect bone marrow suppression, especially a potent, but short-lived neutropenia (33%), but they rarely develop febrile neutropenia (3%).

Oncologists observe nail changes and sensory neuropathy in a third of patients. Retention of fluid, especially swollen feet, is reported in 20% of patients. About one in five patients have problems with alteration of taste and anorexia. Excessive tearing is seen in 10% of patients. Docetaxel can cause liver damage; therefore, in patients with hepatic dysfunction, oncologists should be cautious with its administration when serum bilirubin and serum liver enzymes are elevated.

5. **Complications of bisphosphonate therapy.** In initial studies, when zolendronate was administered intravenously, renal failure was common, but was uncommon when given over 15 to 20 minutes. Serial serum creatinine and blood urea nitrogen (BUN) should be monitored and zolendronate dosing may be titrated according to creatinine clearance. Pamidronate may be safer to give in patients with significant renal dysfunction.

V. **BACKGROUND.** Prostate cancer is the most common malignancy and the second most common cause of cancer-related death in men in the United States. The lifetime risk of a prostate cancer diagnosis is approximately 16%, but the lifetime risk of prostate cancer death is only 3.4%. With the unproven, yet widespread use of PSA screening, the clinical presentation of prostate cancer has changed from advanced to localized disease in more than 80% at the time of diagnosis. The current challenge of research is to use this lead-time bias to our advantage to achieve better overall survival and QOL with new treatments. However, the price of early detection and screening is "overdiagnosis," which results in diagnosis, treatment, side effects, and anxiety in tens of thousands of men who would not have manifested symptoms of prostate cancer within their lifetime.

With improved understanding of the molecular aberrations and their influence on clinical outcomes, it is likely that we will individualize therapy for this common malignancy.

Suggested Readings

Albertsen PC, Fryback DG, Storer BE, et al. Long-term survival among men with conservatively treated localized prostate cancer. *JAMA*. 1995;274:626–631.

Bianco FJ Jr, Scardino PT, Eastham JA. Radical prostatectomy: long-term cancer control and recovery of sexual and urinary function ("trifecta"). *Urology* 2005;66(5 suppl):83–94.

Bolla M, Gonzalez D, Warde P, et al. Improved survival in patients with locally advanced prostate cancer treated with radiotherapy and goserelin. *N Engl J Med* 1997;337:295–300.

Catalona WJ, Carvalhal GF, Mager DE, et al. Potency, continence and complication rates in 1,870 consecutive radical retropubic prostatectomies. *J Urol* 1999;162:433–438.

Catalona WJ, Partin AW, Slawin KM, et al. Percentage of free PSA in black versus white men for detection and staging of prostate cancer: a prospective multicenter clinical trial. *Urology* 2000;55:372–376.

D'Amico AV, Huy-Chen M, Renshaw AA, et al. Identifying men diagnosed with clinically localized prostate cancer who are at high risk for death from prostate cancer. *J Urol* 2006;176:S11–S15.

D'Amico AV, Moul JW, Carroll PR, et al. Surrogate end point for prostate cancer-specific mortality after radical prostatectomy or radiation therapy. *J Natl Cancer Inst* 2003;95:1376–1383.

Konety BR, Allareddy V, Modak S, et al. Mortality after major surgery for urologic cancers in specialized urology hospitals: are they any better? *J Clin Oncol* 2006;24(13): 2006–2012.

Medical Research Council Prostate Cancer Working Party Investigators Group. Immediate versus deferred treatment for advanced prostatic cancer: initial results of the Medical Research Council Trial. *Br J Urol* 1997;79:235–246.

Messing EM, Manola J, Sarosdy M, et al. Immediate hormonal therapy compared with observation after radical prostatectomy and pelvic lymphadenectomy in men with node-positive prostate cancer. *N Engl J Med* 1999;341:1781–1788.

Pilepich MV, Caplan R, Byhardt RW, et al. Phase III trial of androgen suppression using goserelin in unfavorable-prognosis carcinoma of the prostate treated with definitive radiotherapy: report of Radiation Therapy Oncology Group Protocol 85-31. *J Clin Oncol* 1997;15:1013–1021.

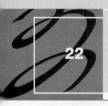

22 GENITOURINARY CANCER: PENILE

Steven Brandes and Joel Picus

I. PRESENTATION. Patients typically ignore penile lesions until they reach considerable size and delay seeking medical attention (15% to 50% of patients delay presentation longer than 1 year). On presentation, 30% to 60% of patients have enlarged/palpable inguinal nodes.

A. Signs and symptoms

1. Signs. Penile cancer (squamous cell carcinoma [SCC] of the penile skin) typically originates on the glans (48%), followed by the prepuce (21%), both prepuce and glands (9%), coronal sulcus (6%), and penile shaft (2%).

Tumor presentation is widely variable. SCC can be papillary and exophytic, flat and ulcerative, or extensively destructive. Patients typically have a long history of phimosis (more than 50%), in which tumors of the glans or prepuce can be concealed, and allow tumor progression. Lesions also can be subtle, as in patchy erythema or cutaneous induration. Such subtle lesions are typically carcinoma *in situ* (CIS), and are typically subdivided into erythroplasia of Queyrat, a velvety, red lesion with ulcerations, localized to the glans penis or prepuce, and Bowen disease, a red plaque with encrustations that involves the remaining genitalia or perineum.

Each penile tumor should be assessed for size, location, mobility, and/or corporal body involvement. Examine the penile base and scrotum for tumor extension. Rectal and bimanual examination can help determine the presence of a pelvic mass, as well as prostatic, urethral, or perineal body tumor involvement.

Careful examination of both groins for any palpable inguinal adenopathy is essential. Nodal size, location, fixation, and involvement should be noted. Reexamine after 4 to 6 weeks of antibiotic therapy to rule out infection due to enlargement.

2. Symptoms. Lesions are typically painless and often secondarily infected. Lesions can also occur as itching or burning of the glans, under the prepuce, which can progress to ulceration. Chronic penile infection can result in fatigue, weight loss, and general malaise.

II. WORKUP AND STAGING

A. Initial diagnosis is by punch, incisional, or excisional biopsy of all suggestive penile lesions for pathologic evaluation. Histologic diagnosis usually does not require special stains. An adequate biopsy is essential, since this will determine the treatment of the primary lesion and stratify the risk for metastases.

The status of palpable inguinal adenopathy versus no adenopathy is assessed by careful physical examination. Both groins can be involved. Of the initially palpable inguinal nodes, 50% to 70% are inflammatory in nature. After 4 to 6 weeks of antibiotic therapy, the groins should be reexamined for persistence of adenopathy.

B. Imaging. Radiographic staging includes a chest radiograph and computed tomography (CT) of the abdomen and pelvis. The CT assesses for the status of the pelvic, common iliac, periaortic, and abdominal lymph nodes, and any other potential metastases. CT-guided biopsy of significant inguinal or pelvic adenopathy can help guide the planning of lymphadenectomy or chemotherapy. Magnetic resonance imaging (MRI) can be helpful in delineating penile shaft (corpora) and adjacent tissue involvement and extent. Nanoparticles of iron oxide in combination with MR have shown recent promise in identifying occult groin metastases.

TABLE 22.1	Jackson Staging of Penile Cancer

Stage 1 (A)	Tumor confined to the glans and/or prepuce
Stage 2 (B)	Tumor extending into the penile shaft/corpora
Stage 3 (C)	Tumors with inguinal metastases amenable to surgery
Stage 4 (D)	Tumors involving adjacent structures or inoperable inguinal metastases (fixed nodes on examination), pelvic node metastases, or distant metastases

To help evaluate for occult inguinal region metastases, recent studies from the Netherlands and Italy have demonstrated the promising technique of injecting the lesion with radioactive tracer and blue dye and then performing a dynamic sentinel biopsy of the blue and/or "hot" node. For excised nodes positive for cancer, a lymph node dissection is performed. Intraoperative lymph node mapping is technically feasible for penile cancer, but false negative rates are high (20%) and the optimal technique is still to be defined. The technique is also difficult to learn for reliable results. A novel fluorescence assay to detect occult inguinal metastasis has also been recently detailed.

C. **Laboratory testing.** Laboratory testing includes a complete blood count (CBC) and electrolytes, including LFTs. Hypercalcemia can occasionally occur, even without evidence of bony metastases.

D. **Staging.** The most commonly used staging system, until recently, has been the Jackson staging for penile cancer (Table 22.1). The tumor, node, metastasis (TNM) staging system, as updated in 1987, has become the standard staging system (Table 22.2).

Histologically, penile SCCs demonstrate keratinization, epithelial pearl formation, and varying degrees of mitoses. Most are low grade.

III. THERAPY AND PROGNOSIS

A. **Prognosis.** Overall, 5-year cancer-specific survival is roughly 55%. Survival is directly related to tumor stage and grade. Overall, the strongest indicator for survival from penile cancer depends largely on the presence or absence of inguinal

TABLE 22.2	TNM Staging of Penile Cancer

Primary tumor (T)	
Tx	Primary tumor cannot be assessed
T0	No evidence of tumor
Tis	Carcinoma *in situ*
Ta	Noninvasive verrucous carcinoma
T1	Tumor invasion into subepithelial connective tissue
T2	Tumor invasion into corpus spongiosum and/or cavernosum
Regional Lymph Nodes (N)	
Nx	Nodes cannot be assessed
N0	No metastases
N1	Metastasis in single superficial inguinal node
N2	Metastases in multiple and/or bilateral superficial nodes
N3	Metastases in deep inguinal or pelvic nodes
Distant Metastases (M)	
Mx	Distant metastases cannot be assessed
M0	No distant metastasis
M1	Distant metastasis

node metastases and/or pelvic node metastases. Prognosis is poor when the diagnosis is late, with deep infiltrating tumors, ilioinguinal node metastases, or pelvic node metastases.

Penile cancer is one of the few malignancies in which regional lymphadenectomy can be curative. The indications and timing for ilioinguinal and/or pelvic lymphadenectomy are controversial. Patients without palpable inguinal adenopathy have a 65% to 80% 5-year survival rate. The 5-year survival rates, however, are 20% to 50% when the palpable inguinal nodes are positive for malignancy. When inguinal node dissection is pathologically negative, survival rates approach 90%.

B. Therapy

1. **Carcinoma *in situ*.** Treatment begins with excisional biopsy to confirm diagnosis and depth of invasion. Local excision is used when the defects will not be overly deforming or do not involve the meatus or urethra. Circumcision is performed for preputial lesions. Other treatments are topical 5-fluorouracil, neodymium/yttrium aluminum garnet (Nd:YAG), or CO_2 laser fulguration, imiquimod cream, and Mohs micrographic surgery.

2. **Invasive squamous cell carcinoma**

   a. **Surgical therapy**

      i. **Primary lesion.** Initial treatment consists of excision of the primary tumor. Depending on the size and location of the tumor, treatment may be circumcision, partial penectomy, or total penectomy. Local wedge resection has more than 50% local recurrence rate. Traditionally, a 2-cm surgical margin proximal to the tumor has been advocated. However, recent studies have questioned the need for such a large margin, particularly for well or moderately differentiated tumors. Selected tumors confined to the prepuce can typically be treated with circumcision. Traditionally, tumors involving the glans or penile shaft require either a partial or total penectomy. In patients in whom a partial penectomy will not leave sufficient penile length to void while standing, or cannot provide a sufficient surgical margin, then total penectomy and perineal urethrostomy is preferred. Recent reports of penile preservation instead of partial penectomy are promising in the short term for local control and survival. Such surgeries attempt to preserve glans sensation, or at least to maximize penile shaft length, without compromising cancer control.

      ii. **Inguinal and pelvic lymph nodes.** Indications for inguinal and pelvic lymphadenectomy are outlined and detailed in Fig. 22.1. Of patients with clinically negative nodes at diagnosis, 20% harbor occult metastases. Because the primary tumor is commonly infected at the time of diagnosis, inguinal lymph node enlargement and lymphangitis is common. Before inguinal lymphadenectomy, all penile cancer patients should be treated with 4 to 6 weeks of antibiotic therapy (i.e., cephalexin, for good gram-positive coverage). After the course of antibiotics, the groins should be carefully examined for adenopathy. Low-grade tumors in which enlarged nodes normalize after antibiotic therapy are candidates for expectant management. Of the persistently palpable nodes, 30% to 50% will harbor metastases. When metastases are present in one groin, 50% to 60% will also have contralateral groin metastases, due to lymphatic crossover. In such cases, then, contralateral inguinal lymphadenectomy is warranted. When inguinal nodes are positive for malignancy, the iliac nodes are involved in 30% to 40% of cases.

      Tumor grade correlates to survival. In a recent U.S. study, 5-year cancer-specific survival for low-grade penile cancers was 84%, and for high-grade tumors, it was 42%. Inguinal nodal metastases were present in 1 (4%) of 52 low-grade and 43 (82%) of 52 high-grade tumors. Similar findings have been reported in series from Brazil and Holland.

   b. **Noninvasive cancers (Tis, Ta, T1 N0 M0).** Grade I (low-grade), noninvasive tumors (Tis, T0, Ta, or T1) with palpably negative inguinal lymph

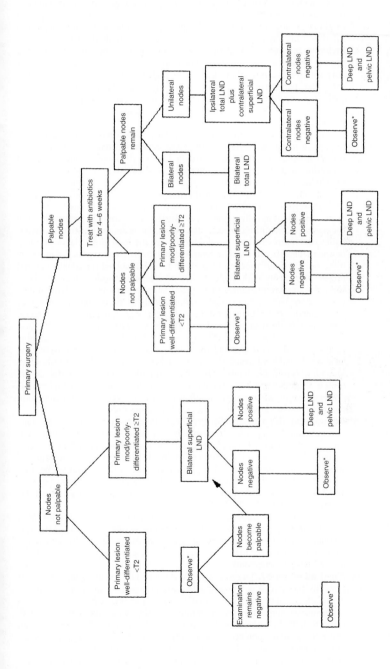

Figure 22.1. Management of inguinal nodes for squamous carcinoma of the penis. (Reproduced from Lynch DF Jr, Schellhammer PF. Tumors of the penis. In: Walsh PC, Retik AB, Vaughn ED, et al. eds. *Campbell's urology*, 7th ed. Philadelphia: WB Saunders, 1998:2474. with permission.)

nodes have a low incidence of nodal metastasis (<6%), and can therefore be safely managed expectantly, as long as frequent and periodic groin examinations can be performed. Such patients are better candidates for organ-sparing or glans-sparing surgery. Unreliable patients or those who cannot be monitored periodically are recommended for inguinal lymphadenectomy.

c. **Invasive cancers (T2).** Patients with moderate or poorly differentiated tumors (grade 2 or 3) or with invasion into the corpus spongiosum or corpora (stage greater than T2) are at high risk for local recurrence and for nodal metastasis (59% by meta-analysis). Vascular invasion is another pathologic positive predictor for inguinal metastases (roughly 75% nodal metastases for T2 tumors with vascular invasion, and 25% for those without).

When the groins have no adenopathy or normalize after antibiotic therapy, such patients have up to 68% occult metastases, and therefore should undergo a prophylactic modified bilateral superficial inguinal groin dissection with frozen-section analysis, as detailed by Catalona et al. A prophylactic groin dissection is performed because of potential survival benefit and the lack of effective alternative treatments. Bilateral superficial node dissections are performed because of the lymphatic crossover. If the nodes are histologically negative, no further dissection is performed, and the patient is monitored expectantly. When the nodes are positive for malignancy, the limits for the groin dissection are extended into a classic inguinal lymphadenectomy and pelvic lymphadenectomy. Deep inguinal and pelvic dissections are performed only on the side with involved superficial inguinal nodes. In patients with clinically negative inguinal nodes, there has been some debate as to the timing of surgery (delayed or immediate). For patients with T2 to T4 and no palpable nodes, there is mounting evidence that prophylactic lymphadenectomy improves survival. For immediate surgery, most reports show that 3 and 5-year survival rates approach 84% and 57% to 88%, respectively. Delaying surgery until the nodes are palpable reduces 3 and 5-year survival to 35% and 8% to 38%, respectively. The lack of effective adjuvant therapies further supports a low threshold to immediate groin dissection. Moreover, complications from nodal dissections are significantly less when performed for occult disease. Metachronous presentation of unilateral groin adenopathy after primary tumor resection demands lymphadenectomy of the involved groin only.

d. **Adenopathy (N1 to N3, M0).** Patients with primary tumors of any stage and persistently palpable and mobile lymph nodes after a course of antibiotic therapy should also undergo classic ilioinguinal lymphadenectomy, if potentially resectable. For unilateral palpable adenopathy, a contralateral superficial node dissection is first performed; 50% will be negative. Because lymphatic drainage is sequential, when the superficial nodes are negative and a pelvic CT scan is negative, ipsilateral deep and pelvic node dissections are not necessary.

Patients with common iliac or para-aortic metastases have poor (5%) 5-year cancer-specific survival rates. Therefore, before any inguinal surgery, fine-needle biopsy or aspiration of suggestive nodes should be performed. Confirming pelvic or distant metastasis avoids unnecessary and potentially morbid lymphadenectomy.

e. **Fixed adenopathy.** Jackson stage IV disease (i.e., fixed inguinal nodes) is typically thought to be unresectable and the prognosis poor; and therefore lymphadenectomy is not warranted. In young patients with such penile cancer, however, heroic surgery and multimodal therapies have been advocated. In up to half the number of such patients, neoadjuvant chemotherapy can make fixed nodes potentially surgically resectable. Some stage IV disease also requires palliation. Lymphadenectomy is typically needed here to prevent or alleviate groin pain, infection, bleeding (by tumor invasion into the femoral vessels), or skin erosion.

f. Surgical techniques for regional metastases

i. Sentinel lymph node biopsy.

On the basis of the work of Cabanas, there is a postulated node or group of nodes in which inguinal metastases from penile cancer typically first occur. A negative sentinel node biopsy was thought to indicate that formal node dissection was not necessary. However, there are numerous reports of regional metastases (10% to 50% of patients) after a negative sentinel node biopsy. Therefore, sentinel node biopsy is unreliable and should not be used. Dual mapping techniques to improve the yield of sentinel node dissections are promising new modalities.

ii. Lymphadenectomy.

A clear knowledge and understanding of the lymphatic drainage pattern of the penis is essential in determining penile cancer management. The prepuce and shaft skin drain into the superficial inguinal nodes (superficial to the fascia lata). The glans and corporal bodies drain into both the superficial and the deep inguinal nodes (deep to the fascia lata). Penile lymphatics cross-communicate, and therefore drainage is bilateral to both groins. Drainage is first to the superficial inguinal nodes, which are anterior and medial to the saphenofemoral junction between Scarpa fascia and the fascia lata. The next group of drainage nodes are the deep inguinal nodes, medial and lateral to the femoral vein and deep to the fascia lata. Subsequent drainage from the inguinal nodes is into the pelvic nodes.

For cartoons of the differing incisions and the margins for resection for the classic inguinal and ilioinguinal lymphadenectomy, see Daeseler et al. (1948). For details of the modified superficial inguinal lymphadenectomy, see Catalona WJ (1988). In brief, in the modified version, the skin incisions are shorter, the saphenous vein preserved, transposition of sartorius muscle eliminated, and there is less node dissection laterally and inferiorly.

g. Alternative therapies

i. Mohs micrographic surgery.

This is the surgical technique of serial resections that maximizes tissue preservation and function, best suited for small and distal tumors. Local control is excellent for tumors smaller than 1 cm and poor (50%) for tumors larger than 3 cm.

ii. Laser therapy.

KTP, Nd:YAG, argon, and CO_2 lasers have been used to treat penile cancers. CO_2 is ideal for treating CIS and superficial disease, but results in poor cancer control and high recurrence when treating T1 or T2 disease.

h. Chemotherapy.

The role of chemotherapy in penile cancer is difficult to evaluate, as most published studies have had small numbers of patients, and patient-selection factors and extents of disease treated have varied. SCC of the penis is relatively responsive to chemotherapy; however, effective treatment combinations are yet to be defined. Single-agent therapy lacks sufficient benefit, and the results of combination regimens are often limited by small sample size and unfavorable toxicity profiles. Currently the role of chemotherapy in penile cancer remains investigational, and there are three basic clinical settings in which this treatment modality may be beneficial: in the presence of metastatic disease, in the neoadjuvant setting to render unresectable disease resectable, and in the setting of pathologically proven lymph node metastases.

Limited experiences suggest that adjuvant chemotherapy can improve long-term survival of patients with radically resected positive nodes. It is also suggested that primary chemotherapy can allow 50% of cases with fixed inguinal lymph nodes to be resectable. A combination of vincristine, bleomycin, and methotrexate has been effective as both neoadjuvant and adjuvant chemotherapy. Regimens containing cisplatin and 5-fluorouracil or cisplatin, methotrexate, and bleomycin also have been effective, with reported response rates as high as 32%.

   i. **Radiotherapy.** SCC is characteristically radioresistant. For small primary lesions that are superficial, exophytic, and on the glans, in patients refusing surgical resection of the primary tumor, radiation therapy (XRT) may be effective. Even if there is an initial response, local recurrence rates after brachytherapy or external-beam radiotherapy are typically high. Prophylactic groin irradiation in patients with clinically negative inguinal nodes has not proved effective in reducing subsequent regional metastases. Irradiation makes physical examination of the groins difficult and makes any future lymphadenectomy surgically challenging and problematic for poor wound healing. After XRT, penile fibrosis is difficult to distinguish from recurrent tumor. Radiation, however, may have a palliative role for patients with unresectable tumor or in those with poor performance status precluding surgery.

IV. COMPLICATIONS

A. **After surgery.** Complications for partial and total penectomy are both psychological and physical. Such patients should receive counseling. Meatal stenosis can occur in up to 20% of partial penectomies. After partial penectomy, roughly one-half of patients are still able to have vaginal intercourse and three fourths are able to ejaculate.

   The severity of complications is influenced by the extent of the nodal tissue removed and the surgical technique. Historically, classic, radical inguinal lymphadenectomy has been associated with high rates of morbidity. Complications include 30% to 50% of patients having long-term disabling morbidity, and mortality rates go up to 3%. Minor complications include mild leg swelling, lymphoceles, and seromas. Major complications typically include the debilitating problems of severe, chronic, and disabling lower extremity and scrotal lymphedema, skin flap necrosis, severe wound infection, and deep venous thrombosis. More contemporary series, however, have lower and more acceptable rates of minor complications (45%) and incapacitating or major complications (5%). Modified inguinal node dissections (after Catalona) are at low risk (17%) for major complications. This is primarily due to the preservation of the saphenous vein and smaller regions of dissection. The best way to avoid complications is to identify those patients who do not require lymphadenectomy and refining surgical staging for those who are shown to not have nodal metastases.

B. **After chemotherapy.** In one phase II evaluation of cisplatin, methotrexate, and bleomycin, there was a high incidence of treatment-related deaths, and a high incidence (17%) of life-threatening toxic episodes. Some of the life-threatening episodes included infections, leukopenias, and pneumonitis. Although chemotherapy in penile cancer appears to have promising results in overall improvement in survival, further emphasis in future research to decrease toxicities would be advantageous.

C. **After radiotherapy.** Severe penile edema and skin maceration, ulceration, and sloughing can result. Urethral fistula, stricture, or meatal stenosis can occur. There are also reports of penile necrosis, pain, edema, and an occasional need for secondary penectomy.

D. **Of the disease.** Anemia, leukocytosis, hypoalbuminemia (from chronic infection of the primary and inguinal sites), azotemia (secondary to urethral obstruction), and hypercalcemia can occur.

V. FOLLOW-UP.
After definitive treatment of the primary tumor, patients whose groins are being monitored expectantly should undergo physical examinations of the groin every 2 months for the first 2 years from diagnosis, then every 6 months for 2 years, and then annually. Equivocal examinations should be further evaluated by groin ultrasonography, CT, or MRI.

   After inguinal lymphadenectomy, patients should be followed up every 3 months for the first 2 years, then every 6 months for 2 years, and then annually. For details of the more intensive European Association of Urology (EAU) guidelines to follow-up schema, see Solsona et al. (2004).

VI. BACKGROUND

A. **Epidemiology.** SCC of the penis is a rare disease in the United States and other developed countries, accounting for less than 1% of all male cancers. In the United

States, for the year 2005, 1,470 new cases of penile cancers (0.2% of male cancers) and 270 deaths occurred from penile cancer (0.1% of male cancer-related deaths). Overall, of the US patients with penile cancer, 23% die of the disease. In the United States, blacks are affected twice as often as whites, as well as are subject to a 2.2-fold increased disease-specific risk of death. When penile cancer is diagnosed in the elderly (older than 65 years), the chance of dying from the disease is 1.5 times higher. In some African and South American countries, penile cancer is common, accounting for up to 20% of male cancers, or incidence of 50 per 100,000. Penile cancer patients are typically in their fifties to seventies, with a mean age of 60. It is rare before age 40.

B. Risk factors. Risk factors for developing penile cancer are poor hygiene, phimosis, uncircumcised penis, chronic irritation of smegma, and viruses. Men with human papilloma virus (HPV) and genital herpes have a higher incidence of penile cancer. HPV strains 16 and 18 have been identified in up to 80% of penile SCC. Sexual behavior, hygiene, and socioeconomic status modulate the above risk factors. Infant circumcision offers protection from future development of penile cancer. Adult circumcision, however, offers no protection. Exposure to cigarette smoking or chewing tobacco has been weakly associated with penile cancer, regardless of circumcision status.

C. Pathophysiology. More than 95% of penile cancers are SCCs. The remaining rare cancers are sarcomas (including Kaposi's sarcoma), melanoma, basal cell carcinoma, leukemia, and lymphoma. Verrucous carcinoma (giant condyloma) is histologically benign and is characterized by aggressive local extension and tissue destruction.

Many benign penile lesions have malignant potential or a close association with cancer development. Up to 30% to 40% of patients with SCC of the penis had a history of a preexisting penile lesion. Penile lesions that are thought to have a malignant potential are **lichen sclerosis et atrophicus** (white patchy lesions of the glans, prepuce, or meatus), **leukoplakia** (whitish plaques usually involving the meatus, more common in diabetic patients), **cutaneous horns** (rare, protuberant, hyperkeratotic lesions), and **pseudoepitheliomatous micaceous,** and **keratotic balanitis.**

D. Natural history. SCC of the penis usually begins as a small lesion on the glans or prepuce. Tumor invasion is usually by direct extension and is capable of destroying adjacent tissues. Exophytic lesions tend to be better differentiated than ulcerative lesions. Ulcerative and flat lesions tend to metastasize earlier. Tumors that metastasize usually spread first to the superficial inguinal nodes, then to the deep inguinal nodes, and then to the pelvic nodes. Skip lesions do not occur. Both groins may be involved because of lymphatic drainage crossover. Distant metastases are rare and tend to involve the abdominal lymph nodes, lung, liver, bones, and brain. Death is usually secondary to inguinal involvement, which can result in skin necrosis, chronic infection, sepsis, or hemorrhage due to tumor erosion into the femoral vessels.

VII. CURRENT FOCUS. Locally recurrent disease can be approached surgically or with local XRT. Patients with nodal recurrences that are not controllable by local measures are candidates for phase I and II clinical trials testing new biologicals (such as cisplatin and IFN-α_{2B}) and chemotherapeutic agents (such as intra-arterial infusion chemotherapy). Other clinical trials using radiosensitizers or cytotoxic drugs are appropriate. Because of the high incidence of microscopic nodal metastases, promising new imaging modalities and minimally invasive methods for accurate sentinel node biopsy are being pursued.

Suggested Readings

Catalona WJ. Modified inguinal lymphadenectomy for carcinoma of the penis with preservation of the saphenous vein: technique and preliminary results. *J Urol* 1988;140:306.

Daesler EH, Anson BJ, Reimann AE. Radical excision of the inguinal and iliac lymph glands: a study based on 150 anatomical dissections and upon clinical observations. *Surg Gynecol Obstet* 1948;87:679.

Haas GP, Blumenstein BA, Galiano RG, et al. Cisplatin, methotrexate, and bleomycin for the treatment of carcinoma of the penis: a Southwest Oncology Group Study. *J Urol* 1999;161:1823.

Ornellas AA, Correia AL, Marota A, et al. Surgical treatment of invasive squamous cell carcinoma of the penis: retrospective analysis of 350 cases. *J Urol* 1994;151:1244.

Pizzacaro G, Piva L. Adjuvant and neoadjuvant vincristine, bleomycin, and methotrexate for inguinal metastases from squamous cell carcinoma of the penis. *Acta Oncol* 1988;27:823.

Sanchez-Ortiz RF, Pettaway CA. The role of lymphadenectomy in penile cancer. *Urol Oncol* 2004;22:236–244.

Solsona E, Algaba F, Horenblas S, et al. EAU guidelines on penile cancer. *Eur Urol* 2004;46:1–8.

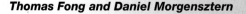

TESTICULAR CANCER AND GERM CELL TUMORS

23

Thomas Fong and Daniel Morgensztern

I. PRESENTATION

A. Subjective. Patients with testicular cancer most commonly present with a painless solid testicular mass. Less frequently, the testicular mass may become painful as the result of bleeding or infarction in the tumor. The presence of acute pain may suggest alternative diagnoses such as testicular torsion, epididymitis, or orchitis. Hydrocele has also been associated with approximately 20% of germ cell tumors (GCTs). Gynecomastia as the first sign of testicular cancer is seen in approximately 10% of patients, whereas infertility as the initial symptom is seen in 3% of patients. Other symptoms such as back pain, nausea, vomiting, constipation, and hemoptysis may be seen in patients with extensive retroperitoneal lymphadenopathy or pulmonary metastasis. Patients with testicular cancer rarely have inguinal lymphadenopathy at presentation, except when they have received surgery to the scrotal area.

B. Objective. A thorough physical examination is essential in patients with suspected testicular cancer. This examination should include evaluation of the external genitalia and scrotum, palpation of each testis by bimanual technique, examination of lymph nodes, with particular attention to the supraclavicular areas, and breast examination for evidence of gynecomastia. If the examination reveals a suggestive scrotal mass, transillumination or ultrasonography should be performed. A solid testicular mass that does not transilluminate should be considered a neoplasm until proved otherwise.

II. WORKUP AND STAGING

A. Practical approach to a new testicular mass. The differential diagnosis for patients presenting with a testicular mass includes malignancy, hernia, hydrocele, and spermatocele. Testicular pain or swelling may suggest epididymitis or orchitis, and an initial trial of antibiotics may be appropriate. Patients with a suspicious testicular mass or persistent testicular tenderness or swelling should have ultrasonographic evaluation. This is highly diagnostic for a testicular tumor, and is performed for most palpable abnormalities to define the lesion. For suspicious testicular masses, further evaluation includes chest x-ray and serum concentrations of α-fetoprotein (AFP), beta-human chorionic gonadotropin (β-hCG), and lactate dehydrogenase (LDH). These tumor markers are useful for diagnosis, prognosis, and assessment of treatment outcome. Referral to urology for suspected testicular malignancy is indicated for radical inguinal orchiectomy. A transscrotal approach is contraindicated due to concerns of tumor seeding. If testicular GCT is confirmed pathologically, computed tomography (CT) scanning of the abdomen and pelvis should be obtained, with chest CT indicated if any retroperitoneal adenopathy is present. Additional imaging such as bone scan or brain magnetic resonance imaging (MRI) may be obtained if suggestive symptoms are present. Sperm banking should be considered before any therapeutic intervention that may compromise fertility, including surgery, radiation therapy, and chemotherapy.

B. Pathologic classification of testicular tumors

1. GCT. Most (95%) of primary testicular tumors originate from germ cells. GCTs carry an excellent prognosis with more than 90% of patients cured, including 70% to 80% of those with advanced disease. GCTs are classified for clinical purposes into two major groups: seminomas or nonseminomas. Nonseminomas include embryonal carcinoma, teratoma, choriocarcinoma, and yolk sac tumor, and frequently contain more than one cell type. Approximately 50% of GCTs are of pure seminoma histology, 35% are nonseminomas, and 15% have features of both. Patients with mixed histology or elevated AFP should be treated as nonseminomas. Pathology reports should also include the presence or absence of vascular/lymphatic invasion (VI) of the primary tumor, which carries prognostic significance in early stage tumors.

a. **Intratubular germ cell neoplasia/carcinoma *in situ* (TIN/CIS).** This is a premalignant germ cell lesion with a 70% probability of progression to GTC within 7 years. It is often found in a normal-appearing testis biopsied for indications such as infertility evaluation, maldescended testis, extragonadal germ cell tumors (EGGCTs), or when a contralateral testis contains a malignant GCT. Contralateral biopsy in patients diagnosed with testicular GCT is not routinely performed due to the low incidence of TIN/CIS (5%) and the infertility that may result from definitive treatment with either orchiectomy or radiation therapy.

b. **Seminomas.** Pure seminoma is the most common testicular tumor, representing approximately 50% of GCTs. They generally have a more favorable prognosis than nonseminomas. Only tumors with pure seminoma histology, and without elevated AFP, are considered seminoma for management purposes. Syncytiotrophoblasts capable of producing hCG are present in roughly 20% of these tumors. Seminoma typically presents in the fourth and fifth decades, but may occur in younger patients. Anaplastic seminoma, i.e., those with a high mitotic index, may have a somewhat poorer prognosis. In these cases, lymphangitic infiltration may also be present.

Spermatocytic seminomas, although often classified as a type of seminoma, are generally benign. They are the most common testicular GCT in the elderly (older than 65 years), but are rare, constituting approximately 3% of all testicular tumors.

c. **Nonseminomas.** These are present in approximately 35% of all testicular tumors, and an additional 15% of GCTs with mixed histology are classified as nonseminoma. They occur most often in the third decade, and occasionally in the latter part of the second decade of life. Nonseminomas often consist of mixed histology in any combination, and may also include histologic features of seminoma.

   i. **Yolk sac tumor.** Yolk sac tumors represent the main source of AFP. This histology is rare as a pure form in adults, but is often seen as a component of a mixed GCT.

   ii. **Choriocarcinoma.** Choriocarcinoma may present with elevated levels of hCG. These tumors occur in three forms: pure, mixed, and placental-site trophoblastic tumor. Mixed trophoblastic tumors contain foci of choriocarcinoma in association with other histologic subtypes. These areas may be associated with hemorrhage. Placental-site trophoblastic tumors are most often seen in children and are often associated with teratomas.

   iii. **Embryonal carcinoma.** Pure embryonal carcinomas usually do not produce AFP, although individual cells may stain positive for this marker. Therefore, increased AFP usually indicates the presence of yolk sac elements. Pure embryonal carcinomas also do not usually produce HCG.

   iv. **Teratomas.** These tumors have elements from one or more germ layers in various stages of maturation. They are most frequent in the first, second, and third decades. Microscopically, teratomas are divided into three subgroups: mature teratoma, immature teratoma, and teratoma with malignant areas. Mature teratoma contains well-differentiated tissue, and may include ectodermal, endodermal, or mesodermal elements (such as cartilage, bone, and muscle). Immature teratomas are characterized by primitive, poorly differentiated tissue.

   v. **Other testicular tumors.** Approximately 5% of testicular tumors are not of germ cell origin. Non-GCT testicular tumors in men older than

50 years are most commonly lymphomas. Other rare tumors include Leydig cell tumors, which produce steroid hormones, Sertoli cell tumors, sarcomas, and embryonal rhabdomyosarcomas of the paratesticular tissues.

    vi. Occult testicular tumor presenting as carcinoma of unknown primary. Metastatic disease alone may be the initial presentation in 5% to 10% of testicular GCTs. The testis may have a small nonsymptomatic tumor, CIS, scar, or residual "burned out" testicular tumor detected only on ultrasonograph. Given the favorable prognosis of testicular cancer, serum tumor markers for GCTs should be part of the diagnostic workup in patients presenting with carcinoma of unknown primary, particularly in cases with midline distribution including retropertitoneal and mediastinal lymphadenopathy.

    vii. Histology of metastases. On occasion, metastases may have different histology as the primary tumor. This may be due to sampling error in the primary tumor or differentiation of the metastasis into another histologic subtype. In a number of patients who have mixed histology, the metastases may show only mature teratoma after chemotherapy. This may occur due to chemotherapy eliminating the sensitive components, leaving behind mature teratoma, or due to differentiation of embryonal carcinoma into teratoma.

C. Serum tumor markers. Serum tumor markers are frequently elevated in GCTs. The three tumor markers which have been established in testicular GCTs are AFP, hCG, and LDH. Elevation of AFP and/or hCG is seen in 80% of metastatic nonseminomas. Most seminomas do not have elevated levels of tumor markers either at diagnosis or relapse, although hCG may occasionally be elevated. In general, elevation of AFP implies the presence of nonseminomatous elements, even if histology is suggestive of pure seminoma.

    1. hCG is produced by syncytiotrophoblasts. Elevation of hCG may be present in either seminoma or nonseminoma, and reflects the tumor burden, not necessarily, clinical aggressiveness. The half-life of hCG is 1 to 3 days. Its persistent elevation after surgery implies metastatic disease. Elevation of hCG is present in approximately 20% of seminomas and 60% of nonseminomas. The absolute elevation before treatment and rate of decline with treatment are of prognostic value.

    2. AFP is produced in nonseminoma only. It is mainly produced by yolk sac elements, and is elevated in approximately 50% of nonseminomas. The half-life of AFP is 5 to 7 days. AFP may also be elevated in hepatocellular disease or due to liver damage from chemotherapy.

    3. LDH is related to bulk and extent of disease, and several large multivariate analyses found it to be an independent prognostic variable. It may also be elevated following treatment resulting from tumor lysis.

    4. Placental alkaline phosphatase (PLAP) is positive by immunohistochemical staining in 90% of seminomas. Serum levels are of unproven value.

    5. Tumor marker decline following orchiectomy is important to monitor. For patients under surveillance for stage I disease, markers should be measured until normalization. During chemotherapy, markers should be checked before each cycle and then every 2 months for the first year, every 3 months for the second, every 4 months for the third year, every 6 months for the fourth year, and yearly thereafter.

D. Imaging studies in testicular cancer

    1. Scrotal ultrasonographic examination is required during the initial physical examination of a testicular mass. A 7.5-MHz transducer should be used, and color Doppler ultrasonography may provide even more useful information regarding blood flow.

    2. CT scans of the abdomen and pelvis with oral and intravenous contrast are required for initial staging investigation. CT scan of the abdomen and pelvis with oral and intravenous contrast are required for initial staging investigation.

MRI of the abdomen and pelvis should be done in patients unable to have intravenous contrast. For patients with a normal CT of the abdomen and pelvis, plain chest x-ray without chest CT is sufficient. If the initial chest radiograph is abnormal, a CT scan of the chest should be obtained. Nevertheless, may oncologists recommend an initial CT scan of the chest.

3. **Other imaging studies** are optional and guided by patient symptoms. Bone scan may be obtained in patients with symptoms suggestive of possible bone metastasis or with elevated alkaline phosphatase levels. Brain imaging, preferably MRI, may be considered in patients with symptoms suggestive of brain metastases such as headache or mental status changes.

E. **Staging.** In addition to traditional TNM (Tumor, Node, Metastasis) classification which assesses the primary tumor, lymph node involvement, and metastatic disease, the American Joint Committee on Cancer (AJCC) guidelines include measurement of serum tumor markers (S) in testicular GCT staging. Stage I is defined as disease limited to the testis; stage II, disease limited to regional (i.e., retroperitoneal) lymph nodes; stage III, disease involving nonregional lymph nodes, distant metastases, or markedly elevated tumor markers (Table 23.1).

All patients with advanced disease requiring chemotherapy as initial treatment should be classified according to their risk status using the International Germ Cell Cancer Consensus Group (IGCCCG) classification system (Table 23.2). Patients with seminoma or nonseminoma are stratified into risk prognostic groups based on the primary site of tumor, presence of nonpulmonary metastatic disease, and serum tumor markers. Risk status is used to predict prognosis and to determine the appropriate first-line chemotherapy.

F. **Management of retroperitoneal lymph nodes: staging and treatment.** Retroperitoneal lymph node dissection (RPLND) is frequently used for staging and therapy in nonseminomas, which predictably spread to the retroperitoneal lymph nodes. This enables determination of pathologic stage, and also removes viable tumor from regional lymph nodes. A transthoracic or transabdominal approach may be used. Nerve-sparing surgery is performed to minimize the complications of retrograde ejaculation and subsequent infertility.

G. **Fertility issues and sperm banking.** Fertility problems are associated with GCT and its treatment. Approximately 50% of patients have impaired spermatogenesis at diagnosis. Following treatment, approximately one third of patients who attempt to conceive will be unsuccessful. Because testicular cancer commonly occurs in young patients who have not conceived any children, cryoconservation can be offered before initiation of any therapy that may compromise fertility (e.g., surgery, radiation therapy, chemotherapy). Baseline fertility assessment should be performed, including determination of total testosterone level, luteinising hormone (LH), follicle-stimulating hormone (FSH), and semen analysis.

In patients with bilateral orchiectomy, lifelong testosterone replacement should be offered. For patients with unilateral orchiectomy, clinical symptoms and serum testosterone levels ought to guide decisions regarding the need for testosterone supplementation.

III. **PROGNOSIS.** Overall prognosis is excellent in testicular GCTs, with more than 90% cure in all patients diagnosed, including a 70% to 80% cure rate in patients with advanced disease treated with chemotherapy. Certain prognostic factors have been identified in clinical early stage tumors which are predictive of higher stage or disease relapse.

A. **Prognostic factors in clinical stage I disease.** For stage I seminoma, the size of the primary tumor (greater than 4 cm) and infiltration of the rete testis provide independent prognostic information regarding potential for occult metastases. The presence of VI and patient age (younger than 34 vs. older than 34 years) are of equivocal prognostic significance.

The main prognostic factors in nonseminomas are the presence of VI and the histology of the primary tumor. Choriocarcinoma has the worst prognosis, followed by embryonal carcinoma. The presence of malignant teratoma increases the potential for metastasis, and the presence of embryonal carcinoma may predict

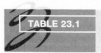

TABLE 23.1 | **Testicular Cancer Staging System of the American Joint Committee on Cancer and the International Union Against Cancer**

Definition of TNM

Primary tumor (T)

pTX	Primary tumor cannot be assessed (if no radical orchiectomy has been performed, TX is used)
pT0	No evidence of primary tumor (e.g., histologic scar in testis)
pT$_{is}$	Intratubular germ cell neoplasia (carcinoma *in situ*)
pT1	Tumor limited to the testis and epididymis and no vascular/lymphatic invasion; tumor may invade the tunica albuginea, but not the tunica vaginalis
pT2	Tumor limited to the testis and epididymis with vascular/lymphatic invasion or tumor extending throughout the tunica albuginea with involvement of tunica vaginalis
pT3	Tumor invades the spermatic cord with or without vascular/lymphatic invasion
pT4	Tumor invades the scrotum with or without vascular/lymphatic invasion

Regional lymph nodes (N)

Clinical

NX	Regional lymph nodes cannot be assessed
N0	No regional lymph node metastasis
N1	Lymph node mass ≤2 cm in greatest dimension; or multiple lymph node masses, none >2 cm in greatest dimension
N2	Lymph node mass >2 cm, but ≤5 cm in greatest dimension; or multiple lymph node masses, any one mass >2 cm, but ≤5 cm in greatest dimension
N3	Lymph node mass >5 cm in greatest dimension

Pathologic

pN0	No evidence of tumor in lymph nodes
pN1	Lymph node mass ≤2 cm in greatest dimension and ≤5 nodes positive, none 2 cm in greatest dimension
pN2	Lymph node mass >2 cm, but ≤5 cm in greatest dimension; >5 nodes positive, none >5 cm; evidence of extranodal extension of tumor
pN3	Lymph node mass >5 cm in greatest dimension; more than five nodes positive, none >5 cm; evidence of extranodal extension of tumor
pN3	Lymph node mass >5 cm in greatest dimension

Distant metastases (M)

M0	No evidence of distant metastases
M1	Nonregional nodal or pulmonary metastases
M2	Nonpulmonary visceral metastases

Serum markers (S)	LDH	hCG (mIU/mL)	AFP (ng/mL)
S0	≤N	≤N	≤N
S1	<1.5 × N	>5,000	<1,000
S2	1.5–10 × N	5,000–50,000	1,000–10,000
S3	>10 × N	>50,000	>10,000

Testis cancer

Stage grouping	T	N	M	S
Stage 0	pT$_{is}$	N0	M0	S0
Stage I	T1–T4	N0	M0	SX
IA	T1	N0	M0	S0
IB	T2	N0	M0	S0
	T3	N0	M0	S0
	T4	N0	M0	S0
IS	Any T	N0	M0	S1–S3

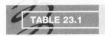

TABLE 23.1 *(Continued)*

Stage grouping	T	N	M	S
Stage II	Any T	Any N	M0	SX
IIA	Any T	N1	M0	S0
	Any T	N1	M0	S1
IIB	Any T	N2	M0	S0
	Any T	N2	M0	S1
IIC	Any T	N3	M0	S0
	Any T	N3	M0	S1
Stage III	Any T	Any N	M1	SX
IIIA	Any T	Any N	M1	S0
	Any T	Any N	M1	S1
IIIB	Any T	Any N	M0	S2
	Any T	Any N	M1	S2
IIIC	Any T	Any N	M0	S3
	Any T	Any N	M1a	S3
	Any T	Any N	M1b	Any S

LDH, lactate dehydrogenase; AFP, α-fetoprotein; hCG, human chorionic gonadotropin.

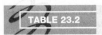

TABLE 23.2 **International Germ Cell Cancer Collaborative Group Risk Classification**

Risk status	Nonseminoma	Seminoma
Good risk	Testicular and retroperitoneal primary tumor and No nonpulmonary visceral metastases and Good markers — all of: AFP <1,000 ng/mL hCG <5,000 iu/L LDH <1.5 × upper limit of normal	Any primary site and no nonpulmonary visceral metastases and, any marker level
Intermediate risk	Testicular and retroperitoneal primary tumor and no nonpulmonary visceral metastases and Intermediate markers — any of: AFP 1,000–10,000 ng/mL hCG 5,000–50,000 iu/L LDH 1.5–10 × upper limit of normal	Any primary site, the presence of nonpulmonary visceral metastases, and any marker level
		Any LDH
Poor risk	Mediastinal tumor or Nonpulmonary visceral metastases or Poor markers — any of: AFP >10,000 ng/mL hCG >50,000 iu/L LDH >10 × upper limit of normal	No patients with seminomas are classified as poor prognosis

AFP, α-fetoprotein; hCG, human chorionic gonadotropin; LDH, lactate dehydrogenase.

an increased risk for pathologic stage (PS) II disease. The presence of yolk sac tumor in the primary tumor decreases the likelihood of progression.

B. **Prognostic factors in clinical stage II disease.** The size and number of lymph nodes found in an RPLND have important prognostic implications. Most studies have shown that fewer than six positive nodes and a size of 2 cm or less is associated with a 35% or less incidence of relapse. Patients with more than six nodes or nodes larger than 2 cm have a recurrence rate of at least 50%. For seminoma, retroperitoneal lymph nodes greater than 10 cm are of prognostic importance, with higher incidence of radiation failure.

C. **Risk classification in advanced testicular GCTs.** Identification of subsets of patients at good, intermediate, or poor risk is important in selection of therapy and prognosis. A consensus classification system developed by the IGCCCG uses pretreatment serum tumor markers, metastases to organs other than lung, and site of primary (mediastinal vs. testis or retroperitoneal) as prognostic factors (Table 23.2). Good-risk patients are defined as having seminomas with no nonpulmonary visceral metastases or nonseminomas with testicular or retroperitoneal primary tumor, no nonpulmonary metastases, and good tumor markers. Intermediate-risk patients include those with seminoma with metastases other than lung or nonseminoma with testicular or retroperitoneal primary tumor, no nonpulmonary visceral metastases, and intermediate tumor markers. High-risk patients are those with nonseminoma of mediastinal origin or metastases other than lung or poor tumor markers. Cure rates for patients with good risk, intermediate risk, and poor risk are 90%, 70% to 80%, and 45% respectively.

IV. THERAPY

A. **Testicular seminoma**

1. **Treatment options for stage I seminoma.** In spite of normal CT scans, there is a 20% risk of occult metastatic disease in locoregional lymph nodes with subsequent disease progression if no adjuvant treatment is given after orchiectomy in stage I seminoma. With adjuvant radiation or adjuvant carboplatin chemotherapy, the relapse rate decreases to approximately 3% to 4%. However, the cure rate in clinical stage I seminoma patients is greater than 99% regardless of management strategy, and adjuvant radiation, adjuvant chemotherapy, or surveillance with subsequent salvage therapy in the event of relapse representing acceptable standard management options.

   a. **Radiation therapy.** Adjuvant radiation therapy is the most frequently used treatment modality, with a relapse rate of 3% to 4%. Radiation therapy is administered with a linear accelerator, with a total dose of 20 Gy given in 2 Gy fractions. The radiation field includes the para-aortic and paracaval lymph nodes extending from T11 to L5 and the ipsilateral hemipelvis. Radiation toxicity is relatively low and includes dose-related gastrointestinal toxicity, impaired fertility, and possibly late malignancies. Limited target volume reduces treatment-related side effects, such as infertility due to scatter radiation doses to the remaining testicle. The few patients who relapse almost always have recurrent disease outside the radiation field, typically within 18 months of diagnosis of the primary, and may still be salvaged with chemotherapy. Contraindications to adjuvant radiation include pelvic or horseshoe kidney, inflammatory bowel disease, or previous radiation, due to risk for excessive toxicity.

   b. **Surveillance.** A surveillance strategy is a reasonable approach given the fact that 80% of patients are cured with orchiectomy alone, and that almost all patients with relapsed disease are ultimately cured with salvage therapy. Patients with stage I seminoma not treated with adjuvant therapy following inguinal orchiectomy require close follow-up, and surveillance is only recommended in patients for whom reliable and committed follow-up is feasible. History and physical examination, serum tumor markers, and CT of the abdomen and pelvis should be performed every 3 to 4 months for the first 3 years, every 6 months from 4 to 7 years , and then annually. Chest x-ray should be obtained every other visit.

Relapse risk may be higher if the primary tumor size is at least 4 cm or if the tumor has infiltrated the rete testis. Given the typical lack of tumor marker elevation and the long natural history of untreated seminoma, prolonged follow-up is required. Fifteen to 20% of patients will develop stage II or III disease within 3 to 4 years, and require salvage radiation for local relapse or chemotherapy for systemic disease. Relapses occur predominantly in the retroperitoneal or high iliac lymph nodes.

c. **Adjuvant carboplatin chemotherapy.** A third alternative is adjuvant chemotherapy with one cycle of carboplatin at area under the curve (AUC) of 7. A large prospective trial (MRC TE 19/EORTC 30982) comparing adjuvant radiation to one cycle of single-agent carboplatin AUC7 showed no significant difference in relapse, time to relapse, and overall survival after a median follow-up of 4 years' in stage I seminoma. The pattern of relapse differs (more retroperitoneal lymph node relapse with carboplatin versus more pelvic lymph node relapse with radiation), but the more rapid completion of adjuvant therapy and lower incidence of contralateral testicular cancer with carboplatin may be advantageous.

2. **Treatment options for stage II seminoma.** The standard treatment in Stage IIA or IIB seminoma following orchiectomy is radiation therapy. This results in a relapse-free survival rate of 95% for stage IIA and 89% for stage IIB at 6 years. The target field includes the para-aortic and ipsilateral iliac lymph nodes, from T11 superiorly to the upper border of the acetabulum inferiorly. Generally 30 Gy for stage IIA and 36 Gy for stage IIB are administered with single doses of 2 Gy at five fractions per week. The remaining testicle is shielded to reduce the risk of infertility from scattered radiation doses.

Chemotherapy with four cycles of etoposide and cisplatin EP is an alternative treatment for patients with larger bulky retroperitoneal disease or who are not willing to undergo radiation therapy (Table 23.3). Patients who relapse after radiation therapy are also salvaged with platinum-based therapy.

3. **Treatment of stage IIC and III seminoma.** These patients with advanced seminoma require chemotherapy similar to that recommended for nonseminoma. Risk status determination based on the IGCCCG classification system is recommended. Patients are considered good-risk if nonpulmonary visceral metastases are not present, and intermediate-risk if present. No seminoma system is recommended. Either three cycles of BEP (bleomycin, etoposide, and cisplatin) or four cycles of EP (etoposide and cisplatin) are considered standard of care, as these are equivalent treatments in good-risk patients. For intermediate-risk patients, four cycles of BEP is considered standard of care. (Table 23.3)

4. **Management of residual mass.** Following chemotherapy for seminoma, reassessment of serum tumor markers and CT scan of the chest, abdomen, and pelvis is recommended. Residual mass on imaging with normal tumor markers is occasionally noted, and this may consist of fibrotic tissue and/or viable tumor cells. Positron emission tomography (PET) scan may be useful in this scenario, with positive results prompting surgical removal of residual masses or adjuvant radiation therapy. Surgical removal or adjuvant radiation should also be considered in patients with residual masses greater than 3 cm, as these patients may have higher local failure rates. Observation with close follow-up including serial CT scans and serum tumor markers is an alternative approach, with salvage chemotherapy given in the case of growing mass or rising tumor markers.

5. **Follow-up.** In general, patients with advanced disease (stage IIC or III, or any stage II treated with chemotherapy) should have follow-up with chest x-ray and tumor markers at each visit every 2 months during the first year, 3-month intervals in the second year, 4-month intervals during the third year, 6-month intervals in the fourth year, and then annually. CT scan of the abdomen and pelvis should be obtained 4 months following surgery, or every 3 months until resolution or stabilization of retroperitoneal disease. Patients who have a

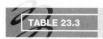

TABLE 23.3	Combination Chemotherapy Regimens Commonly Used in Testicular Germ Cell Cancer

BEP
 Bleomycin, 30 units i.v. weekly on d 2, 9, and 16
 Etoposide (VP-16), 100 mg/m^2 i.v. d 1–5
 Cisplatin, 20 mg/m^2 i.v. daily d 1–5
 21-d cycles
EP
 Etoposide (VP-16), 100 mg/m^2 d 1–5
 Cisplatin, 20 mg/m^2 i.v. d 1–5
 21-d cycles
VelP
 Vinblastine 0.11 mg/kg i.v. d 1–2
 Ifosfamide 1,200 mg/m^2 i.v. d 1–5
 Cisplatin 20 mg/m^2 i.v. d 1–5
 Mesna 400 mg/m^2 i.v. daily every 8 h on d 1–5
 21-d cycles
VIP
 Etoposide 75 mg/m^2 d 1–5
 Ifosfamide 1,200 mg/m^2 d 1–5
 Cisplatin 20 mg/m^2 d 1–5
 Mesna 400 mg/m^2 i.v. daily every 8 h on d 1–5
TIP
 Paclitaxel, 250 mg/m^2 i.v. on d 1
 Ifosfamide, 1,500 mg/m^2 i.v. daily on d 2–5
 Mesna, 500 mg/m^2 i.v. before, and then 4 and 8 h after each dose of ifosfamide
 Cisplatin, 25 mg/m^2 i.v. daily on d 2–5
 21-d cycles

relapse after radiotherapy are usually treated with chemotherapy, except for an isolated inguinal relapse which may be managed surgically.

Patients with stage IIA or IIB disease treated with adjuvant radiation therapy should have chest x-ray and tumor markers obtained at follow-up visits every 3 to 4 months in the first 3 years, every 6 months in the fourth year, then annually. CT scan of the abdomen and pelvis should be obtained 4 months following radiation therapy.

6. **Management of relapsed seminoma.** Approximately 70% of patients who relapse after radiation for seminoma can obtain long-term disease-free survival with chemotherapy. These lower response rates compared with untreated patients are usually explained by the myelosuppression seen in previously irradiated patients, which may prevent the administration the timely administration of chemotherapy at full doses. Recommended therapy for patients with seminoma that relapses following radiation therapy is the same as that for advanced seminoma, namely, three cycles of BEP or four cycles of EP in good-risk patients, and four cycles of BEP for intermediate-risk patients.

B. **Testicular nonseminoma**
   1. **Treatment options for stage I nonseminoma.** The cure rate of patients with clinical stage I nonseminoma is 99% regardless of strategy if performed properly. VI is the most important prognostic factor for relapse, as risk of developing metastatic disease is 48% for patients with VI and only 14% to 22% for patients without VI. Patients are stratified as low-risk for relapse (no VI) or high risk (VI present).
      a. **Low risk.** Patients with low risk should be managed by surveillance, as most of the patients will need no further treatment following orchiectomy. This

approach requires patient compliance with diligent follow-up. Tumor markers should be obtained every 1 to 2 months in the first year, every 2 months in the second year, every 3 months in the third year, every 4 months in the fourth year, every 6 months in the fifth year, and then annually. CT scans are recommended every 3 months during the first 2 years, every 4 months during the third year, every 6 months in the fourth year, and then annually. For patients who relapse under surveillance, chemotherapy results in a cure rate of approximately 100%. If surveillance is not a suitable option, nerve-sparing retroperitoneal lymph node dissection (NS-RPLND) may be performed.

   b. High risk. Adjuvant chemotherapy with two cycles of BEP may be given to patients with high risk of relapse. With this strategy, the relapse rate is less than 5%, the cure rate is approximately 100%. Surgery with NS-RPLND is also an acceptable and highly successful. This surgery makes recurrence in the retroperitoneum extremely rare, and may reduce the risk of late recurrence, although risk for relapse outside of the retroperitoneum is not eliminated. Surveillance is also an acceptable option in compliant patients, although relapses may be detected later and need more intensive treatment. However, patients may experience psychological distress given the significant relapse rate.

2. **Management of clinical stage IIA or IIB nonseminoma.** Patients with clinical stage IIA with elevation in tumor markers, or clinical stage IIB regardless of tumor markers, should be treated with three cycles of BEP or four cycles of EP chemotherapy. If residual mass is present on CT scan following chemotherapy, resection with NS-RPLND should be performed.

   In patients with clinical stage IIA nonseminoma without elevated tumor markers, options include staging NS-RPLND, surveillance, or adjuvant chemotherapy with three cycles of BEP. If In patients undergoing RPLND, further treatment will be dictated by the final PS. For PS IIA/B, further options after lymph node dissection include surveillance or adjuvant chemotherapy with two cycles of EP or BEP. Chemotherapy is recommended if six or more nodes are involved, extranodal extension is present, lymph node dissection is incomplete, or if tumor markers are increasing or persistently elevated.

3. **Management of clinical stage IIC disease.** Stage IIC patients are considered good-risk advanced GCT in the IGCCCG classification system, and should be treated with three cycles of BEP or four cycles of EP chemotherapy as per guidelines for advanced GCT. This should be followed by debulking surgery if residual tumor is present.

4. **Management of clinical stage III (metastatic) or advanced disease requiring chemotherapy.** These patients should be classified according to the IGCCCG criteria as having either good, intermediate, or poor-prognosis disease (Table 23.2).

   a. Good-risk patients. The recommended treatment is four cycles of EP or three cycles of BEP, which may cure approximately 90% of patients. This results in cure in approximately 90% of patients with good-risk. Clinical trials have shown that three cycles of BEP are equivalent to four cycles of BEP in patients with good-risk. The substitution of carboplatin for cisplatin in either EP or BEP was found to be inferior in a prospective trial.

   b. Intermediate/poor-risk patients. Patients should be treated with four cycles of BEP chemotherapy. Patients with intermediate risk have a 70% to 80% cure rate with this regimen. Clinical trials, if available, should be considered for poor-risk patients, as only approximately 45% of these are cured with conventional treatment. If brain metastases are present, cranial irradiation should be offered prior to chemotherapy. Surgery may also be considered when indicated. The use of high-dose chemotherapy with stem cell rescue does not improve treatment outcomes in the first-line setting for patients with intermediate or poor-prognosis GCT in comparison to conventional chemotherapy.

5. **Management of postchemotherapy masses.** CT scan should be obtained following chemotherapy for advanced nonseminoma, and all residual masses detected on CT should be resected in patients with normalization of the tumor markers. Residual masses in the retroperitoneum often represent necrotic or fibrous tissue or teratoma, in which case no further therapy is required following resection. Approximately 10% to 20% of these masses will be found to have viable GCT on pathologic examination, for which two further cycles of EP are recommended.

6. **Management of recurrent disease after initial therapy.** Patients with advanced nonseminoma who have persistent elevation in AFP or hCG following chemotherapy should be considered to have an incomplete response. Approximately one third of patients with advanced disease will not achieve complete remission, or relapse after initial therapy.

Favorable prognosis features for these patients include low serum tumor markers, low volume disease, primary tumor in testis, and complete response to initial therapy. Standard salvage chemotherapy for these patients are either VeIP (vinblastine, ifosfamide, and cisplatin) or TIP (paclitaxel, ifosfamide, and cisplatin) (Table 23.3). In these patients, complete response is obtained in 50% and long-term cure in approximately 25%. Postchemotherapy surgery is often needed, as viable tumor is present in approximately 50% of residual masses following salvage chemotherapy or incomplete response or relapse following salvage chemotherapy either as incomplete responses or at relapse.

Unfavorable prognostic features include incomplete response to first-line therapy, high tumor markers, high volume disease, extratesticular primary, and late relapse. For these patients, high-dose chemotherapy with autologous stem cell support should be evaluated as salvage therapy due to the poor overall survival with conventional salvage chemotherapy. Other options include clinical trials or best supportive care.

C. **Therapy-related complications.** Complications from therapy may be related to surgery, radiation therapy, or chemotherapy. Inguinal orchiectomy is generally a safe and well-tolerated procedure. Nerve-sparing RPLND minimizes the risk of impotence and retrograde ejaculation more commonly seen when nerve dissection is not performed, although these risks are not altogether eliminated. Complications of radiation therapy include gastrointestinal toxicities such as nausea, vomiting, and diarrhea, risk of developing second malignancies in the remaining testicle, and impaired fertility from scatter radiation doses. Chemotherapy side effects from commonly used regimens include myelosuppression, infertility, neuropathy, nephropathy, late cardiotoxicity, and risk of secondary malignancy such as acute leukemia. Bleomycin is associated with the risk of pulmonary fibrosis in approximately 5% of patients.

V. **BACKGROUND AND EPIDEMIOLOGY.** There were 8,250 new cases of testicular cancer in the United States in 2006. While testicular GCTs account for only 2% of all cancers overall, they are the most common solid tumors in men between the ages of 15 and 34 years. The incidence worldwide has more than doubled in the last 40 years. The incidence of testicular GCTs are lower in African American and Asian populations than in Caucasians. Incidence rates climb rapidly and peak in young adults, followed by a decline and leveling off in the elderly. Nonseminoma commonly presents in the third decade of life, and seminoma is more commonly diagnosed in the fourth and fifth decades. Testicular GCTs are a highly curable malignancy, even in advanced disease. Since the advent of cisplatinum-based chemotherapy, the 5-year survival for all patients with GCTs is more than 90%. Patients with advanced stage are cured in 70% to 80% of cases.

Several risk factors have been associated with the development of testicular cancer, including prior testicular cancer, family history, cryptorchidism (maldescended testis), and Klinefelter's syndrome. All abdominal cryptorchid testes should be surgically removed, whereas inguinal cryptorchid testes can be observed. Surgical correction of the undescended testis before the age of 5 years decreases the risk of cancer. Nevertheless, 25% of patients with cryptorchidism will develop cancer in the normally descended testis. Approximately 2% of patients with a history of testicular cancer will develop a second primary in the opposite testis.

VI. CURRENT FOCUS OF RESEARCH. Most patients with testicular cancer are cured with cisplatin-based chemotherapeutic regimens even after relapse, and strategies to minimize late toxicities while maintaining efficacy are being evaluated. Research efforts are also being directed toward developing regimens for salvage purposes, as treatment failure is still frequently observed in high-risk patients. As with many other solid tumors, targeted biologic therapies are being investigated. Activating mutations in the c-KIT proto-oncogene has been described in patients with treatment-refractory nonseminomas. Mutations in K- and N-*ras* have also been described in GCTs. EGFR expression has been investigated as well, with conflicting data regarding its significance in its association with sensitivity to chemotherapy. Clinical investigation regarding the possible role of EGFR inhibitors or tyrosine kinase inhibitors is still preliminary at this time.

VII. EGGCT. An EGGCT is defined as a tumor histologically associated with gonadal origin but found outside the testis, without a detectable testicular mass. These tumors are generally located in the anterior mediastinum, and may include teratomas. Patients with EGGCTs often have greater tumor bulk than with primary testicular tumors, and have a distinctly worse prognosis. These tumors occur mostly in young men, and are classified as poor-risk nonseminomas. Isochrome 12p karyotypic abnormality is often demonstrated. Immature teratomas have a higher incidence of malignant transformation, whereas seminomas have a better prognosis. Patients are often initially seen at an advanced stage including presentations requiring emergent intervention such as superior vena cava syndrome or tracheal compression. Central nervous system disease may also occur in the absence of retroperitoneal or nodal disease.

Suggested Readings

Albers P, Albrecht W, Algaba F, et al. Guidelines on testicular cancer. *Eur Urol* 2005;48:885–894.

Einhorn LH, Williams SD, Loeher PJ, et al. Evaluation of optimal duration of chemotherapy in favorable-prognosis disseminated germ cell tumors: a Southwestern Cancer Study Group protocol. *J Clin Oncol* 1989;7:387–391.

Herr HW, Sheinfeld J, Puc HS, et al. Surgery for a post-chemotherapy residual mass in seminoma. *J Urol* 1997;157:860–862.

Horwich A, Shipley J, Huddart R. Testicular germ cell cancer. *Lancet* 2006;367:754–765.

International Germ Cell Cancer Collaborative Group (IGCCCG). International germ cell consensus classification: prognostic factor-based staging system for metastatic germ cell cancers. *J Clin Oncol* 1997;15:594–603.

Jones RH, Vasey PA. Part I: testicular cancer—management of early disease. *Lancet Oncol* 2003;4:730–737.

Jones RH, Vasey PA. Part II: testicular cancer—management of advanced disease. *Lancet Oncol* 2003;4:738–747.

Miller KD, Loehrere PM, Goin R, et al. Salvage chemotherapy with vinblastin, ifosfamide, and cisplatin in recurrent seminoma. *J Clin Oncol* 1997;15:1427–1431.

Motzer RJ, Mazumdar M, Bajorin DF, et al. High-dose carboplatin, etoposide, and cyclophosphamide with autologous bone marrow transplantation in first-line chemotherapy for patients with poor-risk germ cell tumors. *J Clin Oncol* 1997;15:2546–2552.

Motzer RJ, Sheinfeld J, Mazumdar M, et al. Paclitaxel, ifosfamide, and cisplatin second-line therapy for patients with relapsed testicular germ cell cancer. *J Clin Oncol* 2000;18:2413–2418.

de Santis M, Bokemeyer C, Becherer A, et al. Predictive impact of 2-18-fluoro-2-deoxy-D-glucose positron emission tomography (FDG ET) for residual post-chemotherapy masses in patients with bulky seminoma. *J Clin Oncol* 2001;19:3740–3744.

Shelley MD, Burgon K, Mason MD. Treatment of testicular germ cell cancer: a cochrane evidence-based systematic review. *Cancer Treat Rev* 2002;28:237–253.

Schmoll HJ, Souchon R, Krege S, et al. European consensus on diagnosis and treatment of germ cell cancer: a report of the European Germ Cell Cancer Consensus Group (EGCCCG). *Ann Oncol* 2004;15:1377–1399.

Warde P, Specht L, Horwich A, et al. Prognostic factors for relapse in stage I seminoma managed by surveillance. *J Clin Oncol* 2002;20:4448–4452.

de Wit R, Roberts JT, Wilkinson PM, et al. Equivalence of three or four cycles of bleomycin, etoposide, and cisplatin chemotherapy and of a 3- or 5-day schedule in good-prognosis germ cell cancer: a randomized study of the European Organization for Research and Treatment of Cancer Genitourinary Tract Cancer Cooperative Group and the Medical Research Council. *J Clin Oncol* 2001;19:1629–1640.

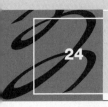

24 GYNECOLOGIC CANCER: OVARIAN
Ashley S. Case and Matthew A. Powell

I. EPITHELIAL OVARIAN CANCER
A. Epidemiology and etiology. Approximately 20,000 new cases of ovarian cancer are diagnosed each year in the United States and 15,310 deaths were estimated to occur in 2006 as a result of this disease. Ovarian cancer remains the fifth most common cause of cancer death in women and the leading cause of death from gynecologic cancer. It has been estimated that 1 woman in 70 in the United States will develop ovarian cancer in her lifetime and 1 in 100 will die from this disease. Most of the (85% to 90%) malignant ovarian tumors are epithelial in origin. The median age at diagnosis is 63 years and incidence is higher in women of white race. Risk factors include a strong family history, nulliparity, early menarche, late menopause, increasing age, white race, and residence in North America and Europe. Oral contraception usage and pregnancy are associated with a decreased risk suggesting that continuous ovulation may lead to malignant changes. The etiology of malignant changes of the ovarian epithelium, which is contiguous with the peritoneal mesothelium, is unknown and likely a combination of genetic, environmental, and endocrine effects.

B. Genetics/familial syndromes. Familial ovarian cancer may be related to a breast-ovarian cancer syndrome caused by an inherited mutation in one of two genes, *BRCA1* and *BRCA2* on chromosome 17 and 13 respectively. Certain ethnic groups such as Ashkenazi Jewish women have an increased risk of a mutation in one of these two genes. Women with a *BRCA1* mutation are reported to have a 16% to 44% lifetime risk of ovarian cancer whereas those with *BRCA2* mutations have a lower risk at 10%. Women with ovarian cancer due to these mutations tend to have a more indolent course than those with sporadic disease. Site-specific familial ovarian cancer and Lynch syndrome II in which multiple individuals within a family develop tumors in the colon, endometrium, and ovary are other types of familial ovarian cancer. Inheritance in familial ovarian cancer is in an autosomal dominant manner with multiple members in successive generations affected. There is sufficient evidence for prophylactic oophorectomy in women with a known mutation in *BRCA1* or *BRCA2* after completion of childbearing or 35 years of age in order to prevent the development of both ovarian and breast cancer.

C. Clinical presentation. Women present with vague, nonspecific symptoms of abdominal bloating, distension, dyspepsia, early satiety, anorexia, weight loss, or constipation. Women are often treated for gastrointestinal problems such as gastritis, irritable bowel syndrome, and gall bladder disease. Physical examination findings may include ascites, pleural effusion, or an umbilical mass. Most patients with early-stage disease are asymptomatic and given the vague nature of the symptoms, approximately 80% present with advanced stage (metastatic) disease. The National Cancer Institute (NCI) does support annual screening through both CA-125 measurements and transvaginal ultrasonography for women at high genetic risk based on family history; however in the general population no data exists that screening is effective in improving length and quality of life in women with ovarian cancer. Several biomarkers with potential application to ovarian cancer screening are under development but have not yet been validated or evaluated regarding their efficacy for early detection and mortality reduction.

Women found to have a mass or ascites on examination or by radiographic or ultrasonographic imaging should be evaluated to assess the possible risk of abnormality representing a malignancy. Appearance and size on ultrasonography or computed tomography (CT) scan combined with patient age and family history are factors that help determine the need for surgical evaluation. A complex mass with both solid and cystic components with septations and internal echoes is suggestive of cancer. Benign-appearing and indeterminate lesions can be followed for a brief period to evaluate for progression of disease. Serum CA-125 cancer antigen can occasionally be of aid in postmenopausal patients. CA-125 is elevated in more than 80% of patients with ovarian cancer but this test is neither sufficiently sensitive nor specific enough to be diagnostic as this may be elevated in a number of other benign and malignant conditions. CA-125 is most useful in following response to postoperative chemotherapy and detecting disease recurrence. No definitive tests are currently available and definitive diagnosis is often only possible with surgical evaluation.

D. Surgical treatment. Surgery is typically performed for histologic diagnosis, staging, and tumor debulking. Exceptions to an immediate surgical approach are patients who are poor surgical candidates secondary to other comorbid diseases or performance status. In these patients, a confirmatory biopsy or cytology is obtained in order to establish a diagnosis followed by chemotherapeutic treatment. Preoperatively patients should undergo all age-appropriate cancer screening (Pap smear, mammogram, colorectal cancer screening) as well as additional tests depending on the clinical scenario (barium enema, colonoscopy, and/or cystoscopy). Laboratory assessment should include complete blood count, type and screen, electrolytes, renal and hepatic panel, electrocardiogram, and chest x-ray. Additional studies depend on the patient's medical condition(s). Given the likelihood of large and small bowel involvement requiring resection, a thorough bowel preparation is recommended. Staging of ovarian cancer is surgical and proper staging procedures should typically consist of the following: (a) midline abdominal incision; (b) evacuation of ascites or peritoneal washings for cytologic analysis; (c) resection of the primary ovarian tumor through total abdominal hysterectomy with bilateral salpingoophorectomy; (d) biopsies of omentum or omentectomy, (e) biopsies of the pelvic and abdominal peritoneum, including pericolic gutters; and (f) retroperitoneal nodal sampling (pelvic and para-aortic) if indicated by lack of abdominal disease greater than 2 cm or if grossly involved with tumor. The surgical staging system established by the International Federation of Gynecology and Obstetrics is depicted in Table 24.1. Tumor debulking is a critical component of initial surgical management as women with residual disease of less than 1 cm have survival rates higher than those with residual disease.

Five-year survival in patients with early-stage disease (stage I or II) is often as high as 80% to 95%; however, patients with advanced disease (stage III or IV) have much lower survival rates of 30% to 40%.

E. Post-operative treatment

   1. Epithelial tumors of low malignant potential (LMP). Also called borderline tumors, this subgroup represents approximately 10% to 15% of all epithelial ovarian tumors. The tumors are usually stage I (80%+) and are characterized pathologically by epithelial cell stratification, increased mitoses, nuclear abnormalities, and atypical cells without stromal invasion. Surgical staging is usually recommended, but given these tumors tend to occur in younger patients, conservation of fertility is often possible. Treatment is simple surgical resection. Chemotherapy does not appear to have a role in treating most of these tumors. However, LMP tumors are on rare occasions found to have invasive implants (metastasis) in which case the patient should be treated similarly to frankly invasive disease with adjuvant chemotherapy. Although by convention the tumor is still considered LMP as the diagnosis is based on the primary tumor only. Recurrent disease is usually treated with repeat surgical debulking. The prognosis for patients without invasive implants is excellent with very few patients dying of disease. The average time to recurrence is 10 years and patients can recur with invasive disease. Patients are often followed with serum CA-125 determinations every 3 to 12 months, but it is unclear if this provides any survival benefit.

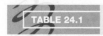

TABLE 24.1 **FIGO Ovarian Cancer Staging.**

FIGO stage	Tumor characteristics
I	Growth limited to the ovaries
IA	Growth limited to one ovary; no ascites; no tumor on the external surface; capsule intact
IB	Growth limited to both ovaries; no ascites; no tumor on the external surfaces; capsule intact
IC	Tumor either stage IA or IB but with tumor on surface of one or both ovaries; or with capsule ruptured; or with ascites present containing malignant cells; or with positive peritoneal washings
II	Growth involves one or both ovaries with pelvic extension
IIA	Extension or metastases to the uterus or tubes
IIB	Extension to other pelvic tissues
IIC	Tumor either stage IIA or IIB, but with tumor on surface of one or both ovaries; or with capsule ruptured; or with ascites present containing malignant cells; or with positive peritoneal washings
III	Tumor involves one or both ovaries with peritoneal implants outside the pelvis and/or positive retroperitoneal or inguinal nodes; superficial liver metastasis equals stage III; tumor is limited to the true pelvis but the histologically proven malignant extension to small bowel or omentum
IIIA	Tumor grossly limited to the true pelvis with negative nodes but histologically confirmed microscopic seeding of abdominal peritoneal surfaces
IIIB	Tumor of one or both ovaries with histologically confirmed implants of abdominal peritoneal surfaces, none exceeding 2 cm in diameter; nodes are negative
IIIC	Abdominal implants >2 cm in diameter or positive retroperitoneal of inguinal nodes
IV	Growth involves one or both ovaries, with distant metastases; if pleural effusion is present, there must be positive cytology to allot a case to stage IV; parenchymal liver metastasis equals stage IV

2. **Early-stage disease.** Patients with stage IA or IB, grade 1 or 2 disease are considered low –risk, with excellent survival chances (90% to 95%). Surgical treatment with careful staging alone followed by close follow-up is typically all the treatment that is required. With adequate staging, a unilateral salpingoophorectomy may be considered in some patients with stage IA grade 1 disease who wish to preserve fertility. Patients with stage IC disease, stage I grade 3 disease, stage I grade 2, or stage II disease are considered at high risk for recurrence and are treated with platinum-based adjuvant chemotherapy to reduce the risk of relapse. With chemotherapy, disease-free survival is approximately 80%. The number of chemotherapeutic cycles for treatment of early-stage disease is debatable and (Gynecology Oncology Group [GOG] 157) recently showed that, compared to three cycles, six cycles of carboplatin and paclitaxel do not significantly alter the recurrence rate in high-risk, early-stage ovarian cancer but are associated with more toxicity; however, some question the statistical power as there was a strong trend toward decreased recurrence in stage I disease with six cycles ($p = .073$).

F. **Advanced disease.** Most of the patients present with advanced stage disease (stage III and IV). Maximal efforts for surgical cytoreduction of the tumor before chemotherapy should be made as studies have consistently demonstrated improved survival in those patients with an "optimal" cytoreduction. Optimal cytoreduction has been defined a variety of ways in the literature. Currently, the GOG defines optimal cytoreduction as no residual tumor nodules with a diameter greater than or equal to 1 cm. Optimally cytoreduced patients have a median progression-free survival (PFS) and overall survival (OS) of 22 months and 50 months, respectively (GOG 158); versus suboptimally cytoreduced patients with an 18-month PFS and 38-month OS (GOG 111). Chi et al. recently assessed survival rates at specific residual disease diameters to determine the optimal goal of primary cytoreduction and found that patients with no gross disease or less than 1 mm had significantly longer overall median survival compared with patients with macroscopic residual disease greater than 1mm (*Gynecol Oncol* 2006). Patients with advanced stage disease will require postoperative adjuvant chemotherapy in order to treat residual disease. Taxane- and platinum-based chemotherapy is the current standard of postoperative care. This combination of chemotherapy extends PFS as well as OS. The current "standard" therapy is based on clinical trials demonstrating similar efficacy of carboplatin/paclitaxel to cisplatin/paclitaxel with less chemotherapy-related toxicity and a shorter administration time. The regimen consists of intravenous administration of paclitaxel (175 mg/m^2) given over 3 hours and carboplatin dosed with an area under the curve (AUC) of 5 to 7.5 (Jeliffe formula to estimate creatinine clearance and Calvert formula to determine AUC). This regimen is given every 3 weeks for a total of six cycles. Response rates (complete response [CR] + partial response [PR]) are approximately 80% with this combination. More than 50% of the patients will have a complete clinical response, with 30% demonstrating a complete pathologic response at second look laparotomy. Recent clinical trials are investigating the success of maintenance chemotherapy in improving both PFS and OS; however; no clear evidence exists for an OS benefit at the present time. Intravenous chemotherapy has been the standard treatment in the past; however, intraperitoneal chemotherapy (IP) has also been investigated over the last several decades. Three recent large prospective trials have shown survival improvements for those patients treated with IP (*N Engl J Med* 2006;354(1):34–43; *N Engl J Med* 1996;335:1950–1955; *J Clin Oncol* 2001;19:1001–1007). Most recently, GOG 172 reported a PFS of 23.8 months for combination IP and intravenous chemotherapy versus 18.3 months for intravenous (IV) alone. Similarly, OS was longer with the combined IP/IV therapy (65.6 months vs. 49.7 months). Patients who receive IP therapy do experience greater toxicity and even report worse quality of life in some studies; therefore, many oncologists are still slow to utilize this method of treatment. Although most patients tolerate platinum- and taxane-based chemotherapy relatively well, some develop severe peripheral neuropathy and the use of docetaxel has been shown to result in less neuropathy with similar efficacy (*J Natl Cancer Inst* 2004;96(22):1682–1691).

Second-look laparotomies are not recommended unless the patient is enrolled in a protocol as these studies have shown no impact on survival. Less commonly, radiation of the abdomen and pelvis is employed as treatment for advanced stage and/or recurrent disease. Following adjuvant chemotherapy, patients are monitored with physical examination, CA-125 measurements, and imaging studies (CT, magnetic resonance imaging [MRI], positron emission tomography [PET]) as clinically indicated for recurrent disease.

G. Recurrent disease. Despite standard treatment with cytoreductive surgery and chemotherapy, up to 75% of patients experience recurrence and will eventually succumb to disease. Median survival following relapse from initial therapy is approximately 2 years. Patients found to progress with upfront therapy or with a recurrence should be offered additional treatments that will hopefully allow for control of their disease and maintain the best quality of life possible. One must realize that very few of these patients are ultimately cured of their disease. The usual first sign of recurrence is a rising CA-125, which is usually followed by evidence of recurrence on examination or by a CT scan of the abdomen and pelvis. It is not clear if early retreatment (before the onset of symptoms or radiographic evidence of disease) of a patient with an elevating CA-125 has any effect on disease control or OS. Treatment of recurrent or persistent disease is based on the timing and location of the recurrence. Because recurrent disease is typically not curable, symptom palliation and prevention of complications such as bowel obstruction remain the goals of management. Radiation and/or surgical resection have been used to successfully treat localized disease. Indications for repeat surgery (secondary debulking) are highly controversial and decisions must be individualized. In general, if the progression-free interval is greater than 1 year and the mass appears isolated, or if it is symptomatic (obstruction of bowel or kidney), surgical resection can result in prolonged survival. "Platinum-sensitive" patients have a recurrence more than 6 months from the time of their initial CR. These patients can be successfully retreated with platinum-based regimens with reasonable responses (20% to 40%). ICON IV showed that in patients with platinum-sensitive disease, combination chemotherapy (platinum plus paclitaxel) led to higher complete or PRs (66% vs. 54%) as well as PFS (13 months vs. 10 months) compared to platinum therapy alone for recurrent disease. Patients with a treatment-free interval of greater than 12 months received the greatest benefit from retreatment with combination platinum, paclitaxel therapy. Patients having a recurrence before 6 months ("platinum-resistant") can be treated with a variety of agents. Many authorities recommend that single-agent therapy be used in this setting to minimize toxicity and to more easily identify nonresponding agents. Given there is no ideal second-line salvage agent(s), patients should be encouraged to participate in available study protocols. Second-line (salvage) agents will have an approximate response rate of 15% to 40%, depending on agent and amount of previous chemotherapeutic treatments. Treatment is usually continued until the CA-125 normalizes, toxicity precludes further therapy, or disease progression. Patients with progressive disease are then offered a different regimen usually with a differing side effect profile to minimize toxicity.

Complications of therapy are primarily related to continued growth of the tumor (bowel obstruction) and toxicities of the chemotherapy. Bowel obstructions should initially be managed conservatively with intravenous fluids and gastric decompression. Studies such as abdominal plain films, small bowel follow-through, contrast enemas, and abdominal/pelvic CT may be necessary to further evaluate cause of obstruction. Persistent obstructions can be managed with chronic decompression (G-tube) or surgical exploration in cases where the imaging studies suggest a limited focus of obstruction. Toxicities of chemotherapy are related to the specific agents and are covered elsewhere in this text.

H. Future directions. A great deal of attention has been focused on identification of the genetic factors involved with ovarian cancer tumorigenesis with identification of potentially useful biomarkers. Inhibition of epidermal growth factor receptor (EGFR) and vascular epithelial growth factor (VEGF) has been studied both alone and in combination with chemotherapy. Recently the GOG reported promising results with bevacizumab (VEGF antibody) therapy in patients with recurrent ovarian cancer and is currently recruiting patients for a randomized prospective trial investigating combination chemotherapy with the addition of bevacizumab. Identification of more specific tumor markers could potentially be used to identify disease at earlier more treatable stages. Microarray gene expression profiles hold promise as prognostic tools for identification of gene targets and may shed light on mechanisms of drug resistance. Current clinical studies are examining new chemotherapeutic agents and novel combinations of known agents in efforts to improve survival of this devastating disease.

II. FALLOPIAN TUBE CARCINOMA. Fallopian tube carcinoma is a rare gynecologic malignancy that behaves biologically like serous epithelial ovarian carcinoma. Fallopian tube carcinoma is staged and treated in a manner similar to ovarian carcinoma. The classic presentation is intermittent, profuse, watery vaginal discharge (hydrops tubae profluens). The diagnosis is seldom made preoperatively but has been detected by Pap smear. Prognosis is related to stage of disease with long-term survival of approximately 50% for stages I and II. As with ovarian carcinoma, long-term survival is rare with advanced disease.

III. GERM CELL OVARIAN CANCERS. These cancers typically occur in young women, are highly curable, and account for approximately 3% of ovarian cancers. The majority present as early-stage lesions confined to one ovary except for dysgerminomas, which are bilateral in 15% of cases. Dysgerminoma, endodermal sinus tumor (yolk sac tumor), embryonal carcinoma, choriocarcinoma, immature (embryonal) teratoma, and malignant mixed germ cell tumors are the cell types seen. Fertility-sparing surgery is nearly always possible. Surgical cytoreduction appears to be important and is likely associated with increased survival. Most of these tumors will have a tumor marker available to follow (human chorionic gonadotropin [HCG], α-fetoprotein [AFP], lactate dehydrogenase [LDH], CA-125, or neuron-specific enolase [NSE]). Following surgery, most tumors are treated with chemotherapy except some well-staged IA/IB cancers. The BEP regimen is the most commonly used and consists of a 5-day regimen, although a 3-day has also been studied (cisplatin 20 mg/m^2 IV days 1 to 5, bleomycin 30 units IV weekly, etoposide 100 mg/m^2 IV days 1 to 5—cycle repeated every 3 weeks). Some support observation only for localized, completely resected malignant germ cell tumors based on French survival data and pediatric oncology group trials.

IV. STROMAL TUMORS OF THE OVARY. Stromal tumors are classified by the World Health Organization (WHO) into five main classes: (a) granulosa-stromal cell tumors (adult and juvenile granulosa cell tumor and tumors in the thecoma/fibroma group); (b) Sertoli-stromal cell tumors (Sertoli, Leydig, or Sertoli-Leydig cell tumor); (c) gynandroblastoma; (d) sex cord tumor with annular tubules; and (e) unclassified. These tumors are rare and are usually of early stage and low grade, which make them readily curable with simple surgical resection. Primary metastatic or recurrent disease is usually treated with surgical cytoreduction followed by combination chemotherapy. The BEP regimen is most often used; however, recent data from Brown et al. suggest that taxanes demonstrate activity against ovarian stromal tumors and have less toxicity than BEP regimens.

Suggested Readings

Armstrong DK, Bndy B, Wenzel L, et al. Intraperitoneal cisplatin and paclitaxel in ovarian cancer. *N Engl J Med* 2006;354(1):34–43.

du Bois A, Luck HJ, Meier W, et al. A randomized clinical trial of cisplatin/paclitaxel vs. carboplatin/paclitaxel as first-line treatment of ovarian cancer. *J Natl Cancer Inst* 2003;95:1320–1330.

Brown J, Shvartsman HS, Deavers MT, et al. The activity of taxanes compared with bleomycin, etoposide, and cisplatin in the treatment of sex cord-stromal ovarian tumors. *Gynecol Oncol* 2005;97(2):489–496.

Disaia PJ, Creasman WT. *Clinical gynecologic oncology,* 6th ed. Elsevier Health Sciences, 2001.

Ford D, Easton DF, Bishop DT, et al. Risks of cancer in *BRCA1* mutation carriers. *Lancet* 1994;343:692–695.

Hoskins, Perez CA, Young RC, et al. *Principles and practice of gynecologic oncology,* 4th ed. Philadelphia: Lippincott Williams & Wilkins, 2004.

Kauff ND, Satagopan JM, Robson ME, et al. Risk reducing salpingoophorectomy in women with a *BRCA1* or *BRCA2* mutation. *N Engl J Med* 2002;346(21):1609–1615.

Ozols RF. Challenges for chemotherapy in ovarian cancer. *Ann Oncol* 2006;17(5):v181–v187.

Ozols RF, Bundy BN, Greer BE, et al. Phase III trial of carboplatin and paclitaxel compared with cisplatin and paclitaxel in patients with optimally resected stage III ovarian cancer. *J Clin Oncol* 2003;21:3194–3200.

Rubin SC, Benjamin I, Behbakht K, et al. Clinical and pathological features of ovarian cancer in women with germ-line mutations of *BRCA1*. *N Engl J Med* 1996;335:1413–1416.

Young RC. Early-stage ovarian cancer: to treat or not to treat. *J Natl Cancer Inst* 2003;95:94–95.

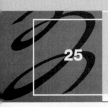

25 GYNECOLOGIC CANCER: UTERINE, CERVICAL, FALLOPIAN, AND VULVAR
Rebecca A. Brooks, Matthew A. Powell, and David G. Mutch

I. UTERINE NEOPLASIA
A. Premalignant disease of the endometrium
1. **Presentation.** Patients usually have abnormal or postmenopausal bleeding. Normal menstrual cycles occur every 28 days (range, 21 to 35 days) with a normal duration of 2 to 7 days and an average blood loss of less than 80 mL. Bleeding outside of these ranges or any postmenopausal bleeding should be evaluated. Any age group can be affected, but one should be especially concerned with abnormal bleeding in patients aged 35 and older. Obesity, a history of irregular periods, and use of an exogenous estrogens without concurrent progestational agents are known risk factors.
2. **Workup and staging.** Typically the diagnosis can be made with an office endometrial (Pipelle) biopsy. If this is nondiagnostic or technically not feasible, a dilation and curettage (D&C), with or without hysteroscopy can be performed. Pathologic specimens demonstrating hyperplasias are classified by the International Society of Gynecological Pathologists (1984) into the following four groups: simple hyperplasia with and without atypia, and complex hyperplasia with and without atypia.
3. **Therapy and prognosis**
   a. **Simple and complex hyperplasias without atypia** are usually caused by anovulation. Treatment is usually conservative and depends on the fertility desires of the patient. If untreated and monitored, 3% of patients with complex hyperplasias without atypia would be expected to develop endometrial cancer over a 13- to 15-year period. Only 1% of patients with simple hyperplasias would be expected to develop cancer; therefore this is likely not considered a premalignant condition. (Table 25.1)
      i. **Treatment for those considering pregnancy** is ovulation induction with clomiphene citrate. Medroxyprogesterone acetate (Provera), 10 mg p.o. per day for 5 to 10 days (after a negative pregnancy test) should be given. Then begin clomiphene citrate, 50 mg p.o. on day 5 of bleeding (which usually begins 2 to 3 days after the completion of the medroxyprogesterone acetate) and continue for a total of 5 days. If patient does not menstruate within a month, repeat the pregnancy test, and if negative, give another 5 days of medroxyprogesterone acetate, 10 mg, and increase the clomiphene citrate by 50 mg per month to a maximum of 750 mg/cycle until ovulation occurs. Limit use to no more than 6 to 12 months.
      ii. **If pregnancy is currently not desired,** cycle the patient with medroxyprogesterone acetate, 10 mg p.o. for 10 days/month or any other progestational therapy (depo-medroxyprogesterone acetate, 100 to 150 mg i.m. injection every month or combination oral contraceptives) or megestrol (Megace) 80 to 160 mg/day.
   b. **Atypical hyperplasia (simple or complex).** Patients with atypical hyperplasia should undergo a fractional D&C. There is a 17% to 25% incidence of concurrent endometrial cancer with atypical hyperplasia. If untreated and followed up for 11 years, 23% of patients would be expected to develop an endometrial cancer (*Cancer* 1985;56:403). In a recent prospective cohort study of women with atypical endometrial hyperplasia (**Gynecologic Oncology Group** [GOG] 167), the rate of concurrent endometrial cancer was 43% for analyzed specimens, with 31% of these demonstrating myoinvasion (at

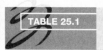

TABLE 25.1	Comparison of Follow-up of Patients with Simple and Complex Hyperplasia and Simple and Complex Atypical Hyperplasia (170 Patients)

Histology	No. of patients	Regressed no. (%)	Persisted no. (%)	Progressed to carcinoma no. (%)
Simple hyperplasia	93	74 (80%)	18 (19%)	1 (1%)
Complex hyperplasia	29	23 (80%)	5 (17%)	1 (3%)
Simple atypical hyperplasia	13	9 (69%)	3 (23%)	1 (8%)
Complex atypical hyperplasia	35	20 (57%)	5 (14%)	10 (29%)

Kurman RJ, Kaminski PF, Norris HJ. The behavior of endometrial hyperplasia: a long-term study of "untreated" hyperplasia in 170 patients. *Cancer* 1985;56:403–412.

least stage Ib), and 11% invading the outer 50% of the myometrium (at least stage Ic). Among women with cancer, the study biopsy panel consensus was widely varied, and it was not possible to accurately predict which patients would show cancer on hysterectomy specimen (*Cancer* 2006;106:812–819).

   i. Patients who desire pregnancy. Ovulation induction should be done as described. Patients should be closely monitored and periodic biopsies taken (every 6 to 12 months).

   ii. Patients not desiring pregnancy. Medical treatment: (approximately 90% to 95% success rate) medroxyprogesterone acetate, 40 mg p.o. per day in divided doses, or megestrol acetate (Megace), 20 to 40 mg p.o. twice daily. Treatment is 40 mg q.i.d. 160 mg to 320 mg/day and the dose can be gradually tapered. **Surgical treatment:** extrafascial hysterectomy with gross inspection of the endometrium for gross evidence of endometrial cancer.

4. Complications are rare and related mainly to abnormal uterine bleeding.

5. Follow-up. Medically managed patients should be resampled after several months (4 to 6) of treatment. Those with normal histology can then either be taken off therapy or be cycled with progestational agents and should undergo periodic endometrial sampling. Follow-up interval for patients after hysterectomy is not well established, but annual examinations should be adequate.

6. Background. Endometrial hyperplasias are proliferative disorders primarily of the endometrial glands, and to a lesser extent, the stroma. Unopposed estrogen (i.e., without progesterone or progesterone-like compounds) is thought to be the etiologic factor for endometrial hyperplasia. This often results from chronic anovulation (polycystic ovarian syndrome), obesity (high peripheral conversion of androstenedione to estrone), estrogen-producing ovarian neoplasms (granulosa cell tumor), or exogenous unopposed estrogen administration.

7. Current focus. The Gynecologic Oncology Group (GOG) is currently evaluating medical versus surgical management of atypical hyperplasias.

B. Endometrial cancer

1. Presentation. More than 90% of patients are first seen with abnormal uterine bleeding. Patients with any amount of postmenopausal bleeding deserve evaluation. Patients with abnormal pre- or perimenopausal bleeding, especially those older than 35 or morbidly obese warrant evaluation as well. Papanicolaou (Pap) smears with atypical glandular cells of undetermined significance (AGUS) in patients of any age, especially those with a history of anovulation or women older than 35 years, should be evaluated with a colposcopy, endocervical curettage, and endometrial biopsy.

2. Workup and staging. An office endometrial biopsy (Pipelle) is an extremely sensitive method of obtaining a tissue diagnosis. A recent meta-analysis of 39 studies involving 7,914 women demonstrated a detection rate for endometrial cancer of 91% and 99.6% in pre- and postmenopausal women respectively

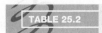

	FIGO Surgical Staging of Endometrial Cancer, 1988

Stage/grade	Description
IA G123	Tumor limited to endometrium
IB G123	Invasion to less than half of the myometrium
IC G123	Invasion to more than half of the myometrium
IIA G123	Endocervical glandular involvement only
IIB G123	Cervical stromal invasion
IIIA G123	Tumor invades serosa and/or adnexal, and/or positive peritoneal cytology
IIIB G123	Vaginal metastasis
IIIC G123	Metastasis of pelvic and/or para-aortic lymph nodes
IVA G123	Tumor invasion of bladder and/or bowel mucosa
IVB G123	Distant metastases including intra-abdominal and/or inguinal lymph nodes

FIGO, International Federation of Gynecology and Obstetrics.

(*Cancer* 2000;89:1765–1772). Patients with a nondiagnostic office biopsy, persistent bleeding abnormality despite a normal office biopsy, or those who are unable to undergo a biopsy in the office should undergo a fractional D&C, with or without hysteroscopy. All patients should be screened for other malignancies as appropriate for age and family history (Pap smear, mammogram, colorectal cancer screening). Cystoscopy, proctoscopy, and radiologic imaging may be necessary, as clinically indicated, if advanced stage endometrial cancer is suspected. Surgical staging of endometrial carcinoma was adopted by the International Federation of Gynecologists and Obstetricians (FIGO) in 1988 and is summarized in Table 25.2. All patients who are medically able should undergo surgical exploration with appropriate staging. Extrafascial hysterectomy with bilateral salpingo-oophorectomy, collection of peritoneal cytology, pelvic and para-aortic lymph node dissection, and biopsy of any suggestive areas are necessary for staging, except in well-differentiated tumors without myometrial invasion. Omentectomy or omental biopsy is also indicated for high-grade tumors.

3. **Therapy and prognosis.** Adjuvant treatment after primary surgical management of endometrial cancer is controversial in many areas. Table 25.3 summarizes current treatment recommendations after surgery for endometrial cancer. **Hormonal** therapy is often used for patients with advanced/recurrent disease who test positive for estrogen and progesterone receptors. In the absence of receptor levels, usually only grade 1 and 2 tumors are treated in this manner. Grade 3 tumors are unlikely (fewer than 25%) to express hormone receptors. Response rate with either medroxyprogesterone acetate, 200 mg daily, or megestrol acetate, 160 mg daily, is approximately 20%. When indicated, **cytotoxic chemotherapy for endometrial cancer** includes the following agents (response rate): cisplatin (20% to 35%), carboplatin (30%), doxorubicin (Adriamycin; 20% to 35%), and epirubicin (25%). The current "standard" combination is doxorubicin, 60 mg/m^2 plus cisplatin 50 mg/m^2 every 3 weeks. A response rate of 42%, progression-free interval of 6 months, and median overall survival of 9 months were noted with this regimen in a randomized trial by the GOG (*J Clin Oncol* 2004;22:3902–3908). Combination of doxorubicin (60 mg/m^2 × seven cycles) and cisplatin (50 mg/m^2 × eight cycles) (AC) was recently shown to be superior to whole-abdominal radiation (WAI, 30 Gy in 20 fractions with a 15-Gy boost) in a phase III GOG trial of 202 randomized patients (GOG 122). Progression-free survival was 38% in the WAI arm as compared to 50% in the AP arm. Overall survival was 42% in the WAI arm as compared to 55% in the AP arm. Patients

TABLE 25.3   **Treatment of Endometrial Cancer**

Condition	Possible therapies to consider
Stage IA or IB and grade 1 or 2	No further therapy or vaginal brachytherapy
Stage IB and HIR (see subsequent text)	Adjuvant external pelvic RT
Any stage I grade 3 or IC of any grade	No further therapy vs. whole pelvic RT vs. vaginal brachytherapy
Stage IC and HIR (see subsequent text)	Adjuvant external pelvic RT
Stage II	Vaginal brachytherapy vs. pelvic RT
	Adjuvant external pelvic RT if HIR (see subsequent text)
Stage IIIA (positive peritoneal cytology)	Treat based on uterine disease risk factors as above vs. progestins vs. intraperitoneal P 32
Stage IIIA (adnexal and/or serosal involvement)	Systemic chemotherapy vs. whole-abdominal RT with pelvic boost (see text)
Stage IIIB (vaginal involvement)	Pelvic RT with vaginal boost
Stage IIIC (microscopic nodal involvement)	Pelvic RT with extended-field radiation to para-aortic region, if indicated
Stage IIIC (macroscopic nodal), stage IV, and recurrent disease (extrapelvic)	Whole-abdominal radiation vs. palliative RT vs. systemic chemotherapy (see text) vs. hormonal therapy (see text) vs. combinations
Recurrent disease (pelvic)	Radiotherapy in the patient without earlier RT vs. possible surgical resection (exenteration) vs. chemotherapy (see text)
High intermediate risk	*Risk factors:*
Any age with three risk factors	*1. Moderately to poorly differentiated tumor*
Age >50 with two risk factors	*2. Lymph vascular space invasion*
Age >70 with one risk factor	*3. Outer 1/3 myometrial invasion*

RT, radiation therapy; HIR, high–intermediate risk.

in the AP arm demonstrated higher treatment-related toxicity, mostly related to hematologic and gastrointestinal (GI) problems. Treatment likely contributed to death in five patients in the WAI arm (2%) and eight patients in the AP arm (4%)(*J Clin Oncol* 2006;24:36–44). Adjuvant radiation therapy (RT) is also recommended in patients with stage Ib, Ic, and II (occult) endometrial cancer, who fall into the high–intermediate risk (HIR) category. Cumulative 2-year incidence of recurrence after surgical staging was only 6% in these patients treated with adjuvant external pelvic RT as compared to 26% in those who received no adjuvant treatment (*Gynecol Oncol* 2004;92:744–751). A recent GOG trial demonstrated improved survival in patients with advanced or recurrent endometrial cancer treated with TAP (paclitaxel, doxorubicin, cisplatin) as compared to cisplatin and doxorubicin alone, although with increased toxicity (*J Clin Oncol* 2004;22:2159–2166). A phase III trial comparing TAP and PT (carboplatin/paclitaxel) is currently underway, and although the TAP regimen may be superior, PT is frequently used.

4. **Complications.** Complications of staging surgery are generally minimal. Lymphocysts and lymphedema of the lower extremities are rare complications of lymphadenectomy. Immediate and late effects of radiation are usually related to bowel and bladder dysfunction. Complications of chemotherapy most commonly include hematologic, GI, and infectious.

5. **Follow-up.** Typically patients are evaluated with physical examination, Pap smear, and pelvic examination every 3 months for the first 2 years, and then every 6 months for 2 years, and then annually.

6. **Background.** Endometrial cancer is the most common gynecologic malignancy in the United States, with approximately 41,200 cases reported annually, and more than 7,300 of these women dying of disease. Five-year survival for localized disease is 96%, whereas relative survival for all stages is approximately 86%. Risk factors include unopposed estrogenic stimulation (either estrogens or tamoxifen), chronic anovulation, obesity (especially truncal), diabetes mellitus, nulliparity, and late age of menopause (older than 52 years).

7. **Current focus.** Endometrial cancer tumorigenesis is rather poorly understood. The genetic and epigenetic factors responsible are slowly being elucidated. Current efforts include identification of tumor suppressor genes, identification of epigenetic changes (DNA methylation), and better understanding of estrogen-driven tumorigenesis. Clinical studies relate to identification of more effective therapies for metastatic and recurrent endometrial cancers. Prevention with levonorgestrel-secreting intrauterine devices is also being investigated. Total laparoscopic staging is being performed with increasing frequency for suspected early-stage endometrial cancer, and lymph node count and survival appear similar when compared to laparotomy. Although laparoscopic staging is associated with shorter hospital stays, smaller blood loss, less perioperative pain, and improved quality of life, the laparoscopic approach is limited by a higher operative complication rate, longer operative time, a steep learning curve, and a theoretical risk of port site metastases. A significant number of laparoscopic cases also result in conversion to open laparotomy (12% to 25%). Randomized prospective studies comparing these two approaches are currently under way (*JSLS* 2005;9:442–446).

C. **Sarcomas**

1. **Presentation** is similar to that of endometrial cancers. A rapidly growing fibroid uterus is only rarely indicative of a uterine sarcoma (0.3%) (*Obstet Gynecol* 1994;83:414–418). Uterine sarcomas are often incidental diagnoses on hysterectomy specimens, and reoperation for complete surgical staging is usually not recommended (*Gynecol Oncol* 2006;100:166–172).

2. **Workup and staging.** Uterine sarcomas have been classified in many different ways, but most commonly they are subdivided into the following four types: (a) leiomyosarcomas, (b) endometrial stromal sarcomas, (c) malignant mixed mesodermal tumors (MMMTs) with homologous or heterologous elements (also called mixed müllerian mesodermal tumors or carcinosarcomas), and (d) other uterine sarcomas. Homologous elements contain stromal tissue components, whereas heterologous sarcomas contain stromal elements from other tissues (e.g., rhabdomyosarcoma and chondrosarcoma). As more is discovered about the biology and activity of these rare cancers, uterine carcinosarcomas may be considered more closely related to poorly differentiated carcinomas and not sarcomas at all. There is no accepted staging system for uterine sarcomas, but the FIGO system used for endometrial cancers is most commonly used (see Table 25.2). Patients should be treated primarily with surgical exploration with appropriate staging, as primary radiotherapy and chemotherapy have very disappointing results.

3. **Therapy and prognosis.** Although each histologic subtype of sarcoma behaves differently, in general, survival is poor, with more than half the number of patients dying of their disease. Adjuvant therapy for **stage I and II** disease in the form of RT often improves local recurrences but has little impact on long-term survival. Cytotoxic chemotherapy may have a role in the adjuvant setting, but currently there is no definitive proof of a survival benefit. Hormonal therapy with high-dose progestin therapy (megestrol acetate, 240 to 360 mg p.o. daily) has shown activity against endometrial stromal sarcomas, especially those that are low grade. **Advanced stage** (III/IV) and **recurrent disease** have been treated with radiotherapy with minimal success. Chemotherapy is most often used in this setting. For the MMMTs, ifosfamide plus MESNA, with or without cisplatin, is most often used (ifosfamide, 1.2 to 1.5 g/m^2 i.v. qd $\times$ 5 days, or ifosfamide, 1.2 to 1.5 mg/m^2 i.v. qd $\times$ 4 days, with cisplatin, 20 mg/m^2/day i.v. $\times$ 4 days, repeated

every 3 weeks (response rates, 30% to 50%). In a randomized GOG study, combination therapy produced higher response rates but greater toxicity and no survival advantage over single-agent ifosfamide. Single agents, doxorubicin (60 mg/m^2 i.v. q3 weeks) or ifosfamide (similar dosing as for MMMTs), have shown activity against leiomyosarcomas (approximate response rates, 25% and 20%, respectively). Surgical resection of recurrent sarcoma has shown beneficial in other soft tissue sarcomas, and may provide a survival advantage in uterine sarcomas as well, although this data is limited.

4. **Complications.** See Section I.B.4.
5. **Follow-up.** See Section I.B.5.
6. **Background.** Two percent to 3% of uterine tumors are sarcomas with the following histologic subtypes: mixed müllerian mesodermal sarcomas (50%), leiomyosarcomas (40%), and endometrial stromal sarcomas (8%).
7. **Current focus.** Patients with optimally debulked MMMTs of any stage are being studied to evaluate WAI versus chemotherapy with ifosfamide and cisplatin in a randomized manner (GOG no. 150). Recent chemotherapy trials for advanced or recurrent leiomyosarcoma have included doxorubicin, 40 mg/m^2; mitomycin, 8 mg/m^2; and cisplatin, 60 mg/m^2 q3 weeks; results not yet available (GOG no. 87-I); liposomal doxorubicin (Doxil), 50 mg/m^2 i.v. q4 weeks (GOG no. 87-J), recently activated; and paclitaxel, 175 mg/m^2 i.v. over a 3-hour period q3 weeks, results not yet available (GOG no. 131-C).

D. **Gestational trophoblastic disease**
1. **Presentation.** Most cases of malignant/persistent gestational trophoblastic disease (GTD) are seen after a hydatidiform mole. Hydatidiform moles usually present with vaginal bleeding and a positive pregnancy test. Nearly all hydatidiform moles are now diagnosed with ultrasound examination, demonstrating the "snow-storm" appearance of the vesicle-filled intrauterine cavity. Occasionally, patients will have symptoms of pre-eclampsia, hyperthyroidism, and/or severe hyperemesis. Physical examination demonstrates uterine size inconsistent with estimated gestational dates, bilateral ovarian enlargement (due to thecal lutein cysts), and usually an absence of fetal heart sounds. GTD can also occur after a normal pregnancy, abortion (spontaneous or induced), or ectopic pregnancy, and the diagnosis is often easily missed in these patients. Presentation is the same in these patients, although the delay in diagnosis may lead to widely metastatic disease.
2. **Workup and staging.** After diagnosis of a molar pregnancy (usually by ultrasound), the patient should undergo chest radiograph (CXR; if positive, a metastatic workup should follow; see later), type and cross-matching of blood, quantitative β-human chorionic gonadotropin (HCG) evaluation, and a suction D&C, followed by sharp curettage. Intravenous (i.v.) oxytocin, 20 to 40 units/L or other uterotonic agents should be used shortly after the beginning of the procedure and continued for several hours to avoid excessive bleeding. Patients with Rh-negative blood should receive Rh immune globulin (RhoGAM), as indicated to prevent isoimmunization in future pregnancies. Patients are followed up after surgery with quantitative pregnancy tests (β-HCG) weekly until normal and then monthly for 1 year. Eighty percent of moles will resolve with D&C alone. **Persistent gestational trophoblastic neoplasia (GTN)** is diagnosed with any of the following conditions (note that histologic verification is not required): (a) after evacuation of a hydatidiform mole, the HCG level does not decrease appropriately (plateau or 2 consecutive weeks with an increasing titer); (b) metastatic disease is discovered; or (c) pathologic diagnosis of choriocarcinoma or placental site trophoblastic tumor. Once the diagnosis of persistent GTN is made, a further metastatic workup should include a complete history and physical examination and computed tomography (CT) of the chest, abdomen, pelvis, and possibly head, if indicated. A pelvic ultrasound should also be performed to rule out an early pregnancy in patients with possible inadequate contraception. Complete blood count (CBC) and metabolic panel (hepatic and renal) are also indicated. An anatomic staging system (FIGO, 1992) does exist but is seldom clinically used.

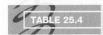

TABLE 25.4	Prognostic Classification of Gestational Trophoblastic Neoplasia

I. Nonmetastatic disease
II. Metastatic disease
    A. Low risk
        1. Short duration since last pregnancy event (<4 mo)
        2. Low pretreatment HCG (<40,000 mIU/mL serum)
        3. No brain or liver metastasis
        4. No prior chemotherapy
        5. Pregnancy event is not a term delivery
    B. High risk
        1. Long duration since last pregnancy event (>4 mo)
        2. High pretreatment HCG (>40,000 mIU/mL serum)
        3. Brain or liver metastasis
        4. Prior chemotherapy failure
        5. Antecedent term pregnancy

NIH, National Institutes of Health; HCG, human chorionic gonadotropin.

Prognosis and subsequent therapy are usually based on the World Health Organization (WHO) scoring system (not shown) or the National Institutes of Health (NIH) system used by most U.S. trophoblastic disease centers (Table 25.4).

3. **Therapy and prognosis.** Therapy is directed by the NIH class or the WHO score. Prognosis is generally excellent, and the key is to limit toxicity of the therapy as much as possible. Therapy should be started immediately, as delays can be devastating. The primary therapy of malignant GTD is chemotherapy. Surgery is used to decrease the amount of chemotherapy required for remission or to remove resistant foci of disease. Treatment of nonmetastatic GTN includes hysterectomy for those no longer desiring fertility and for all with placental site trophoblastic tumors. Chemotherapy is recommended for all

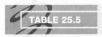

TABLE 25.5	Chemotherapeutic Regimens for Persistent Gestational Trophoblastic Neoplasia (GTN)

Nonmetastatic and low-risk metastatic GTN
    Methotrexate, 0.4 mg/kg i.v./i.m. qd × 5 days, repeat every 2 weeks
    Methotrexate, 30–50 mg/m^2 i.m. qwk (preferred method)
    Methotrexate, 1–1.5 mg/kg i.m., days (1, 3, 5, 7) + folinic acid, 0.1–0.15 mg/kg i.m., days
        (2, 4, 6, 8), repeat every 15–18 days
    Actinomycin D, 10–13 μg/kg i.v./day × 5 days, repeat every 14 days
    Actinomycin D, 1.25 mg/m^2 i.v. q14 days
High-risk metastatic GTN: EMA-CO regimen
    Day 1, etoposide, 100 mg/m^2 i.v. (over 30 min); actinomycin D, 0.5-mg i.v. push;
        methotrexate 100 mg/m^2 i.v. push, then 200 mg/m^2 i.v. infusion over 12 h
    Day 2, etoposide, 100 mg/m^2 i.v. over 30 min; actinomycin D, 0.15-mg i.v. push; folinic acid,
        15 mg i.m. or p.o. q12 h × four doses
    Day 8, vincristine, 1 mg/m^2 i.v., plus cyclophosphamide, 600 mg/m^2 i.v.
    Repeat entire cycle every 2 weeks. Patients with CNS metastasis should also receive
        radiation therapy and intrathecal methotrexate (12.5 mg on day 8) (*Gynecol Oncol*
    1989;31:439)

CNS, central nervous system.

patients, even if hysterectomy is performed, and is usually given as a single agent. Table 25.5 summarizes the chemotherapeutic regimens used to treat GTN. **Low-risk metastatic GTN** is treated primarily with single-agent chemotherapy; both methotrexate and actinomycin D should be used individually before resorting to multiagent chemotherapy. **High-risk metastatic disease** is treated with multi-agent chemotherapy with the addition of radiation if a brain metastasis is present and surgery to remove resistant foci in the uterus or chest, as needed. All patients receiving chemotherapy should be evaluated with appropriate laboratory studies (CBC, hepatic and/or renal panel) for the specific regimens plus a serum β-HCG every cycle. Treatment should continue until three consecutive normal HCG levels are obtained. At least two courses should be given after the first normal HCG.

4. **Complications.** Complications are related mainly to the specific chemotherapeutic regimen used. Single-agent therapy is normally well tolerated with minimal side effects.

5. **Follow-up.** Patients should be monitored with serum HCG monthly for 1 year. Contraception is needed for a minimum of 6 months, but 12 months is preferred. If pregnancy should develop, an early ultrasound should be performed to document an intrauterine pregnancy.

6. **Background.** Abnormal growth of the human trophoblast is called *GTD*. GTD encompasses a spectrum of abnormalities of trophoblastic tissue including classic (complete) hydatidiform moles, partial hydatidiform moles, invasive hydatidiform moles, choriocarcinoma, and placental site trophoblastic tumors. The most common abnormality, the hydatidiform mole, has two pathologic varieties—complete and partial mole. Complete moles are the most common subtype of GTD and typically occur as a result of dispermy, with both chromosomes paternal in origin resulting from fertilization of an empty ovum (46,XX). Partial moles are the result of fertilization of a normal egg by two sperms (69,XXY), resulting in an abnormal pregnancy with fetal parts usually identifiable. The reported incidence of mole varies widely throughout the world, with 1:1,500 pregnancies affected in the United States. Invasive mole is a pathologic diagnosis of a benign tumor that invades the uterine myometrium or on occasion metastasizes. The incidence is estimated at 1:15,000 pregnancies. Choriocarcinoma is a malignant tumor that has a propensity for early metastasis and an aggressive course, arising in 1:40,000 pregnancies. Fifty percent of choriocarcinomas develop after a molar gestation, 25% after a term pregnancy, and 25% after an abortion or an ectopic pregnancy. Placental-site trophoblastic tumor is the rarest variant, arising from the intermediate trophoblast, and is relatively chemotherapy resistant. The tumors often secrete human placental lactogen (HPL), which can be used as a tumor marker. GTD is more common in extremes of reproductive age (teenagers and women aged 40 to 50).

7. **Current focus.** Chemotherapy for low-risk GTN is currently being studied by the GOG (no. 174) in a randomized manner with methotrexate (30 mg/m^2 i.m. q week—maximum, 60 mg) versus dactinomycin (1.25 mg/m^2 i.v. push q2 weeks—maximum, 2 mg). A trial for patients who failed earlier methotrexate therapy using dactinomycin (same dosing as earlier) is also enrolling patients (GOG no. 176). Different dosing regimens of MTX as well as the use of concurrent folic acid has been looked at retrospectively, although no prospective trials have been completed establishing one regimen as superior. Repeat evacuation for persistent disease is controversial and may be beneficial (*Gynecol Oncol* 2004;95:423–429).

II. UTERINE CERVIX NEOPLASMS: PREINVASIVE LESIONS OF THE CERVIX

A. **Presentation.** Preinvasive lesions of the cervix are asymptomatic and are reliably detected only with cytology or biopsy. The American Cancer Society and the American College of Obstetrics and Gynecology recommend that annual cervical cytology screening (Pap smear) and pelvic examination be initiated within 3 years of the onset of sexual activity or by age 21. Women younger than 30 should undergo annual screening. After a woman older than age 30 has had three or more consecutive satisfactory annual examinations with normal findings, the Pap smear

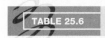

TABLE 25.6	2001 Bethesda System of Categorizing Epithelial Cell Abnormalities

Squamous cell
    Atypical squamous cells
        Of undetermined significance
        Cannot exclude high-grade squamous intraepithelial lesions
    Low-grade squamous intraepithelial lesions
        Encompassing moderate and severe dysplasia, carcinoma *in situ*, CIN 2, and CIN 3
        Squamous cell carcinoma
    High-grade squamous intraepithelial lesions
        Encompassing moderate and severe dysplasia, carcinoma *in situ*, CIN 2, and CIN 3)
    Squamous cell carcinoma
Glandular cell
    Atypical glandular cells
        (Specify endocervical, endometrial, or not otherwise specified)
    Endocervical adenocarcinoma *in situ*
    Adenocarcinoma

CIN, cervical intraepithelial neoplasia.

may be performed less frequently, at the discretion of her physician (if no history of **cervical intraepithelial neoplasia** [CIN] 2 or greater, immunocompetent, human immunodeficiency virus [HIV] negative, and no diethylstilbestrol (DES) exposure). Pap screening is recommended at least annually for women at high risk (HR). Human papillomavirus (HPV) testing can also be used as a screening tool, the nuances of which are beyond the scope of this chapter (see suggested readings). In 1988, the Bethesda system for the reporting of cervicovaginal cytologic results was developed in an effort to simplify and bring uniformity to the reporting of cytology results. This was revised in 1991 and 2001 for clearer terminology and larger application. Specimens are now specifically described in regard to specimen adequacy, ("satisfactory" or "unsatisfactory"), presence of the transformation zone ("present" or "absent"), and evaluation of epithelial cell histology ("negative for intraepithelial lesion or malignancy" or abnormal) (Table 25.6).

B. Workup. The following is a highly simplified approach to managing the abnormal Pap smear and will not apply to all situations, including adolescent patients who may represent a slightly different group. For **atypical squamous cells of undetermined significance (ASCUS),** HR HPV DNA testing is at least 80% effective in detecting CIN 2 or 3 and therefore HPV testing is commonly performed. Patients with ASCUS who are HR HPV positive should undergo colposcopy, whereas ASCUS HR HPV-negative patients may be screened again in 1 year. Alternative triage approaches for ASCUS include immediate colposcopy or repeat paps at 6 and 12 months. If the patient already has had a previously abnormal Pap or is considered "high risk," then colposcopy is indicated. **Atypical squamous cells that cannot exclude HSIL (ASC-H)** represents approximately 15% of ASCUS paps with a much higher predictive value for detecting CIN 2 to 3, and these patients need colposcopic examination. Pap smears with **low-grade squamous intraepithelial lesion (LGSIL) and high-grade squamous intraepithelial lesion (HGSIL)** need colposcopic examination. HR HPV testing is not indicated for ASC-H, LGSIL, and HGSIL pap smears since the test is almost always positive and management decisions will not be affected (a colposcopy is needed for these groups regardless of HPV results). Follow-up evaluation of **AGUS** is more controversial. Colposcopy with endocervical curettage should be performed on all patients. Women older than 35 years or any women with abnormal menstrual bleeding also need sampling of the endometrium. **Colposcopy** is performed with a colposcope that allows magnification of the cervix, which is treated with a 4% acetic acid solution. Colposcopic characteristics of dysplasia include acetowhite changes, punctations, and abnormal vascularity (mosaicism). Biopsies are performed of abnormal areas, and a histologic diagnosis is made (normal, inflammation, or CIN 1, 2, or 3). Endocervical curettage is part of most routine colposcopic examinations, especially those with high-grade cytologic abnormalities or if no ectocervical abnormalities are appreciated on colposcopy. Diagnostic cervical conization (a large cervical biopsy performed with scalpel, laser, or electrosurgical device) may be necessary to evaluate the following further: inadequate colposcopy (lesion extends into the canal or the entire transformation zone is not seen), the endocervical curettage is positive for CIN, there is a high-grade lesion on Pap smear not accounted for by colposcopy, a biopsy suggesting microinvasion, or adenocarcinoma *in situ* of the endocervix. Cervical conizations are also sometimes therapeutic procedures depending on the extent of dysplasia or histologic abnormality.

C. **Therapy and prognosis.** Treatment of CIN is dependent on biopsy results. **Cervical intraepithelial neoplasia I (CIN I)** can safely be monitored with screening Pap smear every 3 to 6 months in a compliant patient. After three consecutive negative pap smears, routine screening guidelines may be resumed. More than 60% of these abnormalities will spontaneously resolve. Repeated colposcopy should be performed if high-grade lesions are suggested or after 1 year of LGSIL on Pap. Low-grade disease that persists may be treated (see treatments later) or continue to be closely monitored. All biopsies showing high-grade lesions should be treated, as progression from CIN 3 to invasive cancer has been reported in up to 36% of cases. Treatment of cervical dysplasia consists of ablative (cryotherapy and laser) and resective techniques (loop electrosurgical excisional procedure [LEEP] and "cold" knife conization). The LEEP procedure has gained widespread acceptance and use; it is a well-tolerated office procedure that results in a pathologic specimen.

D. **Complications.** Cervical stenosis or incompetence as well as decreased fertility have been reported but generally affect fewer than 2% of patients. Hemorrhage after LEEP or cold-knife conization can occur in 3% to 5% of patients.

E. **Follow-up.** After treatment for CIN, patients should be monitored with Pap smears every 3 to 6 months. Repeated colposcopy is needed if recurrent CIN develops.

F. **Background.** More than 2.5 million women in the United States have Pap smear abnormalities, with more than 200,000 new cases of dysplasia diagnosed annually. Risk factors for the development of cervical dysplasia all relate to the likelihood of acquisition of HPV such as early age at first intercourse, smoking, immunocompetence, and number of lifetime partners. HPV DNA has been detected in more than 90% of preinvasive and invasive carcinomas, and there is convincing evidence that HPV is the etiologic factor in the vast majority of dysplasias and cervical cancers. HPV subtypes 16, 18, 45, and 56 are considered HR; 31, 33, 35, 51, 52, and 58 are of intermediate risk; and 6, 11, 42, 43, and 44 are of low risk for progression to cancer. The number of lifetime sexual partners and smoking are the most often cited independent risk factors for the development of dysplasia and cervical cancer. Communities that implement cervical cancer screening programs reduce deaths from cervix cancer by approximately 90%, making it one of the most successful cancer screening programs. Most women in whom cervix cancer develops in the United States have been inadequately screened.

G. **Current focus.** New technologies for Pap smear collection (liquid-based methods), computer-aided evaluation, and molecular testing (HPV) are continuing to be developed. Vaccine and other immune-modulating medications directed at HPV are currently being developed and tested. In June 2006, the U.S. Food and Drug Administration (FDA) approved a new prophylactic vaccine (GARDASIL,Merck) targeted against HPV subtypes 16/18 (responsible for 70% of cervical cancers worldwide) and 6/11 (responsible for 90% of genital warts). This vaccine is administered intramuscularly in a three-dose regiment at 0, 2, and 6 months and was approved for females aged 9 to 26, although it is effective only in women who have never been exposed to the virus. The recombinant vaccine is a mixture of virus-like particles derived from the L1 capsid proteins of the HPV types it is targeted against. Merck recently reported preliminary phase III results demonstrating 0 cases of CIN 2/3 or adenocarcinoma *in situ* in 5,736 vaccinated patients (100% efficacy) as compared to 21 cases in 5,258 patients receiving placebo over an average of 17 months. Long-term follow-up of a similar bivalent vaccine by Glaxo Smith Kline (GSK) demonstrated 98% seropositivity against serotypes HPV 16/18 and 100% efficacy against incident infection and incident CIN at 12 months. The vaccine is anticipated to have a dramatic effect on the incidence of HPV and cervical cancer in the long term.

III. CERVIX CANCER: INVASIVE DISEASE

A. Presentation. Most patients are first seen with abnormal vaginal bleeding or discharge, usually of a serosanguinous or yellow color, often foul smelling. Invasive cancer detected by Pap smear screening is much less common. Visually, cervix cancer lesions are exophytic (most common), endophytic, or ulcerative. Lesions are usually very vascular and bleed easily. Biopsies should be performed on all lesions, with pathologic confirmation of disease before initiation of therapy.

B. Workup and staging. Women with biopsies suggesting microinvasive cervical cancer without a gross lesion on the cervix should undergo a large cone biopsy to evaluate and stage the cancer appropriately. FIGO staging of cervical cancer is clinical and is determined mainly by physical examination, CXR, intravenous pyelography (IVP), cystoscopy, proctosigmoidoscopy, and results of the cone biopsy (if necessary). CT, magnetic resonance imaging (MRI), lymphangiography, and positron emission tomography (PET) scans are used to guide treatment of the patient with cervix cancer but cannot be used to change the stage. Table 25.7 summarizes FIGO staging of cervix cancer, 1995.

C. Therapy and prognosis. In general, all cancers of the cervix can be treated with RT. Specifics of therapy as well as the surgical alternative are as follows: **Stage IA1** may be treated with extrafascial hysterectomy or cervical cone biopsy alone in a patient strongly desirous to preserve her fertility. The risk of lymph node metastasis is very rare (0.2%), and prognosis is excellent, with very few deaths due to disease. Lesions with lymph–vascular space involvement should be treated similar to stage IB cancers. **Stage IA2, IB1, and IIA** can be treated with either radical hysterectomy with pelvic lymphadenectomy or RT, both with similar efficacy. Although controversial, lesions larger than 4 cm should be managed with primary radiotherapy, except when on a study protocol or if a contraindication to RT exists (adnexal mass, inflammatory bowel disease, or earlier RT). Surgically managed patients with positive margins, positive lymph nodes, or other high-risk factors should be offered adjuvant RT. Other high-risk factors include lymphovascular space involvement plus one of the following: (a) deep one-third penetration of tumor, (b) middle-third penetration and clinical tumor larger than 2 cm, or (c) superficial penetration and larger than 5 cm; *or* absence of lymph–vascular space involvement plus middle and deep one-third invasion and clinical tumor larger than 4 cm. Sensitizing chemotherapy (cisplatin) also should be added for patients with positive margins or lymph nodes or whenever radiotherapy is used. **Stage IB2, IIB–IVA** lesions are treated primarily with RT, usually with whole-pelvis radiation with 5,040 cGy, given as 180- to 200-cGy daily fractions with one to three brachytherapy applications. Patients should be given weekly cisplatin chemotherapy as a radiation-sensitizing agent. Our weekly regimen is cisplatin, 40 mg/m^2 i.v. given every Monday during RT. A CBC with differential, basic metabolic panel (electrolytes and renal panel), and magnesium levels are usually obtained weekly before administration of the chemotherapy. **Stage IVB** is usually treated with palliative doses of radiation to minimize symptoms of pain or vaginal bleeding. Chemotherapy in this setting has been disappointing, and no agents or combinations have made a significant effect on survival. Recurrent disease is treated on the basis of site of recurrence and previous therapies. Surgical resection (pelvic exenteration) if the disease is central and not extending to the sidewall, radiation (if outside a previously irradiated area), or chemotherapy can be used. The optimal chemotherapeutic regimen is not known. Single-agent cisplatin (50 to

70 mg/m^2 i.v. q3 weeks) has reported response rates of 20% to 30% and is currently the standard with which other agents/combinations are compared. Prognosis (5-year survival) by stage is as follows: IB, 85% to 90%; IIA, 73%; IIB, 65% to 68%; III, 35% to 44%; and IV, 15%. **Adenocarcinoma of the cervix** is treated in a similar manner as squamous cell carcinoma. **Other histologic variants (small cell: neuroendocrine, carcinoid, oat cell; verrucous carcinoma; sarcoma; lymphoma; and melanoma)** are very rare and are beyond the scope of this text (see Suggested Readings).

D. Complications. Surgical complications of radical hysterectomy are prolonged bladder dysfunction (4%), fistula formation (1% to 2%), lymphocyst requiring drainage (2% to 3%), pulmonary embolism (fewer than 1%), and operative mortality (fewer than 1%). Complications of RT include vaginal stenosis with sexual dysfunction (30% to 60%), serious small- and large-bowel injury (3% to 4%), and urinary fistula formation (2%).

E. Follow-up. In more than one third of patients, the cancer will recur, with more than 80% recurring in the first 2 years after therapy. Patients are seen every 3 months for the first 2 years. Special attention should be paid to weight loss, abdominal pain, leg pain, and lower extremity edema. Examination should include a complete physical examination with attention to the supraclavicular and inguinal lymph nodes. A pelvic examination with Pap smear and rectovaginal examination are performed. The presence of nodularity of the cervix, vagina, or rectum should prompt biopsies.

F. Background. Cervix cancer is the third most common gynecologic malignancy in the United States, with approximately 15,000 cases diagnosed annually, with

 TABLE 25.7   **FIGO Staging of Cervix Cancer, 1995**

Stage	Description
0	Carcinoma *in situ*, intraepithelial carcinoma
I	The carcinoma is confined to the cervix
IA	Invasive cancer identified only microscopically. All gross lesions, even with superficial invasion, are stage IB
IA1	Measured invasion of stroma ≤3 mm in depth, and ≤7 mm width
IA2	Measured invasion of stroma >3 mm and ≤5 mm in depth, and ≤7 mm width
IB	Clinical lesion confined to the cervix or preclinical lesion greater than stage IA
IB1	Clinical lesions ≤4 cm
IB2	Clinical lesions >4 cm
II	The carcinoma extends beyond the cervix but has not extended to the pelvic wall. The carcinoma involves the vagina but not so far as the lower one third
IIA	No obvious parametrial involvement
IIB	Obvious parametrial involvement
III	The carcinoma has extended to the pelvic wall. On rectal examination, there is no cancer-free space between the tumor and the pelvic wall. The tumor involves the lower one third of the vagina. All cases of hydronephrosis or nonfunctioning kidney are included, unless they are known to be due to other causes
IIIA	No extension to the pelvic wall
IIIB	Extension to the pelvic wall and/or hydronephrosis or nonfunctioning kidney
IV	The carcinoma has extended beyond the true pelvis or has clinically involved the mucosa of the bladder or rectum. A bullous edema as such does not permit a case to be allotted to stage IV
IVA	Spread of the growth to adjacent organs
IVB	Spread to distant organs

FIGO, International Federation of Gynecology and Obstetrics.

approximately 5,000 deaths. Worldwide, it is the second most common cancer among women, with approximately 200,000 deaths annually. Areas of the world that have implemented screening and treatment programs for preinvasive cervical lesions have decreased the mortality by approximately 90%. Risk and etiologic factors are summarized in section II.F.

G. Current focus. PET to assess for the presence of metastatic disease and help guide RT is currently being studied and is frequently performed at many institutions. Neoadjuvant chemotherapy with cisplatin and vincristine for stage IB2 lesions followed by surgery is currently being studied by the GOG. Radical trachelectomy with lymph node dissection may be an alternative option in appropriate patients with early-stage disease desiring future fertility, who have been extensively counseled (*Gynecol Oncol* 2006;[E-pub ahead of print]). Laparoscopic radical hysterectomy is another procedure being refined and explored. Multiple chemotherapeutic agents and combinations including cisplatin, carboplatin, liposomal doxorubicin, bevacizumab, topotecan, ifosfamide, and paclitaxel have been investigated for advanced stage, recurrent, or progressive disease, as these patients typically do very poorly. In a recent phase III trial of 280 patients with stage IVb, recurrent, or persistent squamous cell cervical carcinoma, combination cisplatin (50 mg/m2) plus paclitaxel (135 mg/m2) demonstrated improved progression-free survival (4.8 mo) as compared to single-agent cisplatin (2.8 mo) but no difference was found in overall median survival, and grade 3 to 4 neutropenia was more common in the combination arm (*J Clin Oncol* 2004;22:3113–3119). Combination cisplatin and topotecan has shown a survival advantage in patients with advanced or recurrent disease over single-agent platinum agents, and a phase III trial is currently under way comparing these two regimens (GOG 209). Though patients in the combination arm have demonstrated greater hematologic toxicity, quality of life was similar in patients followed up to 9 months after randomization (*J Clin Oncol* 2005;23:4617–4625).

IV. VULVAR CANCER

A. Presentation. The vast majority of patients are first seen with complaints of vulvar pruritus. The presence of a mass, ulcer, bleeding, swelling, and pain with urination also are often noted.

B. Workup and staging. A biopsy should be taken of any gross lesion and especially any new lesion on the vulva. There are a wide variety of appearances of vulvar cancers: raised, ulcerative, exophytic, white, red, and pigmented. Application of 4% acetic acid solution or toluidine blue to the vulva can help define the extent of some lesions. Use of the colposcope is only rarely helpful. A biopsy is performed under local anesthesia, using a 3- to 5-mm Keyes punch biopsy to sample the worst-appearing areas. Hemostasis is obtained with direct pressure, silver nitrate, or suture ligature. More than 90% of vulvar cancers are squamous cell carcinomas, and the other cell types (melanoma, extramammary Paget's disease, basal cell carcinoma, adenocarcinoma, verrucous carcinoma, and sarcoma) are all very rare and are beyond the scope of this text (see Suggested Readings). The trend for surgical management of all vulvar cancers has become more conservative over the last decade. The treatment for invasive vulvar cancer is radical vulvectomy with bilateral groin node dissection (usually through separate skin incisions). Two exceptions to this recommendation are (a) with biopsies demonstrating less than 1 mm of invasion, a radical (down to the level of the underlying fascia) excision with at least 1 cm margin should be performed. If the final pathology confirms only microinvasion, the groin lymph nodes need not be sampled; and (b) invasive lesions (larger than 1 mm) that are less than 2 cm in diameter and more than 2 cm from the midline may be staged with ipsilateral groin node dissection alone. FIGO staging is summarized in Table 25.8.

C. Therapy and prognosis. Surgical resection in patients with pathologically negative groin nodes is curative in more than 90% of patients. More than half of all patients with positive groin nodes will die of their disease. Currently it is recommended that patients with two or more positive groin nodes undergo inguinal and pelvic irradiation after primary surgery.

| TABLE 25.8 | FIGO Staging of Vulvar Carcinoma with TNM Classification |

TNM	Classification	Stage	Description
T	*Primary tumor*	Stage 0	Carcinoma *in situ,* intraepithelial carcinoma
T$_{is}$	Preinvasive carcinoma (carcinoma *in situ*)	Tis	
T1	Tumor confined to the vulva and/or the perineum, ≤2 cm in greatest dimension	Stage I T1 N0 M0	Tumor confined to the vulva and/or perineum, ≤2 cm in greatest dimension, nodes are negative
T2	Tumor confined to the vulva and/or perineum, >2 cm in greatest dimension	Stage II T2 N0 M0	Tumor confined to the vulva and/or perineum, >2 cm in greatest dimension, nodes are negative
T3	Tumor invades any of the following: lower urethra, vagina, or anus	Stage III T3 N0 M0 T3 N1 M0 T1 N1 M0	Tumor of any size with adjacent spread to the lower urethra and/or the vagina, or the anus, and/or unilateral regional lymph node metastasis
T4	Tumor of any size infiltrating the bladder mucosa and/or the rectal mucosa, including the upper part of the urethral mucosa and/or fixed to the bone	Stage IVA T1 N2 M0 T2 N2 M0 T3 N2 M0 T4 any N M0	Tumor invades any of the following: upper urethra, bladder mucosa, rectal mucosa, pelvic bone, and/or bilateral regional node metastasis
N	*Regional lymph nodes*		
N0	No lymph node metastasis		
N1	Unilateral regional lymph node metastasis	Stage IVB Any T, Any N, M1	Any distant metastasis including pelvic lymph nodes
N2	Bilateral regional lymph node metastasis		
M	*Distant metastasis*		
M0	No clinical metastasis		
M1	Distant metastasis (including pelvic lymph node metastasis)		

FIGO, International Federation of Gynecology and Obstetrics.

- **D. Complications.** Wound infections with skin breakdown are very common after surgery, so proper wound care is critical. Lymphocysts and lymphedema are also quite common. Diligent surgical technique and the use of negative-pressure drains help minimize this complication.
- **E. Follow-up.** Most (70% to 80%) recurrences occur in the first 2 years after the initial surgery. Patients should be examined every 3 to 6 months during this period, and biopsies should be liberally performed.
- **F. Background.** Vulvar cancer is the fourth most common gynecologic malignancy, with fewer than 3,000 cases diagnosed annually in the United States. The average age at presentation is in the mid-sixties, but there appears to be a bimodal age distribution. There is an increasing incidence of younger patients developing vulvar cancer, and this is thought to be HPV mediated. The etiology of vulvar cancer is not

well understood. HPV infection, environmental/industrial toxins, chronic irritants, chronic infections, and vulvar non-neoplastic disorders (vulvar dystrophies) may all have an etiologic role. Knowledge of the anatomy of the vulva with special attention to the lymphatic drainage is vital to understanding disease progression.

G. **Current focus.** Current study is under way to investigate the role of chemotherapy (cisplatin) as a radiation-sensitizing agent combined with standard RT for patients requiring adjuvant RT (see Section III.C. for specifics on chemoradiation with cisplatin). Neoadjuvant chemotherapy (cisplatin and 5-FU) or radiotherapy may reduce tumor size and improve operability and allow avoidance of pelvic exenteration in some patients, although this must be balanced with effects on quality of life, and data in this area is limited (*Gynecol Oncol* 2006;100:53–57).

V. VAGINAL CANCER

A. **Presentation.** Vaginal bleeding, either spontaneous or after coitus, and vaginal discharge are most common. Patients may also have an abnormal Pap smear, pelvic pain, dyspareunia, and/or bowel and bladder complaints.

B. **Workup and staging.** Biopsies of gross lesions should be performed to confirm the diagnosis of invasive cancer. A patient with an abnormal Pap smear who has previously undergone hysterectomy or in whom evaluation of the cervix showed no disease should undergo colposcopy of the vagina with biopsies. It is important to realize that tumors of the vagina represent metastatic disease from other sites more often than primary vaginal cancer. Other gynecologic cancers or colorectal carcinomas are the most common tumors metastatic to the vagina, although other metastatic cancers including renal cell have been described. Staging of vaginal cancer (Table 25.9) is similar to that of cervix cancer in that it is a clinical staging system. Stage 0 or vaginal intraepithelial neoplasia (VAIN) is preinvasive disease and is graded in a manner similar to that of CIN, from I to III. Patients with invasive disease should be evaluated with a complete history and physical examination with special attention to supraclavicular and inguinal lymph nodes. CXR and IVP are indicated as part of staging. Location and size of the tumor will dictate the necessity of cystoscopy and proctosigmoidoscopy to complete staging.

C. **Therapy and prognosis. Squamous cell carcinoma** of the vagina is by far the most common primary vaginal cancer, and stage-based treatment is as follows: **Stage 0** (intraepithelial disease) lesions have an unclear malignant potential, and usually only VAIN III lesions are treated. The lesions are often multifocal, so the method of treatment should be tailored to the given lesion(s). Simple surgical excision and/or laser vaporization are most often used. Topical 5-fluorouracil (5-FU) is also used (5 g intravaginally at nighttimes for 5 days; repeated every 2 to 3 months) but can cause significant irritation and burning. All invasive lesions (**stage I to IV**) can be treated with some form of RT; specifics of therapy as well as possible exceptions are as follows: also **stage I** lesions that are next to the cervix may be treated with radical hysterectomy, upper vaginectomy, and pelvic lymphadenectomy. Thereby,

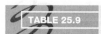

Stage	Characteristics
0	Carcinoma *in situ* (intraepithelial carcinoma)
I	Carcinoma is limited to the vaginal mucosa
II	Carcinoma has involved the subvaginal tissue but has not extended into the pelvic wall
III	Carcinoma has extended into the pelvic wall
IV	Carcinoma extension with involvement of the mucosa of the bladder or rectum or extension beyond the true pelvis

TABLE 25.9   FIGO Staging of Vaginal Cancer

FIGO, International Federation of Gynecology and Obstetrics.

the patient can often avoid radiation and preserve ovarian function. Lesions of the lower one third of the vagina, although staged similarly to upper vaginal lesions, clinically behave more like vulvar carcinomas. For these lesions, bilateral inguinal–femoral lymphadenectomy is recommended to direct possible RT. Patients also may receive RT tailored to the specific lesion(s). RT consists of brachytherapy alone (tandem and ovoids, intracavitary vaginal cylinder, or interstitial implants) or in conjunction with external-beam radiation to treat the pelvic and/or inguinal lymph nodes. **Stage II to IV** lesions are usually treated first with external-beam radiation (5,000 to 6,000 cGy) to treat the pelvic lymph nodes and to shrink the primary tumor, allowing easier application of brachytherapy. Brachytherapy with interstitial needles usually provides the best tumor dosing. **Long-term survival** in patients treated with definitive irradiation by stage at our institution is as follows: I, 75%; II, 49%; III, 32%; and IV, 10%. **Clear cell adenocarcinomas, melanomas, rhabdomyosarcomas,** and **endodermal sinus tumors** are rare tumors of the vagina and are beyond the scope of this text—refer to Suggested Readings.

D. **Complications.** Major complications of therapy (primarily radiation) are seen in 10% to 15% of patients and are directly related to the dose of radiation. Vaginal stenosis, fistulas (large or small bowel, bladder, and ureteral), bowel and ureteral obstruction, and bowel perforation are not uncommon.

E. **Follow-up.** Patients are usually seen every 3 to 6 months for the first 2 years after therapy and are evaluated with pelvic examination with Pap smear. Recurrences can be treated successfully with pelvic exenteration.

F. **Background.** Vaginal cancers are very rare, forming only 1% to 2% of gynecologic malignancies. Squamous cell carcinoma is the most common primary tumor, but metastatic disease from other sites is more common. Squamous cancers are most often located on the anterior wall of the upper third of the vagina and are usually multifocal. The specific etiology is unclear, but as with cervical cancer, HPV appears to have a role.

G. **Current focus.** The combination of chemotherapy (cisplatin) with radiation, although not well studied in vaginal squamous cancer, will likely become the preferred method of treatment, although the literature so far demonstrates conflicting results (cisplatin, 40 mg/m^2 i.v. q week for six cycles given concurrently with RT—see Section III.C.). Improved sensitivity of PET as compared to CT for detection of the vaginal lesions and positive lymph nodes has also been demonstrated at our institution (*Int J Radiat Oncol Biol Phys* 2005;62:733–737).

VI. **FALLOPIAN TUBE CARCINOMA.** Fallopian tube carcinoma is an extremely rare gynecologic malignancy that behaves biologically like serous epithelial ovarian carcinoma. Fallopian tube carcinoma is staged and treated in a manner similarly to ovarian carcinoma. The classic presentation is intermittent, profuse, watery vaginal discharge (hydrops tubae profluens). The diagnosis is seldom made preoperatively but has been detected by Pap smear in rare cases. Prognosis is related to stage of disease, with long-term survival of approximately 50% for stages I and II. As with ovarian carcinoma, long-term survival is rare with advanced disease. This disease entity is discussed further in Chapter 24.

Suggested Readings

Abu-Rustum NR, Aghajanian C, Barakat RR, et al. Salvage weekly paclitaxel in recurrent ovarian cancer. *Semin Oncol* 1997;24:62.

Ahlgren JD, Ellison NM, Gottlieb RJ, et al. Hormonal palliation of chemoresistant ovarian cancer: three consecutive phase II trials of the Mid-Atlantic oncology program. *J Clin Oncol* 1993;11:1957.

American College of Obstetricians and Gynecologists. Cervical cytology screening. ACOG Practice Bulletin No. 45. *Obstet Gynecol* 2003;103:417–427.

American College of Obstetricians and Gynecologists. Management of abnormal cervical cytology and histology. ACOG practice bulletin no. 66. *Obstet Gynecol* 2005;106: 645–664.

ASCUS-LSIL Triage Study (ALTS) Group. Results of a randomized trial on the management of cytology interpretations of atypical squamous cells of undetermined significance. *Am J Obstet Gynecol* 2003;188:1383–1392.

Ball HG, Blessing JA, Lentz SS, et al. A phase II trial of paclitaxel in patients with advanced or recurrent adenocarcinoma of the endometrium: a Gynecologic Oncology Group study. *Gynecol Oncol* 1996;62:278.

Berkowitz RS. Gestational trophoblastic diseases: recent advances in the understanding of cytogenetics, histopathology, and natural history. *Curr Opin Obstet Gynecol* 1992;4:616–620.

Berkowitz RS, Goldstein DP. Chorionic tumors. *N Engl J Med* 1996;335:1740–1748.

du Bois A, Lueck HJ, Meier W, et al. Cisplatin/paclitaxel vs. carboplatin/paclitaxel in ovarian cancer: update of an Arbeitsgemeinschaft Gynaekologische Onkologie (AGO) study group trial. *Proc Am Soc Clin Oncol* 1999;18:356a.

Bolis G, Bonazzi C, Landoni F, et al. EMA/CO regimen in high-risk gestational trophoblastic tumor (GTT). *Gynecol Oncol* 1988;31:439.

Cohn DE, Herzog TJ. Gestational trophoblastic diseases: new standards for therapy. *Curr Opin Oncol* 2000;12:492–496.

Cohn DE, Rader JS. Gynecology. In: Norton JA, Bollinger RR, Chang AE, et al. eds. *Surgery: basic science and clinical evidence.* New York: Springer-Verlag New York, 2001.

Dijkhuizen FP, Mol BW, Brolmann HA, et al. The accuracy of endometrial sampling in the diagnosis of patients with endometrial carcinoma and hyperplasia: a meta-analysis. *Cancer* 2000;89:1765–1772.

Doherty MG, Copeland LJ, Powell MA. Clinical anatomy of the pelvis. In: Copeland LJ, ed. *Textbook of gynecology.* Philadelphia: WB Saunders, 2000.

Fanning J, Evans MC, Peters AJ, et al. Adjuvant radiotherapy for stage I, grade 2 endometrial adenocarcinoma and adenoacanthoma with limited myometrial invasion. *Obstet Gynecol* 1987;70:920–922.

Fleming GF, Brunetto VL, Cella D, et al. Phase III trial of doxorubicin plus cisplatin with or without paclitaxel plus filgrastim in advanced endometrial carcinoma: a Gynecologic Oncology Group Study. *J Clin Oncol* 2004;22:2159–2166.

Gal D. Hormonal therapy for lesions of the endometrium. *Semin Oncol* 1986;13:33.

Geisler JP, Manahan KJ, Buller RE. Neoadjuvant chemotherapy in vulvar cancer: avoiding primary exenteration. *Gynecol Oncol* 2006;100:53–57.

Hertel H, Kohler C, Grand D, et al. The German Association of Gynecologic Oncologists (AGO). Radical vaginal trachelectomy (RVT) combined with laparoscopic pelvic lymphadenectomy: prospective multicenter study of 100 patients with early cervical cancer. *Gynecol Oncol* 2006;103(2):506–511.

Herzog TJ, Williams S, Adler LM, et al. Potential of cervical electrosurgical excision procedure for diagnosis and treatment of cervical intraepithelial neoplasia. *Gynecol Oncol* 1995;57:286–293.

Hicks ML, Piver MS. Conservative surgery plus adjuvant therapy for vulvovaginal rhabdomyosarcoma, diethylstilbestrol clear cell adenocarcinoma of the vagina, and unilateral germ cell tumors of the ovary. *Obstet Gynecol Clin North Am* 1992;19:219–233.

Homseley HD, Blessing JA, Rettenmaier M, et al. Weekly intramuscular methotrexate for non-metastatic gestational trophoblastic disease. *Obstet Gynecol* 1988;72:413.

Keys HM, Bundy BN, Stehman FB, et al. Cisplatin, radiation, and adjuvant hysterectomy compared with radiation and adjuvant hysterectomy for bulky stage IB cervical carcinoma. *N Engl J Med* 1999;340:1154–1161.

Keys HM, Roberts JA, Brunetto VL, et al. A phase III trial of surgery with or without adjunctive external pelvic radiation therapy in intermediate risk endometrial adenocarcinoma: a Gynecologic Oncology Group Study. *Gynecol Oncol* 2004;92:744–751.

Koutsky LA, Ault KA, Wheeler CM, et al. Proof of Principle Study Investigators. A controlled trial of a human papillomavirus type 16 vaccine. *N Engl J Med* 2002;347:1645–1651.

Krebs H-B. Premalignant lesions of the cervix. In: Copeland LJ, ed. *Textbook of gynecology.* Philadelphia: WB Saunders, 2000.

Kurman RJ, Kaminski PF, Norris HJ. The behavior of endometrial hyperplasia: a long-term study of "untreated" hyperplasia in 170 patients. *Cancer* 1985;56:403–412.

Lamoreaux WT, Grigsby PW, Dehdashti F, et al. FDG-PET evaluation of vaginal carcinoma. *Int J Radiat Oncol Biol Phys* 2005;62:733–737.

von Minckwitz G, Bauknecht T, Visseren-Gurl CM, et al. Phase II study of gemcitabine in ovarian cancer. *Ann Oncol* 1999;10:853–855.

Monk BJ, Huang HQ, Cella D, et al. Quality of life outcomes from a randomized phase III trial of cisplatin with or without topotecan in advanced carcinoma of the cervix: a Gynecologic Oncology Group Study. *J Clin Oncol* 2005;23:4617–4625.

Moore DH, Blessing JA, McQuellon RP, et al. Phase III study of cisplatin with or without paclitaxel in stage IVB, recurrent, or persistent squamous cell carcinoma of the cervix: a Gynecologic Oncology Group Study. *J Clin Oncol* 2004;22:3113–3119.

Moore DH, Valea F, Crumpler LS, et al. Hexamethylmelamine/altretamine as second-line therapy for epithelial ovarian carcinoma. *Gynecol Oncol* 1992;46:326.

Morris M, Eifel PJ, Lu J, et al. Pelvic radiation with concurrent chemotherapy compared with pelvic and para-aortic radiation for high-risk cervical cancer. *N Engl J Med* 1999;340:1137–1143.

Muggia FM, Hainsworth JD, Jeffers S, et al. Phase III study of liposomal doxorubicin in refractory ovarian cancer: antitumor activity and toxicity modification by liposomal encapsulation. *J Clin Oncol* 1997;15:987–993.

Mutch DG, Soper JT, Baker ME, et al. Recurrent gestational trophoblastic disease: experience of the Southeastern Regional Trophoblastic Disease Center. *Cancer* 1990;66:978.

Neijt JP, Engelholm SA, Tuxen MK, et al. Exploratory phase III study of paclitaxel and cisplatin versus paclitaxel and carboplatin in advanced ovarian cancer. *J Clin Oncol* 2000;18:3084–3092.

Ozols RF. Carboplatin and paclitaxel for the treatment of advanced ovarian cancer. *Int J Gynecol Cancer* 1994;4:13–18.

Ozols RF, Bundy BN, Fowler J, et al. Randomized phase III study of cisplatin (CIS)/paclitaxel (PAC) versus carboplatin (CARBO/PAC) in optimal stage III epithelial ovarian cancer (OC): a Gynecologic Oncology Group trial (GOG 158). *Proc Am Soc Clin Oncol* 1999;18:356a.

Parker WH, Fu YS, Berek JS. Uterine sarcoma in patients operated on for presumed leiomyoma and rapidly growing leiomyoma. *Obstet Gynecol* 1994;83:414–418.

Perez CA, Camel HM, Galakatos AE, et al. Definitive irradiation in carcinoma of the vagina: long-term evaluation of results. *Int J Radiat Oncol Biol Phys* 1988;15:1283.

Perez CA, Gersell DJ, McGuire WP, et al. eds. *Principles and practice of gynecologic oncology*, 3rd ed. Philadelphia: Lippincott Williams & Wilkins, 2000.

Peters WA, Liu PY, Barrett RJ, et al. Concurrent chemotherapy and pelvic radiation therapy compared with pelvic radiation therapy alone as adjuvant therapy after radical surgery in high-risk early-stage cancer of the cervix. *J Clin Oncol* 2000;18:1606–1613.

Pezeshki M, Hancock BW, Silcocks P, et al. The role of repeat uterine evacuation in the management of persistent gestational trophoblastic disease. *Gynecol Oncol* 2004;95:423–429.

Piccart MJ, Green JA, Jimenez Lacave A, et al. Oxaliplatin or paclitaxel in patients with platinum pretreated advanced ovarian cancer: a randomized phase II study of the European Organization for Research and Treatment of Cancer Gynecology Group. *J Clin Oncol* 2000;18:1193–1202.

Powell MA, Mutch DG. Tumors of the vulva. In: Edlich RF, ed. *Advances in medicine.* Arlington: ABI Professional Publications, 2000.

Randall ME, Filiaci VL, Muss H, et al. Randomized phase III trial of whole-abdominal irradiation versus doxorubicin and cisplatin chemotherapy in advanced endometrial carcinoma: a Gynecologic Oncology Group Study. *J Clin Oncol* 2006;24:36–44.

Roberts JA, Aaino R, Keys H. A phase III randomized study of surgery versus surgery plus adjunctive radiation therapy in intermediate risk endometrial adenocarcinoma. *Proc Soc Gynecol Oncol* 1998;68:258.

Rose PG, Blessing JA, Mayer AR, et al. Prolonged oral etoposide as a second-line therapy for platinum-resistant and platinum-sensitive ovarian carcinoma: a Gynecologic Oncology Group Study. *J Clin Oncol* 1998;16:405–410.

Rose PG, Bundy BN, Watkins EB, et al. Concurrent cisplatin-based radiotherapy and chemotherapy for locally advanced cervical cancer. *N Engl J Med* 1999;340: 1144–1153.

Sedlis A, Bundy BN, Rotman MZ, et al. A randomized trial of pelvic radiation therapy versus no further therapy in selected patients with stage IB carcinoma of the cervix after radical hysterectomy and pelvic lymphadenectomy: a Gynecologic Oncology Group Study. *Gynecol Oncol* 1999;73:177–183.

Silverberg SG, Major FJ, Blessing JA, et al. Carcinosarcoma (malignant mixed mesodermal tumor) of the uterus: a Gynecologic Oncology Group pathologic study of 203 cases. *Int J Gynecol Pathol* 1990;9:1.

Society of Gynecologic Oncologists. Clinical practice guidelines: uterine corpus: sarcomas. *Oncology* 1998;12:1–19.

Society of Gynecologic Oncologists. Clinical practice guidelines: gestational trophoblastic disease. *Oncology* 1998;12:455–458.

Society of Gynecologic Oncologists. Clinical practice guidelines: uterine corpus: endometrial cancer. *Oncology* 1998;12:122–126.

Solomon D, Darvey D, Kurman R, et al. The 2001 Bethesda system: terminology for reporting results of cervical cytology. Forum Group Members; Bethesda 2001 Workshop. *JAMA* 2002;287:2114–2119.

Sorensen P, Hoyer M, Jakobsen A, et al. Phase II study of vinorelbine in the treatment of platinum-resistant ovarian carcinoma. *Gynecol Oncol* 2001;81:58–62.

Stehman FB, Perez CA, Kurman RJ, et al. Uterine cervix. In: Hoskins WJ, Perez CA, Young RC, eds. *Principles and practice of gynecologic oncology*, 3rd ed. Philadelphia: Lippincott Williams & Wilkins, 2000:841–918.

Sutton G, Brunetto VL, Kilgore L, et al. A phase III trial of ifosfamide with or without cisplatin in carcinosarcoma of the uterus: a Gynecologic Oncology Group Study. *Gynecol Oncol* 2000;79:147–153.

Swisher EM, Mutch DG, Rader JS, et al. Topotecan in platinum- and paclitaxel-resistant ovarian cancer. *Gynecol Oncol* 1997;66:480–486.

Thigpen JT, Blessing J, Homesley H, et al. Phase III trial of doxorubicin ± cisplatin in advanced or recurrent endometrial carcinoma: a Gynecologic Oncology Group (GOG) Study. *Proc Am Soc Clin Oncol* 1993;12:261.

Thigpen JT, Brady MF, Homesley HD, et al. Phase III trial of doxorubicin with or without cisplatin in advanced endometrial carcinoma: a Gynecologic Oncology Group Study. *J Clin Oncol* 2004;22:3902–3908.

Trimble CL, Kauderer J, Zaino R, et al. Concurrent endometrial carcinoma in women with a biopsy diagnosis of atypical endometrial hyperplasia: a Gynecologic Oncology Group Study. *Cancer* 2006;106:812–819.

Verschraegen CR, Sittisomwong T, Kudelka AP, et al. Docetaxel for patients with paclitaxel-resistant mullerian carcinoma. *J Clin Oncol* 2000;18:2733–2739.

Villa LL, Costa RL, Petta CA, et al. Prophylactic quadrivalent human papillomavirus (types 6, 11, 16, and 18) L1 virus-like particle vaccine in young women: a randomised double-blind placebo-controlled multicentre phase II efficacy trial. *Lancet Oncol* 2005;6:271–278.

Whitney CW, Sause W, Bundy BN, et al. Randomized comparison of fluorouracil plus cisplatin versus hydroxyurea as an adjunct to radiation therapy in stage IIB-IVA carcinoma of the cervix with negative para-aortic lymph nodes: a Gynecologic Oncology Group and Southwest Oncology Group study. *J Clin Oncol* 1999;17:1339–1348.

Williams SD, Birch R, Einhorn LH, et al. Treatment of disseminated germ cell tumors with cisplatin, bleomycin and either vinblastine or etoposide. *N Engl J Med* 1987;316:1435.

Wu T, Chang T, Hsueh S, et al. Prognostic factors and impact of adjuvant chemotherapy for uterine leiomyosarcoma. *Gynecol Oncol* 2006;100:166–172.

Young RC, Walton LA, Ellenberg SS, et al. Adjuvant therapy in stage I and stage II epithelial ovarian cancer: results of two prospective randomized trials. *N Engl J Med* 1990;322:1021.

Zorlu CG, Simsek T, Ari ES. Laparoscopy or laparotomy for the management of endometrial cancer. *JSLS* 2005;9:442–446.

Zullo F, Palomba S, Russo T, et al. A prospective randomized comparison between laparoscopic and laparotomic approaches in women with early stage endometrial cancer: a focus on the quality of life. *Am J Obstet Gynecol* 2005;193:1344–1352.
http://www.cancer.org/docroot/PRO/content/PRO_1_1_2002_Fact_Sheets.asp
https://www.merckvaccines.com/gardasilProductPage_frmst.html

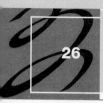

26 HEMATOLOGIC MALIGNANCIES: LYMPHOMA

Nancy L. Bartlett and Nina D. Wagner-Johnston

I. HODGKIN'S LYMPHOMA
A. Presentation
1. **Subjective.** Classical Hodgkin's disease or Hodgkin's lymphoma (HL) usually presents as painless lymphadenopathy in the cervical and/or supraclavicular regions. Isolated subdiaphragmatic lymphadenopathy or organ involvement is rare. Although staging studies reveal mediastinal adenopathy in more than 85% of patients, symptoms of cough, chest pain, dyspnea, and superior vena cava (SVC) syndrome are uncommon, even in patients with bulky mediastinal disease. Systemic symptoms or "B" symptoms, including fevers (temperature greater than 38°C), drenching night sweats, or weight loss (more than 10% of baseline body weight in the preceding 6 months) occur in 30% to 40% of patients with stage III or IV disease, but in fewer than 10% of patients with stage I or II disease. In most series, the presence of B symptoms portends a worse prognosis. Generalized, severe pruritus occurs in approximately 25% of patients with HL, often precedes the diagnosis by months, can be a presenting symptom of both early and advanced-stage disease, and has no known prognostic significance. Alcohol-induced pain in involved lymph nodes is a rare symptom of HL (less than 1%). B symptoms and pruritus usually subside within a few days of initiating therapy. When HL presents in older patients or patients with the human immunodeficiency virus (HIV), B symptoms and intra-abdominal and extranodal involvement including lung, bone marrow, liver, or bone are more common. HL as well as non-Hodgkin's lymphoma (NHL) should always be considered in the differential diagnosis of fever of unknown origin in an older patient, even without evidence of adenopathy.

   Nodular lymphocyte–predominant Hodgkin's lymphoma (LPHL), which represents less than 5% of cases of HL in the United States and Europe, is often first seen as a solitary cervical, axillary, or inguinal lymph node. In LPHL, the mediastinum is generally spared, and in contrast to the contiguous pattern of lymph node involvement in classic HL, there is no consistent pattern of spread.

2. **Objective.** Although computed tomography (CT) scans and positron emission tomography (PET) scans have replaced the physical examination in staging, thorough examination of all lymph node–bearing areas in patients with HL remains pertinent. Occasionally small supraclavicular and infraclavicular nodes can be missed on neck and chest CT scans. In addition, chest CT scans do not always include the entire axillae, especially in larger patients. Physiologic uptake in the sternocleidomastoid muscles on PET scan may decrease the sensitivity of this test in the cervical and supraclavicular regions. Identification of all involved nodal areas is especially important in early-stage patients who may receive limited chemotherapy and "involved field" radiotherapy (IFRT).

B. Workup and staging.
HL is nearly always diagnosed by an excisional lymph node biopsy, although rarely, biopsy of an extranodal site may be the source of diagnostic tissue. Diagnosis requires the presence of Hodgkin's or Reed–Sternberg cells (HRS) within an appropriate cellular background of inflammatory cells. Despite improved diagnostic techniques, needle biopsies should not be used as the sole source of diagnosis in HL. The most recent classification system proposed by the World Health Organization (WHO) classifies HL as either "classical" HL or nodular LPHL. This distinction is essential because LPHL and classical HL have different natural histories, prognoses, and treatments. Immunohistochemical studies

accurately distinguish LPHL from classical HL and should be performed if histology is equivocal. In classical HL, the large atypical cells generally express CD15 and CD30, whereas other T- and B-cell–associated antigens are usually negative. In contrast, the tumor cells of LPHL are CD20$^+$ (a pan–B-cell antigen), CD45$^+$ (leukocyte common antigen), CD15$^-$, and variably reactive for CD30, an immunophenotype often seen in B-cell NHL.

Pathologists continue to describe four patterns of classical HL, including nodular sclerosis, mixed cellularity, lymphocyte rich, and lymphocyte depletion. Nodular sclerosis Hodgkin's lymphoma (NSHL) is the most common type (60% to 80%), accounting for most cases of HL in young adults and those with mediastinal involvement. With current therapies, these subtypes have little prognostic significance.

Additional workup after a diagnostic lymph node biopsy includes a history and physical examination, laboratory evaluations, radiographic studies, and in some cases, a bone marrow biopsy. Necessary laboratory tests include a complete blood count (CBC), alkaline phosphatase, calcium, albumin, and erythrocyte sedimentation rate (optional). A significant minority of patients have a mild leukocytosis, neutrophilia, lymphopenia, and rarely eosinophilia. Elevated alkaline phosphatase is common and does not necessarily signify liver or bone involvement. Anemia and decreased albumin are usually seen only in patients with B symptoms and stage III or IV disease.

The Ann Arbor staging system for HL is detailed in Table 26.1. The designation E applies to extranodal involvement, which is limited in extent and contiguous with lymph node disease. Since the inception of the classification system in 1971, subtle modifications have been suggested but never universally adopted. Proper staging requires CT scans of the chest, abdomen, and pelvis. CT scans of the neck are optional and probably add little to a thorough physical examination. The mediastinal mass ratio (MMR), defined as the ratio of the maximal transverse diameter of the mediastinal mass to the maximal transverse intrathoracic diameter, is an important prognostic factor and should be calculated in all patients with significant mediastinal adenopathy. An MMR greater than 0.33 by chest radiograph (CXR) or 0.35 by CT portends a worse prognosis and may influence treatment recommendations. PET/CT upstages 10% to 15% of patients with HL compared to CT alone and should be considered in the initial staging of patients with early-stage disease. Bilateral bone marrow biopsies are recommended in patients with B symptoms, known stage III or IV disease, or a subdiaphragmatic presentation of stage I or II disease. Laparotomy with splenectomy, gallium scans, and lymphangiograms are no longer used to stage HL.

C. **Therapy and prognosis.** The treatment of HL has been a true success story, with approximately 80% of all patients having durable remissions. Current efforts are

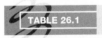

TABLE 26.1	Ann Arbor Staging System

Stage	Description
Stage I	Involvement of a single lymph node region (I) or a single extralymphatic organ or site (IE)
Stage II	Involvement of two or more lymph node regions on the same side of the diaphragm (II) or localized involvement of an extralymphatic organ or site (IIE)
Stage III	Involvement of lymph node regions on both sides of the diaphragm (III) or localized involvement of an extralymphatic organ or site (IIIE) or spleen (IIIS) or both (IIISE)
Stage IV	Diffuse or disseminated involvement of one or more extralymphatic organs with or without associated lymph node involvement

aimed at minimizing therapy for low-risk patients in an effort to avoid both short- and long-term complications.

1. **Stage I/II classical Hodgkin's disease: low risk.** Early-stage HL is usually considered "favorable" or low risk if there are no B symptoms and no sites of bulky disease, with bulk commonly defined as an MMR greater than 0.33 or a nodal mass greater than 10 cm. Extended-field radiotherapy (RT) is no longer the appropriate therapy for these patients due to long-term complications. Debate continues regarding the best approach to treatment. Several trials demonstrate equivalent survivals for chemotherapy alone versus chemotherapy followed by IFRT (*J Clin Oncol* 2005;23:4634–4642; *Blood* 2004;104:3483–3489). In most studies, chemotherapy alone is associated with a slightly inferior event-free survival (EFS) compared to combined-modality therapy. However, many investigators agree that this modest increase in relapses will be counterbalanced by a significant reduction in fatal radiation-induced complications during long-term follow-up. Both approaches are acceptable alternatives while we await mature results of randomized trials. Chemotherapy alone is particularly appealing in women aged 15 to 30 years, a subgroup particularly susceptible to second breast cancers after mediastinal and axillary radiation; smokers, due to a marked increase risk of lung cancer after mediastinal RT; and patients with a strong family history of cardiovascular disease. Trials are also ongoing to determine if lower doses of radiation (20 Gy) in combination with chemotherapy are equivalent to currently prescribed doses of 35 to 40 Gy (*J Clin Oncol* 2005;23:561s, Abst. 6506). The impact of these changes on the frequency of serious long-term complications will not be realized for at least two decades.

2. **Stage I/II classical Hodgkin's disease: high risk.** Patients with less favorable limited-stage disease, including those with B symptoms or bulky disease, should receive combined-modality therapy. At least 75% of patients are cured with this approach. Standard therapy is four to six cycles of ABVD followed by IFRT. Because most of these patients have bulky mediastinal disease, there is at least a theoretic concern about the overlapping cardiopulmonary toxicities of RT, doxorubicin, and bleomycin with this approach. Consequently, regimens that limit the cumulative doses of doxorubicin and bleomycin should be considered in this subset of patients. For example, excellent preliminary results have been reported with the Stanford V regimen plus IFRT (*J Clin Oncol* 2002;20:630–637). Chemotherapy is administered weekly for 12 weeks, alternating myelosuppressive and nonmyelosuppressive drugs, including doxorubicin, vinblastine, mechlorethamine, vincristine, bleomycin, etoposide, and prednisone (Table 26.2). The cumulative doses of doxorubicin and bleomycin, respectively, in the Stanford V regimen, are 50% and 25% of those in six cycles of ABVD. The 5-year failure-free survival (FFS) rate with Stanford V chemotherapy and IFRT was 96% for stage II patients with bulky mediastinal disease. A large cooperative group trial for bulky stage I or II HL and good prognosis stage III or IV HL comparing ABVD with the Stanford V regimen was recently completed and results are pending.

3. **Stage III/IV classical HL.** Approximately 60% to 70% of patients with advanced-stage HL can be cured with six cycles of ABVD chemotherapy, the current standard of care. The older MOPP (nitrogen mustard, vincristine, procarbazine, prednisone) chemotherapeutic regimen is inferior to ABVD, whereas the seven- to eight-drug regimens such as MOPP/ABV and MOPP/ABVD are equally efficacious but more toxic.

   The International Prognostic Factors Project on advanced HL identified seven independent prognostic factors in 1,618 patients with advanced-stage HL (*N Engl J Med* 1998;329;1506–1514). These included serum albumin less than 4 g/dL, hemoglobin less than 10.5 g/dL, male sex, aged 45 years or older, stage IV disease, leukocytosis (white blood corpuscles [WBC] greater than 15,000/mm[3]), and lymphocytopenia (lymphocyte count less than 600/mm[3] and/or lymphocyte count less than 8% of the WBC). The HL prognostic score showed that patients at the lowest risk with zero to two high-risk features had a 67% to 84% freedom

TABLE 26.2	**Chemotherapeutic Regimens**			

ABVD				
Doxorubicin	25	mg/m^2	i.v.	d1, 15
Bleomycin	10	mg/m^2	i.v.	d1, 15
Vinblastine	6	mg/m^2	i.v.	d1, 15
Dacarbazine	375	mg/m^2	i.v.	d1, 15
Cycles are repeated every 28 days				
Stanford V				
Mechlorethamine	6	mg/m^2	i.v.	wk 1, 5, 9
Doxorubicin (Adriamycin)	25	mg/m^2	i.v.	wk 1, 3, 5, 7, 9, 11
Vinblastine	6	mg/m^2	i.v.	wk 1, 3, 5, 7, 9, 11
Vincristine	1.4	mg/m^2	i.v.	wk 2, 4, 6, 8, 10, 12 (max, 2 mg)
Bleomycin	5	mg/m^2	i.v.	wk 2, 4, 6, 8, 10, 12
Etoposide	60 × 2	mg/m^2	i.v.	wk 3, 7, 11
Prednisone	40	mg/m^2	p.o.	wk 1–10 qod, taper wk 11, 12
G-CSF	5	mcg/kg	s.c.	Dose reduction or delay
Escalated BEACOPP				
Bleomycin	10	mg/m^2	i.v.	d8
Etoposide	200	mg/m^2	i.v.	d1–3
Doxorubicin (Adriamycin)	25	mg/m^2	i.v.	d1
Cyclophosphamide	1,250	mg/m^2	i.v.	d1
Vincristine	1.4	mg/m^2	i.v.	d1 (max, 2 mg)
Procarbazine	100	mg/m^2	p.o.	d1–7
Prednisone	40	mg/m^2	p.o.	d1–14
G-CSF	5	mcg/kg	s.c.	d8+
Cycles are repeated every 21 days				

G-CSF, granulocyte–colony-stimulating factor.

from progression (FFP) at 5 years, whereas those at highest risk with four to seven adverse risk factors had a 42% to 51% FFP. Efforts to minimize toxicity in low-risk patients and improve outcomes in high-risk patients are under way.

The German Hodgkin's Study Group also reported encouraging results of a more intense regimen, dose-escalated BEACOPP (bleomycin, etoposide, doxorubicin [Adriamycin], cyclophosphamide, vincristine, procarbazine, and prednisone) for patients with advanced-stage HL (Table 26.2). In a randomized trial, dose-escalated BEACOPP resulted in a 2-year FFS rate of 89% compared with 70% for standard COPP/ABVD chemotherapy (*N Engl J Med* 2003;348:2386–2395). Compared with ABVD, dose-escalated BEACOPP results in sterility in nearly all patients and is associated with a higher incidence of secondary acute leukemia. These added toxicities may be acceptable in the highest-risk patients if improved cure rates can be confirmed.

4. **LPHL.** Nodular LPHL is characterized by its indolent nature and favorable prognosis with 5- and 10-year overall survival (OS) rates of approximately 88% and 80%, respectively. Although, approximately 20% of patients with LPHL eventually relapse, the prognosis after recurrence does not change greatly, with approximately 80% and 70% OS rates at 5 and 10 years, respectively. At least half of all deaths in patients with LPHL are potentially treatment related, primarily cardiac disease and second malignancies. Unlike classical HL, LPHL does not have a contiguous pattern of spread. This, in combination with long-term complications, rules out any role for extended-field or even "regional" (involved-field

plus contiguous sites) RT in this disease. Most physicians currently recommend IFRT alone for treatment of early-stage LPHL. Because most patients are first seen with stage I disease in the neck, axilla, or groin, exposure of normal tissues would be quite limited with IFRT. Treatment for the rare patient with stage III to IV disease continues to be combination chemotherapy.

5. **Recurrent Hodgkin's disease.** All patients younger than 70 years who relapse after chemotherapy or combined-modality therapy should be considered for autologous hematopoietic cell transplant (HCT). Initially patients should receive one of several effective salvage regimens for two to four cycles to reduce tumor burden. Non–cross-resistant regimens such as ESHAP (etoposide, methylprednisolone, high-dose cytarabine, cisplatin) and ICE (ifosfamide, cisplatin, etoposide) are associated with response rates of 73% to 88% in relapsed HL. Those patients who respond to salvage chemotherapy have a better prognosis with HCT, but even patients with stable disease or minor responses following standard salvage regimens should be considered for high-dose therapy. Several studies have shown that at least 20% to 30% of these patients will achieve long-term remission with HCT. Patients with frank progression on salvage therapy should be considered for investigational approaches, as the results with autologous transplant are unacceptable in this small subset of patients.

Overall, high-dose chemotherapy with HCT is associated with progression-free survival (PFS) rates of 40% to 50%. Salvage therapy is most likely to be successful in patients whose initial remission is longer than 12 months, whose relapse is confined to limited sites including no bone marrow or pulmonary involvement at relapse, and who are without constitutional symptoms. The best approach for patients with favorable early-stage disease, treated with chemotherapy alone, who relapse in initial sites of disease must still be determined. RT or standard-dose salvage chemotherapy followed by RT may be adequate in patients with a first remission lasting more than 12 months and relapse limited to the initial site(s) of disease.

Patients who are ineligible for HCT or relapse after transplant are candidates for investigational drugs. Palliation for months or years is often possible with sequential use of single-agent chemotherapy after failure of HCT, especially in those relapsing more than 6 months after transplant. Vinblastine, chlorambucil, oral etoposide, and newer agents such as vinorelbine and gemcitabine have all shown activity in this setting.

D. **Complications**

1. **Acute complications of therapy.** ABVD chemotherapy can cause nausea, vomiting, pulmonary toxicity, fever, neutropenia, peripheral neuropathy (secondary to vinca alkaloids), hair loss, occasionally chemical phlebitis related to DTIC, and very rarely acute cardiac toxicity due to doxorubicin. All cycles require premedication with a serotonin antagonist antiemetic and dexamethasone. Central venous access for drug administration is occasionally needed because of marked pain during DTIC infusion through a peripheral vein. Bleomycin can cause acute lung injury, manifested by shortness of breath and a cough. A CXR and pulmonary-function tests should be obtained for any pulmonary symptoms developing while receiving therapy. Bleomycin should be discontinued immediately if there are new pulmonary parenchymal abnormalities or a significant decrease in the carbon dioxide diffusion in the lung (DLCO). Severe or life-threatening infections are rare with ABVD, occurring in approximately 2% of patients. Consequently, there is no role for prophylactic growth factors with this regimen. A significant minority of patients will have dose delays due to inadequate counts on day 1 of each cycle. Use of growth factors in this setting to maintain dose intensity is common practice, but not of proven clinical benefit. Small retrospective studies have shown that full dose ABVD therapy can be safely administered on schedule without growth factor support regardless of the neutrophil count on the day of therapy (*J Clin Oncol* 2006;24: Abst. 7515). Small studies of patients treated with ABVD have shown an increased risk of pulmonary toxicity with the use of growth factors presumably related to some interaction between growth factors

and bleomycin. Acute toxicities related to RT usually include mild esophagitis, dry mouth, nausea if abdominal field is radiated, fatigue, and occasionally radiation pneumonitis occurring 2 to 6 months after treatment.

2. **Late complications of therapy.** The devastating late complications of HL therapy, including second cancers and life-threatening cardiovascular disease, have led to a reconsideration of our approach to this disease. After 15 years, the actuarial risk of death from other causes surpasses deaths due to HL. Most series attribute most of the excess deaths after treatment for HL to long-term effects of radiation. Currently, there are limited data on the long-term effects of chemotherapy alone, the dose effect of radiation, and the use of more limited field radiation. These studies will be essential for evaluating new approaches to HL.

   The elimination of MOPP-like drugs from most HL-treatment regimens has dramatically decreased the incidence of treatment-related acute leukemia. Second solid tumors generally have a long latent period and continue to increase more than 30 years after therapy. Examples of the approximate relative risk (RR) of developing second solid cancers after treatment for HL include lung (10.3), breast (4.1), malignant melanoma (11.6), soft tissue sarcoma (24.3), salivary gland (37.9), and thyroid (10.6). An increase in nearly every solid tumor has been reported. The RR of breast cancer is highly dependent on the patient's age at the time of treatment, with a 40-fold increased risk in women treated before the age of 20 and only a slightly elevated risk for those older than 30 years at the time of treatment. The RR of lung cancer increases with higher doses of radiation to the lung. Importantly, there also appears to be a multiplicative effect between the carcinogenic effects of smoking and radiation.

   Cardiac disease has been responsible for approximately 20% of deaths from causes other than HL itself. After mediastinal RT, there is a more than threefold increase in the risk of cardiac deaths compared with that in a control population. Most of the deaths are due to myocardial infarction and the remainder are from congestive heart failure, pericarditis, cardiomyopathy, or valvular heart disease. Of note, the RR of cardiac deaths appears to decrease substantially when mediastinal RT doses are 30 Gy or less. Modern treatment techniques including lower doses per fraction, restricted doses to the whole heart, and delivery of RT equally from back and front should substantially decrease the risk of cardiac complications, but further follow-up is needed.

   Thyroid diseases are common after neck irradiation, with an actuarial risk of 67% at 26 years after therapy. In most of these patients, hypothyroidism develops, but the risk of Graves' disease is 7 to 20 times greater than for healthy subjects. Infertility is uncommon with modern chemotherapy and the near-complete elimination of pelvic RT.

3. **Complications of the disease.** Significant or life-threatening complications of HL are infrequent at diagnosis. Problems related to bulky mediastinal disease are most common, including cough, dyspnea, pleural effusion, and rarely SVC syndrome. Symptoms resolve rapidly after initiation of therapy. Paraneoplastic syndromes are rare and include case reports of nephropathy, cerebellar degeneration, limbic encephalopathy, opsoclonus–myoclonus, intrahepatic cholestasis, hypercalcemia, and immune thrombocytopenia. Paraneoplastic manifestations have been reported months or years before the diagnosis of HL and in many cases do not resolve, despite successful treatment of the underlying disease. HL is also associated with a poorly understood decrease in cell-mediated immunity. Patients with advanced disease exhibit lymphopenia and a depressed $CD4^+/CD8^+$ ratio. Uncommonly, patients with HL experience opportunistic infections including *Listeria* sp., mycobacteria, herpes zoster, and cytomegalovirus. The decreased $CD4^+/CD8^+$ ratio is exacerbated by therapy and is slow to recover.

E. **Follow-up.** The goals of follow-up are to provide reassurance to the patient, detect recurrent HL, and monitor for long-term complications of therapy. Anxiety and depression, often related to fear of recurrence, are common in the early follow-up period. Individual counseling, support groups, and occasionally short-term use of antidepressants may be needed.

Seventy percent of all relapses occur in the first 2 years after therapy, and fewer than 10% occur after 5 years. History and physical examination alone detect 70% to 80% of all recurrences, with at least half of these identified at appointments arranged by the patient for evaluation of symptoms, not at routine follow-up. A common practice is to perform a history and physical examination every 3 to 4 months for the first 2 years, and then every 4 to 6 months for the following 3 years. A routine annual CXR for the first 3 years detects most of the remainder of the asymptomatic recurrences. Additional routine laboratory tests and radiographs rarely detect asymptomatic recurrences. An annual thyroid-stimulating hormone (TSH) test should be done in all patients who received mediastinal or neck irradiation. CT scans should probably not be performed more often than annually for the first 2 years after therapy, if at all, and only for evaluation of symptoms thereafter. After 5 years, a history and physical examination should be obtained annually to screen for late complications; follow-up with either an oncologist or a primary care physician is appropriate at this time.

Greater emphasis should be placed on patient education, rather than on routine follow-up testing. Patients should be familiar with symptoms and patterns of relapse as well as signs and symptoms of late complications, including thyroid disease, second cancers, and cardiac disease. Education about the need to minimize sun exposure, avoid smoking, and reduce cardiovascular risk factors is essential. Women who received mediastinal or axillary irradiation should be encouraged to do breast self-examinations, and annual mammograms should be initiated 5 to 8 years after completion of treatment.

F. Background

1. **Epidemiology and risk factors.** Approximately 7,500 cases of HL are diagnosed annually in the United States. HL has a bimodal age distribution in developed countries, with the first peak occurring in the third decade of life and the second peak occurring after the age of 50 years. Men have a slightly higher incidence than women. There is an association between HL and factors that decrease exposure to infectious agents at an early age, including advanced maternal education, early birth order, decreased number of siblings, and living in a single-family residence. A history of infectious mononucleosis increases the risk of HL two- to threefold and suggests the Epstein–Barr virus (EBV) as an etiologic agent. Although, approximately 50% of patients with HL have detectable EBV DNA in the HRS cells, there is no direct evidence of a causative role. There is a slightly increased risk of HL in patients infected with HIV, but not in other conditions associated with chronic immunosuppression. An increased incidence among first-degree relatives, a significant concordance rate among identical, but not fraternal twins, and linkage with certain human leukocyte antigen (HLA) types suggest a genetic predisposition for HL.

2. **Molecular biology.** The amplification and analysis of genes of single HRS cells has provided overwhelming evidence that at least 95% of HL cases represent monoclonal B-cell disorders. Clonal immunoglobulin gene rearrangements are present in the HRS cells of both classical HL and LPHL.

3. **Genetics.** Cytogenetic analysis in lymph nodes involved by HL is limited because of the low number of obtainable mitoses from lymph node suspensions and the inability to attribute abnormalities to the malignant cells. A specific chromosomal marker of HL has not been identified, but a variety of numeric and structural abnormalities have been found in approximately half of the HL cases analyzed.

G. Current focus

1. **Ongoing research efforts include the following:**
   - Tailoring treatments based on prognostic factors, with identification of the minimal effective treatment for the most favorable patients and the role of dose intensity in high-risk patients.
   - Development of better prognostic models that incorporate potential biologic markers of HL such as soluble CD30 levels, soluble IL-2 receptors, IL-10 levels, adhesion molecules, CD44, and EBV.

■ Effective ways to incorporate new active agents such as vinorelbine and gemcitabine into the treatment of HL.

II. NHL

A. Presentation

1. **Subjective.** Presenting symptoms of NHL vary substantially depending on the pathologic subtype of NHL and the site(s) of disease. Indolent lymphomas such as follicular lymphoma (FL) or small lymphocytic (SLL) lymphomas usually present with painless peripheral adenopathy or occasionally with abdominal pain, bloating, or back pain related to bulky mesenteric or retroperitoneal adenopathy. Because spontaneous regressions occur in up to 20% of patients with FL, the patient may describe a history of waxing and waning adenopathy. Most patients with indolent lymphoma feel well at presentation, and B symptoms, including fevers, drenching night sweats, and weight loss, are unusual. MALT (mucosa-associated lymphoid tissue) lymphomas and indolent lymphomas occurring in extranodal sites, most commonly stomach and lung, usually have mild symptoms referable to the site of involvement. Indolent lymphomas are uncommon before the age of 50 years.

Many aggressive lymphomas, the most common being diffuse large B-cell (DLC), also often occur as painless, peripheral adenopathy without other associated symptoms. Fevers, night sweats, or weight loss occur in approximately 20% of patients with advanced-stage disease. Bulky retroperitoneal nodes are common and may be asymptomatic or associated with mild abdominal pain, bloating, or back pain. Mediastinal adenopathy occurs in only a few patients, usually young women with DLC lymphoma with sclerosis, and can present with cough, dyspnea, chest pain, or rarely, SVC syndrome.

Primary extranodal large cell lymphomas are common, accounting for 15% to 20% of all large cell lymphomas. NHL should remain in the differential diagnosis of a mass in any organ until pathology is confirmed. Approximately half of the extranodal lymphomas occur in the gastrointestinal tract, including stomach, bowel, tonsils, nasopharynx, and oropharynx. Other sites include bone, testis, thyroid, skin, orbit, salivary glands, sinuses, liver, kidney, lung, and central nervous system (CNS).

The very aggressive lymphomas, lymphoblastic, and small noncleaved (Burkitt's), are rare in the adult population, but can occur with acute symptoms and can be life threatening without rapid intervention. In adults, lymphoblastic lymphomas occur most commonly in young men, and frequently occur with acute respiratory compromise due to bulky mediastinal adenopathy, and pleural or pericardial effusions. Burkitt's lymphomas often present with abdominal pain and occasionally bowel obstruction related to bulky abdominal adenopathy and intestinal involvement.

Patients with HIV-associated lymphomas (usually DLC or Burkitt's subtypes) often have advanced disease, B symptoms, and involvement of liver, bone marrow, or CNS. A unique presentation of HIV-associated lymphomas is primary effusion, or body cavity–based lymphomas, which are characterized by the presence of NHL along serous membranes in the absence of identifiable tumor masses and with ascites or pleural effusions. Primary effusion lymphomas and CNS lymphomas are extremely rare in patients on appropriate retroviral therapy.

Less common subtypes of NHL often have a unique clinical presentation. Examples include, but are not limited to, mycosis fungoides, a primary cutaneous T-cell NHL characterized by pruritic patches and plaques; mantle cell lymphoma (MCL), seen most often in older men with marked hepatosplenomegaly; and primary splenic lymphoma with villous lymphocytes seen as isolated splenomegaly.

2. **Objective.** Despite the availability of CT scans, physical examination with accurate documentation of the size and location of all enlarged lymph nodes, tonsillar enlargement, hepatosplenomegaly, and skin involvement is important at the time of initial diagnosis in patients with NHL. Comparable physical examinations during and after therapy will allow evaluation of ongoing response without the need for frequent scans. Patients with active, indolent lymphomas

are often observed without therapy at diagnosis. Regular repeated physical examinations are essential to allow for intervention before significant symptoms develop. A thorough neurologic examination should be performed in all patients with lymphoblastic or Burkitt's lymphoma, looking for subtle signs of CNS involvement. Active involvement of the cerebrospinal fluid, meninges, or brain parenchyma would require a more intensive approach to the CNS.

B. Workup and staging. An adequate tissue biopsy is critical to the evaluation and treatment of all patients with NHL. The most recent WHO classification includes more than 25 subtypes of NHL, with B-cell neoplasms representing 80% to 90% of cases (Table 26.3). Optimal therapy requires accurate subclassification.

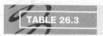

TABLE 26.3	Proposed World Health Organization Classification for NHL

B-cell neoplasms
  Precursor B-cell lymphoblastic leukemia/lymphoma[a]
  Mature B-cell neoplasms
    B-cell chronic lymphocytic leukemia/small lymphocytic lymphoma
    B-cell prolymphocytic leukemia
    Lymphoplasmacytic lymphoma (*lymphoplasmacytoid lymphoma*)[b]
    Mantle cell lymphoma
    Follicular lymphoma[c] (*follicle center lymphoma*)
    Marginal zone B-cell lymphoma of mucosa-associated lymphoid tissue (MALT) type
    Nodal marginal zone lymphoma ± monocytoid B cells
    Splenic marginal zone B-cell lymphoma
    Hairy cell leukemia
    Diffuse large B-cell lymphoma[c]
    Subtypes: mediastinal (thymic), intravascular, primary effusion lymphoma
    Burkitt lymphoma
    Plasmacytoma
    Plasma cell myeloma
T-cell neoplasms
  Precursor T-cell lymphoblastic leukemia/lymphoma[a]
  Mature T-cell and NK-cell neoplasms
    T-cell prolymphocytic leukemia
    T-cell large granular lymphocytic leukemia
    NK-cell leukemia
    Extranodal NK/T-cell lymphoma, nasal-type (*angiocentric lymphoma*)
    Mycosis fungoides[c]
    Sézary syndrome
    Angioimmunoblastic T-cell lymphoma
    Peripheral T-cell lymphoma (unspecified)[c]
    Adult T-cell leukemia/lymphoma (HTLV1+)[c]
    Systemic anaplastic large cell lymphoma (T-and null cell types)[c]
    Primary cutaneous anaplastic large cell lymphoma[c]
    Subcutaneous panniculitis-like T-cell lymphoma
    Enteropathy-type intestinal T-cell lymphoma
    Hepatosplenic γ/δ T-cell lymphoma

NHL, non-Hodgkin's lymphoma; NK, natural killer.
[a]The classification of acute lymphoid leukemias will expand on the classification of precursor B-cell and T-cell malignancies, incorporating both immunophenotypic and genetic features.
[b]Terms shown in italics have been altered in the WHO classification. The italicized version represents the term as it was used in the REAL (Revised European American Lymphoma) classification. If no italicized term appears, the REAL and WHO terms are essentially equivalent.
[c]Morphologic and/or clinical variants of these diseases are not listed, for the purpose of clarity and ease of presentation.

Historically, diagnosis and subclassification required an excisional lymph node biopsy or alternatively a surgical biopsy of an extranodal site. Although this is still the preferred approach, accurate diagnosis by core needle biopsy is now a realistic possibility in some cases of NHL, for example, small lymphocytic lymphoma, MCL, lymphoblastic lymphoma, and occasionally, DLC lymphomas. Lymphomas with a unique immunophenotype are those most likely to be diagnosed accurately with limited material. In patients without easily accessible tissue, it is reasonable to start with a radiographically guided core needle biopsy.

Immunohistochemistry (IHC), now routinely performed in most new cases of NHL, is often necessary for accurate subclassification. Common examples include the differentiation of small lymphocytic lymphoma (CD5$^+$, CD23$^+$) and mantle cell NHL (CD5$^+$, CD23$^-$), identification of peripheral T-cell lymphomas with aberrant expression of one or more of the T-cell markers CD3, CD4, CD5, CD7, and CD8, verification of lymphoblastic lymphoma with deoxynucleotidyl transferase (TdT) stains, and the presence of cyclin D1 in MCLs. Even with the aid of IHC, peripheral T-cell lymphomas can be difficult to diagnose because many have a histologic appearance similar to that of a benign, reactive lymph node and do not have a unique immunophenotype. Biopsies on patients in which the clinical history is suggestive of lymphoma, but initial histologic review as well as IHC by flow cytometry or on paraffin-embedded tissue sections is nondiagnostic, should be tested for T-cell receptor and immunoglobulin heavy-chain gene rearrangements. Cases in which the pathologic diagnosis seems inconsistent with the clinical history should be reviewed by an expert hematopathologist.

Additional workup after a diagnostic biopsy includes a history and physical examination with documentation of adenopathy, hepatosplenomegaly, performance status, the presence of B symptoms, laboratory evaluations, radiographic studies, and in most cases, a bone marrow biopsy. Necessary laboratory tests include a CBC, liver-function tests, calcium, creatinine, and lactate dehydrogenase (LDH). Cytopenias usually signify bone marrow involvement or less commonly hypersplenism. LDH is an important prognostic factor in the International Prognostics Factor Index, and patients with an elevated LDH should be considered for more aggressive therapies.

The Ann Arbor staging system, initially developed for HL, is also used to stage NHL (Table 26.1). Alternative staging systems have been proposed but never adopted. Proper staging requires CT scans of the chest, abdomen, and pelvis, as well as bilateral bone marrow biopsies. Marrow evaluation is not always necessary in asymptomatic, older patients with indolent lymphomas if a CBC is normal, as the findings are unlikely to alter management of the disease. Patients with lymphoblastic or Burkitt's lymphoma should have a lumbar puncture. If Waldeyer ring is involved, an upper gastrointestinal (GI) or upper endoscopy should be considered, given the increased incidence of gastric involvement in these patients.

PET and PET/CT scans have improved the accuracy of initial staging and response assessment, especially in patients with aggressive subtypes of NHL. As initial staging, they are most useful in patients with equivocal CT findings and in patients who appear to have localized disease at presentation, where finding additional sites of involvement could potentially alter management.

C. Therapy and prognosis

1. **Indolent lymphomas.** The approach to patients with indolent lymphomas has changed significantly in the last 5 years, due to the publication of several randomized trials showing a significant improvement in remission duration and survival with the combination of rituximab (a chimeric anti-CD20 antibody specific for B lymphocytes) and chemotherapy compared to chemotherapy alone. Despite the marked improvement in outcomes, there is still no plateau in the EFS curves with the use of chemoimmunotherapy and "cures" are unlikely. The Follicular Lymphoma International Prognostic Index (FLIPI) includes five independent poor prognostic factors, including age equal to or greater than 60, stage III or IV, greater than four involved nodal areas, elevated serum LDH, and hemoglobin less than 12 gm/dL (*Blood* 2004;104:1258–1265). The 10-year OS rate for patients with three or more risk factors according to the FLIPI is 35%

compared to 70% for patients with none or one high-risk feature. Importantly, this index was developed using data from patients treated before rituxiamb was in widespread use and these numbers likely underestimate expected survivals for all risk-groups.

a. **Stages I or II.** Given the improved sensitivity of staging studies including CT scans, PET scans, and the use of flow cytometry to evaluate bone marrow specimens, the diagnosis of limited-stage indolent lymphoma is uncommon. Observation, IFRT, single-agent rituximab, a combination of rituximab and chemotherapy, and combined-modality therapy with rituximab plus or minus chemotherapy with IFRT are all options for patients with this unusual presentation. There are no randomized trials comparing these approaches and treatment decisions should be based on the site and bulk of disease and patients' age, with the more aggressive approaches being preferred for younger patients and those with bulky stage I and stage II disease.

Gastric and other extranodal MALT lymphomas commonly present with early-stage disease. Gastric MALT lymphomas appear to occur as a direct result of antigenic stimulation from *Helicobacter pylori* infection. Most of the patients with gastric MALT lymphoma will have complete regression of disease with appropriate therapy for *H. pylori*, including antibiotics and proton-pump inhibitors (*J Natl Cancer Inst* 1997;89:1350–1355). Longer-term follow-up is needed to determine the durability of these remissions. For the subset of patients with gastric MALT lymphoma who do not respond to or relapse after *H. pylori* therapy, or are *H. pylori* negative, results with IFRT are excellent with one series of 17 patients reporting a 100% EFS at a median follow-up of 2 years (*J Clin Oncol* 1998;15:1110–1117). Other isolated extranodal presentations such as salivary gland, thyroid, breast, conjunctiva, or a unifocal skin site are also effectively treated with low-dose IFRT (30 Gy). Transformation of MALT lymphomas to aggressive, large cell lymphomas occurs in a minority of patients, but can be resistant to therapy.

b. **Stage III or IV disease.** The current standard of care for patients with indolent lymphomas requiring therapy is a combination of rituximab (R) and chemotherapy. Following the improvement in outcomes with chemoimmunotherapy, the role of observation or "watch and wait" has been questioned. However, despite many effective, but to date "noncurative" therapies, there has never been any objective evidence that early intervention improves OS in asymptomatic patients (*Lancet* 2003;362:516–522). There remains a subset of patients with indolent lymphomas that have no indications for therapy more than 15 years after diagnosis. Asymptomatic, older patients with low volume disease may still be best served by close observation until progression. Retrospective data suggesting a decreased risk of transformation with initial anthracycline-based therapy has been used as an argument in favor of early therapy (*J Clin Oncol* 2006;24:424s, Abst. 7510). Importantly, this series showed no difference in 10-year OS despite a higher incidence of transformation with nonanthracycline-based therapy and a dismal prognosis following transformation.

Several randomized trials show a significant improvement in EFS and OS with the addition of rituximab to combination chemotherapy (*Blood* 2005;105:1417–1423; *J Clin Oncol* 2004;22:558s, Abst. 6502; *Blood* 2003; 102:104a, Abst. 352). Three- to 5-year EFS rates range from 50% to 77% in recent series of combination therapy. There is no clear advantage of one chemotherapeutic regimen over another and excellent results have been reported with R-CVP (cyclophosphamide, vincristine, prednisone), R-CHOP (cyclophosphamide, doxorubicin, vincristine, and prednisone), R-FND (fludarabine, mitoxantrone, dexamethasone), and R-fludarabine. An ongoing European study (PRIMA trial) comparing R-CHOP, R-CVP, and R-FCM (fludarabine, cyclophosphamide, mitoxantrone) will help define the role of anthracycline-based chemotherapy as first-line treatment of indolent lymphoma. Currently the choice of regimen should be based on patient age and comorbid conditions. Nonanthracycline-based approaches should be considered in patients older than 65 and those with underlying cardiac disease. Fludarabine-based regimens are associated with an increased risk of opportunistic infections, particularly Varicella zoster, due to a marked, prolonged decrease in the CD4 count (*J Clin Oncol* 2005;23:694–704). Trimethoprim–sulfamethoxazole and antiviral prophylaxis should be considered during purine analog therapy and for 6 to 12 months after discontinuation of treatment to prevent *Pneumocystis carinii* pneumonia and Varicella zoster, respectively. Investigators testing R-FND in patients with newly diagnosed FL reported an alarming 4% incidence of myelodysplasia and acute myeloid leukemia (*Blood* 2005;105:4573–4575).

The question of maintenance rituximab following first-line chemoimmunotherapy is under investigation. Two large studies have shown a significant improvement in remission duration and OS with maintenance rituximab following chemoimmunotherapy for relapsed FL (*Blood* 2006;108:3295–3301; *J Clin Oncol* 2006;24:422s, Abst. 7502). Previous studies utilized a variety of maintenance schedules including one dose every 3 months for 2 years, four weekly doses every 6 months for 2 years, four weekly doses at 3 and 9 months after completion of chemoimmunotherapy and one dose every 2 months for 8 months. No data is available on continuing maintenance rituximab beyond 2 years. There are no known long-term effects of prolonged rituximab therapy.

An alternative approach for patients with low volume disease, older patients, and patients with serious comorbid conditions is single-agent rituximab. Toxicities of rituximab are mild and are limited primarily to infusion-related reactions such as fevers, chills, myalgias, transient hypotension, and rarely bronchospasm. Maintenance rituximab following an initial course of four weekly doses improves remission durations, but does not improve survival or increase the time for requiring chemotherapy compared to retreatment with rituximab at relapse (*Blood* 2004;103:4416–4423; *J Clin Oncol* 2005;23:1088–1095).

Studies of mAbs conjugated with radioisotopes are promising. Response rates of approximately 80% have been reported with both the [^{131}I]-anti-CD20 mAb, Bexxar, and the [yttrium-90]-anti-CD20 mAb, Zevalin. Side effects are modest and self-limited. The current U.S. Food and Drug Administration (FDA) approval is for patients with relapsed indolent lymphomas; however, encouraging results have been reported incorporating Bexxar into front-line therapy, either as a single agent or as consolidation following chemotherapy. Kaminski et al. reported a 95% response rate, a 75% complete response rate, and a 6-year PFS in 76 patients with previously untreated indolent lymphoma following a single dose of Bexxar (*N Engl J Med* 2005;352:441–449). Press et al. reported a 67%, 5-year PFS rate for CHOP followed by Bexxar as initial therapy of FL. (*J Clin Oncol* 2006;24:4143–4149). Larger series with longer follow-up are required before approaches incorporating radioimmunotherapy become standard of care.

c. **Relapsed disease.** Multiple effective options are available for recurrent indolent lymphoma. If the first remission lasted longer than 1 to 2 years, patients often respond to the same regimen given as first-line therapy. However, remission durations are usually shorter with each subsequent treatment. All of the agents described earlier have activity in relapsed disease. In patients younger than 70 years who relapse less than 1 year after initial treatment, or have evidence of transformation to an aggressive lymphoma, high-dose therapy with peripheral blood stem cell rescue should be considered. Most studies of autologous stem cell transplantation for relapsed indolent lymphoma show longer remission durations compared to historical controls. The only randomized trial of autologous transplant versus standard chemotherapy for relapsed indolent lymphoma showed both a PFS and OS advantage to transplant. Small series evaluating allogeneic transplant for patients with refractory disease show encouraging results. Treatment-related mortality rates have decreased significantly with the use of reduced intensity conditioning but serious complications of both acute and chronic graft versus host disease continue to restrict this approach to patients with short remissions or refractory disease following standard approaches.

2. **Aggressive NHL.** Large cell, mantle cell, Burkitt's, and lymphoblastic lymphomas compose most of the aggressive lymphomas. Standard approaches and prognosis vary for these subtypes of lymphoma and are addressed separately.

   a. **Stage I to II large cell lymphoma.** The current standard of care for limited-stage nonbulky large cell lymphoma is three cycles of R-CHOP followed by IFRT. A phase II study of this approach showed 2-year PFS and OS rates of 94% and 95%, respectively (*Blood* 2004;104:48a; abstr 158). A recent randomized trial showed no advantage to four cycles of CHOP plus RT over four cycles of CHOP alone for the treatment of low-risk localized large cell in patients older than 60 years (*J Clin Oncol* 2007;25:787–792). Long-term follow-up of a previous trial comparing limited chemotherapy plus IFRT to eight cycles of CHOP alone also showed no survival advantage to RT beyond 9 years because an excess of late lymphoma relapses in the RT arm. These results have resulted in recommendations to consider six cycles of R-CHOP plus or minus IFRT as an alternative approach, especially in older patients and those with other high-risk features such as an elevated LDH.

   Several small retrospective studies have shown a potential advantage to the 12-week chemotherapeutic regimen, VACOP-B (etoposide, doxorubicin, cyclophosphamide, vincristine, bleomycin, prednisone) followed by IFRT, compared with CHOP plus IFRT in the small subset of patients with stage I or II primary mediastinal large B-cell lymphoma with sclerosis. Because of the rarity of this disease, these treatments will not be compared in a randomized, prospective trial. R-VACOP-B plus IFRT and R-CHOP plus IFRT are both reasonable choices for these primary mediastinal large cell lymphomas.

   b. **Stage III or IV large cell lymphoma.** Two large randomized trials confirmed the superiority of R-CHOP over CHOP as first-line therapy for advanced-stage disease. In patients over the age of 60, R-CHOP was associated with 5-year EFS and OS rates of 54% and 58% respectively compared to 30% and 45% for CHOP alone (*J Clin Oncol* 2005;18:4117–4126). The second large trial in patients older than 60 also showed a marked difference in 2-year time to treatment failure (77% with R-CHOP vs. 45% with CHOP), but has not yet shown a difference in OS (*Blood* 2004;104:40a, Abst. 127). In contrast to indolent lymphomas, there is no improvement in remission duration or survival when maintenance rituximab is administered following R-CHOP. The benefit of adding rituximab to chemotherapy in patients with large cell lymphoma is most significant in tumors that overexpress bcl-2, bcl-6, or p53.

   In addition to systemic chemotherapy, the use of prophylactic intrathecal therapy should be considered for patients with testicular, orbital, epidural, paranasal sinus, or extensive bone marrow involvement. These presentations are known to carry an increased risk of CNS relapse, usually meningeal. Despite this increased risk of CNS disease, the benefits of intrathecal therapy are not proved. Specialized protocols using high-dose methotrexate and cytosine arabinoside (ara-C) should be used for patients with primary CNS lymphoma (*J Clin Oncol* 2000;18:3144–3150).

   The International Prognostic Index (IPI) helps predict prognosis for individual patients with advanced-stage large cell lymphoma. The presence or absence of five independent poor prognostic features (age older than 60 years, stage III or IV disease, more than one extranodal site, performance status two or more, and elevated serum LDH) effectively predicts an individual's risk of relapse and death from lymphoma after standard chemotherapy. For patients treated with R-CHOP, 4-year OS rates according to the IPI are approximately 86% for patients with zero to one risk factor, 81% for patients with two risk factors, and 54% to 58% for those with three or more factors (*Blood* 2005;106:147a, Abst. 492).

c. **Burkitt's lymphoma.** Burkitt's lymphomas have a poor prognosis with standard CHOP chemotherapy, and several specialized centers have developed more aggressive chemotherapeutic regimens. All stages of disease are approached similarly, although patients with stage I or II disease, who also have a normal LDH and a good performance status, have an excellent prognosis, and standard-dose therapies, such as those used for large cell lymphoma, may be appropriate for this small subset of patients. For all other patients, short-duration intensive therapies are indicated. Most current protocols prescribe four to six cycles of chemotherapy including intensive doses of alkylating agents such as cyclophosphamide or ifosfamide, vincristine, anthracyclines, and high-dose methotrexate alternating with high-dose ara-C and etoposide. Two-year EFS rates of 50% to 90% are reported with this approach. CNS prophylaxis with intrathecal methotrexate and ara-C is an essential component of therapy. Prophylactic cranial irradiation has been associated with significant intellectual impairment and is not recommended. Patients with an elevated LDH and bulky disease should be treated with allopurinol and vigorous hydration during initiation of therapy to minimize the risk of tumor lysis.

d. **Lymphoblastic lymphoma.** Treatment for this rare, highly aggressive lymphoma must include intensive combination chemotherapy and CNS prophylaxis. Most centers now use therapies modeled after acute lymphoblastic leukemia (ALL) regimens including induction, consolidation, and maintenance with total treatment duration of 2 to 3 years. Five-year survival rates with this approach are approximately 50%.

e. **MCL.** More aggressive approaches, such as those used for acute leukemia and Burkitt's lymphoma have resulted in improved outcomes for patients with MCL. Although remissions and survivals are substantially longer with intensive therapy, no study has yet reported a plateau in the PFS rate with more than 5 years of follow-up. In addition, the improved results are likely biased by patient selection, with aggressive regimens most feasible for younger patients without significant comorbidites. MCL occurs most frequently in men older than 60 years. Historical series of standard chemotherapeutic regimens such as CVP or CHOP include substantial numbers of older patients. Investigators at the MD Anderson Cancer Center reported 3-year FFS and OS rates of 64% and 82%, respectively, with R-hyperCVAD (rituximab, high-dose cyclophosphamide, vincristine, doxorubicin, dexamethasone) alternating with high-dose methotrexate and ara-C (*J Clin Oncol* 2005;23:7013–7023). The role of consolidative autologous stem cell transplant in first remission is unproven but this approach is widely used.

f. **HIV–associated lymphoma.** Treatment approaches have changed with the advent of highly active antiretroviral therapy (HAART). Previously, most clinicians favored low-dose chemotherapy because studies comparing low-dose and standard-dose therapy showed similar response and survival rates and more toxicity with standard-dose therapy. However, a study in which all patients received HAART, in addition to chemotherapy, showed a lower response rate (30% vs. 48%) and no difference in toxicity for low-dose chemotherapy compared with standard-dose chemotherapy with granulocyte–colony-stimulating factor (*J Clin Oncol* 2001;19:2171–2178). In contrast to non—HIV-related aggressive lymphomas, a small phase III study comparing R-CHOP to CHOP showed no significant difference in response rate, time to progression or OS (*Blood* 2005;106:1538–1543). Treatment-related infectious deaths occurred in 14% of patients receiving R-CHOP compared to 2% in the chemotherapy alone, group ($p = 0.035$). Of the deaths, 60% occurred in patients with CD4 counts less than $50/mm^3$. CNS prophylaxis should be considered in all patients with HIV-related lymphomas.

g. **Relapsed disease.** Patients younger than 70 to 75 years without significant concurrent illnesses should be considered for high-dose therapy and autologous or allogeneic stem cell transplantation at relapse. Several effective salvage regimens are available as cytoreduction before transplant, includ-ing most commonly ICE (ifosfamide, carboplatin, and etoposide) or ESHAP (etoposide, methylprednisolone [Solu-Medrol], high-dose ara-C, cisplatin). In patients with chemosensitive relapse, the 5-year disease-free survival (DFS) rate after transplant is approximately 40%, whereas in patients with refrac-tory relapse; it is less than 10%. Allogeneic stem cell transplant should be considered for patients with a remission duration less than 1 year after initial therapy, refractory disease at relapse, and all patients with relapsed Burkitt's or lymphoblastic lymphoma.

D. Complications

1. Therapy related.
Most first-line therapies for indolent lymphomas are well tolerated, with minimal risk of severe toxicity. Oral alkylating agents rarely cause hair loss, nausea, or significant cytopenias. Purine analogs are also not associated with hair loss or nausea, but can cause significant myelosuppression, a marked reduction in CD4 counts, and an increased risk of opportunistic infections. Rare cases of hemolytic anemia and immune thrombocytopenia have been reported with fludarabine. Most patients experience moderate to severe infusion-related symptoms, including fevers, chills, dyspnea, and hypotension, during administration of the first dose of rituximab. These side effects are uncommon with subsequent doses.

Potential complications of CHOP chemotherapy include hair loss, a moder-ate risk of fever and neutropenia, minimal nausea and vomiting if serotonin-antagonist antiemetics are used, peripheral neuropathy secondary to vinca alkaloids, cardiomyopathy related to anthracyclines, and rarely, hemorrhagic cystitis related to cyclophosphamide. The current American Society of Clinical Oncology (ASCO) guidelines recommend prophylactic hematopoietic colony-stimulating factors for patients older than 65 treated with CHOP (*J Clin Oncol* 2006;24:3187–3205). Another clinical scenario that may justify the use of pro-phylactic growth factors is a patient with extensive marrow involvement and cytopenias at diagnosis.

First-line regimens for Burkitt's and lymphoblastic lymphomas, as well as most salvage regimens for relapsed aggressive NHL, have significant toxicities associated with them, most commonly, severe pancytopenias and increased risk of life-threatening infection. Prophylactic growth factors should be used with these regimens. Renal insufficiency and mucositis occur frequently with regimens containing high-dose methotrexate. Cerebellar toxicity, somnolence, and rarely, coma are reported with high-dose ara-C, particularly in older patients. These reg-imens should usually be administered in a hospital setting with close monitoring of electrolytes, creatinine, and fluid balance.

Patients with advanced-stage Burkitt's or lymphoblastic lymphoma are at significant risk of acute tumor lysis during initiation of therapy. Patients with an elevated LDH or creatinine are at greatest risk. Complications of tumor lysis include hyperkalemia, hyperphosphatemia, hyperuricemia, renal failure, hypocal-cemia, and death. Vigorous intravenous hydration (250 to 500 mL/hour) should be given for 2 to 3 days. Bicarbonate should be avoided. While urinary alkalin-ization improves uric acid excretion, systemic alkalinity increases the chance of hypocalcemia, potentially resulting in tetany and cardiac arrhythmias. Allopurinol or rasburicase should be given before initiation of chemotherapy and continued for 10 to 14 days. If a high urine flow cannot be maintained, urgent hemodialysis may be necessary to treat and prevent life-threatening biochemical abnormalities.

Therapy-related myelodysplastic syndrome (MDS) and secondary acute myelogenous leukemia (AML) are rare but are the devastating late complications of therapy for NHL. These complications can occur in patients with indolent lymphomas as a consequence of years of intermittent alkylator therapy. There is also an increased risk of MDS/AML after stem cell transplantation with as many as 12% of patients developing this complication, a median of 4 years after transplant. Most have complex karyotypes with deletions in chromosomes 5 and 7. The prognosis is dismal. New radioimmunotherapy drugs such as Bexxar and Zevalin may also be associated with an increased risk of MDS and AML, particularly in heavily pretreated patients.

2. **Disease related.** Most patients with indolent lymphomas are asymptomatic at presentation and have no significant complications of the disease until the terminal stages. Occasionally, lymphedema related to pelvic adenopathy or hydronephrosis related to retroperitoneal adenopathy can require urgent therapy. Both RT and chemotherapy are effective modalities in this setting.

Patients with aggressive histologies occasionally have serious disease-related complications, particularly those with Burkitt's or lymphoblastic histologies. Such complications include airway obstruction secondary to paratracheal adenopathy, cardiac tamponade, paraplegia secondary to spinal cord compression, gastrointestinal bleeding, bowel obstruction or perforation, SVC syndrome, ureteral obstruction, cranial neuropathies, or radiculopathies related to meningeal involvement, and very rarely hypercalcemia or uric acid nephropathy. When these complications occur at initial presentation or first relapse, rapid initiation of chemotherapy is imperative. In patients with late-stage or refractory disease, these complications are often fatal and supportive care is appropriate.

E. **Follow-up.** The goals of follow-up are to provide reassurance to the patient, to detect recurrent or progressive NHL, and to monitor for long-term complications of therapy. Anxiety and depression, often related to fear of recurrence, are common in the early follow-up period. Individual counseling, support groups, and occasionally short-term use of antidepressants may be needed.

As described earlier, asymptomatic patients with indolent lymphoma are often observed without therapy. Appropriate follow-up for these patients includes a history and physical examination every 3 to 4 months, and a CBC, LDH, and creatinine levels check once or twice a year. Patients with significant intra-abdominal disease, but no peripheral adenopathy, need an abdominal and pelvic CT scan annually. In addition to close monitoring, patients must be educated to report potential symptoms of progression including new or enlarging lymph nodes, abdominal or back pain, bloating, lower extremity edema, or B symptoms. Because of the recurring nature of the disease, most patients with indolent lymphoma need life-long follow-up with an oncologist.

For patients with aggressive lymphomas who achieve remission with initial therapy, definitive recommendations regarding the optimal follow-up strategy are not available. A retrospective study of 36 patients with large cell lymphoma who relapsed after achieving a complete remission with combination chemotherapy revealed that 89% of these relapses were detected during unscheduled evaluations prompted by symptoms. Only 3 of 36 relapses were detected by routine screening procedures, 2 by physical examination and 1 by routine CT scan. All of these patients had physical examinations every 2 to 3 months the first year and every 4 to 6 months thereafter, a routine CBC and LDH at most visits, and radiographs every 3 months during the first year and every 6 months for the next 1 to 2 years. Most of the aggressive NHL recurrences happen in the first 2 years after treatment, and rarely after 5 years. Sites of recurrence include at least one previously involved site in 75% of cases and only new sites in 25% of cases. A reasonable approach to follow-up of these patients might include a history and physical examination every 3 months for 2 years and every 6 months for the next 3 years, with a CBC and LDH at each visit. Scans should probably not be performed more than annually for the first 2 years, and only to evaluate new symptoms during 3 to 5 years. Routine CT scans might not be indicated at all for patients at low risk for recurrence, including those with no high-risk features at diagnosis.

F. **Background**
1. **Epidemiology and risk factors.** Between 1970 and 1995, the annual incidence rate of NL increased by 3% to 4% per year. Interestingly, over the last 10 years the incidence has plateaued. The cause for the sustained increase is incompletely understood. The HIV epidemic and the increase in NHL after solid-organ transplants account for only a minority of the new lymphomas. The incidence of NHL is slightly higher in men than women, and increases exponentially with age. The most reproducible environmental risk factors include exposure to

certain pesticides or herbicides. Inconsistent associations have been reported with hair dyes, certain occupations, smoking, consuming foods high in animal fat, and receiving blood transfusions. Infectious agents, including EBV, HIV, human T-cell leukemia virus (HTLV)-1, *H. pylori, chlamydia psittaci*, hepatitis C, HHV8, and *borrelia burgdorferri* have been proposed as etiologic agents in the pathogenesis of some cases of NHL. Other factors associated with a significant increased risk of NHL include autoimmune disorders, most commonly Sjögren syndrome and rheumatoid arthritis, although it is difficult to separate the effects of immuno-suppressive drugs used to treat these diseases and the underlying autoimmune disease.

2. **Molecular biology.** Tremendous advances in our understanding of the biology of lymphomas, particularly B-cell lymphomas, have occurred since 1980. Most cases of FL contain a t(14;18) chromosomal translocation resulting in dysregulation of the bcl-2 gene, one of many important genes thought to play a role in apoptosis. Overexpression of bcl-2 appears to inhibit cell death. Extended cell survival may increase the opportunity of cells to acquire additional genetic defects in growth and proliferation genes. Multiple additional translocations and abnormalities of gene expression have been reported in NHL and are beyond the scope of this chapter. Examples of the better-characterized abnormalities include the t(8;14) translocation in most Burkitt's lymphomas, resulting in dysregulation of the c-*myc* oncogene, and a t(11;14) translocation in most MCLs with dysregulation of bcl-1, and overexpression of cyclin D1. The new DNA microarray technology will allow for rapid evaluation of gene expression in a variety of lymphomas and perhaps provide clues to the pathogenesis of this disease (*Nature* 2000;403:503–511).

3. **Genetics.** Familial aggregations of lymphoma are uncommon but reported. The molecular basis of a predisposition for lymphoma is not known. Malignant lymphomas are part of the spectrum of Li–Fraumeni syndrome (LFS), but p53 germline mutations have not been found in familial lymphomas outside the setting of LFS.

G. **Current focus of research.** Examples of ongoing research efforts aimed at improving the therapy include the following:

1. Development of adjuvant vaccine therapies for patients with FL who achieve a remission with chemotherapy. Results of two large randomized trials testing the use of "consolidative" idiotype vaccines following chemotherapy or rituximab as first-line therapy for follicular NHL are pending.

2. Development of additional mAbs directed at targets other than CD20.

3. Randomized trials to determine the efficacy of mAbs versus radioimmunoconjugates in combination with standard chemotherapy are ongoing. Trials designed to determine how best to incorporate mAbs and radioimmunoconjugates into high-dose therapy approaches are also under way.

4. Development of new prognostic indices that build on the IPI by adding biologic factors such as the molecular classification of tumors on the basis of gene expression.

5. Clarification of the role of PET/CT in interim restaging of aggressive NHLs may result in a better outcome for high-risk patients if inadequate therapies are identified early in the course of treatment and alternate approaches applied.

Suggested Readings

Alizadeh AA, Eisen MB, Davis RE, et al. Distinct types of diffuse large B-cell lymphoma identified by gene expression profiling. *Nature* 2000;403:503–511.

Blum KA, Lozanski G, Byrd JC. Adult Burkitt leukemia and lymphoma. *J Clin Oncol* 2004;104:3009–3020.

Bonadonna G, Bonfante V, Viviani S, et al. ABVD plus subtotal nodal versus involved-field radiotherapy in early-stage Hodgkin's disease: long-term results. *J Clin Oncol* 2004;22(14):2835–2841.

Coiffier B, Lepage E, Briere J, et al. CHOP Chemotherapy plus rituximab compared with CHOP alone in elderly patients with diffuse large-B-cell lymphoma. *N Engl J Med* 2002;346(4):235–242.

Czuczman MS, Weaver R, Alkuzweny B, et al. Prolonged clinical and molecular remission in patients with low-grade or follicular non-Hodgkin's lymphoma treated with rituximab plus CHOP chemotherapy: 9-year follow-up. *J Clin Oncol* 2004;22(23):4711–4716.

Diehl V, Franklin J, Pfreundschuh M, et al. Standard and increased-dose BEACOPP chemotherapy compared with COPP-ABVD for advanced Hodgkin's disease. *N Engl J Med* 2003;348(24):2386–2395.

Ghielmini M, Schmitz S-FH, Cogliatti SB, et al. Prolonged treatment with rituximab in patients with follicular lymphoma significantly increases event-free survival and response duration compared with the standard weekly × 4 schedule. *Blood* 2004;103(12):4416–4423.

Hainsworth JD, Litchy S, Shaffer DW, et al. Maximizing therapeutic benefit of rituximab: maintenance therapy versus re-treatment at progression in patients with indolent non-Hodgkin's lymphoma--a randomized phase II trial of the Minnie Pearl Cancer Research Network. *J Clin Oncol* 2005;23(6):1088–1095.

Harris NL, Jaffe ES, Diebold J, et al. World Health Organization classification of neoplastic diseases of the hematopoietic and lymphoid tissues: report of the Clinical Advisory Committee meeting, Arlie House, Virginia, November 1997. *J Clin Oncol* 1999;17:3835–3849.

Hasenclever D, Diehl V. A prognostic score for advanced Hodgkin's disease. *N Engl J Med* 1998;329:1506–1514.

Marcus R, Imrie K, Belch A, et al. CVP chemotherapy plus rituximab compared with CVP as first-line treatment for advanced follicular lymphoma. *Blood* 2005;105(4):1417–1423.

Meyer RM, Gospodarowicz MK, Connors JM, et al. Randomized comparison of ABVD chemotherapy with a strategy that includes radiation therapy in patients with limited-stage Hodgkin's lymphoma: National Cancer Institute of Canada Clinical Trials Group and the Eastern Cooperative Oncology Group. *J Clin Oncol* 2005;23(21):4634–4642.

van Oers MHJ, Klasa R, Marcus RE, et al. Rituximab maintenance improves clinical outcome of relapsed/resistant follicular NHL in patients both with and without rituximab during induction: results of a prospective randomized phase 3 intergroup trial. *Blood* 2006;108(10):3295–3301.

Press OW, Unger JM, Braziel RM, et al. Phase II trial of CHOP chemotherapy followed by Tositumomab/Iodine I-131 tositumomab for previously untreated follicular non-Hodgkin's lymphoma: five-year follow-up of Southwest Oncology Group Protocol S9911. *J Clin Oncol* 2006;24(25):4143–4149.

Rosenwald A, Wright G, Chan WC, et al. The use of molecular profiling to predict survival after chemotherapy for diffuse large-B-cell lymphoma. *N Engl J Med* 2002;346(25):1937–1947.

Straus DJ, Portlock CS, Qin J, et al. Results of a prospective randomized clinical trial of doxorubicin, bleomycin, vinblastine, and dacarbazine (ABVD) followed by radiation therapy (RT) versus ABVD alone for stages I, II, and IIIA nonbulky Hodgkin's disease. *Blood* 2004;104(12):3483–3489.

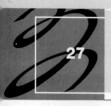

27 HEMATOLOGIC MALIGNANCIES: ACUTE LEUKEMIAS
Amanda Cashen

I. PRESENTATION
A. Subjective. Acute leukemia often presents with symptoms or signs related to pancytopenia or organ infiltration. Severe neutropenia (absolute neutrophil count [ANC] less than 100/μL) predisposes to fever and infection, especially in the sinuses, perirectal area, skin, lungs, and oropharynx. Thrombocytopenia is associated with purpura, petechiae, gingival bleeding, epistaxis, and retinal hemorrhage. Anemia can cause fatigue, shortness of breath, chest pain, or lightheadedness.

Less common presenting symptoms include lymphadenopathy, splenomegaly, and hepatomegaly, which occur more often with acute lymphoblastic leukemia (ALL) than acute myeloid leukemia (AML). Five percent to 10% of patients with ALL have involvement of the central nervous system (CNS), causing headache, confusion, and/or focal neurologic deficits. Monocytic subtypes of AML can infiltrate the skin (leukemia cutis) or gingiva, leading to purple, nontender papules or gingival hyperplasia, respectively. Tumors composed of myeloid blasts, known as *granulocytic sarcomas* or *chloromas*, can involve almost any organ and may precede bone marrow involvement by AML.

A syndrome called **leukostasis** (see Chapter 35) occurs in up to 50% of patients with AML and an absolute blast count (white blood cell [WBC] count × percent circulating blasts) exceeding 100,000/μL. Symptoms include respiratory compromise and CNS manifestations such as headache or confusion. Emergency leukapheresis can be lifesaving. Transfusion of packed red cells may increase blood viscosity and should be minimized until leukapheresis can be performed.

B. Objective. Approximately half of patients present with an elevated white count, and most have blasts circulating in the peripheral blood. Thrombocytopenia, anemia, and neutropenia are due to suppression of normal hematopoiesis in the bone marrow. Hyperuricemia, hyperphosphatemia, and hypocalcemia may indicate tumor lysis syndrome (TLS). Elevated lactate dehydrogenase (LDH) is found in most patients with ALL and many with monocytic variants of AML. Spurious laboratory values associated with hyperleukocytosis (WBC more than 100,000/μL) and blast cell metabolism can include falsely prolonged coagulation tests, hypoxemia, and hypoglycemia. Disseminated intravascular coagulation (DIC) is common in acute promyelocytic leukemia (APL) and is associated with microangiopathic hemolytic anemia, thrombocytopenia, hypofibrinogenemia, elevated fibrin split products, and prolongation of the prothrombin time.

The presence of a mediastinal mass on chest radiograph is suggestive of T-cell ALL. Osteopenia or lytic lesions may be seen in up to 50% of patients with ALL.

II. WORKUP AND STAGING.
The recommended workup of patients with newly diagnosed acute leukemia is shown in Table 27.1. A thorough history and physical examination is aimed at identifying the duration and severity of symptoms, evidence of extramedullary (including CNS) leukemia, and presence of risk factors like prior exposure to chemotherapeutic agents. Factors that will impact therapeutic decisions include coexisting medical problems, infection with human immunodeficiency virus (HIV) or hepatitis viruses, and presence of full siblings. Comprehensive laboratory testing can uncover organ dysfunction, TLS, DIC, or infection. It is also important to send a peripheral blood specimen for human leukocyte antigen (HLA) typing, as many patients will be future candidates for stem cell transplantation. A multiple-gated acquisition (MUGA) scan or other test of cardiac function is routinely performed before the patient begins anthracycline containing therapy.

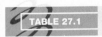

| **TABLE 27.1** | **Approach to the Newly Diagnosed Patient with Acute Leukemia** |

History/examination
  Infection: Fever; localizing symptoms, especially sinus, mouth, anogenital, skin, and lungs
  Hemorrhage: Petechiae, ecchymosis, epistaxis, oral/GI bleeding, visual complaints
        Symptoms of intracranial bleed, including headache and neurologic deficits
  Anemia: Exertional dyspnea, CHF, angina, orthostasis, syncope
  CNS leukemia: Headache, confusion, neurologic deficits
  Leukostasis: Dyspnea, headache, confusion
  Monocytic leukemia: Gingival hyperplasia and/or nontender cutaneous nodules
  Other
        Long-standing symptoms suggest preceding myelodysplasia
        Full siblings, Allergies, Major medical problems,
        HIV risk factors, Previous hepatitis,
        Previous chemotherapy, Exposure to benzene,
Routine laboratory testing
  Before treatment: blood chemistry, LFT, CBC/manual differential, PT/PTT, FDP, fibrinogen,
        uric acid, LDH, pregnancy test, HIV, HLA class I/II, urinalysis, type/cross
  During treatment: CBC daily and blood chemistry/LFT twice weekly
Radiographic studies
  Chest radiograph
  MUGA scan
Procedures
  Placement of central venous access
  Lumbar puncture if CNS leukemia is suspected
  Leukapheresis if leukostasis is present
Management of a febrile patient
  Culture blood, urine, suspected sites of infection
  Inspect indwelling line
  Initiate broad-spectrum antibiotics promptly
    Cefepime or ceftazidine or imipenem
    Vancomycin if line infection suspected
    Allergic to β-lactams: ciprofloxacin or levaquin and vancomycin
    Clinically septic: add gentamicin
    Oral or possible intraabdominal infection: add anaerobic coverage

GI, gastrointestinal; CHF, congestive heart failure; CNS, central nervous system; HIV, human immunodeficiency virus; LFT, liver function tests; CBC, complete blood count; PT, prothrombin time; PTT, partial thromboplastin time; FDP, fibrin degradation products; LDH, lactate dehydrogenase; HLA, human leukocyte antigen; MUGA, multiple-gated acquisition.

Other initial workup focuses on determining the subtype of acute leukemia. The classification of acute leukemia is based on morphology, cytochemistry, flow cytometry, and cytogenetics. Although recently supplanted by the World Health Organization (WHO) classification, the French–American–British (FAB) classification remains a commonly used system for the description of acute leukemias. The FAB classification relies on morphology, cytochemistry, and flow cytometry to define subtypes of AML (M0 through M7) and ALL (L1 through L3). Application of these criteria requires a thorough examination of the peripheral blood and bone marrow aspirate with enumeration of blasts, which are characterized by a high nucleus/cytoplasm ratio with fine nuclear chromatin and one or more nucleoli. The FAB criteria define AML when greater than 30% blasts are present in the bone marrow aspirate; greater than 20% blasts define AML in the WHO classification. Cytochemistry can be helpful in the diagnosis of acute leukemia (for instance, myeloid blasts are positive for myeloperoxidase), but now flow cytometry is the primary method for determining the leukemia subtype. Lymphoid cells are identified by the presence of CD10, CD19, and

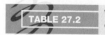

TABLE 27.2	**World Health Organization Classification of Acute Myeloid Leukemia**

AML with recurrent genetic abnormalities
   t(8;21); (*AML1/ETO*)
   inv(16) or t(16;16); (*CBFβ/MYH11*)
   APL (AML with t(15;17) and variants)
   11q23 (*MLL*) abnormalities
AML with multilineage dysplasia
   With a preceding MDS or myeloproliferative disorder
   Without a preceding MDS or myeloproliferative disorder
Therapy-related AML and MDS
   Related to an alkylating agent
   Related to a topoisonerase II inhibitor
AML not otherwise categorized
   Minimally differentiated
   Without maturation
   With maturation
   Acute myelomonocytic leukemia
   Acute monoblastic and monocytic leukemia
   Acute erythroid leukemia
   Acute megaloblastic leukemia
   Acute basophilic leukemia
   Acute panmyelosis with myelofibrosis
   Myeloid sarcoma

AML, acute myeloid leukemia; APL, acute promyelocytic leukemia; MDS, myelodysplastic syndrome.

CD20 (B cell) or CD2, CD3, CD4, CD5, and CD8 (T cell). Myeloid markers include CD13, CD33, and CD117/c-Kit; CD14 and CD64 (monocytic markers); glycophorin A (erythroid); and CD41 (megakaryocytic).

Subtypes of AML and ALL as defined by the FAB system are of limited prognostic or therapeutic importance. The WHO classification, on the other hand, incorporates cytogenetic and clinical features of known prognostic significance. In the WHO system, AML subtypes are organized into four categories: AML with recurrent genetic abnormalities, AML with multilineage dysplasia (often associated with a preceding myelodysplastic syndrome [MDS]), therapy-related AML, and AML not otherwise categorized (Table 27.2). Therapy-related AML and AML with multilineage dysplasia have a generally poor prognosis, and patients with these subtypes may be candidates for early allogeneic stem cell transplantation. In the WHO classification, ALL is categorized as precursor B-cell ALL or precursor T-cell ALL. Burkitt lymphoma/leukemia is grouped with the mature B-cell neoplasms.

It must be emphasized that cytogenetics is crucial for the prognosis and treatment of acute leukemia. Therefore, cytogenetics should be obtained on an initial bone marrow and/or peripheral blood sample. Early recognition of APL (FAB-M3, AML with t[15;17]) is particularly important, as these patients are at risk of DIC, and optimal initial treatment includes all-*trans*-retinoic acid (ATRA; see Section III.B.). Advantages and pitfalls of diagnostic tools commonly used in the diagnosis of APL are summarized in Table 27.3. Molecular techniques (Southern blot, real-time polymerase chain reaction reverse transcriptase [RT-PCR]) and fluorescence *in situ* hybridization (FISH) can detect important chromosomal rearrangements that are not apparent by routine cytogenetics. These techniques will assume greater importance as additional molecular abnormalities are described that are not accompanied by abnormal cytogenetics.

III. THERAPY AND PROGNOSIS. In the absence of antileukemic therapy, the median survival of newly diagnosed patients is 2 to 4 months. Chemotherapy induces responses

TABLE 27.3	Advantages and Pitfalls of Diagnostic Tools Commonly Used in the Diagnosis of Acute Promyelocytic Leukemia				
Methods	**Markers**	**Time**	**Advantages**	**Drawbacks**
Morphology	Dysplastic promyelocytes	30 min	Diagnostic >90%	M3 variant difficult
Immunophenotype	CD13$^+$, CD33$^+$, CD9$^+$, HLA-DR$^-$, CD34	2–3 h	Informative for uncertain morphology, detects CD56$^+$ cases	Specificity, 95%
Karyotyping/FISH	t(15, 17)	48 h	Specific for APL	Quality of mitosis, false negatives
RT-PCR/Southern blot	PML/RAR-α	6–12 h	Hallmark of APL	Qualified laboratory

FISH, fluorescence *in situ* hybridization; APL, acute promyelocytic leukemia; RT-PCR, real time–polymerase chain reaction; PML, promyelocytic leukemia; RAR, retinoic acid receptor.

in most patients with acute leukemia, although for many patients remission is short-lived. The goal of induction chemotherapy is complete remission (CR), which is a prerequisite for cure. CR is defined as normalization of blood counts (ANC more than 1,500/μL, platelet more than 100,000/μL), with bone marrow aspirate/biopsy demonstrating fewer than 5% blasts. Postremission therapeutic options include additional chemotherapy or stem cell transplantation. Chemotherapy given during CR can include consolidation (intensity similar to that for induction) and maintenance (reduced intensity administered for 18 to 36 months).

A. AML. As stated above, the prognosis for patients with AML is largely determined by the cytogenetic risk group. Translocation between chromosomes 8 and 21 (AML-ETO, t[8;21]), present in some patients with FAB-M2 AML, and inversion 16, present in most patients with FAB-M4Eo, have a favorable prognosis with chemotherapy alone. Unfavorable cytogenetics, found in 30% to 40% of AML patients, include monosomies or deletions of chromosomes 5 and 7 (−5, −7, 5q−, 7q−) and equal to or greater than three chromosomal abnormalities. Half the number of patients with AML have intermediate-risk cytogenetics, primarily a normal karyotype. In a large series from the cancer and leukemia group B (CALGB), the 5-year survival rate was 55%, 24%, and 5% for patients with favorable, intermediate, and unfavorable cytogenetics, respectively.

An active area of investigation is the identification of molecular prognostic factors that can guide therapeutic decisions in patients with normal cytogenetics. One such abnormality is an internal tandem duplication (ITD) or mutation of the *FLT3* gene, which is associated with a high WBC and a worse prognosis. For instance, among 224 AML patients with normal cytogenetics, 5-year survival was 20% for patients with an *FLT3* ITD or mutation, versus 42% for those with normal *FLT3*.

For more than 20 years, standard remission induction chemotherapy for AML has included treatment with cytarabine (cytosine arabinoside, ara-C) and an anthracycline. The most common regimen combines 7 days of continuous infusion cytarabine (100 to 200 mg/m^2/day) with 3 days of daunorubicin or idarubicin (7 + 3; Table 27.4). A bone marrow examination is repeated 14 to 21 days after starting treatment, and patients with bone marrow cellularity 20% or greater and more than 5% blasts are considered to have residual disease. Patients with persistent disease may achieve a remission after a second, usually abbreviated, course of cytarabine and daunorubicin (5 + 2). Sixty percent to 70% of patients achieve a CR after standard induction chemotherapy, with neutrophil (ANC more than 500/μL)

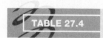

TABLE 27.4	Acute Myelogenous Leukemia Chemotherapeutic Regimens

7 and 3 chemotherapeutic regimen for newly diagnosed AML[a]

   Ara-C, 100 mg/m^2/day, as a continuous infusion for 7 days

   Daunorubicin, 45 mg/m^2/day × 3 on days 1, 2, 3 of ara-C

   Administration of additional chemotherapy: Perform bone marrow on day 14 of chemotherapy; if cellularity is >20% and blasts are >5%, administer second cycle of chemotherapy (5 and 2): same doses as above with 5 days of araC and 2 days of daunorubicin

High-dose araC consolidation regimen[b]

   Cytosine arabinoside: 3.0 g/m^2 in 500-mL D5W infused i.v. over 3-h period every 12 h twice daily, days 1, 3, 5 (total, six doses)

   Before each dose, patients must be evaluated for cerebellar dysfunction; if present, stop drug and do not resume; one way to monitor cerebellar function is to have patients sign name on sheet of paper before each dose; for significant change in signature, physician should evaluate patient before any further therapy is given

   To avoid chemical keratitis, administer dexamethasone eye drops, 0.1% 2 drops OU q6 h starting 1 h before first dose and continued until 48 h after last dose

Use of Gemtuzumab (Mylotarg)

   Dose is 9 mg/m^2; a second dose is usually given ~14 days later; each dose is given as a 2-h i.v. infusion; fever, which may be delayed, is the most common immediate reaction

   Premedication: acetaminophen (Tylenol) and diphenhydramine (Benadryl), 50 mg, are given p.o. 1 h before; repeat Tylenol 4 and 8 h later; observe for a minimum of 4 h after dose

AML, acute myelogenous leukemia; araC, cytosine arabinoside.
[a]From Bloomfield CD, James GW, Gottlieb A, et al. Treatment of acute myelocytic leukemia: a study by cancer and leukemia group B. *Blood* 1981;58:1203–1212, with permission.
[b]From Mayer RJ, Davis RB, Schiffer CA, et al. Intensive postremission chemotherapy in adults with acute myeloid leukemia. *N Engl J Med* 1994;331:896, with permission.

and platelet (more than 20,000/μL) recovery occurring an average of 21 to 25 days after the start of therapy. Failure to achieve CR with induction chemotherapy can result from resistant leukemia or early death. Therapy-related mortality increases with age, poor performance status, and underlying organ dysfunction and can be as high as 30% to 40% in elderly patients. Resistant leukemia is associated with a preceding hematologic disorder and adverse cytogenetics, both of which are found more commonly in elderly patients.

Patients will invariably relapse if they do not receive additional therapy after achieving CR. Commonly used consolidation strategies include high-dose cytarabine (HDAC), autologous stem cell transplantation, or allogeneic stem cell transplantation. HDAC (Table 27.4) can overcome resistance to conventional doses of the drug, producing CR in approximately 40% of patients with resistant leukemia. On this basis, trials of HDAC consolidation for AML in first CR (CR1) were carried out. The value of HDAC consolidation was demonstrated in a CALGB trial, which randomized 596 patients in CR1 to consolidation with four cycles of conventional-dose (100 mg/m^2/day × 5 days), intermediate-dose (400 mg/m^2/day × 5 days), or high-dose (3.0 g/m^2, total of six doses over 5 days) cytarabine. Among patients less than or equal to 60 years old, 4-year progression-free survival was 44% for HDAC consolidation versus 24% for conventional-dose cytarabine. Patients older than 60 did poorly regardless of the type of consolidation they received, with fewer than 20% achieving durable remission. The subgroup analysis of this trial underlines the critical role of cytogenetics for predicting the outcome of consolidation therapy for AML. The estimated likelihood of cure among patients with favorable cytogenetics (t[8;21] and inv16) who received HDAC was 84% versus less than 25% for patients with unfavorable cytogenetics.

HDAC can produce significant neurotoxicity, primarily cerebellar dysfunction and less commonly somnolence or confusion. Cerebellar function should be assessed before each dose, and the drug should be stopped if there is evidence of neurotoxicity. A sensitive way to assess cerebellar function is to ask the patient to sign his or her name on a signature record before each dose. Another unique toxicity of HDAC is keratitis, which can be prevented by administration of dexamethasone eye drops, 0.1%, two drops to each eye every 6 hours, from the time treatment is started until 48 hours after HDAC ends. Other potential toxicities of HDAC include an erythematous rash, often worse on the palms and soles, and hepatic dysfunction.

Several trials have examined the role of consolidation with allogeneic or autologous transplantation for patients younger than 55 to 60 years with AML in CR1. In these studies, transplantation was associated with improved leukemia-free survival compared with chemotherapy. However, overall survival was not significantly improved, probably because transplantation is associated with higher treatment-related mortality and because some patients who relapse after consolidation chemotherapy can be salvaged with transplantation. These trials also found that cytogenetic risk group was the major determinant of survival, regardless of whether consolidation was with chemotherapy or transplantation.

The available data from clinical trials allows therapeutic recommendations to be made for some groups. Because 60% to 70% of patients with AML and favorable cytogenetics achieve 3-year survival with intensive consolidation that includes HDAC, chemotherapy is the treatment of choice for this group. On the other hand, patients with adverse cytogenetics have a very poor outcome with conventional chemotherapy. For these patients, allogeneic transplant in CR1 is the treatment of choice, if a matched sibling or matched unrelated donor (MUD) can be identified. For patients with adverse cytogenetics who do not have a histocompatible donor or who could not tolerate the toxicity of an unrelated donor transplant, autologous transplant is an option. Optimal treatment for patients with intermediate-risk cytogenetics is not clear.

When patients with AML relapse after conventional chemotherapy, they generally do so within 3 years. The risk of relapse more than 5 years after diagnosis is 5% or less. For patients with relapsed AML and for those who do not achieve CR despite optimal induction chemotherapy, the only treatment option with curative potential is stem cell transplantation. For patients with an HLA-identical sibling, allogeneic transplant is the treatment of choice among those younger than 60. Recent results with reduced intensity regimens suggest that, in the absence of major medical problems, older patients can safely undergo allogeneic transplant. However, relapse is common, and only 20% to 30% of those transplanted in second CR (CR2) are cured. Disease status at transplant (CR2 vs. relapse) and the presence or absence of graft-versus-host disease are the most important prognostic factors. For relapsed patients (younger than 60) who lack an HLA-identical sibling, MUD transplant is the treatment of choice. However, durable remission occurs in fewer than 10% of patients who undergo MUD transplant in overt relapse.

Because outcomes are poor when patients are transplanted with active AML, an attempt is often made to achieve CR before transplant. Salvage chemotherapeutic regimens for relapsed or refractory disease include HDAC $\pm$ an anthracycline, etoposide with mitoxantrone, or fludarabine containing regimens. Participation in a clinical trial is strongly recommended.

Another treatment option for recurrent AML is gemtuzumab ozogamicin (Mylotarg), a recombinant, humanized anti-CD33 antibody conjugated to the cytotoxic agent calicheamicin. CD33 is present on leukemic blasts in more than 80% of patients with AML and is also expressed by committed hematopoietic progenitors. When the antibody binds to CD33, calicheamicin is internalized, leading to cell death. Gemtuzumab ozogamicin is approved for the treatment of resistant AML in patients 60 years or older, based on data from three single-arm, multicenter trials that included 142 patients with AML in first relapse. The overall response rate in these trials was 30% (16% CR and 14% CR but with a platelet count less than 100,000/μL). Most patients went on to receive additional chemotherapy or stem cell transplant. Median relapse-free survival was 7 months. The role of gemtuzumab ozogamicin in remission consolidation and in front-line therapy is being explored in a number of ongoing trials.

Gemtuzumab ozogamicin is given as a 2-hour infusion at a dose of 9 mg/m^2, and most patients receive at least two doses, 14 to 28 days apart. Most patients experience an infusion-related symptom complex which includes chills, fever, nausea, and vomiting. Anaphylaxis is rare. Because of these side effects, patients should be premedicated with acetaminophen and diphenhydramine (Benadryl) with careful observation and frequent vital signs taken for at least 4 hours after the infusion begins. Essentially all patients treated with gemtuzumab ozogamicin develop grade 3 or 4 neutropenia or thrombocytopenia, and the median time to ANC more than 500/μL and platelet greater than 25,000/μL is approximately 40 days from the first dose. Although gemtuzumab ozogamicin lacks chemotherapy-related side effects such as stomatitis and enteritis, the severe pancytopenia it causes is similar to that produced by intensive chemotherapy. Patients must be followed carefully for infectious complications.

B. APL. APL is a distinct clinical and pathologic subtype of AML, characterized by a reciprocal translocation between the long arms of chromosomes 15 and 17. The breakpoint on chromosome 17 disrupts a gene that encodes a nuclear receptor for retinoic acid (RAR-α), and its translocation, most commonly to chromosome 15, results in a fusion protein, PML-RAR-α. Detection of PML-RAR-α is associated with a good prognosis. Indeed, patients with APL who achieve CR have better long-term survival than do other patients with AML. Given its unique response to specific therapy, rapid and accurate diagnosis is crucial. It is now commonly accepted that molecular evidence of the PML/RAR-α rearrangement is the hallmark of this disease, as it may be found in the absence of t(15,17).

As soon as the diagnosis of APL is entertained, it is critical to identify and manage **APL-associated coagulopathy.** Five percent to 10% of patients with APL die of hemorrhagic complications during induction chemotherapy, and approximately half these deaths occur within the first week of diagnosis. Consequently, monitoring DIC with twice-daily serum fibrinogen levels and aggressive replacement with cryoprecipitate (5 to 10 units for fibrinogen less than 100 mg/dL) is common clinical practice during the first weeks of treatment of APL. Patients may also require liberal transfusion of fresh frozen plasma. If coagulopathy or bleeding is present, the platelet count should be maintained greater than 30 to 50,000/μL.

A distinguishing feature of APL is its sensitivity to ATRA. The advantage of including ATRA in the front-line therapy for APL has now been clearly established in several randomized trials, with CR rates ranging from 72% to 95%, and a 3- to 4-year disease-free survival of 62% to 75%. These studies also found that disease-free survival is improved when ATRA is given concurrently with chemotherapy. Furthermore, the addition of maintenance therapy with ATRA and/or chemotherapy after two cycles of intensive postremission consolidation is associated with improved disease-free and overall survival. However, many questions remain unanswered. In some studies, cytarabine was omitted inconsequently from induction and/or consolidation regimens. Given the lack of randomized trials, long-term results of these trials are needed to clarify the role cytarabine plays in the management of APL. Additionally, the optimal maintenance regimen is still unknown. In one study, the combination of ATRA (45 mg/m^2/day, 15 days every 3 months) with 6-mercaptopurine (90 mg/m^2/day, orally) and methotrexate (15 mg/m^2/week, orally) was associated with the lowest relapse rates, especially for APL patients with a high WBC. An approach for the treatment of patients with newly diagnosed APL is summarized in the algorithm in Fig. 27.1.

Because abnormal promyelocytes may be found in the bone marrow several weeks after the initiation of induction therapy, without any prognostic significance, early evaluation for persistent disease is not helpful, as it is with other subtypes of AML. Rather, the first morphologic and cytogenetic evaluation should be performed 5 to 6 weeks after induction. At that point, patients who have achieved

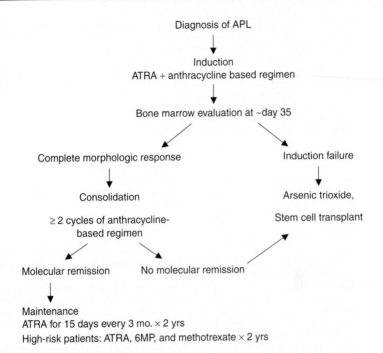

Figure 27.1. Proposed algorithm for patients with newly diagnosed APL (acute promyelocytic leukemia), ATRA, all-*trans*-retinoic acid.

a cytogenetic remission should proceed to consolidation therapy. Approximately half the number of patients in CR will still have PML-RARα detected by RT-PCR at the end of induction, and the persistence of the PML-RARα transcript at this time point does not necessitate a change in therapy. However, patients who have not achieved a molecular remission (polymerase chain reaction [PCR] negative) at the completion of consolidation should receive salvage therapy (discussed in the subsequent text). RT-PCR should be used to monitor for disease relapse, and the emergence of a detectable PML-RARα transcript is reason to consider salvage therapy.

The two most important factors affecting CR rates and survival in patients with APL are age and the WBC at diagnosis. Age younger than 30 and WBC less than 5,000 to 10,000/μL are favorable prognostic factors. In contrast, several other biologic features such as the type of PML-RARα isoform, additional karyotypic abnormalities, and expression of the reciprocal RARα-PML transcript do not appear to influence outcome. Recent data suggest that the expression of CD56 antigen on promyelocytes is associated with an increased risk for relapse.

Although ATRA is usually well tolerated, some patients develop a unique complication called **retinoic acid syndrome** (RAS). RAS occurs usually early after initiation of ATRA (7 to 12 days) and is diagnosed on clinical grounds. It is characterized by unexplained fever (80%), weight gain (50%), respiratory distress (90%), lung infiltrates (80%), pleural (50%) or pericardial effusion (20%), hypotension (10%), and renal failure (40%). RAS is the most serious toxicity of ATRA and is often, but not always, associated with the development of hyperleukocytosis. Its incidence varies from 6% to 25%, and mortality is variable (7% to 27%). The best approach to predict, prevent, or treat this syndrome has not been established. Early institution of corticosteroids (dexamethasone, 10 mg i.v. twice daily) simultaneous with cytoreduction (induction chemotherapy or hydroxyurea) is associated with rapid resolution of the syndrome in most patients. Discontinuation of ATRA is common practice after onset of RAS. RAS has not been observed when ATRA was given as maintenance therapy.

Approximately 10% to 25% of patients treated with ATRA-based therapy ultimately relapse. The duration of first CR and the achievement of a second PCR-negative remission after reinduction have been shown to be prognostic determinants. The first choice for salvage therapy is usually arsenic trioxide (ATO). In a U.S. trial, 85% of patients treated with relapsed APL treated with ATO achieved a CR, 91% of whom had a molecular remission. However, most patients will relapse without additional therapy, which may include additional course of ATO, chemotherapy, and/or autologous or allogeneic stem cell transplantation. Toxicities of ATO include QT prolongation, which rarely may lead to torsades de pointes, and APL differentiation syndrome, which is similar to RAS.

Patients with APL who undergo autologous stem cell transplantation while in second remission have a 30% 7-year leukemia-free survival. However, after stratification according to PCR status of the grafted marrow, it appears that patients transplanted with PML-RARα−negative marrow cells are more likely to have prolonged clinical and molecular remissions. In contrast, relapse after autologous transplant is inevitable in patients with persistently positive PCR after reinduction and consolidation therapy. Allogeneic stem cell transplantation may be the preferable treatment modality in this setting.

C. **ALL.** For ALL, clinically meaningful subtypes are defined by immunophenotype (B-progenitor, B cell, and T cell) as determined by flow cytometry. As for AML, cytogenetics is of critical prognostic and therapeutic value. Translocation between chromosomes 12 and 21 (TEL-AML, t[12;21]), found in 25% of pediatric ALL but rarely in adult ALL, is associated with a good prognosis. Cytogenetics associated with a poor prognosis include abnormalities of 11q23 (mixed lineage leukemia (MLL)) and presence of the Ph chromosome (BCR-ABL, t[9;22]).

Accurate subtyping of ALL is essential for appropriate treatment. Approximately 70% to 75% of patients have B-precursor, 20% to 25% have T-cell, and approximately 5% have mature B-cell ALL. **Mature B-cell ALL** expresses surface-membrane immunoglobulin and is characterized by the t(8;14), which results in fusion of the *myc* oncogene with part of the immunoglobulin heavy-chain gene. Variant translocations involve *myc* and light-chain genes (t[2;8], t[8;22]). Mature B-cell ALL is the leukemic equivalent of Burkitt's lymphoma and is arbitrarily defined by the presence of more than 25% blasts in the bone marrow. B-cell ALL/Burkitt is the most rapidly proliferating neoplasm, and treatment is often complicated by TLS. Treatment for mature B-cell ALL differs from that for other types of ALL in that intensive chemotherapy is given over a relatively short period (2 to 8 months) without maintenance chemotherapy. Important components of this therapy include high total doses of cyclophosphamide and/or ifosfamide given in fractions over several days along with HDAC and high-dose methotrexate. Addition of the anti-CD20 monoclonal antibody rituximab to the chemotherapeutic regimen appears to improve CR rate and disease-free survival. Intrathecal chemotherapy is included in the therapy of mature B-cell ALL, because without adequate prophylaxis, CNS relapse is common. With an aggressive combination of chemotherapy and intrathecal therapy, 50% to 70% of patients achieve long-term disease-free survival.

Treatment of **B-progenitor and T-cell ALL** in adults was adapted from regimens developed for high-risk childhood ALL. Therapy is comprised of four components: induction, consolidation, and maintenance, as well as CNS prophylaxis. For induction, combinations of vincristine, prednisone or dexamethasone, L-asparaginase, and an anthracycline result in CR rates of 75% to 90%. Inclusion of cyclophosphamide and cytarabine appears to increase CR rate and remission duration, particularly among patients with T-cell ALL. Standard consolidation therapy includes treatment with several cycles of chemotherapy that include agents used during induction, along with antimetabolites such as 6-mercaptopurine and methotrexate. Recent trials have examined the role of intensive consolidation including HDAC and high-dose methotrexate. Patients with Ph+ ALL probably benefit from the incorporation of the BCR-ABL inhibitor imatinib into the treatment regimen.

Whereas CNS relapse is very uncommon in AML, in the absence of CNS prophylaxis, the risk of CNS relapse in ALL exceeds 10%; therefore consolidation therapy has usually included intrathecal chemotherapy and cranial radiation. However, cranial radiation may be associated with long-term neurologic sequelae including impaired cognition. Recent studies indicate that the combination of intrathecal prophylaxis and CNS-penetrating chemotherapy is associated with a risk of CNS relapse similar to that achieved with intrathecal prophylaxis and cranial radiotherapy.

For patients with B-progenitor and T-cell ALL, induction and consolidation usually occupy the first 6 months after diagnosis. Patients then go on to receive maintenance chemotherapy. The most commonly used regimen includes daily oral 6-mercaptopurine, weekly oral methotrexate, a single intravenous dose of vincristine monthly, and 5 days of prednisone/month. Maintenance therapy is continued until 24 to 36 months after diagnosis. With this approach, the likelihood of 5-year disease-free survival is approximately 25% to 50%.

In addition to the importance of cytogenetics in determining the outcome of ALL, presenting white count and age demonstrate independent prognostic significance in multivariate models. Another important factor is the rate of clearance of blast cells; patients who achieve CR more rapidly are more likely to achieve durable remission. On the basis of data from CALGB, adult B-progenitor and T-cell ALL can be divided into three prognostic groups. Good-risk patients are characterized by all of the following: absence of adverse cytogenetics; age less than 35 ; presenting WBC less than $30,000/\mu$L; and remission achieved within 4 weeks of diagnosis. These patients have a 50% to 75% likelihood of 3-year disease-free survival with chemotherapy, so that transplant is reserved for relapse. Poor-risk patients are characterized by any of the following: adverse cytogenetics (particularly t[9;22]); for B progenitor, presenting WBC greater than $100,000/\mu$L; more than 4 weeks to achieve CR; and age older than 60 . For these patients, 3-year disease-free survival is 0% to 20% with conventional chemotherapy, so that allogeneic transplant is the treatment of choice for patients younger than 60 with histocompatible donors. Older patients may be candidates if they are in good health. The remaining intermediate-risk patients represent approximately one third of all cases of ALL and primarily include patients younger than 60 with B-progenitor ALL. For these patients, chemotherapy appears to be the treatment of choice, because transplantation has not been proven to improve survival.

Most adult patients with ALL will experience disease relapse. Reinduction is most successful if the patient has been in CR for more than 1 year before relapse. Salvage chemotherapeutic regimens can include HDAC, mitoxantrone, or fludarabine. The araguanosine analog nelarabine is active in relapsed T-cell ALL. As for patients with relapsed AML, allogeneic stem cell transplantation is the only potentially curative therapy for patients with relapsed ALL, and eligible patients who achieve a second remission should proceed as quickly as possible to transplantation.

D. CNS involvement with acute leukemia. Patients with acute leukemia who develop neurologic symptoms or signs should be evaluated with computed tomography (CT) or magnetic resonance imaging (MRI) of the head and, in the absence of a mass lesion, proceed to lumbar puncture. Cerebrospinal fluid (CSF) should be sent for glucose, protein, routine cultures, Gram's stain, cryptococcal antigen, cell count with differential, and cytology. In the absence of contamination with peripheral blood, patients with blasts in the CSF should receive intrathecal chemotherapy, preferably through an Ommaya reservoir. Cranial radiotherapy can also be considered. Intrathecal therapy may include methotrexate, 12 to 15 mg, or cytarabine, 50 to 100 mg. Drugs must be preservative-free and sterile. Cytology and cell count with cytospin differential should be repeated with each intrathecal treatment until blasts have cleared. Intrathecal therapy is given twice weekly until blasts have cleared and then monthly for 6 to 12 months.

The sudden onset of unexplained cranial nerve palsy in a patient with acute leukemia is usually due to CNS leukemia, regardless of whether the CSF shows blasts. Such patients should be treated as described above. Because isolated CNS relapse of leukemia is generally followed soon thereafter by systemic relapse, salvage chemotherapy followed by allogeneic transplant should be considered if patients relapse with CNS involvement.

IV. COMPLICATIONS AND SUPPORTIVE CARE

A. Transfusions. Essentially all adults with acute leukemia will require support with multiple platelet and red cell transfusions. In the absence of bleeding, platelet transfusions can safely be withheld until the platelet count is less than or equal to $10,000/\mu L$. Patients who are bleeding or need a surgical procedure should have their platelet count maintained at greater than $50,000/\mu L$ (greater than $100,000/\mu L$ for CNS bleeding). Menstruation should be suppressed to reduce uterine blood loss. The threshold for routine transfusion of red blood cells may vary from patient to patient. The policy at Washington University is to transfuse blood to maintain hemoglobin at greater than 8.0 g/dL. However, younger patients may tolerate lower levels, whereas older patients and those who are critically ill may require a higher threshold value for red cell transfusion. Hypofibrinogenemia, usually the result of DIC or treatment with L-asparaginase, should be treated with cryoprecipitate when the fibrinogen decreases to less than 100 mg/dL. All blood products must be irradiated (2,850 cGy), in order to prevent transfusion-related graft-versus-host disease.

Poor response to platelet transfusions may occur when leukocyte contamination of blood products results in alloimmunization. Platelet refractoriness can be reduced by transfusing leukoreduced products and minimizing the number of transfusions a patient receives. Patients with poor increments to platelet transfusions may respond to HLA-matched products. Family members are a potential source of HLA-matched products, although the use of products from related donors may increase the risk of rejecting a subsequent sibling-donor allogeneic stem cell transplant.

An effort should be made to prevent transfusion-related infection with cytomegalovirus (CMV) in any patient who is a potential candidate for allogeneic transplant, as reactivation of CMV after allogeneic transplant can result in life-threatening or fatal disease. To this end, CMV-seronegative patients should receive products that have been collected from seronegative donors. If such products are not available, then the risk of CMV transmission may be reduced by leukoreduction of platelet products. Patients who are CMV seropositive may receive blood products from seropositive or seronegative donors.

B. Infection. Infection is a major cause of death in patients with acute leukemia. These patients are at high risk of infection primarily due to prolonged periods of neutropenia. In addition, indwelling catheters and compromised mucosal barriers (mucositis or enteritis from chemotherapy) provide portals of entry for infectious agents. Because most infections arise from the patient's own microbial flora, rigorous isolation procedures are not necessary. However, good hand washing is always important, and patients should wear a mask when in crowds. Food-borne infection is very uncommon, and it is reasonable to prohibit only consumption of uncooked meat.

Antimicrobial prophylaxis during periods of neutropenia and/or immunosuppression can reduce the incidence of some viral, fungal, and bacterial infections. Acyclovir (400 PO t.i.d. or 125 mg/m^2 i.v. b.i.d.) is recommended for patients with a history of cold sores or herpes simplex seropositivity. Patients with ALL are treated with a long course of steroids and are therefore at risk of *Pneumocystis* pneumonia. They should receive *Pneumocystis* prophylaxis with either trimethoprim/sulfamethoxazole 1 double strength (DS) b.i.d. 2 days/week, dapsone 100 mg daily, or aerosolized pentamidine, 300 mg monthly. During periods of neutropenia or prolonged steroid use, nystatin (15 mL, swish and swallow 5 times a day) or clotrimazole troche (5 times daily) can reduce oral candidiasis. The use of other antibiotics for infection prophylaxis is controversial. Oral fluoroquinolones reduce the risk of infection with gram-negative organisms, but they are associated with an increased risk of gram-positive bacteremia and fluoroquinolone-resistant *Pseudomonas aeruginosa*. Because prophylaxis with systemic antifungals has not been shown to reduce the risk of treatment-related mortality, their routine use during induction chemotherapy is not recommended.

Fever greater than $38.3°C$ in a neutropenic patient (ANC less than $500/\mu L$) requires prompt evaluation and treatment, as bacterial infections can become rapidly life-threatening. Blood and urine should be cultured, and empiric broad-spectrum antibiotics (cefepime or ceftazidime, 1 g i.v.) should be administered. Vancomycin should be added for the following indications: severe mucositis, evidence of a catheter-related infection, fever equal to or greater than $40°C$, hypotension, or known colonization with resistant streptococci or staphylococci. Patients with allergy to β-lactams may receive aztreonam or a fluoroquinolone with vancomycin. Febrile patients with hypotension or respiratory distress should receive at least one dose of an aminoglycoside antibiotic (gentamicin 5 mg/kg i.v.). When fevers and neutropenia persist for more than 3 days and no source of infection has been identified, empiric antifungal coverage can be added (caspofungin 70 mg i.v. loading dose × 1 then 50 mg i.v. qd or fluconazole 400 mg i.v. qd). Febrile patients with newly diagnosed or relapsed acute leukemia should receive empiric broad-spectrum antibiotics whether or not they are neutropenic.

Once antibiotics are begun, they are continued until neutrophil recovery (ANC greater than $500/\mu L$), even if fever resolves. Otherwise, the choice and duration of antimicrobial therapy is dictated by the source of infection. Bacteremia is treated with a 10- to 14-day course of antibiotics. Indwelling catheters should be removed for fungemia, persistent bacteremia, or *Staphylococcus aureus* or *Pseudomonas* bacteremia. Patients with a history of *Aspergillus* or *Mucor* sp. infection should receive prolonged antifungal therapy, especially if profound neutropenia is likely during subsequent courses of chemotherapy.

Typhlitis (neutropenic enterocolitis) is a syndrome of right-sided colonic inflammation in neutropenic patients. It presents with fever, abdominal pain, and tenderness that can mimic appendicitis. The etiology is unclear. Treatment is with broad-spectrum antibiotics, including anaerobic coverage, and nasogastric suction. Surgical intervention is reserved for patients with bowel perforation or suspected bowel necrosis.

C. **Growth factors.** The use of myeloid growth factors in acute leukemia remains controversial despite multiple randomized trials. Treatment with granulocyte colony-stimulating factor (G-CSF) or granulocyte–macrophage colony-stimulating factor (GM-CSF) after induction chemotherapy shortens the duration of ANC less than $500/\mu L$ by 3 to 6 days. The duration of hospitalization and antibiotic use are also shortened by treatment with growth factors. Although the effectiveness of chemotherapy is not compromised by the use of these agents, most evidence indicates that growth factors do not improve the likelihood of CR or long-term survival. Often, growth factors are reserved for older patients or for those with life-threatening infection.

D. **Intravenous access.** All patients with acute leukemia should have a central venous catheter placed. Temporary catheters, such as the Hohn catheter, are usually chosen because fever, coagulopathy, or poor increments with platelet transfusion represent relative contraindications to placement of a more permanent, tunneled catheter.

E. **Tumor lysis syndrome.** TLS (see Chapter 35) is a complication of rapid tumor breakdown after chemotherapy. Clinically it is marked by hyperuricemia, hyperkalemia, hyperphosphatemia, hypocalcemia, and acute oliguric renal failure. Risk factors for TLS include B-cell ALL, WBC greater than $50,000/\mu L$, LDH greater than 1,000 IU/L, renal dysfunction, and elevation of the uric acid or phosphorus before treatment. All patients with newly diagnosed acute leukemia should be vigorously hydrated to maintain urine output at more than 2.5 L/day, and volume status should be closely monitored. If the patient's renal function is normal, allopurinol, 600 mg, is given the day before chemotherapy, followed by 300 mg daily until the WBC is less than 1,000/μL. If the pretreatment uric acid is more than 9 mg/dL, rasburicase can be used in place of allopurinol to reduce the uric acid level rapidly. Patients at high risk for TLS should have electrolytes, calcium, magnesium, and phosphorus monitored two to three times daily for the first 2 to 3 days of induction chemotherapy.

V. FOLLOWUP. Patients who are in a CR after induction and consolidation therapy require close follow-up. The highest risk for relapse of acute leukemia is within the first 3 years of completion of treatment. During that time, patients should be evaluated with history, physical examination and complete blood count (CBC) every 2 to 3 months. Bone marrow biopsy should be repeated routinely every 3 to 6 months, or if the blood counts fall or blasts are observed in the peripheral blood. Because patients may have disease relapse at extramedullary sites, suspicious skin or soft tissue lesions should be biopsied to rule out granulocytic sarcoma, and new neurologic deficits should be evaluated by brain imaging and lumbar puncture to rule out CNS leukemia. Molecular monitoring of APL (i.e., RT-PCR for PML-RARα) should be performed every 2 to 3 months for 3 years' postconsolidation for patients at high risk of relapse, particularly those with a presenting WBC more than 10,000/μl. Relapse of acute leukemia is very uncommon after approximately 5 years, and follow-up can become less frequent after that.

VI. EPIDEMIOLOGY AND RISK FACTORS. Approximately 13,000 new cases of acute leukemia are diagnosed in the United States each year. The annual incidence of AML is approximately 3.5 per 100,000 and of ALL is approximately 1.5 per 100,000 persons. Although acute leukemia represents only 5% of all new cancer cases, acute leukemia is the most common cause of cancer death for persons younger than 35 years. ALL has a bimodal age distribution. Most cases occur in childhood, with a peak incidence at approximately age 5 years, and there is a second increase in incidence after 60 years of age. The incidence of AML increases steeply beyond 50 years, and the median age is approximately 65 years.

Fewer than 5% of cases of acute leukemia can be attributed to prior exposure to a leukemogenic agent. Ionizing radiation and benzene are clearly associated with an increased risk of acute AML, with an average latency of approximately 5 years. Two classes of chemotherapeutic agents are associated with an increased risk of acute leukemia (secondary leukemia). Alkylating agents can cause AML approximately 4 to 8 years after exposure. AML that arises in this setting is often associated with a preceding MDS and adverse cytogenetics, particularly abnormalities of chromosomes 5 and 7. Topoisomerase II inhibitors such as etoposide or anthracyclines are associated with AML or mixed lineage leukemia with a short (1- to 2-year) latency without a preceding hematologic disorder. The most common cytogenetic abnormalities associated with topoisomerase II inhibitors involve the MLL gene at 11q23. Given the poor prognosis of treatment-related leukemia, allogeneic transplantation in first complete remission (CR) should be considered if a donor is available.

Rare families with a genetic predisposition to acute leukemia have been described, but in the vast majority of cases, there is no clear hereditary risk. However, acute leukemia does occur more frequently in family members than would be expected by chance. Full siblings have an approximately twofold increase in risk, and the concordance rate of infantile leukemias in identical twins has been reported to be as high as 25%. The only infectious agent associated with acute leukemia is human T-lymphocyte leukemia virus (HTLV)-1, which causes T-cell adult leukemia/lymphoma. Congenital disorders that have an increased risk of acute leukemia include Down syndrome, disorders associated with increased chromosomal fragility (Bloom syndrome and Fanconi's anemia) and those associated with immunodeficiency (X-linked agammaglobulinemia and ataxia telangiectasia).

VII. FUTURE DIRECTIONS

    A. Monitoring of minimal residual disease. After remission induction, most patients with acute leukemia receive several additional courses of aggressive chemotherapy with the goal of eliminating subclinical leukemia. A sensitive and specific technique for detection of minimal residual disease (MRD) could provide important prognostic information, allowing for rational treatment decisions. As discussed earlier, detection of MRD has already an important role in the therapy of APL: detection of the PML-RARα fusion transcript after consolidation therapy identifies patients at high risk of clinical relapse. Monitoring MRD in other AML subtypes is difficult because molecular rearrangements amenable to PCR have been found in a relatively small proportion of patients. Monitoring MRD in ALL is facilitated by the presence of clonotypic T cell–receptor gene or immunoglobulin heavy-chain gene rearrangement. Also, BCR-ABL can be followed in patients with Ph+ ALL. However, the role of MRD monitoring and the necessity of obtaining an MRD negative status remains to be defined for AML and ALL.

B. Identification of molecular prognostic factors. Although cytogenetics have proved to be extremely valuable for the risk stratification of patients with acute leukemia, there remains a significant proportion of patients who fall into the "intermediate" or indeterminant group. Additional molecular markers are being sought to distinguish which intermediate risk patients would benefit from more aggressive therapy such as stem cell transplantation. Gene expression profiling using microarray technology may better classify patients into risk groups, as well as identify new therapeutic targets.

C. New therapies. Given the high rate of relapsed and resistant disease among adults with acute leukemias, the need for new, effective therapies is significant. Recently approved drugs for the treatment of relapsed acute leukemia include clofarabine, a purine nucleoside with activity in both AML and ALL and the araguanosine analog nelarabine, which is active in relapsed T-cell ALL. Imatinib and other inhibitors of the BCR-ABL tyrosine kinase have activity in Ph+ ALL and are being investigated as part of upfront therapy or for treatment of relapsed disease. Promising agents for the treatment of AML include the hypomethylating agents azacitidine and decitabine, histone deacetylase inhibitors, farnesyl transferase inhibitors, *FLT3* inhibitors, and an antisense oligonucleotide against the apoptosis inhibitor BCL-2. Many of these new agents are being investigated for the treatment of elderly AML patients, for whom current therapies are particularly toxic and generally ineffective.

Suggested Readings

Burnett AK, Goldstone AH, Stevens RM, et al. Randomised comparison of addition of autologous bone-marrow transplantation to intensive chemotherapy for acute myeloid leukaemia in first remission: results of MRC AML 10 trial. *Lancet* 1998;351(9104): 700–708.

Byrd JC, Mrozek K, Dodge RK, et al. Pretreatment cytogenetic abnormalities are predictive of induction success, cumulative incidence of relapse, and overall survival in adult patients with de novo acute myeloid leukemia: results from Cancer and Leukemia Group B (CALGB 8461). *Blood* 2002;100(13):4325–4336.

Fenaux P, Chastang C, Chevret S, et al. A randomized comparison of all transretinoic acid (ATRA) followed by Chemotherapy and ATRA plus chemotherapy and the role of maintenance therapy in newly diagnosed acute promyelocytic leukemia. *Blood* 1999;94(4):1192–1200.

Fenaux P, Le Deley M, Castaigne S, et al., European APL 91 Group. Effect of all transretinoic acid in newly diagnosed acute promyelocytic leukemia. Results of a multicenter randomized trial. *Blood* 1993;82(11):3241–3249.

Frohling S, Schlenk RF, Breitruck J, et al. Prognostic significance of activating FLT3 mutations in younger adults (16 to 60 years) with acute myeloid leukemia and normal cytogenetics: a study of the AML Study Group. *Blood* 2002;100(13):4372–4380.

Hoelzer D, Thiel E, Loffler H, et al. Prognostic factors in a multicenter study for treatment of acute lymphoblastic leukemia in adults. *Blood* 1988;71(1):123–131.

Jabbour EJ, Estey E, Kantarjian HM. Adult acute myeloid leukemia. *Mayo Clin Proc* 2006;81:247–260.

Jabbour EJ, Faderl S, Kantarjian HM. Adult acute lymphoblastic leukemia. *Mayo Clin Proc* 2005;80:1517–1527.

Jaffe ES, Harris NL, Stein H, et al., eds. *World health organization classification of tumours: pathology and genetics of tumours of haematopoietic and lymphoid tissues.* Lyon: IARC Press, 2001.

Larson RA, Boogaerts M, Estey E, et al. Antibody-targeted chemotherapy of older patients with acute myeloid leukemia in first relapse using Mylotarg (gemtuzumab ozogamicin). *Leukemia* 2002;16(9):1627–1636.

Larson R, Dodge R, Burns C, et al. A five-drug remission induction regimen with intensive consolidation for adults with acute lymphoblastic leukemia: Cancer and Leukemia Group B study 8811. *Blood* 1995;85(8):2025–2037.

Mayer RJ, Davis RB, Schiffer CA, et al. Intensive postremission chemotherapy in adults with acute myeloid leukemia. *N Engl J Med* 1994;331(14):896–903.

Pui CH, Evans WE. Acute lymphoblastic leukemia. *N Engl J Med* 1998;339:605–615.

Rebulla P, Finazzi G, Marangoni F, et al. The threshold for prophylactic platelet transfusions in adults with acute myeloid leukemia. *N Engl J Med* 1997;337(26):1870–1875.

Sanz MA, Tallman MS, Lo-Coco FL. Tricks of the trade for the appropriate management of newly diagnosed acute promyelocytic leukemia. *Blood* 2005;105:3019–3025.

Sievers EL, Larson RA, Stadtmauer EA, et al. Efficacy and safety of gemtuzumab ozogamicin in patients with CD33-positive acute myeloid leukemia in first relapse. *J Clin Oncol* 2001;19(13):3244–3254.

Soignet SL, Frankel SR, Douer D, et al. United states multicenter study of arsenic trioxide in relapsed acute promyelocytic leukemia. *J Clin Oncol* 2001;19(18):3852–3860.

Suciu S, Mandelli F, de Witte T, et al. Allogeneic compared with autologous stem cell transplantation in the treatment of patients younger than 46 years with Acute Myeloid Leukemia (AML) in first complete remission (CR1): an intention-to-treat analysis of the EORTC/GIMEMAAML-10 trial. *Blood* 2003;102(4):1232–1240.

Tallman MS, Gilliland DG, Rowe JM. Drug therapy for acute myeloid leukemia. *Blood* 2005;106:1154–1163.

Wetzler M, Dodge RK, Mrozek K, et al. Prospective karyotype analysis in adult acute lymphoblastic leukemia: The Cancer and Leukemia Group B Experience. *Blood* 1999;93(11):3983–3993.

Wheatley K, Burnett AK, Goldstone AH, et al. A simple, robust, validated and highly predictive index for the determination of risk-directed therapy in acute myeloid leukaemia derived from the MRC AML 10 trial. *Br J Haematol* 1999;107(1):69–79.

HEMATOLOGIC MALIGNANCIES: CHRONIC LEUKEMIAS

Todd A. Fehniger, John S. Welch, and Timothy J. Pluard

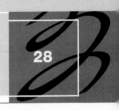

28

I. INTRODUCTION. Chronic leukemias are malignancies of the myeloid or lymphoid hematopoietic lineages that have historically been characterized as having an indolent course when compared to their acute counterparts. While the indolent nature of these diseases results in a relatively long median survival as compared to other cancers, chronic leukemias have not typically been considered curable, except in some cases following allogeneic stem cell transplantation (SCT). Here we review clinical features and current treatment approaches to the most common chronic leukemias, chronic myelogenous leukemia (CML) and chronic lymphocytic leukemia (CLL).

CML is the most frequent chronic leukemia of myeloid derivation and is categorized as a clonal myeloproliferative disorder within the World Health Organization (WHO) classification. This disease is characterized by peripheral blood leukocytosis resulting from an expansion of normally differentiated myeloid cells and typically presents incidentally on routine laboratory testing. CML is notable as the first leukemia identified with a causative clonal chromosomal rearrangement, t(9;22) or the Philadelphia chromosome (Ph), which juxtaposes the *ABL* tyrosine kinase next to the break point cluster (*BCR*) region, yielding the BCR-ABL fusion protein. The management of CML has been revolutionized over the past 6 to 8 years through targeted inhibition of BCR-ABL by the oral tyrosine kinase inhibitor imatinib mesylate (Gleevec), which has provided the first proof-of-principle for small molecule targeted therapy of cancer. CML therapy continues to rapidly evolve with the advent of new generations of small molecular inhibitors of BCR-ABL, and current challenges include defining the optimal approach to utilize these drugs.

CLL is the most common lymphoid leukemia, and is combined with small lymphocytic lymphoma (SLL) as a mature B-cell neoplasm in the WHO classification. Advances in our understanding of the pathophysiology of CLL have yielded an updated view on the natural history and important prognostic factors in this disease. Improvements in the initial therapy of CLL include combining chemotherapeutic agents with monoclonal antibodies, and expanded treatment options now exist for patients with disease refractory to purine analogs such as fludarabine.

II. CHRONIC MYELOGENOUS LEUKEMIA (CML)

    A. Epidemiology. CML accounts for 14% of all leukemias and 20% of adult leukemias with an annual incidence of 1.6 cases per 100,000 adults. Since the advent of imatinib, the annual mortality has decreased to 1% to 2%. The median age at presentation is 65 and incidence increases with age. The etiology is unclear; no correlation with monozygotic twins, geography, ethnicity or economic status has been observed. However, a significantly higher incidence of CML has been noted in survivors of the atomic disasters at Nagasaki and Hiroshima, in radiologists, and in patients treated with radiation to the spine for ankylosing spondylitis.

    B. Pathogenesis. Historically, CML was the first disease in which a specific chromosomal abnormality was linked to the pathogenesis of the disease: the foreshortened chromosome 22, named the *Philadelphia (Ph) chromosome.* Subsequently the *BCR-ABL* fusion gene resulting from the common t(9;22) translocation has been noted in almost all patients with CML and is now considered pathognomonic. This fusion of the *BCR* (breakpoint cluster region) serine kinase with the human homologue *ABL1* of the Abelson murine leukemia virus oncogene results in constitutive tyrosine kinase activity of ABL and thereby dysregulated activity of multiple signal-transduction pathways controlling cell proliferation and apoptosis. BCR-ABL may also play a direct role in signals leading to independence from external growth signaling, cell adhesion modulation, and DNA repair.

C. **Clinical and laboratory features.** In most patients, CML is diagnosed incidentally. Symptomatic constellations typically result from concurrent anemia and splenomegaly: fatigue, early satiety and sensation of abdominal fullness, but may also include weight loss, bleeding, or bruising in advanced disease. Leukocytosis with a myeloid shift is universal. In contrast to cases of acute leukemia, in which an arrest in maturation is the rule, granulocytes at all stages of maturation are observed on the peripheral smear. Anemia and thrombocytopenia are common although basophilia (more than 7%) occurs in only 10% to 15% of patients. Leukocyte alkaline phosphatase (LAP) activity is usually reduced, but can be increased with infections, stress, on achievement of remission, or on progression to blast phase (BP). The diagnosis is confirmed by the detection of the Ph chromosome t(9;22)(q34.1;q11.21). In 5% of patients, a *BCR-ABL* fusion can be detected without classic Ph chromosomal cytogenetics and rarely translocations can involve three or more chromosomes. The bone marrow is typically hypercellular and devoid of fat. All stages of myeloid differentiation are present and megakaryocytes may be increased, suggesting that chronic-phase CML is a disease of discordant maturation, where a delay in myeloid maturation results in increased myeloid cell mass.

D. **Natural history.** The natural history of CML is a triphasic process. Most patients present in chronic phase, characterized by an asymptomatic accumulation of differentiated myeloid cells in the bone marrow, spleen, and peripheral blood. CML usually progresses through a transient accelerated phase, lasting 4 to 6 months and then inevitably to BP, an incurable acute leukemia that is fatal within 3 to 6 months. In the 2 years after initial diagnosis of CML, 5% to 15% of untreated patients will enter blast crisis. In subsequent years, the annual rate of progression increases to 20% to 25% with progression commonly occurring between 3 and 6 years after diagnosis.

The definition of accelerated phase CML relies on several clinical and laboratory features and is characterized by increasing arrest of maturation. Current WHO criteria include at least one of the following: 10% to 19% blasts in peripheral blood or bone marrow, equal to or more than 20% peripheral basophils, thrombocytopenia less than $100,000/\mu L$ and unresponsive to therapy, increasing spleen size and increasing white blood cell (WBC) count unresponsive to therapy, or cytogenetic evidence of clonal evolution. Once either accelerated phase or blast crisis occurs, the success of any therapy declines dramatically.

Several prognostic models (Sokal score, Hasford, MD Anderson Cancer Center staging system) have been developed to stratify patients into groups with different average survival using variables such as age, spleen size, platelet count, percentage of peripheral blood blast count, hematocrit, cytogenetic clonal evolution, and gender. Although these scoring systems were developed before imatinib, post hoc analysis of the IRIS (International Randomized Study of Interferon vs. STI-571) study provided an initial validation of the Sokal score in this imatinib treated population. Other predictors of outcome derived from the IRIS study include response to imatinib at 3, 12 and 18 months. Future models will likely incorporate cytogenetics and *BCR-ABL* mutational analysis.

E. **Treatment of chronic myeloid leukemia: tyrosine kinase inhibitors**

1. **Imatinib mesylate (Gleevec).** Imatinib revolutionized the treatment of CML with its phase I trial in 2001. Imatinib is a targeted tyrosine kinase inhibitor, which antagonizes the activity of the *ABL* tyrosine kinase as well as c-Kit, and platelet-derived growth factors α and β. At nanomolar concentrations, imatinib binds to the adenosine triphosphate (ATP)-binding pocket of the BCR-ABL fusion protein while in the inactive conformation, resulting in competitive inhibition. This nearly completely abolishes autophosphorylation of BCR-ABL, inactivates dysregulated downstream signaling through multiple pathways including JAK-STAT, PI3K, RAS, AKT, and ERK, thereby specifically inhibiting the growth of *BCR-ABL* positive bone marrow progenitor cells.

The optimal dose of imatinib remains under study. In the initial dose-escalation trial, few patients responded to doses lower than 250 mg/day, whereas

98% of patients receiving at least 300 mg/day achieved a complete hematologic response. During follow-up of the phase III IRIS trial, an initial dose of 400 mg every day followed by escalation to 400 mg b.i.d. if needed results in 98% complete hematologic response and 87% complete cytogenetic response (CCgR) at 60 months with an estimated 5-year survival of 90%. Higher dosing schedules of 600 mg and 800 mg have been shown to be tolerable, although it is not clear if they result in longer-duration CCgR or simply a quicker achievement of this goal.

Side effects of imatinib mesylate are generally mild, but include hematologic suppression (neutropenia, thrombocytopenia, and anemia), constitutional symptoms (diarrhea, edema, and rash) and rare organ damage (transaminitis, hypophosphatemia, and potential cardiotoxicity). These can usually be managed with growth factors or dose reduction, but occasionally require discontinuation, either briefly or permanently.

2. **Goal-directed therapy.** Increased risk of progression to accelerated phase and BP has been demonstrated if imatinib does not help patients achieve specific clinical goals. These currently include complete hematologic response with normal peripheral counts and more than 1-log reduction in *BCR-ABL* transcripts by quantitative polymerase chain reaction (qPCR) at 3 months; cytogenetic response with less than 35% Ph chromosome–positive bone marrow cells at 6 months; CCgR with undetectable Ph chromosome at 12 months; and major molecular remission with 3-log reduction by qPCR of peripheral *BCR-ABL* at 18 months (Table 28.1). Failure to reach any of these goals warrants close follow-up, ABL tyrosine kinase domain mutation analysis, dose escalation, or change to second-line tyrosine kinase inhibitor and consideration for hematopoietic stem cell transplant.

Follow-up during initial treatment requires monthly complete blood count (CBC) and peripheral *BCR-ABL* qPCR every 3 months with bone marrow biopsy every 6 months until major molecular remission is achieved. Once molecular remission is documented, *BCR-ABL* transcripts should still be followed up every 3 months with annual bone marrow examination for cytogenetics. Rising *BCR-ABL* transcripts should be quickly reevaluated and treatment altered accordingly.

3. **Imatinib resistance.** Resistance to imatinib has been noted in 2% to 4% of patients annually for the first 3 years of imatinib therapy and may decrease thereafter. Mechanisms proposed include the acquisition of point mutations in the *BCR-ABL* kinase SH1 domain, over expression of BCR-ABL, activation of BCR-ABL–independent pathways including SRC kinases, increased imatinib efflux through the multidrug resistance (MDR) pump and progressively abnormal cytogenetics. Of these, point mutations in the SH1 kinase domain likely play the most prominent role and more than 50 distinct mutations have been documented in 42% to 90% of resistant cases with increasing prevalence in accelerated phase and blast crisis. Mutations have also been found *de novo* in untreated chronic-phase patients suggesting they may exist before treatment and are slowly selected out during therapy. As rates of progression decline over time, imatinib therapy is not currently thought to induce new mutations. These mutations act by either decreasing the affinity for imatinib binding in the ATP-binding pocket or shifting the kinetics of BCR-ABL to prefer the active conformation, to which imatinib will not bind.

Imatinib resistance can be overcome either with increasing doses or a second-line tyrosine kinase inhibitor such as dasatinib. Dasatinib inhibits BCR-ABL in either active or inactive conformation, providing sensitivity to most imatinib resistant point mutations with the exception of T315I, which confers a high degree of resistance to both drugs. Mutational analysis is therefore critical in determining clinic course after resistance is noted. Multiple novel multitarget kinase inhibitors are in development, which promise improved response against imatinib resistant BCR-ABL.

4. **Treatment duration.** Treatment length continues to be defined, but we recommend indefinite tyrosine kinase inhibition. Recent data suggest tyrosine kinase

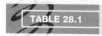

TABLE 28.1	Chronic Myelogenous Leukemia Treatment Goals with Imatinib	

Time	Workup	Inadequate treatment response[a]
Diagnosis	CBC, peripheral qPCR, Bone marrow cytogenetics.	At risk: high risk by Sokal score, abnormal cytogenetics in Ph + cells, Del 9q+
3 mo	CBC, peripheral qPCR	Failure: persistent disease At risk: incomplete hematologic response (WBC count >10, Plt >450, immature cells)
6 mo	CBC, peripheral qPCR, Bone marrow cytogenetics	Failure: incomplete hematologic response (WBC count >10, Plt count >450, immature cells) At risk: partial cytogenetic response (>35% Ph + cells on BMBx)
12 mo	CBC, peripheral qPCR, Bone marrow cytogenetics	Failure: partial cytogenetic response (>35% Ph + cells on BMBx) At risk: incomplete cytogenetic response (Persistent Ph + cells on BMBx)
18 mo	CBC, peripheral qPCR, BMBx if not in complete cytogenetic remission at 12 mo	Failure: incomplete cytogenetic response (persistent Ph + cells on BMBx) At risk: No major molecular response (< 3-log reduction in qPCR level)
Follow-up	Q3 mo: CBC and peripheral qPCR Q12 mo: bone marrow cytogenetics	At risk: rise in qPCR transcript level, cytogenetic evolution

CBC, complete blood count; qPCR, q**uantitative polymerase chain reaction;** WBC, white blood cell; PLt, platelet; BMBx, bone marrow biopsy.
[a]Warrants mutational analysis and close follow-up after dose escalation vs. Dasatinib or stem cell transplantation.

inhibitors are not cytotoxic to early, quiescent BCR-ABL positive precursor cells. Multiple small series have been published demonstrating, despite CCgR, rapid molecular recurrence occurs in approximately half of patients after tyrosine kinase inhibition is withdrawn. Once noted, nearly all of these patients respond to tyrosine kinase inhibition reintroduction. Further study will be needed before drug holidays and discontinuation can be general recommended.

5. **Conventional chemotherapy.** Until 1980, hydroxyurea and busulfan were the two most effective anti-CML agents. Both offer mild hematologic control associated with myelosuppression; however, the uniform transformation to the acute phase of the disease is unchanged. Subsequently, interferon α used alone or in combination with cytarabine has demonstrated improved response over chemotherapy with major cytogenetic responses in 40% to 50% of patients. Upwards of 80% of these patients have a durable response resulting in a 10 year survival of 75%. However, interferon α therapy is complicated by significant side effects including flu-like symptoms, anorexia, weight loss, depression, autoimmune (AI) disorders, thrombocytopenia, alopecia, rashes, and neuropathies resulting in discontinuation in approximately a fifth of patients. Given the superior response to tyrosine kinase inhibitors and their relatively benign side-effect profile, conventional chemotherapy and interferon have fallen from common use in CML.

F. **Treatment of chronic myelogenous leukemia: transplant options**

1. **Allogeneic bone marrow transplantation.** Allogeneic BMT from either related or unrelated donors remains the only known curative therapy for CML. Transplantation from a matched-sibling donor during chronic phase is associated with

a 10-year survival of 50% to 70%. Results of transplantation from unrelated donors are somewhat less impressive, but are improving with better matching strategies and supportive care. The objective of BMT is cure of CML by eradication of the leukemic clone with myeloablative chemoradiotherapy, and restoration of hematopoiesis by transplantation of normal donor-derived stem cells. In addition, the donor-derived allogeneic immune cells confer an important graft-versus-leukemia (GVL) effect, which acts to prevent recurrence of disease. GVL has been closely associated with the presence of graft versus host disease (GVHD). GVHD does not develop in patients receiving transplants from identical twin donors. These patients have at least twice the risk of relapse of CML compared with transplant recipients from HLA-identical siblings.

The best results occur when patients are transplanted while in chronic phase. Long-term survival after BMT in accelerated phase is only 20% to 40%, whereas survival after transplants performed in BP further declines to less than 20%. The highest rates of survival for related and unrelated-donor transplantation in the pre-imatinib era are documented in patients transplanted within 1 year of diagnosis.

One third of patients will have a histocompatible donor, and 50% of the population will locate a suitable unrelated donor (70% for whites and 15% for African Americans and other minorities in the United States). Age older than 50 to 60 years has been found to constitute a significant hurdle for transplant success, especially in the unrelated-donor transplant setting, although this is improved with modified intensity and nonmyeloablative transplant. Approximately 76% of patients are older than 60 years at the time of diagnosis. Therefore, when donor availability and age are considered, allogeneic transplantation is an option for only a minority of patients.

Most CML patients transplanted in chronic phase are cured of their disease, although transplant-related morbidity and mortality remain a significant problem. The cumulative incidence of severe GVHD is approximately 20% to 35% in matched-sibling transplantation and 40% to 55% in recipients of transplants from unrelated donors. Infection is a major cause of non-relapse mortality in allogeneic transplantation. GVHD and immunosuppression are predisposing factors for infectious complications.

2. **Allogeneic bone marrow transplantation since imatinib.** The effect of pre-transplant tyrosine kinase inhibitor therapy, which will delay transplant and may thereby increase its risks, is still under study. Initial retrospective studies comparing imatinib treated transplant patients with historical controls show no difference in rates of engraftment and acute or chronic GVHD suggesting delays due to therapy do not adversely affect the transplant itself. However, rates of relapse were higher in imatinib treated patients as these patients were transplanted more often in accelerated phase or blast crisis. Given the high response rates to tyrosine kinase inhibitors, their initial use is still recommended. High-risk patients, who present with cytogenetic changes beyond Ph chromosome, who demonstrate increasing cytogenetic complexity, who do not meet standard goals of therapy at 3, 6, 12, or 18 months, or who have rising qPCR levels of *BCR-ABL* should be evaluated for human leukocyte antigen (HLA) matched siblings and potential unrelated donors. Progressive disease despite appropriate tyrosine kinase inhibition warrants transplant consideration as early as possible.

Relapse following transplant has been successfully treated with both donor lymphocyte infusion and tyrosine kinase inhibition. Mutational analysis of *ABL* kinase domain may help guide appropriate therapy choice.

G. **Accelerated and blast-phase chronic myelogenous leukemia.** Despite profound advances in the treatment of chronic-phase CML, accelerated and blast-phase CML in most cases progress uniformly and there remains no successful standard therapy. Imatinib has been shown to improve survival in accelerated phase with improved hematologic and cytogenetic responses at higher doses (600 to 1,000 mg) compared to typical dosing in chronic phase, but responses are often short lived. *BRC-ABL* mutational analysis should be performed with early consideration for dasatinib, transplant, or clinical trial. However, because most patients now developing accelerated phase have been previously treated with imatinib, mutations in and over expression of *BCR-ABL* are to be expected. Simple dose escalation is rarely sufficient therapy.

Blast phase (BP) is characterized by cytogenetic evolution in approximately 70% of patients. The most common chromosomal abnormalities are trisomy 8 in 30% to 40% of patients, additional Ph chromosome in 20% to 30% and isochromosome 17 in 15% to 20%. Corresponding mutations in p53 are also seen in 20%-30% of patients, amplification of *c-myc* in 20%, and less commonly mutations and deletions of *ras*, *Rb*, or *p16*. As with *de novo* acute myelocytic leukemia (AML), complex cytogenetics are associated with decreased response rates and survival.

Treatment of BP-CML remains a challenge, with survival of only 2 to 4 months in non-responders. Treatment is dictated by hematologic features. Myeloid features are seen in 50% of patients, lymphoid in 25%, and undifferentiated in 25%. Typical AML induction chemotherapy is used for BP-CML with myeloid features and acute lymphoblastic leukemia (ALL) induction chemotherapy for lymphoid features. Each has response rates of only 30%. Myeloid BP-CML is generally treated with cytarabine based regimens or decitabine, both with similar response rates. Lymphoid BP-CML has been treated with HyperCVAD or other regimens including vincristine and prednisone. Studies with imatinib show early hematologic response rates of approximately 70%, but these were short lived. Dasatinib has also demonstrated response rates in imatinib resistant BP-CML with progression-free survival (PFS) of 45% at 12 months in myeloid, but only 20% PFS at 6 months in lymphoid BP-CML. Transplant during BP-CML remains the only curative options, but is associated with an approximately 80% risk of relapse and a 5-year survival only ~5%.

III. CHRONIC LYMPHOCYTIC LEUKEMIA (CLL)

A. **Epidemiology.** CLL is the most common form of leukemia in adults, and accounts for ~30% of adult leukemia in Western countries. Approximately 10,000 new cases are diagnosed annually, and 4,700 deaths are attributed to CLL each year in the US. According to the Surveillance, Epidemiology, and End Results (SEER) cancer database, from 2000 to 2003 the median age at presentation was 72 years, and only 13% of patients were less than 55 years old at the time of diagnosis. The age-adjusted incidence rate for CLL was 3.8 per 100,000 men and women per year, with an approximately 2:1 male:female ratio. There are no clear environmental or occupational risk factors that predispose to CLL, and patients who are exposed to radiation do not appear to have an increased frequency of CLL. Interestingly, the incidence of CLL is much lower (~10% that of Western countries) in Asian countries such as China and Japan, which is attributed to genetic rather than environmental factors. CLL (and other malignancies) occur at a higher than predicted frequently among first degree relatives of patients with CLL (relative risk of approximately 1.5 to 7.5), the highest familial risk of all hematologic malignancies, suggesting an inherited predisposition. Studies of familial cohorts with CLL are ongoing, and the future identification of genes involved in familial CLL may provide insights into the pathogenesis of CLL. Of note, clonal B cells with a CLL phenotype were detected in 3.5% of normal healthy control subjects, and there was a significant increase in the detection of such cells in members of family members of CLL patients (13.5%).

B. **Pathogenesis.** CLL is a clonal lymphoproliferative disorder characterized by the accumulation of neoplastic, functionally incompetent B lymphocytes in the blood, bone marrow, lymph nodes, or spleen. After encountering antigen, a normal B-cell enters the germinal center and proliferates, where the B-cell receptor genes undergo somatic hypermutation, which allows for B-cell receptor affinity maturation and selection of B-cell clones with high affinity for the antigen. Despite their uniform morphologic appearance and immunophenotype, there appears to be significant heterogeneity in CLL patients with regard to the mutational status of the immunoglobulin (Ig) heavy-chain variable region (IgVH), which usually indicates whether the B cell has experienced somatic hypermutation in the germinal center. In CLL, approximately half of patients have a mutated IgVH (M-IgVH) indicative of a post-germinal center B cell, whereas other patients have an unmutated IgVH

(UM-IgVH), a finding that has prognostic significance. The precise normal counterpart(s) of CLL cells during B-cell development has not been definitely identified, however the CLL immunophenotype is similar to that of mature, antigen-experienced, activated B cells. Recent gene expression array experiments indicate that both M-IgVH and UM-IgVH CLL cells resemble memory B cells more than any other identified normal B-cell subset. In addition, over expression of the src tyrosine kinase ZAP-70 in CLL, which is normally expressed in T and natural killer (NK) cells and not B cells, is strongly correlated with UM-IgVH subset. Further advances in defining the relationship between CLL cells and normal B-cell development may yield novel therapeutic targets in CLL.

Unlike many hematologic malignancies, CLL cells do not contain balanced chromosomal translocations, detectable using traditional cytogenetic techniques. However, advances in fluorescence *in situ* hybridization (FISH) technology on nondividing cells (i.e., interphase cytogenetics) has identified recurrent chromosomal abnormalities in ~80% of CLL cases. The most common cytogenetic abnormalities in CLL are del(13q14), del(11q), trisomy 12, and del(17p), which influence prognosis (Table 28.2). The gene(s) involved in 13q14 deletion have not been definitively identified; however, the retinoblastoma (Rb) gene maps close to this region. Recently, two micro-RNAs (miR-15, miR-16) have been mapped to the 13q locus and are also potential candidates for mediating this locus effect in CLL. Del(11q22-23) encompasses the ataxia telangiectasia mutated (ATM) gene locus, and mutations in the ATM gene have been observed in CLL, suggesting that ATM is the target of this deletion. Similarly, del(17p) encompasses the p53 tumor suppressor gene, and point mutations or deletions of p53 are also present in CLL patients with poor prognosis, suggesting p53 is the target gene in del(17p) CLL patients. The gene(s) important for trisomy 12 effects have not been identified. Approximately 95% of CLLs have increased expression of the anti-apoptotic Bcl-2 oncogene, and 70% have expression levels equivalent to follicular lymphoma cells harboring t(14;18). CLL cells utilize other mechanism to increase Bcl-2 expression, and do not typically contain the classic t(14;18) present in follicular non-Hodgkin's lymphoma (NHL). The advances in identifying M/UM-IgVH and ZAP-70+ CLL patient subsets and specific chromosomal abnormalities with prognostic significance are currently being validated in prospective in clinical trials to identify high-risk CLL patients, and to explore risk-stratified treatment strategies.

C. **Clinical presentation, laboratory features, and diagnosis.** Patients with CLL have a wide range of symptoms, signs, and laboratory abnormalities at the time of initial diagnosis. Many patients are asymptomatic, and a routine CBC reveals a lymphocytosis, whereas fewer patients present with extreme fatigue or B symptoms including fevers, night sweats, unintentional weight loss equal to or less than 10% of body weight. Other presentations include painless lymphadenopathy, anemia, thrombocytopenia, and infections. Physical examination findings are normal in

TABLE 28.2   Cytogenetic Abnormalities in Chronic Lymphocytic Leukemia

Aberration	% Patients	Prognosis	Clinical feature	Gene
13q-	55%	Good	Slower progression Lymphadenopathy	?
11q-	18%	Poor	Rapid progression Shorter PFS with Flu-regimens	ATM
12q+	16%	Intermediate		?
17p-	7%	Poor	Shorter PFS with Flu-regimens	p53

ATM, ataxia telangiectasia mutated; PFS, progression-free survival; Flu, fludarabine; ?, not definitvely identified.

20% to 30% of patients, but may include lymphadenopathy, splenomegaly, and hepatomegaly in approximately half the number of patients. Laboratory findings uniformly include a lymphocytosis (greater than 5,000/uL), and may include anemia, thrombocytopenia, elevated lactose dehydrogenase (LDH) levels, elevated B2M levels, positive Coombs' test, polyclonal increase in γ-globulin levels, or hypogammaglobulinemia. The peripheral blood smear typically shows numerous small, mature appearing lymphocytes with clumped chromatin and no nucleolus, with "smudge" cells present as crush artifacts of fragile CLL cells. Bone marrow biopsy shows infiltration with small lymphocytes in nodular, interstitial, or diffuse pattern. The histopathologic lymph node findings in CLL/SLL consist of diffuse effacement of the nodal architecture by small, mature appearing lymphocytes with a low mitotic rate, and few (less than 10%) larger prolymphocytes. Peripheral blood, bone marrow, or lymph node flow cytometry reveals a characteristic immunophenotype (Table 28.3). The essential diagnostic criteria for CLL identified by the CLL international working group (IWG) include an absolute lymphocytosis of more than 5,000/uL with a typical morphology, a bone marrow infiltrated with small lymphocytes accounting for more than 30% of nucleated cells, and a typical immunophenotype (CD5+, CD23+, CD10-, CD19+, CD20$^{+\text{dim}}$, CyclinD1-, CD43±). In addition, the following tests may be useful under certain circumstances: molecular genetic analysis to detect antigen receptor rearrangements, interphase FISH for 17p-, 11q-, 13q-, +12, and determination of CD38 and/or ZAP-70 expression. The differential diagnosis of CLL includes other indolent B-cell lymphomas (mantle cell, follicular, lymphoplasmacytic), hairy cell leukemia, Large granular lymphocytic (LGL) leukemia, prolymphocytic leukemia (PLL), and adult T-cell leukemia/lymphoma. Once the diagnosis is made, initial workup should include physical examination, performance status, assessment of B symptoms, CBC with differential count, LDH, comprehensive metabolic panel, and in certain circumstances quantitative Igs, reticulocyte count, direct Coombs' test, computed tomography (CT) scans of the chest/abdomen/pelvis, B2M, and uric acid.

D. Staging and prognosis. The Rai and Binet clinical staging systems were described in the 1970s provided prognostic information on survival based upon physical examination findings and blood counts (Table 28.4). These clinical staging systems have been extensively validated and are widely used in clinical practice to provide estimates of survival to patients. However, the clinical course of early stage patients is heterogeneous: some patients do not require therapy for many years whereas others have rapid progression and poor responses to therapy. Further, these staging systems provide little information to help predict the clinical outcome of early stage patients or the response to therapy. Additional laboratory parameters have been identified as markers of tumor burden and independent poor prognostic factors

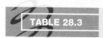

TABLE 28.3	**Immunophenotypic Features of Malignant Conditions Affecting Mature B Lymphocytes**
Disorder	**Common immunophenotype**
CLL	DR+, CD19+, CD20+, CD5+, CD22−, CD23+, CD10−, weak sIg
Prolymphocytic leukemia	DR+, CD19+, CD20+, CD5−, CD22+, CD23−, CD10−, bright sIg
Mantle cell lymphoma	DR+, CD19+, CD20+, CD5+, CD22+, CD23−, CD10−, moderate sIg
Follicular lymphoma	DR+, CD19+, CD20+, CD5−, CD22+, CD23−, CD10+, bright sIg
Hairy cell leukemia	DR+, CD19+, CD20+, CD5−, CD22+, CD23−, CD10−, CD11c+, bright sIg

CLL, chronic lymphocytic leukemia; sIg, surface immunoglobulin.

TABLE 28.4 Chronic Lymphocytic Leukemia Staging Systems

Staging system	Presentation	Median survival (yr)	Patients (%)
Rai			
0	Lymphocytosis	>10	30
I	LN	9	35
II	Splenomegaly	7	25
III	Anemia	5	7
IV	Thrombocytopenia	5	3
Binet			
A	Lymphocytosis, <3 areas of LN	>10	65
B	Lymphocytosis, >3 areas of LN	7	30
C	Anemia, thrombocytopenia, or both	5	5

LN, lymph node enlargement.

including an elevated LDH, a lymphocyte doubling time of less than 12 months, and diffuse bone marrow infiltration pattern. Serum proteins have also been linked to poor prognosis including elevated levels of thymidine kinase (TK), soluble CD23 (sCD23), and B2-microglobulin (B2M). Notably, patients with an elevated B2M level have a shorter survival, and worse responses to traditional chemotherapy approaches. A summary of prognostic factors in CLL is provided in Table 28.5.

The mutational status of the IgVH locus is an important genetic parameter for prognostication in CLL patients, with the mutated IgVH (M-IgVH) associated with slow progression and long survival, whereas the unmutated IgVH (UM-IgVH) associated with an unfavorable course and rapid progression. Surrogate markers of UM-IgVH and poor prognosis include flow cytometry-detected expression of CD38 and ZAP-70 by CLL cells. Recent studies have suggested that more than 20% ZAP-70 expression as assessed by flow cytometry is associated with a median survival of less than 5 years, compared with 10 years in patients with less than 20% expression, and is now widely available. This was superior in predicting outcomes in CLL patients compared to IgVH mutational status testing.

Interphase cytogenetics has identified both favorable (13q-) with a longer treatment-free interval and overall survival, and unfavorable (17p-, 11q-) with short treatment-free interval and overall survival, subsets of CLL patients (Table 28.2).

TABLE 28.5 Prognostic Factors in Chronic Lymphocytic Leukemia

Favorable	Unfavorable
Low Rai or Binet clinical stage	High Rai or Binet clinical stage
Lymphocyte doubling time >12 mo	Lymphocyte doubling time <12 mo
Nodular or interstitial BM infiltrate	Diffuse BM infiltrate
Mutated IgVH	Unmutated IgVH
ZAP-70 negative (low)	ZAP-70 positive (high)
CD38 negative	CD38 positive
13q-	17p-/p53 abnormalities, 11q-/ATM abnormalities, +12
	Increased levels of : B2M, LDH, sCD23

BM, bone marrow; ATM, ataxia telangiectasia mutated; LDH, lactose dehydrogenase; B2M, beta 2 microglobulin.

Consistent with this, subsets of patients with mutations in p53 (17p) or ATM (11q) have a poorer prognosis. When molecular parameters consisting of IgVH mutational status, 17p-, and 11q- were included in a multivariate analysis the clinical stage was not identified as an independent prognostic factor. Four distinct molecular prognostic groups (17p-, 11q-, UM-IgVH, M-IgVH) have been identified, and may provide the frame work for future risk-adapted therapeutic strategies. Laboratory testing by interphase cytogenetics for genetic abnormalities of clinical significance in CLL patients is now widely available. Although these advances in genetic and molecular prognostic factors are promising, the decision to treat patients with CLL based upon them requires validation in prospective, randomized clinical trials.

E. **Complications associated with chronic lymphocytic leukemia**

1. **Richter's transformation.** Richter's syndrome (RS), originally described as the development of an aggressive NHL in patients with CLL/SLL, is now commonly used to describe transformation into any aggressive malignancy including diffuse large B-cell lymphoma (DLBCL), PLL, Hodgkin's lymphoma (HL), lymphoblastic lymphoma, hairy cell leukemia, or aggressive T-cell NHL. RS occurs in 2% to 8% of CLL patients, and results are conflicting on whether purine analog therapy increases the risk for transformation. The malignant clone in RS may develop through transformation of the original CLL clone, or arise as an independent neoplasm. This syndrome is suspected clinically in patients with CLL/SLL that have a rapidly enlarging lymph node group, rapidly progressive splenomegaly or hepatomegaly, elevated LDH and beta 2 microglobulin (B2M), new B symptoms (fever, night sweats, weight loss), or a sudden decline in performance status. Patients with suspected RS should have a tissue biopsy to confirm the diagnosis. Treatment usually involves aggressive chemotherapy combinations utilized in NHL or lymphoblastic lymphoma/ALL sometimes combined with radiation therapy, with response rates of 5% to 43%, and median survival between 5 and 8 months. Allogeneic SCT has produced durable long-term remissions in small subsets of RS patients, and is typically offered to those patients who respond to initial chemotherapy and who are good transplant candidates with an HLA-matched donor. Overall, RS patients have a poor prognosis, and novel treatment strategies are needed.

2. **AI complications.** AI phenomena are common in CLL, occur more frequently in advanced-stage patients and those with UM-IgVH, and include autoimmune hemolytic anemia (AIHA), autoimmune thrombocytopenia (ITP), AI neutropenia, and pure red cell aplasia (PRCA) (Table 28.6). In CLL patients with isolated anemia, laboratory evaluation for hemolysis should be performed including direct Coombs' (direct antiglobulin) testing, LDH, haptoglobin, indirect bilirubin, and reticulocyte count. It is important to note that these tests may not provide consistent findings of hemolysis in CLL patients, as an elevated LDH may be due to other causes in CLL, and a low reticulocyte count could be due to poor bone marrow responses when infiltrated with CLL. In addition, AI complications may be triggered in CLL patients at the time of treatment with fludarabine. Treatment of AIHA is similar to the steroid approach in non-CLL patients, with a typical course of prednisone 1 mg/kg/day until a response is achieved, followed by a prolonged 2- to 3-month taper. If the AI complication is not responsive to steroids, other treatments include intravenous immunoglobulin (IVIG), cyclosporine, splenectomy, and rituximab.

3. **Infectious Complications.** The immune deficiency associated with CLL is multifactorial, and includes hypogammaglobulinemia, T cell dysfunction, and decreased phagocytic function. Infectious complications are frequent and respond to appropriate antimicrobial therapy (Table 28.6). For CLL patients with hypogammaglobulinemia and recurrent infections, treatment with IVIG 400 mg/kg IV every 3 to 4 weeks (goal IgG trough approximately 500 mg/dL) reduces serious bacterial infection rates without altering overall survival. Patients treated with fludarabine or alemtuzumab develop therapy-related T-cell immune defects, and are at a significantly increased risk of cytomegalovirus (CMV) reactivation, pneumocystis, varicella zoster, herpes viruses, listeria, and other opportunistic

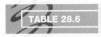

TABLE 28.6	Complications Associated with Chronic Lymphocytic Leukemia

Complication	Patients affected (%)
Autoimmune	
Hemolytic anemia	10–25
Thrombocytopenia	2
Neutropenia	0.5
Pure red cell aplasia	0.5
Hypogammaglobulinemia	20–60
Infections	
Streptococcus, Staphylococcus sp.	
Haemophilus sp.	
Candida, Aspergillus sp.	
Varicella zoster	
Legionella, Pneumocystis, Listeria sp.	
Toxoplasma sp.	
Disease transformation	
Prolymphocytic leukemia	10
Richter's transformation	3–5
Second cancers (lung, skin, GI)	5–15

GI, gastrointestinal.

infections. Prophylaxis against pneumocystis, herpes simplex virus (HSV), and varicella zoster virus (VZV), as well as monitoring for CMV reactivation should be considered when treating CLL patients with these agents.

F. Decision to initiate treatment. Treatment of CLL has historically been palliative as chemotherapeutic regimens have not impacted overall survival to date, and therefore the diagnosis of CLL does not mandate the need for therapy. Indications for treatment include (a) eligibility for treatment on a clinical trial, (b) advanced clinical stage (Rai III/IV), (c) AI cytopenias, (d) recurrent infections, (e) B symptoms, (f) threatened compromise of organ function, (g) cytopenias, (h) bulky disease, (i) rapid progression of disease, (j) histologic transformation, or (k) patient preference for immediate treatment. Observation until an indication for treatment arises does not impact CLL patients' overall survival or response to therapy when initiated. As therapies for CLL become more effective and strategies to monitor for minimal residual disease develop, this paradigm of initial observation may change in the future.

G. Initial treatment of chronic lymphocytic leukemia. The goal of CLL chemotherapy remains palliative; however, these objectives are currently being reevaluated in clinical trials as chemotherapy and monoclonal antibody combinations produce high complete remission rates and in some cases elimination of disease based on sensitive molecular and flow cytometric techniques. Accepted first-line therapy options include clinical trials (preferred as standard therapy is not curative), radiation therapy, alkylating agents (e.g., chlorambucil or cyclophosphamide), purine analogs (fludarabine), or combinations such as fludarabine plus cyclophosphamide (FC), fludarabine plus rituximab (FR), fludarabine plus cyclophosphamide plus rituximab (FCR) (see Appendix for treatment regimens). Randomized clinical trials have established higher complete remission rates and PFS intervals for fludarabine over alkylating agents and FC over fludarabine alone; however, no difference in overall survival has been demonstrated. Treatment duration is clinically aimed at palliating the inciting cause for therapy, and is typically 4 to 8 cycles. Before initiating treatment, consideration should be given to tumor lysis prophylaxis, especially in patients with very high lymphocyte counts or bulky disease. In addition, patients treated with purine analogs should be considered for prophylaxis against pneumocystis and varicella zoster. Ongoing studies are evaluating the role of alemtuzumab in consolidation in the front-line setting, after treatment with rituximab and fludarabine (e.g., Cancer and Leukemia Group B [CALGB] 10101). We currently utilize FR as our standard front-line therapy for CLL patients, and reserve oral chlorambucil and prednisone for patients with poor performance status not related to disease. Clinical research defining the optimal treatment approach for CLL patients continues at a rapid pace, and as new data emerges, these treatment recommendations will also evolve.

H. Treatment of relapsed and fludarabine-refractory chronic lymphocytic leukemia. Patients who relapse longer than 12 months after initial therapy with fludarabine are generally approached in a similar manner as untreated patients and almost 50% will respond to retreatment. Patients who fail to respond initially to a fludarabine-based regimen or progress within 6 months of such therapy remain a significant clinical challenge and their prognosis remains poor with a historical median overall survival of approximately 10 months regardless of therapy. Alemtuzumab (Campath), a humanized anti-CD52 monoclonal antibody, has been approved for fludarabine-refractory CLL patients in the USA. Treatment of heavily pretreated fludarabine-refractory CLL patients with alemtuzumab results in response rates of 29% to 50%, median PFS of 7 to 9 months, and overall survival of 13 to 16 months. Patients with poor performance status or bulky (more than 5 cm) disease have markedly less clinical benefit from alemtuzumab, and its use in patients with these characteristics is not recommended. Toxicities with alemtuzumab therapy are problematic with high rates of infusion reactions when administered intravenously, myelosuppression, opportunistic infections, and CMV reactivation, requiring routine prophylaxis against infectious pathogens and CMV monitoring. Administering alemtuzumab subcutaneously circumvents infusion reactions, for example, 3 mg SQ on day 1, 10 mg SQ on day 3, and 30 mg SQ on day 5 and then thrice weekly for 18 weeks (see Appendix). Interestingly, patients with p53 mutations have been shown to respond to alemtuzumab while being generally resistant to other treatment approaches.

Other treatment strategies for refractory CLL patients include retreatment with various combinations of fludarabine, cyclophosphamide, and rituximab, which yield overall response rates of 29% to 59% in this patient population, but also have significant toxicities. For example, a study from MD Anderson demonstrated that FCR combination yielded a 59% overall response rate and 5% complete response rate in fludarabine-refractory patients, but with high rates of grade 3 to 4 neutropenia and infectious complications. Early clinical studies have also shown promising results in fludarabine-refractory CLL patients using pentostatin in combination with cyclophosphamide and rituximab, and pentostatin-based chemotherapy approaches are being evaluated in additional clinical trials. High-dose steroids, for example, methylprednisolone 1 g/m^2 daily for 5 days repeated monthly, have also provided responses in refractory CLL patients, with response rates up to 77% including patients with p53 or 17p- genetic abnormalities. Life-threatening infections occur in approximately one third of patients treated with this approach and it necessitates routine prophylaxis against infections. Unfortunately, for most of these treatment approaches the duration of remission is typically 8 to 20 months, and most patients ultimately relapse and die from their disease.

Myeloablative allogeneic SCT has historically been used in a limited manner in CLL patients, primarily due to their advanced age. Small single-center and registry studies of selected CLL patients undergoing myeloablative SCT have shown treatment-related mortality rates of 24% to 46%, PFS of 26% to 62%, and overall survival of 31% to 76% at 3 to 10 years of projected follow-up. Recent studies utilizing reduced-intensity or nonmyeloablative allogeneic SCT have shown promising results with treatment-related mortalities of 15% to 22%, PFS of 52% to 67%, overall survival of 60% 80% with a short 2-year projected follow-up. In general, results are superior in younger patients, those with few comorbidities, and those with chemosensitive disease before transplantation. The optimal conditioning regimens, patient age eligible for transplantation, and salvage chemotherapeutic regimens remain under investigation.

Numerous new drugs are being evaluated in early clinical trials for patients with relapsed and fludarabine-refractory CLL, and enrollment on a clinical trial should be considered routinely for these patients. Lenalidomide (Revlimid) is a thalidomide analog with multiple potential mechanisms of action that has shown considerable single-agent clinical activity in multiple hematologic diseases, including multiple myeloma and myelodysplastic syndrome. Two phase II clinical trials have investigated lenalidomide doses of 25 mg daily for days 1 to 21 of a 28-day cycle in relapsed CLL patients, and have shown excellent tolerability and overall response rates of 32% to 65% and a complete response rate of 5% to 9%. Flavopiridol is a synthetic flavone with early clinical activity in a single-institution study that demonstrated overall response rates of 43% (many of which were durable for more than 12 months) as well as responses in patients with high-risk genetic features. The most notable toxicity reported was tumor lysis syndrome, which should be monitored for closely when treating CLL patients with this agent. Clinical trials evaluating lenalidomide and flavopiridol alone and with other agents are ongoing. In summary, depending on patient characteristics, appropriate treatment options for fludarabine-refractory CLL include clinical trials, alemtuzumab, combination chemotherapeutic regimens, high-dose steroids, and, in appropriate candidates, allogeneic SCT.

Suggested Readings

Chronic Myeloid Leukemia

Baccarani M, Saglio G, Goldman J, et al. Evolving concepts in the management of chronic myeloid leukemia: recommendations from an expert panel on behalf of the European LeukemiaNet. *Blood* 2006;108:1809–1820.

Deininger M, Schleuning M, Greinix H, et al. The effect of prior exposure to imatinib on transplant-related mortality. *Haematologica* 2006;91:452–459.

Druker BJ, Guilhot F, O'Brien SG, et al. Five-year follow-up of patients receiving imatinib for chronic myeloid leukemia. *N Engl J Med* 2006;355:2408–2417.

Mauro MJ. Defining and managing imatinib resistance. *Hematology* 2006:219–225.

Mauro MJ, Maziarz RT. Stem cell transplantation in patients with chronic myelogenous leukemia: when should it be used? *Mayo Clin Proc* 2006;81:404–416.

Chronic Lymphocytic Leukemia

An excellent in depth review of all aspects of CLL may be found in Volume 33, Number 2 of the Seminars in Oncology published in April 2006, edited by John C. Byrd and Michael R. Grever, including the following articles:

Byrd JC, Lin TS, Grever MR. Treatment of relapsed chronic lymphocytic leukemia: old and new therapies. *Semin Oncol* 2006;33:210–219.

Calin GA, Croce CM. Genomics of chronic lymphocytic leukemia microRNAs as new players with clinical significance. *Semin Oncol* 2006;33:167–173.

Hamblin TJ. Autoimmune complications of chronic lymphocytic leukemia. *Semin Oncol* 2006;33:230–239.

Seiler T, Dohner H, Stilgenbauer S. Risk stratification in chronic lymphocytic leukemia. *Semin Oncol* 2006;33:186–194.

Tsimberidou AM, Keating MJ. Richter's transformation in chronic lymphocytic leukemia. *Semin Oncol* 2006;33:250–256.

Wadhwa PD, Morrison VA. Infectious complications of chronic lymphocytic leukemia. *Semin Oncol* 2006;33:240–249.

Wierda WG, O'Brien SM. Initial therapy for patients with chronic lymphocytic leukemia. *Semin Oncol* 2006;33:202–209.

Additional Suggested Readings in CLL:

Byrd JC, Peterson BL, Morrison VA, et al. Randomized phase 2 study of fludarabine with concurrent versus sequential treatment with rituximab in symptomatic, untreated patients with B-cell chronic lymphocytic leukemia: results from Cancer and Leukemia Group B 9712 (CALGB 9712). *Blood* 2003;101:6–14.

Chiorazzi N, Rai KR, Ferrarini M. Chronic lymphocytic leukemia. *N Engl J Med* 2005;352:804–815.

Dohner H, Stilgenbauer S, Benner A, et al. Genomic aberrations and survival in chronic lymphocytic leukemia. *N Engl J Med* 2000;343:1910–1916.

Klein U, Tu Y, Stolovitzky GA, et al. Gene expression profiling of B-cell chronic lymphocytic leukemia reveals a homogeneous phenotype related to memory B cells. *J Exp Med* 2001;194:1625–1638.

Krober A, Seiler T, Benner A, et al. V_H mutational status, CD38 expression level, genomic aberrations, and survival in chronic lymphocytic leukemia. *Blood* 2002;100:1410–1416.

Montserrat E, Moreno C, Esteve J, et al. How I treat refractory CLL. *Blood* 2005;107: 1276–1283.

National Comprehensive Cancer Network. *The NCCN guidline on Non-Hodkin's Lymphoma, Clinical Practice Guidelines in Oncology (Version 2.2006).*© National Comprehensive Cancer Network, Inc. Available at: http://www.nccn.org. To view the most recent and complete version of the guideline, go online to www.nccn.org. 2006.

Rai KR, Peterson BL, Appelbaum FR, et al. Fludarabine compared to chlorambucil as primary therapy for CLL. *N Engl J Med* 2000;343:1750–1757.

Rassenti LZ, Huynh L, Toy TL, et al. ZAP-70 compared with immunoglobulin heavy-chain gene mutation status as a predictor of disease progression in chronic lymphocytic leukemia. *N Engl J Med* 2004;351:893–901.

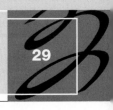

HEMATOLOGIC MALIGNANCIES: PLASMA CELL DYSCRASIAS 29

Tanya Wildes and Ravi Vij

I. MULTIPLE MYELOMA

A. Subjective. Symptoms of multiple myeloma (MM) include bone pain, fatigue, renal insufficiency and recurrent bacterial infections. Fatigue, present in one third of patients, is usually attributable to anemia. One third of MM patients develop hypercalcemia which presents with nausea, constipation, dehydration, and mental status changes. One fourth of patients will present with weight loss. Paresthesias and neuropathy related to the monoclonal paraprotein (M protein) are present in 5% of newly diagnosed MM patients. Tumor fever is rare, and is a diagnosis of exclusion; febrile MM patients are infected until proved otherwise. One third of patients have a prior diagnosis of a plasma cell proliferative process preceding the diagnosis of MM.

B. Objective. Physical examination may reveal pallor, bony tenderness, a subcutaneous mass secondary to a plasmacytoma, or focal neurologic signs due to spinal cord compression. Hepatomegaly, splenomegaly, and lymphadenopathy are rare.

C. Workup and staging

1. **Laboratory.** Anemia is present in three quarters of patients at diagnosis and is generally normochromic and normocytic. White blood cell (WBC) and platelet counts are usually preserved, although marrow replacement by MM may lead to pancytopenia. Examination of the peripheral smear may reveal rouleaux formation. The erythrocyte sedimentation rate (ESR) is generally elevated in MM. Almost 20% of patients will have creatinine more than 2.0 mg/dL at diagnosis. Hypercalcemia due to extensive bone involvement and hyperuricemia can worsen renal function. Albumin has prognostic significance and is a component of the International Staging System. A serum protein electrophoresis (SPEP) and urinary protein electrophoresis (UPEP) should be performed on patients in whom the diagnosis of MM is suspected. Immunofixation is more sensitive than electrophoresis and is done to confirm the presence and type of a paraprotein (M protein). An M protein is detectable in the serum of more than 90% of patients. The paraprotein is an IgG in approximately half the cases and an IgA in 20% of cases. IgD, IgE, and IgM paraproteins are very rare. IgM paraproteins are almost always associated with Waldenstrom's macroglobulinemia (WM). Free light chains are present in approximately 15% of patients. Kappa (κ) light chains are more common than lambda (λ) by approximately 2:1. Bences-Jones proteinuria occurs when light chains are freely filtered at the glomerulus and are excreted in the urine. The light chain will therefore usually be undetected on SPEP, but will be detected on UPEP. If light chains are detected in the urine, a 24-hour urine specimen should be collected to quantify the protein and monitor response to treatment. The serum free light chain (SFLC) assay now allows for quantification of light chains in the serum. Nonsecretory myeloma constitutes less than 5% of patients. These patients have no paraprotein detectable on SPEP, UPEP, and immunofixation. However, a majority will have an abnormal SFLC κ:λ ratio.

2. **Radiographic imaging.** All patients should have a skeletal survey including the skull, spine, pelvis, femurs, and humeri. Almost 80% of patients have at least one abnormality on radiographs; two thirds of patients will have punched-out lytic lesions, whereas pathologic fractures, vertebral compression fractures, or osteoporosis are each present in one fourth of patients. Radionuclide bone scans detect osteoblastic response and are therefore less sensitive than plain

333

radiographs in detecting skeletal involvement. Magnetic resonance imaging (MRI) of the spine is more sensitive than plain radiographs in detecting early lesions. Patients thought to have solitary plasmacytomas should undergo MRI of the spine to exclude systemic disease. The role of ^{18}F-fluorodeoxyglucose positron emission tomography (FDG PET) in the workup of multiple myeloma is evolving. It may have a role in the initial evaluation of nonsecretory MM and subsequent evaluation of response to therapy.

3. **Bone marrow evaluation.** Patients should undergo bone marrow biopsy and aspiration for quantification of bone marrow plasma cells. The malignant plasma cells stain positive for CD138. Monoclonality is established by immunostains which demonstrate κ or λ restricted cytoplasmic immunoglobulin staining. Karyotyping is now recommended as a prognostic tool. Conventional cytogenetic analysis in MM is often difficult because of the low growth fraction and paucity of mitotic cells. However, using a variety of fluorescent *in situ* hybridization (FISH) probes (del 13q, t[4;14], t [11;14], del 17p) on interphase cells, cytogenetic abnormalities are commonly found in MM. The plasma cell labelling index (PCLI) performed on bone marrow biopsy measures the percentage of MM cells that synthesize DNA; an elevated labelling index implies a more aggressive MM and poor prognosis.

D. **Diagnosis.** To meet classic diagnostic criteria for myeloma, patients must have a combination of major and minor criteria as follows: I + b, c, or d; II + b, c, or d; III + a, c, or d; a + b + c; a + b + d (Table 29.1). The International Myeloma Working Group has established simplified criteria for the plasma cells dyscrasias (Table 29.2).

E. **Staging.** The Durie–Salmon staging system is most frequently used (Table 29.3). The International Staging System (Table 29.4) is a new, simplified staging system that utilizes only the β2-microglobulin and albumin.

F. **Treatment**

1. **High-dose therapy (HDT)/autologous transplant.** High-dose chemotherapy with autologous stem cell transplant is considered standard of care for transplant eligible patients with MM. Response rates (RRs) to HDT approach 90% with approximately one third having a complete response. A patient suitable for transplant undergoes induction therapy with 4 to 6 months of a regimen containing thalidomide, bortezomib, or an anthracycline. Alkylating agents should be avoided in these patients because of the stem cell toxicity of this class of drugs. Subsequently, the patient undergoes stem cell collection, consolidative HDT and transplant. Alternatively, patients may undergo harvest and stem cell storage first, and then proceed to alkylator-based treatment, postponing transplant until first relapse. Randomized trials have shown equivalent survival with these two approaches; however, quality of life analysis and total treatment time favor early transplant. Conditioning for transplant with single-agent melphalan is the

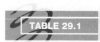

TABLE 29.1   Diagnostic Criteria for Myeloma

Major criteria	Minor criteria
I. Plasmacytosis on tissue biopsy	**a.** Marrow plasmacytosis 10%–30%
II. Marrow plasmacytosis of >30%	**b.** Monoclonal protein present but less than in major criterion III
III. Monoclonal protein >3.5 g/dL for IgG or 2 g/dL for IgA or unequivocal light-chain (Bence Jones) proteinuria	**c.** Lytic bone lesions
	d. Hypoglobulinemia: IgM, <50; IgA, <100, or IgG, <600/dL

Ig, immunoglobulin.

TABLE 29.2   International Myeloma Working Group Classification System

Multiple myeloma	M protein in serum and/or urine
	Bone marrow (clonal) plasma cells or plasmacytoma
	Related organ or tissue impairment[a]
Smouldering myeloma	M protein in serum <30 g/L and/or
	Bone marrow clonal plasma cells <10%
	No related organ or tissue impairment or symptoms[a]
MGUS	M protein in serum <30 g/L
	Bone marrow clonal plasma cells <10% and low level of plasma cell infiltration in a trephine biopsy (if done)
	No evidence of other B-cell proliferative disorders
	No related organ or tissue impairment[a]
Solitary plasmacytoma of bone	No M protein in serum and/or urine[b]
	Single area of bone destruction due to clonal plasma cells
	Bone marrow not consistent with multiple myeloma
	Normal skeletal survey (and MRI of spine and pelvis if done)
	No related organ or tissue impairment (other than solitary bone lesion)[a]
Extramedullary plasmacytoma	No M protein in serum and/or urine[b]
	Extramedullary tumor of clonal plasma cells
	Normal bone marrow
	Normal skeletal survey
	No related organ or tissue impairment[a]

MGUS, monoclonal gammopathy of unknown significance; MRI, magnetic resonance imaging.
[a]**Related organ or tissue involvement (ROTI)** includes bone lesions (lytic lesions or osteoporosis), hypercalcemia, renal insufficiency , anemia, hyperviscosity, amyloidosis or recurrent bacterial infections.
[b]A small M-component may sometimes be present.

standard of care. Although controlled trials of transplant generally excluded patients older than 65 years, improvements in supportive care have allowed the application of high-dose therapy and autologous transplant to elderly patients older than 70. Medicare approves this procedure for patients up to 76 years of age. Toxicities of high-dose therapy include mucositis and infectious complications; overall transplant-related mortality is 1% to 2%. Repeated HDT

TABLE 29.3   Durie–Salmon Staging System

Stage I	All of the following
	Hemoglobin >10 g/dL
	Normal serum calcium
	0 or 1 bone lesions on skeletal survey
	Low quantity of monoclonal paraprotein (IgG, <5 g/dL; IgA, <3 g/dL, or urine light chains <4 g/day)
Stage II	Does not meet criteria for stage I or stage III
Stage III	Any one of the following
	Hemoglobin <8.5 g/dL
	Serum calcium >12mg/dL
	Advanced (>3) lytic bone lesions
	High quantity of monoclonal paraprotein (IgG, >7 g/dL; IgA, >5 g/dL; or urine light chains, >12 g/24 h)

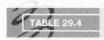

TABLE 29.4	International Staging System for Multiple Myeloma	
	Criteria	**Median survival**
Stage I	β2M <3.5 mg/L and albumin $\geq$3.5 g/dL	62 months
Stage II	Not I or III	45 months
Stage III	β2M $\geq$5.5 mg/L	29 months

β2M, β2microglobulin.

and transplant within 6 months ("tandem transplant") may provide a survival benefit in patients who have less than a very good partial response (less than 90% reduction in paraprotein) after their first transplant.

2. Conventional therapy

   a. Thalidomide has considerable activity in MM. Approximately one third of patients with untreated MM respond to single-agent thalidomide; RRs approach 70% when thalidomide is used in combination with dexamethasone. The RR to single-agent thalidomide is also approximately 30% in relapsed/refractory MM. Thalidomide is also being studied in combination with other agents. Doses of 100 mg/day appear to be as effective as higher doses of 400 mg/day and are better tolerated. Side effects of thalidomide include sedation, peripheral neuropathy, constipation, and thrombosis. Thalidomide is a potent teratogen; women who may conceive and sexual partners of women of child-bearing age are extensively educated on avoiding pregnancy while taking thalidomide. The mechanism of action of thalidomide remains unclear; proposed mechanisms include suppression of angiogenesis, immunomodulation through inhibition of tumor necrosis factor α and decreased NF-κB binding, cell-mediated cytotoxicity, and alteration of expression of cellular adhesion molecules.

   b. Lenalidomide is an immunomodulatory agent that, *in vitro*, has greater potency than thalidomide. In relapsed/refractory MM, lenalidomide plus dexamethasone improves time to progression and overall survival compared to dexamethasone alone; the RR to lenalidomide plus dexamethasone approaches 60%. Lenalidomide is also being studied as initial therapy and in combination with other agents. Myelotoxicity and thromboembolism are lenalidomide's most prominent side effects.

   c. Bortezomib, a proteosome inhibitor, prolongs time to progression and improves overall survival in relapsed myeloma compared to dexamethasone. The RR to bortezomib in relapsed myeloma is almost 40%, with a 6% complete response rate. Bortezomib has also demonstrated impressive RRs as initial therapy and in combination with other agents. The main side effect of bortezomib is neurotoxicity. Although the mechanism of action is not completely understood, its effects may be mediated through direct cytotoxicity and induction of apoptosis, as well as through effects on the bone marrow microenvironment through blockage of cytokines, angiogenesis, and cell adhesion.

   d. Melphalan and prednisone (MP) is a well-tolerated oral treatment option. RRs to MP approach 50%, although fewer than 5% of patients will have a complete response. Response to MP is slow, taking up to 6 months. Treatment should be continued for 1 year or until patients reach a plateau phase. Long-term treatment with melphalan or other alkylating agents make stem cell harvest and autologous transplant difficult; melphalan should not be given to a patient who is a candidate for transplantation.

   e. Vincristine, doxorubicin (Adriamycin), and dexamethasone (VAD) Compared with MP, VAD produces a faster response, which may be helpful in controlling disease-related symptoms. RRs to VAD as initial therapy are 55% to 65%; in the relapsed/refractory setting, RRs are 25% to 50%. VAD is less toxic to hematopoietic stem cells than is alkylator-based chemotherapy and is used for induction before autologous transplant, with the goal of preserving stem cells for later harvest. However, the 4-day infusional regimen of VAD is cumbersome, requiring a central line and either hospitalization or a portable pump. Substitution of infusional adriamycin with bolus liposomal doxorubicin (DVD regimen) offers comparable responses. Toxicities of VAD include cardiotoxicity due to doxorubicin, peripheral neuropathy due to vincristine, and complications related to central venous access required for this infusional regimen, such as catheter-associated bloodstream infections.

f. **Dexamethasone** alone is a very active agent in MM with a RR more than 40% in untreated myeloma. Dexamethasone is not myelosuppressive, and may be especially suited to patients with severe marrow compromise. High-dose dexamethasone may cause gastric ulcers, hyperglycemia, or psychiatric side effects such as agitation or depression. Although the exact mechanism of dexamethasone in MM is unknown, it downregulates gene expression of interleukin 6 (IL-6), a major myeloma growth factor.

g. **Other.** Multiple alkylator regimens such as M2 (vincristine, carmustine, cyclophosphamide, and melphalan) are reserved for patients who relapse after autologous transplant or other special cases. Other agents being studied include arsenic, and regimens containing cytarabine, cisplatin and etoposide that resemble salvage lymphoma regimens.

3. **Maintenance therapy.** A number of agents have been studied in the postconventional therapy or posttransplant maintenance setting. Interest in interferon has waned as no survival benefit has been seen. Prednisone 50 mg PO every other day following conventional therapy improves progression-free and overall survival compared to 10 mg PO every other day. Thalidomide and lenalidomide are also being actively investigated as maintenance therapy.

4. **Allogeneic transplant.** Allogeneic transplant is usually considered for young, fit patients for whom autologous transplant has failed and who have a matched sibling donor. Allogeneic transplant after myeloablative conditioning in MM carries a high treatment-related mortality. Interest in nonmyeloablative allogeneic transplant strategies as part of the initial treatment of MM is increasing as it is recognized that the mortality is lower (100-day mortality less than 10%). However, long-term followup data are lacking currently. Initial data on tandem autologous transplant followed by reduced intensity conditioning allogeneic stem cell transplant are encouraging, but this approach has yet to be shown to be superior in a randomized controlled trial.

G. **Adjunct treatments**

1. **Bisphosphonates** inhibit osteoclastic resorption of bone. In patients with MM, bisphosphonates decrease skeletal-related events, including fractures and hypercalcemia. Pamidronate or zoledronic acid should be administered once a month. Current guidelines recommend indefinite use of bisphosphonates. However, there is increasing recognition that long-term use of these agents is associated with renal toxicity and the rare but potentially very disabling complication of osteonecrosis of the jaw. Recommendations regarding frequency and duration of therapy may change.

2. **Erythropoietin.** Anemia is a common complication of MM. Erythropoietin decreases transfusion requirements in MM patients, including patients with refractory disease.

3. **Radiation.** MM is a radiosensitive tumor. External-beam radiation can effectively palliate discrete areas of bone pain or areas of mass effect such as spinal cord compression.

4. **Surgery.** Radiographs of long bones done for staging or to evaluate pain may reveal lytic lesions concerning for impending fracture. Orthopedic surgery consultation and prophylactic surgical pinning may prevent some of the morbidity

of a fracture. Patients who undergo pinning should generally undergo x-ray therapy (XRT) to the area postoperatively.

5. **Hemodialysis.** Renal failure may occur early in the course of disease. Renal impairment may be reversible if the MM responds to treatment, and support with hemodialysis is appropriate. The value of plasmapheresis to reduce the paraprotein level in this situation is debatable.

6. **Infection prophylaxis.** MM patients have a deficit in humoral immunity due to decreased levels of normal immunoglobulins. The risk of infection is further increased both by direct marrow suppression from chemotherapy as well as immunosuppression associated with long-term, high-dose corticosteroids. All MM patients should be vaccinated against *Streptococcus pneumoniae*.

H. Follow-up. M protein levels in the serum or urine fluctuate with tumor load and can be used as an index to monitor MM response to treatment. However, sometimes paraprotein levels may lose their value for follow-up later in the course of the disease as the myeloma cells may dedifferentiate and grow in the absence of a secreted paraprotein. Other markers such as peripheral blood counts or serum calcium and creatinine levels may correlate with disease progression or response to therapy. It is particularly difficult to follow patients with nonsecretory myeloma. Repeated skeletal surveys are not a viable way to monitor disease response, because even with good responses, lytic lesions may not show healing on radiographs. The patchy nature of bone marrow plasmacytosis also makes serial bone marrow biopsies an unreliable predictor of response. Serial positron emission tomography (PET) scans and SFLC analysis have an evolving role in this subgroup of patients.

I. Natural history

1. **Survival.** Like those with other hematologic malignancies, patients with advanced MM usually die of infection. In MM, conventional chemotherapy ameliorates symptoms and prolongs life from a median of 6 months to 3 years. Recently, in untreated elderly patients, melphalan/prednisone in combination with thalidomide (MPT) was shown to provide superior overall survival compared with MP alone (median overall survival greater than 56 months with MPT versus 30.3 months with MP). High-dose therapy with autologous transplant provides a median overall survival of 5 or more years in most series. Data regarding the impact of agents such as bortezomib and lenalidomide on survival is not yet available.

2. **Prognostic factors.** Serum β_2-microglobulin levels are highly correlated with prognosis. Other poor prognostic factors include high lactate dehydrogenase (LDH), high plasma cell–labeling index, low albumin, plasmablastic features in the bone marrow, circulating plasma cells, and certain chromosomal abnormalities and translocations. Deletion of chromosome 13 on karyotyping is associated with poor response to therapy and shorter overall survival. A number of translocation partners involving the immunoglobulin heavy gene locus on chromosome 14 have prognostic significance. The t(4;14) involving the tyrosine kinase FGFR3 and MMSET genes and the immunoglobulin heavy-chain gene portends a poor prognosis. The t(14;16) causes the upregulation of the transcription factor c-*maf*, resulting in shorter survival. The t(11;14), resulting in dysregulated cyclin D1, appears to have a neutral impact on survival. Deletions of chromosome 17p13, the p53 locus, and hypodiploidy are also associated with poor prognosis.

J. Background

1. **Epidemiology.** The incidence of MM is 4/100,000/year. MM represents 1.1% of all new cancer diagnoses and 2% of all cancer deaths. Incidence in African Americans is double that in the white population. The median age of patients is 65 to 70 years. The etiology of MM is unknown. A prior diagnosis of monoclonal gammopathy of unknown significance (MGUS) is a risk factor for MM. Benzene and radiation exposure appear to be additional risk factors.

2. **Pathophysiology.** Cytokines provide autocrine and paracrine growth signals to myeloma cells. IL-6, insulin-like growth factor-1, stromal cell derived factor-1 and vascular endothelial growth factor have all been shown to be important in

myeloma cell survival and growth. The interaction between MM cells and stromal cells involving adhesion molecules such as intercellular adhesion molecule 1 (ICAM-1) and vascular adhesion molecule 1 (VCAM-1) is thought to provide critical survival signals. There is a growing body of literature on the pathophysiology of myeloma bone disease. Lytic bone lesions are a hallmark of MM. Under normal circumstances, receptor activator of nuclear factor κB ligand (RANKL) on osteoblasts binds to receptor activator of nuclear factor κB (RANK) on osteoclasts, prolonging osteoclast life span. Osteoprotegerin (OPG) blocks the effects of RANKL by acting as a decoy receptor for RANKL, suppressing osteoclast formation. In MM, lytic lesions result from increased RANKL production, decreased OPG production, tumor-derived osteoclast activating factors such as macrophage inflammatory protein-1 α (MIP-1 α), and osteoblast inhibition through MM-derived dickkopf-1 (DKK-1).

   3. Molecular biology. Although the critical genetic events in the pathogenesis of malignant plasma cells are not known, recent karyotypic and gene expression analysis has provided proof of a multistep pathogenesis in MM. IgH translocations, trisomies and 13q deletions are observed in patients with MGUS and are thought to be early genetic events. Activating mutations of *ras, myc* dysregulation, inactivation of Rb and loss/mutation of p53 appear to be critical late events in pathogenesis.

K. Research frontiers. New approaches to therapy will include novel agents either alone or in combination with established agents. Drugs being studied in MM include tyrosine kinase inhibitors, monoclonal antibodies, histone deacetylase inhibitors, mammalian target of rapamycin (mTOR) inhibitors, and heat shock protein 90 (HSP90) inhibitors. Novel proteosome inhibitors and immunomodulatory agents are also under investigation.

II. OTHER PLASMA CELL DISORDERS

A. Monoclonal gammopathy of undetermined significance (MGUS). The term MGUS implies the presence of paraprotein without malignancy (Table 29.2). A paraprotein is present in 2% to 14% of well elderly people, and the incidence increases with age. It is often discovered when the workup for renal insufficiency or anemia reveals the presence of a small amount of paraprotein on SPEP. MGUS patients should be monitored with SPEP every 6 months to assess the level of the paraprotein. One percent of patients with MGUS progress to a more clinically significant plasma cell dyscrasia each year. Risk factors for progression to MM include an abnormal SFLC ratio, which confers a threefold higher risk of progression to MM, and the presence of circulating plasma cells, which doubles the risk of progression.

B. Smouldering myeloma. Patients with smouldering MM are generally observed off therapy until symptoms develop or there is evidence of disease progression. (Table 29.2).

C. Plasma cell leukemia. Plasma cell leukemia occurs when there are greater than 2×10^9/L plasma cells in the peripheral blood or greater than 20% plasma cells in the differential WBC count. When plasma cell leukemia arises *de novo* without an antecedent plasma cell disorder, median survival is 6 months. When plasma cell leukemia occurs as a late terminal event in a patient with known MM, the median survival is only 1 to 2 months. Patients with high-grade plasmacytic malignancies are initially treated with induction regimens used in myeloma, such as VAD.

D. Solitary plasmacytomas of bone. Patients with a solitary plasmacytoma have normal bone marrow and no evidence of systemic disease (Table 29.2). An MRI of the spine should be obtained to exclude additional occult lesions. Radiation provides excellent local control, with 90% free from local recurrence. There is no evidence that chemotherapy during or after radiation provides a benefit to patients with solitary plasmacytoma. Patients with lesions larger than 5 cm have the greatest risk of recurrence after radiotherapy. Survival is excellent, with half the number of patients alive at 10 years. Up to half the number of patients may develop overt MM, which may occur more than a decade later.

E. Extramedullary plasmacytomas. Extramedullary plasmacytomas are clonal proliferations of plasma cells that arise outside of the bone marrow (Table 29.2).

Lesions occur most frequently within the upper respiratory tract, including the sinuses, nasal cavity, nasopharynx, and larynx, but may occur in virtually any organ. They are associated with an IgA monoclonal protein. Extramedullary plasmacytomas are very sensitive to radiation therapy, and chemotherapy does not provide additional benefit. Ten-year overall survival approaches 70%, and only 15% to 30% of patients will develop MM.

III. AMYLOIDOSIS

A. Subjective. Patients with amyloidosis (AL) present with nonspecific complaints such as fatigue, weight loss, and lightheadedness. Orthostasis may result from nephrotic syndrome and intravascular volume depletion, from restrictive cardiomyopathy, or from autonomic instability. Edema may result from nephrotic syndrome or congestive heart failure. Infiltration of soft tissues can cause capillary fragility and purpuric bruising; periorbital ecchymosis is a classic symptom of AL. Less common symptoms include tongue enlargement, endocrine symptoms, neuropathy, and carpal tunnel syndrome.

B. Objective. Physical findings in AL vary depending on which organ systems are affected by amyloid deposits. Examination may reveal macroglossia, periorbital ecchymosis, hepatomegaly, or edema. Nerve involvement can result in sensory, motor, or autonomic deficits. Laboratory evaluation may reveal renal insufficiency or hypoalbuminemia due to nephrotic syndrome. Half the number of patients will have low voltage in the limb leads on electrocardiogram. Amyloid infiltration of the heart may appear on echocardiography as hypertrophic cardiomyopathy with a restrictive filling pattern or with increased "sparkling" echogenicity.

C. Workup. The first step in the workup of AL is to suspect the diagnosis. A clue to the possibility of AL is the discovery of a paraprotein in the serum or urine of the patient. The paraprotein may be a complete immunoglobulin, although only the light-chain component contributes to amyloid formation. Only a small quantity (less than 1 g/dL) of paraprotein may be present. SFLC assays can be utilized in patients with a negative serum immunfixation. The λ light chains are three times more commonly associated with AL, presumably because these more often possess amyloidogenic characteristics. Under polarized light, amyloid shows apple-green birefringence when stained with Congo red stain. Immunoperoxidase stains on tissue specimens can differentiate between different types of amyloid. Biopsy of abdominal fat is often done in an attempt to make a tissue diagnosis while avoiding biopsy of vital organs. The presence of amyloid is 100% specific, but sensitivity varies and can be less than 75%. A bone marrow biopsy will be positive for amyloid deposition in 60% of cases. In most cases of primary AL, clonal plasma cells represent less than 10% of the marrow. MM and AL sometimes coexist: 20% of patients with AL are found on workup to have myeloma, and in 10% to 15% of patients with MM, AL will eventually develop. If fat-pad and bone marrow biopsies are negative, it may be necessary to perform a biopsy of the kidney, myocardium, or other affected organ. Troponin T and N-terminal probrain natriuretic peptide (NT-proBNP) are both powerful predictors of survival in AL patients.

D. Therapy

1. Chemotherapy. There are currently no therapeutic agents that accelerate amyloid destruction. Treatment has been directed at the underlying plasma cell dyscrasia with regimens active in MM. Approximately one third of patients will respond to MP. Melphalan plus dexamethasone (Melph/dex) has produced responses in two thirds of patients. Approximately half the number of patients will respond to VAD or thalidomide plus dexamethasone (Thal-dex).

2. High-dose therapy/autologous transplant. The role of HDT in amyloid remains controversial. Small phase II trials suggest impressive results with autologous transplant following melphalan conditioning. However, a recent prospective randomized trial failed to show a survival advantage to transplant over conventional therapy, but this trial has been criticized for the small number of patients randomized and a higher than expected mortality in the transplant arm.

3. Future directions. Preliminary reports have shown encouraging responses with bortezomib and lenalidomide.

E. Epidemiology and survival. The estimated incidence is 5.1 to 12.8 new cases per million per year. Systemic AL is invariably fatal, although prognosis depends on the organs affected. Median survival is approximately 1 to 2 years in untreated patients, but is less than 6 months in patients with cardiac amyloid. After HDT, median overall survival in some series approaches 5 years, but this effect may be due to selection bias.

F. Pathophysiology. AL is actually a group of syndromes in which symptoms arise from infiltration of tissue with proteinaceous material. In primary amyloid (AL), the amyloid is composed of paraprotein light chains secreted by monoclonal plasma cells in β sheet conformation; the protein is very resistant to proteolysis. Sequence characteristics of the light-chain M protein determine whether it will be cleared or accumulate as amyloid. Other syndromes include secondary amyloidosis (AA) due to chronic inflammation, dialysis-associated AL, and familial AL. In each of these diseases, the amyloid is composed of a different protein, but the microscopic appearance of the depositions is the same.

IV. WALDENSTRÖM'S MACROGLOBULINEMIA. In the World Health Organization (WHO) classification of non-Hodgkin's lymphoma (NHL), WM is a subset of lymphoplasmacytic lymphoma (LPL), a mature B-cell neoplasm closely related to chronic lymphocytic leukemia/small lymphocytic lymphoma (CLL/SLL).

A. Subjective. Patients may present with nonspecific symptoms such as fevers, night sweats, fatigue, anorexia, weight loss, or peripheral neuropathy. Monoclonal IgM may cause the classic triad of hyperviscosity syndrome (HVS) in up to one third of patients: bruising/bleeding, visual changes and neuropsychiatric symptoms. Easy bleeding results from paraprotein interfering with coagulation factors and platelet function. Retinal bleeding or blindness may occur. Neuropsychiatric symptoms include transient ischemic attacks (TIAs), paralysis, seizures, dementia, or coma. IgM deposits in the skin may cause purpuric lesions. Occasionally, the IgM paraprotein is a cryoglobulin and causes Raynaud's syndrome and acral cyanosis.

B. Objective. Many patients with WM have no obvious physical findings. On funduscopic examination, patients may have retinal hemorrhages, exudates, or papilledema. Approximately one third of patients have hepatomegaly, splenomegaly, or lymphadenopathy. IgM can act as an autoantibody against autologous antigens, resulting in autoimmune phenomenon such as demyelinating peripheral neuropathy, cryoglobulinemia, cold agglutinin disease, glomerulonephritis, paraneoplastic pemphigus, or retinitis.

C. Workup and staging. Patients are usually anemic. They may have renal insufficiency or proteinuria. High paraprotein levels can cause pseudohyponatremia. The ESR may be very high or spuriously low. Bone marrow involvement is universal. The diagnosis of LPL may be made on bone marrow biopsy or lymph node biopsy. LPL cells express cytoplasmic immunoglobulin, distinguishing them from CLL/SLL cells, which do not. Other immunophenotypic markers are similar to those of CLL, including expression of CD19 and CD20. During workup of WM, serum viscosity should be measured. Symptomatic hyperviscosity usually does not occur until IgM is greater than 3 g/dL and the serum viscosity is more than 5 cp (normal is 1.4 to 1.8 cp), although symptoms can occur at lower levels of paraprotein and lower serum viscosities.

D. Therapy. Treatment of WM is directed at reducing serum viscosity and treating the underlying lymphoma. Plasmapheresis rapidly reduces circulating IgM, ameliorating symptoms of hyperviscosity. Plasmapheresis alone is sometimes used to palliate refractory or frail patients. Severe neurologic symptoms or intractable bleeding due to hyperviscosity are an oncologic emergency, requiring urgent plasmapheresis. The LPL underlying WM is treated the same as CLL/SLL. Treatment should be reserved for patients who are symptomatic either from the LPL or from high levels of IgM. Fludarabine is often used as first-line treatment alone or in combination with rituximab. RRs to single-agent fludarabine are 40% to 80% with median overall survival of 7 years. Rituximab alone has been shown to be effective in both untreated and relapsed LPL, but may cause an IgM flare. Chlorambucil, pentostatin, and cladribine also have established efficacy. Autologous and allogeneic stem cell transplants have been utilized, but it is unclear whether these confer any benefit over conventional therapy.

   E. **Epidemiology/natural history.** WM is uncommon, occurring in 3.4 per million men and 1.7 per million women. Median age is 65. Unlike MM, WM occurs much more often in white than in African Americans. Median survival is 5 to 6 years. Patients may eventually develop refractory disease or undergo transformation into a higher-grade neoplasm. Advanced age, anemia, hypoalbuminemia and elevated β2-microglobulin are adverse prognostic factors.

V. **POEMS SYNDROME (POLYNEUROPATHY, ORGANOMEGALY, ENDOCRINO-PATHY, M PROTEIN, AND SKIN CHANGES).** These patients present in the sixth decade of life with stocking-glove numbness, paresthesias, weakness, fatigue, or other nonspecific symptoms. Half the number of patients have organomegaly (hepatomegaly, splenomegaly, or lymphadenopathy). Evidence of Castleman's disease (giant lymph node hyperplasia) may be found. Sclerotic bone lesions, present in almost all patients, are composed of collections of clonal plasma cells. Diabetes mellitus and gonadal dysfunction are the most common endocrinopathies in POEMS syndrome. Skin changes include hyperpigmentation, hemangiomas, hair changes, and acrocyanosis. Other associated features are papilledema, effusions, ascites, peripheral edema, clubbing, sclerotic bone lesions, polycythemia, and thrombocytosis. The M protein is generally small and virtually always λ restricted. Bone marrow biopsy generally demonstrates less than 5% plasma cells. Single bone lesions may be irradiated. Systemic therapy with alkylators, combination chemotherapy, or steroids is indicated for patients who are symptomatic. Peripheral blood stem cell transplant following high-dose therapy has been successfully used. The course of POEMS syndrome is extremely indolent, with median survival of almost 14 years.

VI. **LIGHT-CHAIN DEPOSITION DISEASE.** Some patients with the clinical features of AL but without detectable tissue amyloid may have nonamyloid light-chain deposition disease (LCDD). LCDD tends to present with nephrotic syndrome or renal insufficiency. Unlike AL, κ light chains predominate over λ; LCDD deposits do not take on the amyloid structure or stain with Congo red. Most patients have detectable serum or urinary M protein and may have an associated plasma cell dyscrasia or lymphoproliferative disorder. Treatment is similar to that described earlier for AL.

VII. **HEAVY-CHAIN DISEASE.** Rarely an M protein is found to be a truncated heavy chain with no associated light chain. The γ and μ heavy-chain paraproteins are rare and are usually associated with NHL. α-Heavy chain proteinemia is associated with *immunoproliferative small intestinal disease* (IPSID), also called Mediterranean lymphoma. IPSID, now considered to be a mucosa-associated lymphoid tissue (MALT) lymphoma, primarily affects young adults in areas of the Mediterranean, North Africa and the Middle East who suffer from chronic intestinal diseases and malnutrition. Peripheral adenopathy is rare, but retroperitoneal adenopathy may be palpable as an abdominal mass. Diffuse infiltration of the intestine by lymphocytes or plasma cells results in a thickened, hard, pipe-like intestine on endoscopy or imaging. The truncated α-heavy chain M protein associated with IPSID is an abnormal IgA molecule that may be detectable by immunofixation on serum, urine, tissue samples, or jejunal secretions sampled by endoscopy. Electrophoresis is less effective at detecting heavy chains, as they migrate as a smear rather than a discrete band. Biopsy of the intestine or mesenteric nodes is necessary for diagnosis. Patients should be evaluated for intestinal pathogens such as Giardia. Similar to *Helicobacter pylori* –associated gastric MALTomas, early-stage IPSID may respond to antimicrobials directed at any documented intestinal pathogens. More advanced disease may require chemotherapy appropriate for low-grade NHL. IPSID has an indolent course with a 5-year survival rate of approximately two thirds.

Suggested Readings

Blade J. Transplantation for multiple myeloma: who, when, how often? High-dose therapy in multiple myeloma. *Blood* 2003;102(10):3469–3477.

Comenzo RL, Gertz MA. Autologous stem cell transplantation for primary systemic amyloidosis. *Blood* 2002;99(12):4276–4282.

Dimopoulos MA, Kyle RA, Anagnostopoulos A, et al. Diagnosis and management of Waldenstrom's macroglobulinemia. *J Clin Oncol* 2005;23(7):1564–1577.

Dimopoulos MA, Moulopoulos LA, Maniatis A, et al. Solitary plasmacytoma of bone and asymptomatic multiple myeloma. *Blood* 2000;96(6):2037–2044.

Falk RH, Comenzo RL, Skinner M. The systemic amyloidosis. *N Engl J Med* 1997;337(13): 898–909.

Gertz MA, Lacy MQ, Dispenzieri A, et al. Amyloidosis: diagnosis and management. *Clin Lymphoma Myeloma* 2005;6(3):208–19.

Hideshima T, Bergsagel PL, Kuehl WM, et al. Advances in biology of multiple myeloma: clinical applications. *Blood* 2004;104(3):607–618.

Kyle RA, Rajkumar SV. Multiple myeloma. *N Engl J Med* 2004;351:1860–73.

Merlini G, Bellotti V. Molecular mechanisms of amyloidosis. *N Engl J Med* 2003;349: 583–96.

Pozzi C, D'Amico M, Fogazzi GB, et al. Light chain deposition disease with renal involvement: clinical characteristics and prognostic factors. *Am J Kidney Dis* 2003;42(6): 1154–1163.

Rajkumar SV, Dispenzieri A, Kyle RA. Monoclonal gammopathy of undetermined significance, Waldenstrom macroglobulinemia, AL amyloidosis, and related plasma cell disorders: diagnosis and treatment. *Mayo Clin Proc* 2006;81(5):693–703.

Treon SP, Gertz MA, Dimopoulos M, et al. Update on treatment recommendations from the third international workshop on Waldenstrom's macroglobulinemia. *Blood* 2006;107(9):3442–3446.

Witzig TE, Wahner-Roedler DL. Heavy chain disease. *Curr Treat Options Oncol* 2002;3: 247–254.

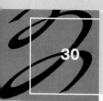

HIV AND CANCER
Lee Ratner and Benjamin Tan

GENERAL CARE OF THE PATIENT WITH HIV AND CANCER

I. **GENERAL.** A malignancy develops in approximately 20% of patients with human immunodeficiency virus (HIV) during their lifetime, and is often the first clinical evidence of HIV infection. It is also responsible for 28% of acquired immunodeficiency syndrome (AIDS) patients' deaths. The most common malignancies in this patient population are non-Hodgkin's lymphoma (NHL), Kaposi's sarcoma, and anogenital carcinoma. Most of these malignancies are associated with oncogenic viruses, including Epstein Barr virus (EBV), human herpesvirus 8 (HHV-8), and human papilloma viruses (HPV). The incidence of other malignancies is also increased in HIV-infected patients, including Hodgkin's lymphoma (HL), lung cancers, multiple myeloma, testicular tumors, and childhood sarcomas.

II. **DIAGNOSTIC STUDIES FOR HIV INFECTION** should be considered in patients who are not known to be HIV infected, but who develop a malignancy that occurs at increased frequency with HIV infection. Many patients with HIV infection are unaware of their risk factors or deny their existence. HIV testing should be recommended to all individuals presenting with aggressive B-cell lymphomas, Kaposi's sarcoma, or anogenital carcinomas, as well as individuals with any malignancy who have higher than average risk for HIV (i.e., IV drug abusers, homosexuals or bisexuals, individuals with large numbers of sexual partners, and individuals from countries in Africa, southeast Asia, or parts of the Caribbean where HIV is especially prevalent). Appropriate pre- and post-testing counseling services should be available for these individuals. The screening HIV test is an enzyme-linked immunosorbent assay (ELISA), which if positive, is confirmed by Western blot analysis or plasma HIV RNA. The rapid, point-of-care, HIV antibody tests are acceptable alternatives to the ELISA and are in wide use; one test is oral and the other two are based on plasma or whole blood. If HIV is diagnosed concurrently with such a malignancy, additional clinical evaluation of their HIV infection may be indicated. Plasma HIV RNA and CD4 should be determined during the evaluation of HIV-associated malignancies. However, it is important to recognize that chemotherapy can cause wide fluctuations of the CD4 count that may not be an accurate measurement of the immune status.

III. **HIGHLY ACTIVE ANTIRETROVIRAL THERAPY (HAART)** will usually be recommended as concurrent therapy for their malignancy, and in some cases, prophylaxis for opportunistic infections (OIs). Although issues of drug–drug interactions and excessive toxicity must be considered, there is now considerable evidence supporting the concurrent use of HAART in individuals with a CD4 count less than 350/mm^3, HIV virus load greater than 100,000 copies/ml, or prior evidence of OI.

A. **HAART regimens** include the use at least three antiretroviral agents with nucleoside or nucleotide reverse transcriptase inhibitors (zidovudine or azidothymidine or Retrovir; didanosine or Videx; didexoycytidine or zalcitabine or HIVID; stavudine or Zerit; lamivudine or Epivir; abacavir or Ziagen; tenofovir or Viread; emtricitabine or Emtriva) combined with nonnucleoside reverse transcriptase inhibitors (nevirapine or Viramune; delaviridine or Rescriptor; efavirenz or Sustiva) or protease inhibitors (indinavir or Crixivan; ritonavir or Novir; nelfinavir or Viracept; saquinavir or Invirase or Fortavase; amprenavir or Agenerase; lopinavir plus ritonavir or Kaletra; atazanavir or Reyataz; tipranvir or Aptivus). Several nucleoside combination pills are available, including Combivir (zidovudine plus lamivudine), Epzicom (lamivudine plus abacavir), Truvada (tenofovir plus emtricitabine), and Atripla (truvada and sustiva). A triple nucleoside regimen without a nonnucleoside or protease inhibitor is not appropriate.

B. **Benefits of HAART** include a lower incidence of development of HIV-associated malignancies, especially primary central nervous system lymphoma (PCNSL) and Kaposi's sarcoma. Moreover, with HAART the onset of malignancies is in individuals at a higher level of CD4, there is improved tolerance of full dose chemotherapy, improved response rates and duration of responses, and improved survival during treatment of their malignancy. Pharmacokinetic studies have suggested that metabolism and clearance of several chemotherapeutic agents is not affected by HAART, but caution is still recommended when high doses of chemotherapy are utilized, for example, during stem cell transplantation studies.

C. **Specific recommendations for combining HAART with chemotherapy** include avoiding the nucleoside analog zidovudine, in light of excessive neutropenia and anemia. Moreover, the protease inhibitor atazanavir, which causes indirect hyperbilirubinemia in almost one third of patients can also be problematic when topoisomerase I inhibitors are utilized. Some authors have also suggested that HAART regimens including protease inhibitors may be associated with more myelosuppression when combined with chemotherapy than those lacking protease inhibitors, but this remains controversial. Caution is recommended in the use of antiretrovirals associated with neurotoxicity (e.g., didanosine, stavudine, dideoxcytidine) together with chemotherapeutic regimens including vinca alkaloids, especially in individuals with pre-existing HIV-associated neuropathy. It should also be recognized that nucleoside inhibitors may cause lactic acidosis, abacavir may cause a multisystem hypersensitivity reaction, emtricitabine occasionally causes hyperpigmentation of the palms and soles, nevirapine may cause liver toxicity, and efavirenz is frequently associated with central nervous side effects. A well tolerated regimen for a HAART-naïve patient who will receive chemotherapy would be once daily Atripla (300 mg tenofovir, 200 mg emtricitabine plus 600 mg efavirenz).

D. **Initiation of HAART therapy** should be accompanied by liver function tests, amylase and lipase as baseline values because several antiretrovirals (e.g., didanosine) can cause pancreatitis, an HIV genotype test to identify drug-resistant mutations, fasting lipid profile because protease inhibitors may cause dyslipidemias, a serologic tests for syphilis, hepatitis A, B, and C viruses, toxoplasmosis, cytomegalovirus (CMV), glucose-6-phosphate dehydrogenase testing in case dapsone will be needed, cervical Papanicolaou smear, opthalmalogy examination, anal and cervical screening for HPV if available, tuberculin skin test, chest radiography, and an electrocardiogram because HIV may be associated with cardiomyopathy. Vaccinations for influenza, hepatitis A and B viruses, and Streptococcus pneumonia should also be considered.

E. **Optimal care** of the HIV-infected patient should be done in collaboration with an infectious disease specialist. During active treatment, repeat HIV RNA levels should be assessed, and after completion of therapy, both HIV RNA and CD4 counts should be obtained.

IV. **PROPHYLAXIS FOR OPPORTUNISTIC INFECTIONS (OIs)** is also indicated in individuals with depressed CD4 count. Since chemotherapy can also transiently affect the CD4 count, it has been suggested that OI prophylaxis recommendations be expanded in individuals receiving chemotherapy. Thus, if it is anticipated that the CD4 count will decline below $200/mm^3$, prophylaxis for *Pneumocystis jiroveci* pneumonia (PCP) is recommended with bactrim thrice weekly, or in allergic patients, dapsone or atovaquone. If the CD4 count is anticipated to decline below $50/mm^3$ prophylaxis for *Mycobacterium avium intracellulare* (MAI) is also indicated with weekly azithromycin. In individuals with prior OI, who have a CD4 count above these cut-off values and have discontinued prophylactic antibiotics, resumption of prophylactic antibiotics concurrent with chemotherapy may be indicated. Special attention is also recommended in evaluating possible clinical signs of OI in the HIV-positive patient receiving chemotherapy as follows: (a) any CD4 count: oral and esophageal Candidiasis, Mycobacteria tuberculosis, bacterial pneumonias, histoplasmosis or coccidiomycosis, (b) CD4 less than 100: MAI, *Toxoplasma* encephalitis, (c) CD4 less than 50: CMV retinitis, pneumonia, or colitis, or progressive multifocal leukoencephalopathy.

V. **EVALUATION OF ANEMIA IN AN HIV-POSITIVE PATIENT WITH A MALIGNANCY** should consider causes other than chemotherapy or antiretrovirals, and should also include other causes of decreased erythropoiesis including (a) drugs (e.g., trimethoprim-sulfamethoxazole, ganciclovir, and dapsone), (b) nutritional deficiency of iron, folate, or vitamin B12, (c) effects of uncontrolled HIV on bone marrow stromal cells, (d) OIs (e.g., parvovirus, atypical or typical mycobacteria, or histoplasmosis, (e) or pre-existing conditions (e.g., sickle cell disease or thalassemia). Alternatively, causes of erythrocyte loss should also be considered, including (a) hemolysis due to thrombotic thrombocytopenic purpura, glucose-6-phosphate dehydrogenase deficiency, autoimmune hemolytic anemia, or drug-induced hemolysis, (b) gastrointestinal (GI) bleeding which may complicate lymphoma, Kaposi sarcoma (KS), or enteric infections due to CMV, Candida, or parasites, or (c) hypersplenism associated with infection, lymphoma, or cirrhosis that may complicate hepatitis B or C virus infections.

VI. **EVALUATION OF NEUTROPENIA IN AN HIV-POSITIVE PATIENT WITH A MALIGNANCY** should consider causes other than chemotherapy or antiretrovirals. These include causes of decreased myelopoiesis from drugs (e.g., ganciclovir, trimethoprim-sulfamethoxazole, pentamidine, rifabutin, dapsone), nutritional deficiencies (e.g., folate or vitamin B12 deficiency), infections (e.g., uncontrolled HIV, atypical or typical mycobacteria, histoplasma), or bone marrow involvement by the malignancy (e.g., lymphoma, multiple myeloma). Increased loss of neutrophils may occur with autoimmune neutropenia or hypersplenism. Granulocyte colony-stimulating factor (G-CSF) has been shown to be safe and effective in HIV-infected patients, although there is controversy about the use of granulocyte-macrophage colony-stimulating factor (GM-CSF), which can potentiate HIV replication in macrophages.

VII. **EVALUATION OF THROMBOCYTOPENIA IN AN HIV-POSITIVE PATIENT WITH A MALIGNANCY** should consider causes other than chemotherapy or antiretrovirals. Causes of decreased thrombopoiesis include (a) drugs (e.g., trimethoprim-sulfamethoxazole, pyrimethamine, ganciclovir, fluconazole, clarithromycin), (b) nutritional deficiency (e.g., folate or vitamin B12), (c) infection (e.g., uncontrolled HIV, mycobacteria, histoplasma, or *Bartonella henselae*), or (d) bone marrow involvement by lymphoma. Causes of decreased platelet survival include (a) immune thrombocytopenic purpura from HIV infection or autoimmune conditions, (b) thrombotic thrombocytopenic purpura, or (c) hypersplenism.

ACQUIRED IMMUNODEFICIENCY SYNDROME-ASSOCIATED DIFFUSE LARGE B-CELL LYMPHOMAS

I. **CLINICAL PRESENTATION**

A. **NHLs** are 100 to 200 more frequent in HIV-positive individuals than the general population, and occur in 5% to 10% of HIV-infected individuals. AIDS-associated lymphomas are generally aggressive B-cell malignancies that present at an advanced stage with extranodal involvement in more than two thirds of individuals.

B. **Pertinent history** should include performance status, duration of HIV infection, treatment of OIs, and current antretroviral regimen.

C. **B symptoms** such as fever, night sweats, and weight loss in excess of 10% of the normal body weight are very common, and should be attributed to AIDS-associated lymphoma, only after exclusion of OI. Extreme fatigue from anemia caused by bone marrow involvement may be seen.

D. **Lymph node enlargement** may be asymptomatic or associated with pain or obstructive symptoms. This should be differentiated from persistent generalized lymphadenopathy (PGL) due to HIV replication or other AIDS-related OI. Splenomegaly is commonly present, and may be related to the cause of lymphadenopathy.

E. **GI involvement** causing anorexia, nausea, vomiting, hemorrhage, change in bowel habits, or obstruction occurs in 10% to 25% of patients. Jaundice and abdominal discomfort may be due to lymphomatous hepatic or pancreatic involvement.

F. **Central nervous system (CNS) or meningeal involvement** resulting in seizures, altered mental status, neurologic defects, or no symptoms occurs in 10% to 30% of patients. Other causes of neurologic defects in this patient population should also be considered, such as HIV-associated encephalopathy.

G. **Pleural or pericardial effusions** may cause dyspnea and chest discomfort.

H. **The physical examination** should include careful examination and measurements of enlarged lymph nodes, spleen, and liver. Pulmonary and cardiac examinations may reveal pleural or pericardial effusions. A thorough neurologic examination should be done to determine the presence of meningismus or focal neurologic defects.

II. DIAGNOSTIC WORKUP AND STAGING

A. **Pathology.** Definitive diagnosis of AIDS-associated NHL is made with identification of lymphoma in lymph node biopsies or other tissues (bone marrow, cerebrospinal fluid [CSF], pleural fluid, liver, etc.,), in an HIV infected individual. Diffuse large B-cell lymphoma (DLBCL) is characterized large noncleaved cells which usually express cell surface pan-B cell marker, CD20, and lymphocyte common antigen, CD45, but not CD3. The transcription factor Bcl-6 is expressed in the centroblastic subtype but not the immunoblastic subtype. In contrast, the immunoblastic subtype is typically characterized by CD138 expression as well EBV latent membrane protein-1 (LMP-1). Centroblastic DLBCL is thought to arise in the germinal center, whereas immunoblastic DLBCL is a postgerminal center lymphoma.

B. **Laboratory tests.** Complete blood counts (CBCs) may reveal anemia, leukopenia, or thrombocytopenia, even if there is no marrow involvement. Serum chemistries may show abnormalities in liver function tests, elevated lactate dehydrogenase (LDH), calcium, or uric acid. Electrolytes and creatinine should also be monitored during therapy.

C. **Radiology/procedures**

1. **Computed tomography (CT) scan** of the chest, abdomen, and pelvis with a CT or magnetic resonance imaging (MRI) scan of the brain is necessary for the staging of AIDS-related NHL. Special note should be given to mesenteric adenopathy, a site not usually affected in PGL.

2. **Positron emission tomography (PET)** scans are helpful in distinguishing adenopathy due to lymphoma which generally show significant uptake of fluorodeoxyglucose (FDG), from that associated with PGL or OI, which show less intense FDG uptake. Alternatively, gallium scanning may be useful for this purpose. PET or gallium scans are useful to detect residual disease after therapy, and to distinguish fibrosis from refractory tumor.

3. **Bone marrow aspiration and biopsies** reveal bone marrow involvement in approximately 20% of patients, and may be associated with increased risk for CSF involvement.

4. **Lumbar puncture** should be performed and CSF sent for cytologic examination. Cell count and protein may be normal or elevated, whereas glucose may be low. Analysis of CSF for EBV DNA by polymerase chain reaction (PCR) may predict lymphomatous meningitis.

D. **The Ann Arbor staging** for NHL also is used for AIDS-related NHL. Prognostic factors correlating with poor survival in patients with AIDS-related NHL include stage IV disease, Karnofsky performance status less than 70%, CD4 count less than 100/mm^3, elevated LDH, and history of OI before lymphoma diagnosis.

III. THERAPY

A. **m-BACOD** (methotrexate, bleomycin, doxorubicin, vincristne, and dexamethasone) was used in AIDS-DLBCL patients in the pre-HAART era. Given in a low dose regimen, this resulted in 41% complete remissions and median survival of 35 weeks, whereas standard dose m-BACOD with GM-CSF resulted in 52% complete remissions with a median survival of 31 weeks, and more grade 3 toxicity (70% vs. 51%). Since the demonstration in the HIV-negative population, that m-BACOD was similar in efficacy to CHOP, the m-BACOD regimen has not been routinely utilized in AIDS-DLBCL.

B. **CHOP** (cyclophosphamide, doxorubicin, vincristine, prednisone) given at the same doses as in the HIV-negative patient population together with HAART and G-CSF, is feasible and effective. In a nonrandomized study, this therapy resulted in a complete response rate of 30% when given in low doses, and 48% when full doses were provided. The chemotherapy had no adverse effect on HAART activity. Moreover, HAART with a protease inhibitor, indinavir, had no effect on doxorubicin clearance, and only a 1.5-fold reduction in cyclophosphamide clearance which did not translate into excessive neutropenia.

C. **R-CHOP** is not significantly more effective than CHOP in AIDS-NHL (complete response rates of 58% and 47%, respectively), but is significantly more toxic (14% and 2% treatment-related toxicities). The increase in mortality with R-CHOP compared to CHOP, in this randomized study was primarily due to infectious deaths, particularly in individuals with CD4 lymphocyte counts less than $50/mm^3$.

D. **The infusional dose-adjusted EPOCH regimen** (etoposide, prednisone, vincristine, cyclophosphamide, and doxorubicin) with growth factor support resulted in complete remission in 74% of 39 patients, with 60% disease-free survival at 53 months. In this trial, antiretrovirals were withheld during chemotherapy, and after reinstitution of HAART, CD4 cells recovered by 12 months and viral load decreased below baseline by 3 months. Important features of this regimen are that it utilizes 5 days of oral prednisone (60 mg/m^2/day), a 4-day infusion of etoposide (50m/m^2/day), vincristine (0.4 mg/m^2/day up to 2 mg total), and doxorubicin (10 mg/m^2/day), and day 5 cyclophosphamide, followed by G-CSF or Neulasta. Cycle 1 cyclophosphamide dose is 187 mg/m^2 for patients with CD4 less than 100 and 375 mg/m^2 for patients with CD4 greater than 100. In subsequent cycles the cyclophosphamide dose is increased by 187 mg/m^2 each cycle up to a maximum of 750 mg/m^2 if grade 3 or 4 neutropenia or thrombocytopenia have not occurred, and decreased by 187 mg/m^2 each cycle if one of these complications has occurred. Thus monitoring of the CBC at days 8, 10, and 12 of each cycle is necessary for guiding subsequent therapy.

E. **CDE** (cyclophosphamide, doxorubicin, and etoposide) is an alternative infusional regimen that has resulted in complete response rates of 46% to 86%, but grade 3 or 4 neutropenia and thrombocytopenia in 75% and 55% of participants, respectively.

F. Indications for **CNS prophylaxis** in AIDS-DLBCL are not well defined. Bone marrow involvement has been suggested as increasing the likelihood of CNS relapse, as well as paraspinal, paranasal, epidural, testicular, or widespread systemic involvement. When CNS prophylaxis is provided, the usual recommendation is 4 weekly treatments of either intrathecal cytarabine (50 mg) or methotrexate (12 mg).

G. **Lymphomatous meningitis** should be treated with intrathecal cytarabine or methotrexate two to three times weekly through Ommaya reservoir until the CSF is clear of malignant cells, and then weekly for 4 weeks, and then monthly. The duration of therapy remains poorly defined, but is often given for 6 to 12 months. Alternatively, liposomal cytarabine (Depocyt) can be given with a 5 day course of decadron 4 mg bid with each treatment, on weeks 1 and 3 for induction, on weeks 5, 7, 9, and 13 for consolidation, and weeks 17, 21, 25, and 29 for maintenance. In patients failing to respond to intraventricular chemotherapy, CSF flow studies can be performed after instilling radioisotope to identify possible blockade.

H. **Radiotherapy** may be given as palliation to bulky, rapidly enlarging, organ compressing, or CNS lesions or as consolidation to patients with localized lymphoma after chemotherapy.

I. **Duration of first-line therapy** for AIDS-DLBCL should be four to eight cycles, unless there is severe toxicity or lymphoma progression. This should include two cycles after obtaining a complete response. However, for patients with stage I disease and good prognostic characteristics, three cycles of therapy followed by involved field radiation is appropriate therapy.

J. **Salvage chemotherapeutic** regimens for AIDS-associated lymphomas are not highly effective (response rates of 10% to 25%) with almost all patients relapsing within months, as in the HIV-negative population. This includes the use of etoposide and high-dose cytosine arabinoside and cisplatin (ESHAP), mitoguazone, or a combination of etoposide, mitoxantrone, and prednimustine. The use of rituximab with ifosfamide, carboplatin, etoposide (ICE) is a reasonable choice for a salvage regimen, but trials in AIDS patients have not yet been reported. There is little reported experience with dexamethasone, cisplatin, cytarabine (DHAP), mesna, ifosfamide, mitoxantrone, etoposide (MINE), or carmustine, etoposide, cytarabine, melphalan (miniBEAM) regimens in this patient population.

K. **Autologous stem cell transplantation** has also been utilized for refractory or relapsed AIDS-associated lymphomas, particularly in the HAART era. In individuals with a good performance status, lacking severe immune compromise, stem cell collections were successful in 80% to 100% of cases, and graft failure was rare. Long-term survivors have been reported from such studies, but the number of patients in each series remains low. Only anecdotal reports have appeared for the use of allogeneic transplants in HIV-infected individuals.

IV. COMPLICATIONS

A. **Complications of disease:** Rapidly enlarging tumors may compromise airways, and other vital organs. Significant hepatic dysfunction, hypercalcemia, and CNS relapse may occur. OI and other AIDS-related illnesses are causes for morbidity and mortality in patients with AIDS-NHL; therefore PCP and mycobacterial prophylaxis should be continued during active lymphoma therapy, if indicated.

B. **Complications of therapy**

1. **Lymphocytotoxic chemotherapy** may cause depletion of CD4 and total lymphocyte counts, increasing the risk of severe myelosuppression and infections. Potential interactions with chemotherapy and HAART may produce substantial and unexpected toxicity that may require dose delay or reduction, possibly compromising optimal antilymphoma therapy.

2. **Tumor lysis syndrome** may occur with chemotherapy. Aggressive hydration, allopurinol, and alkalinization of urine should be instituted during therapy, and electrolytes and renal function monitored carefully. Uricase (Rasburicase) may also be useful in this setting.

3. **Intrathecal chemotherapy** may cause chemical arachnoiditis which is relatively acute, subacute neurologic deficits occurring within days to weeks, or chronic encephalopathy occurring over weeks to months.

4. **Hyperglycemia** may occur with protease inhibitors and prednisone.

5. **Cardiomyopathy** may occur after use of doxorubicin, particularly in individuals receiving cumulative doses of more than 550 mg/m^2, but may occur at lower cumulative doses in individuals who received chest radiotherapy, or have other cardiac disorders, such as HIV-associated cardiomyopathy.

V. FOLLOWUP.
During treatment, intervening history, physical examination, CBC, chemistries, and LDH should be obtained prior to the initiation of each cycle of therapy, and as clinically indicated. With dose-adjusted EPOCH, more frequent measurements of CBC are required to guide the dose level for the subsequent cycle. After completion of therapy, for patients in complete remission, followup visits and laboratory studies are required every 1 to 2 months for 1 year, every 2 to 3 months during the second year, and then every 3 to 6 months. CT scans are usually performed every 3 months for 2 years. It is important to remember that these patients are at risk for relapse of their AIDS-NHL or development of a second AIDS-NHL.

VI. BACKGROUND

A. **EBV infection** occurs in approximately 50% of AIDS-associated DLBCL. In these cases, latency type 3 antigens are expressed, including Epstein Barr virus nuclear antigens 1 and 2 (EBNA-1 and -2), latent proteins (LP) 3A, and 3C, as well as LMP-1. Immunohistochemical stains for LMP-1 or *in situ* hybridization for Epstein Barr virus-associated RNAs (EBERs) are often used to identify EBV in pathologic samples.

B. **Chronic antigen induction** of polyclonal B-cell expansion and cytokine deregulation (especially interleukins 6 and 10) during HIV infection may also contribute to transformation.

VII. CURRENT FOCUS OF RESEARCH. A current study of AIDS-DLBCL is evaluating the combination of EPOCH with HAART and concurrent or sequential rituximab. Future studies of AIDS-DLBCL will include studies of ESHAP followed by consolidative therapy with zevalin, combination of bortezomib and zidovudine, and substitution of liposomal for nonliposomal doxorubicin in CHOP therapy.

ACQUIRED IMMUNODEFICIENCY SYNDROME-ASSOCIATED BURKITT-LIKE LYMPHOMAS

I. CLINICAL PRESENTATION. Burkitt lymphoma (BL) accounts for 15% to 40% of AIDS-NHL cases. The clinical presentations of AIDS-BL patients are similar to those of HIV-negative patients in terms of histology, disease stage, and proportion with bone marrow and CNS involvement.

II. DIAGNOSTIC WORKUP AND STAGING. The **pathology** of AIDS-BL is characterized by a population of small noncleaved lymphocytes, typically exhibiting a "starry-sky" appearance and a cohesive growth pattern, which are generally CD10+, CD20+ and usually express proliferation antigen Ki-67 on almost 100% of malignant cells, transcription factor Bcl-6, and uncommonly antiapoptosis protein Bcl-2. These are classified as high grade lymphomas. Molecular diagnostic or cytogenetic studies can be used to confirm the presence of the 8;14 translocation or the variant translocation 2;8 or 8;22.

III. THERAPY

    A. CHOP therapy was used for AIDS-associated BL, prior to the development of HAART, and responses were similar to those of AIDS-associated DLBCL. However, with HAART therapy, AIDS-BL may have a worse prognosis than AIDS-DLBCL when treated in the same manner, suggesting a need for more aggressive therapy in this setting.

    B. Hyper-CVAD was employed more recently for AIDS-BL. This is a regimen of hyperfractionated cyclophosphamide, vincristine, doxorubicin, dexamethasone, and rituximab given in alternating cycles with high doses of both cytosine arabinoside and methotrexate followed by leucovorin for a total of eight cycles. Antibiotic prophylaxis is provided with a quinolone, fluconazole, and valganciclovir, together with standard prophylactic regimens for PCP, MAI, and CMV, where indicated. In a single center study, 9 of 11 patients achieved complete response, and one patient partial response. Grade 3 or 4 myelosuppression occurred in all patients, and fever or infection during 35% of chemotherapy cycles. Six of seven patients given HAART concurrently with chemotherapy remained in complete remission for a median of 29 months.

    C. CODOX-M/IVAC (cyclophosphamide, doxorubicin, high-dose methotrexate/ifosfamide, etoposide, and high-dose cytarabine) was used for treatment of 14 HIV-positive patients, of whom 63% had complete responses, with a 2 year disease-free survival of 60%. Grade 3 or 4 toxicities included anemia (100%), neutropenia (88%), thrombocytopenia (75%), mucositis (75%), neutropenic fever (63%), sepsis (38%), neuropathy (38%), and nephrotoxicity (24%).

    D. Prophylactic intrathecal chemotherapy with methotrexate or cytosine arabinoside should be given to all AIDS-BL patients, generally 4 to 6 weekly doses of therapy in patients who do not have positive CSF cytology.

IV. COMPLICATIONS. The risks of myelosuppression, tumor lysis syndrome, and neurotoxicity are higher for AIDS-BL patients given more intensive therapies, such as hyper-CVAD or CODOX-M/IVAC than AIDS-DLBCL patients given CHOP.

V. FOLLOWUP is as described for AIDS-DLBCL patients.

VI. BACKGROUND. AIDS-BL is associated with EBV infection in 80% of cases. However, the pattern of latency differs from that of AIDS-DLBCL, with expression of EBNA-1 but not LMP-1 or EBNA2. As in BL not associated with HIV, translocations between immunoglobulin genes and myc are uniformly present. Mutational inactivation of tumor suppressor protein p53 is also prevalent.

VII. CURRENT FOCUS OF RESEARCH. A future study of AIDS-BL will evaluate the CODOX-M/IVAC regimen is a multicenter study.

ACQUIRED IMMUNODEFICIENCY SYNDROME-ASSOCIATED PRIMARY CENTRAL NERVOUS SYSTEM LYMPHOMAS

I. **CLINICAL PRESENTATION.** PCNSL usually presents in severely immunocompromised individuals with CD4 counts less than $50/mm^3$. Thus, with widespread use of HAART, the incidence of AIDS-associated PCNSL has declined significantly. Typical presentations are with confusion, memory loss, lethargy, or focal neurologic signs. Patients may also present with seizures, headaches, or dementia.

II. **DIAGNOSTIC WORKUP AND STAGING**

   A. **Differential diagnosis** includes systemic lymphomas with CNS involvement, toxoplasmosis, HIV encephalopathy, progressive multifocal leukoencephalopathy, and other viral, fungal, or mycobacterial infections.

   B. **Diagnostic workup** should include chest, abdomen, and pelvis CT scans and bone marrow biopsy to exclude systemic lymphoma. Body PET scans may be indicated as well in selected cases.

   C. **Brain MRI or CT scan** typically shows multifocal disease. However, lesions are typically larger, and fewer in number than those associated with *Toxoplasma* encephalitis. Lesions may be ring-enhancing, and often associated with edema and shift of normal brain structures, and may be found at any location in the brain

   D. **PET or single photon emission computer tomography (SPECT)** are helpful in distinguishing PCNSL from other HIV-associated brain lesions, such as toxoplasmosis, which exhibit less uptake of FDG.

   E. **Brain biopsy** is the gold standard for diagnosis, but tumor location and other factors may preclude this procedure. CT-guided stereotactic brain biopsies can produce diagnostic rates with acceptable morbidity, comparable to that of open brain biopsy.

   F. **CSF EBV PCR** is a sensitive (80%) and specific (99%) test for AIDS-associated PCNSL, because EBV infection is uniformly associated with this condition. For patients with positive CSF EBV PCR and PET or SPECT scans showing intense uptake in the brain lesion, biopsy may be obviated.

   G. Some investigators have suggested that in patients with serologic evidence of prior toxoplasma exposure, a 14-day course of antitoxoplasmosis therapy may be indicated to assess response. However, given the other diagnostic modalities available, this approach is rarely utilized now, and the delay in therapy resulting from this approach is potentially risky.

   H. **Pathology** is typically a DLBCL, usually of the immunoblastic subtype, with angiocentric distribution.

III. **THERAPY** for PCNSL should also include HAART, which dramatically improves survival.

   A. **Whole brain radiotherapy alone** was used in the pre-HAART era, because the median survival of patients presenting with PCNSL was only 1 to 3 months as a result of OI. Typically, 4,000 cGy is used in fractions of 267 cGy each. Cranial irradiation alone results in 53% rate of tumor regression and slightly improved survival compared to untreated individuals. Because of the multifocal nature of AIDS-PCNSL, radiation should be directed to the whole brain and meningeal fields to the level of the second cervical vertebra without spinal irradiation. In patients with poor performance status, who are severely immune compromised, and/or patients with multidrug resistant HIV infection, this may be the most appropriate therapy. Autopsy studies showed that patients who did not receive radiotherapy died of lymphoma progression, whereas those that did receive radiotherapy died of OI.

   B. **High-dose methotrexate** (2.5 to 3.5 g/m^2 every 14 days) with leucovorin rescue was reported to produce a complete response rate of 50%, and a median survival of 10 months, and improved quality of life. For patients with a good performance status, who are not severely immunocompromised and are responding to HAART therapy, a chemotherapeutic regimen including high-dose methotrexate may be appropriate, followed by cranial irradiation, as in the HIV-negative

PCNSL population. This therapy requires careful monitoring of methotrexate levels and adjustment of leucovorin doses if delayed methotrexate clearance is found. Methotrexate should not be used with individuals with a third space fluid collection.

   C. Steroids are used to limit edema, but the impact on survival is unclear

   D. Rituximab has been reported to play a role in CNS lymphomas not associated with AIDS, but there are no reports of its use for AIDS-PCNSL.

IV. COMPLICATIONS

   A. Complications of PCNSL include ocular lymphoma which may involve the vitreous, uvea, or retina, and are usually bilateral. Bilateral ocular irradiation, or high-dose cytarabine or methotrexate which penetrate the vitreous may be given. Leptomeningeal lymphoma can be treated with intrathecal methotrexate or cytarabine through Ommaya reservoir.

   B. Complications of therapy of AIDS-associated PCNSL are coincident OIs, and neurologic toxicity from whole brain radiotherapy.

V. FOLLOWUP should be performed monthly in the first year after completion of therapy with MRI brain scans performed every 3 months, and less often thereafter.

VI. BACKGROUND. AIDS-PCNSL occurs in 2% to 11% of HIV-infected patients, representing a 3,600-fold higher incidence of this disease, compared to that of the general population. Latent EBV infected cells develop into malignant clones in the relatively immunoprivileged CNS, secondary to decreased immunosurveillance resulting from HIV-related T-cell depletion.

VII. CURRENT FOCUS OF RESEARCH. A recent trial for AIDS-PCNSL has evaluated the activity of high-dose zidovudine to inhibit nuclear factor κB induced antiapoptotic proteins, combined with ganciclovir.

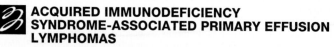

ACQUIRED IMMUNODEFICIENCY SYNDROME-ASSOCIATED PRIMARY EFFUSION LYMPHOMAS

I. CLINICAL PRESENTATION

   A. Primary effusion lymphomas (PEL) account for 1% to 5% of HIV-NHL. PEL presents less common in HIV-negative patients, including elderly individuals or organ transplant recipients. In HIV-positive patients, these lymphomas are uniformly associated with HHV-8.

   B. Classical presentations of PEL are ascites, pleural effusion, or pericardial effusions without infiltrative growth patterns or tumor masses. Some cases of PEL extend into tissues underlying serous cavities, including the omentum, mediastinum, and lung. Other cases of HHV-8-positive solid lymphomas are extracavitary variant of PEL.

   C. PEL occurs primarily in homosexual men, and late stages of HIV infection (mean CD4 count 98/mm^3). In one study, 64% of patients had previous manifestations of AIDS. PEL commonly occurs in patients with previous manifestations of HHV-8 infection, such as Kaposi's sarcoma or Castleman's disease.

II. DIAGNOSTIC WORKUP AND STAGING

   A. Diagnostic thoracentesis, pericardiocentesis, or paracentesis is usually required to diagnose patients with PEL.

   B. PEL is classified as a stage IV NHL

   C. Pathology of PEL usually demonstrates plasma cell differentiation as shown by expression of CD138 or syndecan-1. The cells typically express leukocyte common antigen, CD45, and activation antigens, HLA-DR, epithelial membrane antigen (EMA), CD30, CD38, and CD77. However, they usually are negative for T- and B-cell markers, including CD20, although clonal immunoglobulin gene rearrangements are present. Although the large, pleomorphic malignant cells may resemble Reed-Sternberg cells, they are CD15 negative.

III. THERAPY

   A. CHOP therapy was generally ineffective in the pre-HAART era. However, now that HAART is available, the CHOP regimen is an appropriate choice of therapy for these patients, if they have adequate performance and immune status.

B. **HAART alone** has been reported to be effective for AIDS-PEL, based on anecdotal reports.

C. **Major prognostic** factors for response were good performance status and pre-existing use of HAART therapy. In one study, a variety of different treatment regimens, of which CHOP was the most common, resulted in greater than 3-year survival in 32% of patients.

IV. **BACKGROUND** AIDS-associated PEL are uniformly associated with HHV-8 infection, and frequent coinfection with EBV. It is unclear why PEL arise in body cavities, but there is evidence that viral Bcl-2 is activated by hypoxia, which may contribute to lymphoma development.

 ## ACQUIRED IMMUNODEFICIENCY SYNDROME-ASSOCIATED HODGKIN'S LYMPHOMAS

I. **CLINICAL PRESENTATION.** HL is 10- to 20-fold increased in incidence in the HIV-positive population compared to the HIV-negative population.

A. **At diagnosis,** 74% to 92% of HIV-HL patients present with advanced disease, with frequent extranodal involvement, including the bone marrow, liver, and spleen, but mediastinal involvement is uncommon. Moreover, 70% to 96% of patients have B-symptoms. Bone marrow involvement is present in 40% to 50% of patients, and is the first indicator of disease in 20% of cases. In contrast to the HIV-negative population, noncontiguous nodal spread of lymphoma is common, e.g., liver without splenic involvement, or lung without mediastinal node involvement.

B. **Median CD4** count at presentation is in the range of 275 to 300/mm^3.

II. **DIAGNOSTIC WORKUP AND STAGING**

A. **Lymph node enlargement** may be due to HIV or HL, and PET scans may be helpful in distinguishing the etiology. Other coincident causes of lymph node enlargement should also be excluded, such as mycobacterial or CMV infection, or NHL.

B. **Pathology** shows the mixed cellularity subtype as the most common variant in HIV-infected individuals, as well as an increased frequency of the lymphocyte depleted subtype compared to HIV-negative HL. EBV LMP-1 is expressed in almost all cases in the Reed-Sternberg cells.

C. **Staging evaluation** is as described by AIDS-DLBCL except that brain MRI/CT scans and lumbar puncture may be omitted unless there are neurologic symptoms.

III. **THERAPY**

A. **Full dose chemotherapeutic regimens** are recommended, combined with HAART and G-CSF or Neulasta.

B. **ABVD** (doxorubicin, bleomycin, vinblastine and dacarbazine) given with G-CSF support is the most commonly used regimen, given at the same doses as in the HIV-negative population. In pre-HAART era, this regimen resulted in a complete response rate of 42%.

C. **EBVP** (epirubicin, bleomycin, vinblastine, prednisone) resulted in a complete response rate of 74%, with grade 3 or 4 leukopenia in 32% of patients.

D. **The Stanford V regimen** (doxorubicin, vinblastine, mechlorethamine, etoposide, vincristine, bleomycin, and prednisone) resulted in a complete remission rate of 81%, 3-year overall survival of 51% and disease-free survival of 68%. This regimen maintains or increases the dose-intensity of individual drugs, but reduces the cumulative doses of bleomycin and doxorubicin compared to ABVD, and may reduce the incidence of pulmonary or cardiac dysfunction.

E. **The BEACOPP regimen** (cyclophosphamide, doxorubicin, etoposide, procarbazine, prednisone, bleomycin, and vincristine) resulted in complete remission in all 12 treated patients and 83% 2-year survival, but grade 3 or 4 leukopenia in 75% of cases.

F. **Salvage** therapy studies have not been reported in AIDS patients. However, patients relapsing more than 12 months after obtaining an initial complete remission may be candidates for treatment with one of the first-line regimens described above. Patients relapsing in a shorter period of time may be candidates for similar approaches as described for AIDS-DLBCL patients.

IV. COMPLICATIONS of the disease or treatment are as described for AIDS-DLBCL with the addition of possible pulmonary fibrosis resulting from use of bleomycin. This complication, characterized by acute pneumonitis with fever, congestion, cough, and dyspnea, occurs most commonly after doses of more than 200 to 400 U/m², but may occur at lower doses when chest radiotherapy is also utilized.

V. FOLLOWUP should be as described for AIDS-associated DLBCLs.

VI. BACKGROUND. EBV has been identified in 80% to 100% of HIV-HL cases compared to approximately 50% in the HIV-negative population. The Reed-Sternberg cells of HL from HIV-negative patients are generally derived from germinal center B-cells, whereas those of HIV-HL patients are derived from postgerminal center B-cells.

VII. CURRENT FOCUS OF RESEARCH. Current research is focusing on the possible **substitution of liposomal for nonliposomal doxorubicin** in the ABVD regimen, the use of **stem cell transplantation**, either autologous or allogeneic in the treatment of HIV-HL, as well as **therapeutic strategies targeting EBV infection**.

ACQUIRED IMMUNODEFICIENCY SYNDROME-ASSOCIATED ANAL CARCINOMAS

I. CLINICAL PRESENTATION

A. HIV-infected individuals have a 30- to 120-fold higher rate of anal carcinoma than HIV-negative individuals. These squamous cell carcinomas result from high risk HPV infections. These malignancies do not require immune suppression, and occur in individuals with a wide range of CD4 counts, and are not considered AIDS-defining illnesses. There has been no change in the incidence, clinical features, or overall survival of patients with these cancers since the introduction of HAART.

B. The most common clinical presentation is rectal bleeding. However, larger tumors may interfere with anal sphincter function and lead to incontinence.

C. Clinical examination will identify a mass, and the size and position within the anal canal or anal margin should be documented. Rectal examination may detect enlarged perirectal lymph nodes. A general lymphnode examination is also important for stage determination.

D. Proctosigmoidoscopy should be done in all of these patients.

E. A thorough gynecologic examination should be done in women, especially if the tumor is situated to the anterior or if the perineum is involved. Evidence of vaginal mucosal involvement suggests that rectovaginal fistula might develop during treatment. If pelvic examination can not be performed due to pain, this examination should be done under anesthesia.

II. DIAGNOSTIC WORKUP AND STAGING

A. Screening strategies for anal or cervical dysplasia may be based on CD4 count, and the local expertise.

B. Pathology shows that distal anal tumors tend to be keratinized, whereas more proximal tumors are nonkeratinized and referred to as *cloacogenic or basaloid*. However, the clinical behavior of both types of tumors is similar.

C. Differential diagnosis includes other rare tumors arising in the anal canal that need to be distinguished from squamous cell carcinoma including adenocarcinomas of the anal ducts or glands, melanomas, clear cell sarcomas, and neuroendocrine tumors.

D. Staging evaluations should include endoanal ultrasonography, CT, or MRI

E. Prognosis depends on sex, tumor stage, nodal status, and response to chemoradiation. Patients with well differentiated tumors have a more favorable outcome than those with poorly differentiated cancers.

III. THERAPY is generally with synchronous chemotherapy with radiotherapy.

A. Chemotherapy options may include fluorouracil and mitomycin, as in the HIV-negative patient population, or fluorouracil alone, or fluorouracil with cisplatin. Local control rates are 80% to 90% for tumors less than 4 cm, and 70% to 85% for larger tumors. The addition of mitomycin to fluorouracil improves local control and disease-free survival. HIV-infected patients with CD4 counts greater than $200/mm^3$, generally tolerate therapy similar to that of the HIV-negative patient population. Individuals with CD4 counts less than $200/mm^3$, may tolerate chemotherapy less well, and consideration should be given for withholding mitomycin.

B. Recurrent or residual disease is associated with substantial morbidity, associated with poor wound healing and wound infections or sinuses. Salvage therapy for recurrent local disease in selected cases may include inguinofemoral lymph node dissection or additional radiotherapy if the region has not received the maximum tolerated doses.

C. Distant metastatic disease is managed with palliative intent and active chemotherapeutic agents include cisplatin and fluorouracil. Resection of isolated metastases in the liver or lung may be considered in select cases.

IV. COMPLICATIONS. Late complications of chemoradiotherapy occur in 3% to 16% of patients after 3 to 10 years, and include necrosis of the anus, especially after more than 60 Gy external radiotherapy or interstitial implants. Other complications includes neurogenic bladder, urethral stenosis, small bowel damage, cytopenias, intractable diarrhea, and radiation-induced sarcoma. These complications are more common in patients with CD4 less than $200/mm^3$.

V. FOLLOWUP of treated patients involves digital rectal examination and proctoscopy every 2 months for 1 year, every 3 months in the second year, and then every 6 months thereafter. If persistent thickening is present after 3 months, followup CT or MRI exams and/or biopsies may be indicated.

VI. BACKGROUND. Anogenital squamous cell carcinomas are uniformly associated with HPV infection, particularly high risk strains 16, 18, 31, and 35. The HPV E6 protein binds tumor suppressor protein p53 and promotes its degradation, abrogating its cell cycle arrest and apoptosis functions. The HPV E7 protein binds retinoblastoma family proteins, p105, p107, and p130, and promotes cell cycle transition into the S phase.

VII. CURRENT FOCUS OF RESEARCH is examining the efficacy of vaccines in preventing acquisition of high risk HPV strains, in different populations. Moreover, vaccines expressing epitopes of HPV E6 or E7 are also being examined as therapeutic vaccines. The use of infrared coagulation for treatment of high grade squamous intraepithelial neoplasia of the anal canal is also being studied. In addition the role of cidofovir against HPV for high grade perianal dysplasia will be investigated.

ACQUIRED IMMUNODEFICIENCY SYNDROME-ASSOCIATED KAPOSI SARCOMA

I. CLINICAL PRESENTATION

A. KS occurs 500- to 10,000-fold more commonly in HIV-positive individuals than the general population. Although occurring more commonly in patients with less than 200 CD4 lymphocytes/mm^3, the CD4 count at presentation can be quite variable, and KS may be the first manifestation of AIDS.

B. Clinical presentation depends on the site and degree of KS involvement. Manifestations of disease may range from asymptomatic innocuous cutaneous macules to life-threatening visceral lesions. The clinical course of KS is also highly variable, with rapid increase in number and size of lesions in some patients over the course of weeks to months, or indolent lesions gradually shrinking over years.

C. Pertinent history should include a description of all areas of initial KS involvement, lesion duration and rates of progression, oral lesions, GI and pulmonary lesions, presence of KS-associated edema, and other KS-associated symptoms, AIDS-defining illnesses, other sexually transmitted diseases, OI, and past and current antiretroviral treatment.

D. Physical examination includes evaluation of performance status, complete evaluation of the skin, oral cavity, and lymph nodes, with assessment of the chest, abdomen, and neurologic assessment, and genital and rectal examinations. **Baseline measurements** of at least five indicator lesions, description of whether lesions are flat or raised, and determination of the number of lesions/area (i.e., left leg, torso, head and neck) are necessary for later assessment of rate of progression and response to therapy. Photographs or drawings of sites of KS involvement are helpful for followup evaluations.

1. **Cutaneous manifestations.** Typically KS presents with pigmented skin lesions, from a few millimeters to several centimeters in size, which may be flat or raised, with a pink to purple or brown color. These lesions tend to be painless and nonpruritic, although bleeding and superficial infection or cellulitis may occur. Visceral KS can occur without skin manifestations.

   a. **Facial KS** typically involves the nasal, periorbital, or conjunctival areas. These lesions may be cosmetically unappealing and cause anxiety and social stigmatization.

   b. **Oral KS** occurs in 30% of patients, and often involves the hard and soft palates, and occasionally the gums, tongue, tonsils, and pharynx. The lesions may be macular, nodular, or exophytic, causing dysphagia, odynophagia, or speech difficulties.

   c. **Genital KS** is characterized by irregular erythematous patches on the foreskin or shaft of the penis.

   d. **KS of the feet** may cause pain and ambulation difficulties.

   e. **Lymphedema** may occur because of dermal and lymphatic involvement of KS, resulting in a nonpitting, sometimes wood-like edema of the lower extremities and genitals, sometimes disproprotionally more severe than the degree of KS involvement. Skin breakdown may cause weeping, ulceration, and subsequent superimposed bacterial infections.

2. **Nodal KS** may present with painless lymph node enlargement, caused by focal or total replacement with KS. This should be differentiated from lymphoma, mycobacterial, or HIV lymphadenitis.

3. **Visceral manifestations** most often affect the lungs and GI tract.

   a. **Pulmonary KS** affects 40% of KS patients and is usually associated with dyspnea without fever, cough, or hemoptysis. This may be progressive, debilitating, and rapidly fatal if left untreated.

   b. **GI KS** occurs anywhere in the GI tract in 40% of patients at diagnosis, and is generally asymptomatic, although bleeding, obstruction, or enteropathy can occur.

   c. **Other visceral organs,** such as spleen, bone marrow, liver, heart, and pericardium may be involved with KS. However, CNS involvement with KS is highly unusual.

II. DIAGNOSTIC WORKUP AND STAGING

A. **Diagnosis of KS** should be confirmed in all patients by biopsy on at least one occasion. **Differential diagnosis** of pigmented skin lesions in HIV-infected patients includes ecchymosis, nevi, melanoma, Bartonella henslae-associated skin lesions, and dermatofibromas.

B. **Clinical Evaluations**

1. **Evaluation of cutaneous disease** includes counting the number of lesions if less than 50, or the number of lesions on a single portion of the body, measurement of biperpendicular diameters of 5 lesions, description of the color of the lesions and whether they are raised or flat, whether there is tumor-associated edema, and photographic documentation of the lesions

2. **Evaluation of mucosal lesions** should include description of the size of the lesions and their site of involvement

3. **Evaluation of visceral disease** should be directed primarily at assessing pulmonary and GI tract lesions. Patients should have a baseline and at least annual chest x-ray, or if indicated, chest CT. If GI bleeding, vomiting, pain, or other abdominal symptoms are present, upper or lower endoscopy should be strongly considered.

C. **Pathology.** The diagnosis of KS is made by biopsy and histologic examination of cutaneous lesions, enlarged lymph nodes, or visceral tissues. There is a proliferation of spindle cells that may express endothelial markers such as CD31 and CD34, mixed with endothelial cells, fibroblasts, inflammatory cells, and extravasated erythrocytes. Similar histologic findings are present in non-AIDS-related KS.

D. Radiology and endoscopic procedures
   1. **A baseline chest radiograph** is done for all patients with KS to exclude pulmonary KS and other cardiopulmonary disorders associated with HIV infection. Localized or diffuse interstitial reticulonodular infiltrates with mediasitinal prominence may be seen in patients with pulmonary KS, and should be differentiated from lymphoma or PCP and other typical (i.e., bacterial) and atypical pneumonias (i.e., mycobacterial, CMV, or histoplasma pneumonias). KS may also present with alveolar infiltrates, pleural effusion, or isolated pulmonary nodules
   2. **Bronchoscopy** may reveal endobronchial erythematous KS-like lesions even with radiologically normal studies. Because transbronchial biopsies have poor histologic yield, a presumptive diagnosis of pulmonary KS can be made based of dyspnea without fever, chest radiograph, and bronchoscopic findings after exclusion of other disease processes.
   3. **Chest radiographic findings** of KS include interstitial or alveolar infiltrates, pleural effusion, or isolated pulmonary nodules. KS lesions are generally thallium or PET positive and gallium negative, in contrast to pulmonary infections.
E. Staging of KS utilizes the AIDS Clinical Trials Group (ACTG) classification system, which characterizes patients as good risk or poor risk, based on their tumor burden (T), immune function (I), and presence of systemic illness (S). T0 denotes good risk KS confined to skin and/or lymph nodes and/or minimal oral disease, whereas T1 poor risk lesions are associated with symptomatic lymphedema, tumor ulceration, extensive oral disease, and/or visceral involvement. Immune function is categorized according to whether the CD4 count is less than or greater than $150/mm3$. S0 is defined as no history of OI, B symptoms, other HIV-related illness, and Karnofsky score at least 70%. Good risk KS patients are T0I0S0.
F. Prognosis in the HAART era is largely determined by the T and S stages, and in the era of HAART use, CD4 count does not have a significant impact on survival. The 3-year survival rate is 88% for individuals with T0S0, 81% for T0S1 patients, 80% for T1S0 patients, and 53% for T1S1 patients.
G. Morbidity from KS is associated with painful lesions in the mouth or on the soles of the feet, lymphedema, symptoms associated with visceral KS, or psychologic disturbances resulting from the cosmetic effects of KS lesions.
H. Mortality from KS is associated primarily with pulmonary KS and less commonly with hemorrhage from GI lesions.

III. THERAPY
   A. Patients with good risk KS may be offered local or systemic therapy.
   1. **Local therapies** include electron beam radiotherapy, topical 9-cis retinoic acid (Panretin Gel), intralesional injections or iontophoresis of vinblastine (0.1 mL of 0.1 mg/mL) or 3% sodium tetradodecyl sulfate (0.1 to 0.3 mL), cryotherapy, laser coagulation therapy, or surgical excision. Despite the effectiveness of these procedure, complications can arise. Radiotherapy may result in chronic residual lymphedema, postirradiation telangiectasias, woody skin changes, and reappearance of KS after treatment. It is more toxic for mucosal than skin lesions. Panretin gel can cause local inflammation and lightening of the skin, resulting in inadequate cosmetic results. Photodynamic therapies can result in moderate pain and photosensitivity for a number of weeks after treatment. Intralesional injections cause necrosis or sclerosis of mucocutaneous lesions which may be quite painful. Cryotherapy can result in hypopigmented areas, particularly troublesome for dark-skinned individuals. Surgical excision is not optimal for large lesions due to reappearance of KS at the margins.
   2. **HAART therapy alone** produces a response rate of approximately 80% in patients with T0 lesions, but responses are unusual in patients with T1 lesions. This approach is more likely to be effective in patients naïve to HAART who have previously poorly controlled HIV, and who will be compliant with subsequent use of HAART. The time to response is 3 to 9 months. Protease inhibitor-based and nonnucleoside reverse transcriptase inhibitor-based HAART regimens have

been verified to be similarly effective. It should be noted that progressive KS may also develop in patients who have recently initiated HAART, attributed to an immune reconstitution syndrome.

3. **Thalidomide** has been reported to produce responses in 30% to 50% of patients, at doses of 100 to 1,000 mg/day (200 mg/day is the usual maximal tolerated dose), but is complicated by fatigue, constipation, neuropathy, xerostomia, neutropenia, orthostatic hypotension, risk of birth defects, and less commonly, hyper- or hypoglycemia, hypothyroidism, tremor, elevated serum transaminases, or thrombosis. Use of other thalidomide analogs, such as lenalidomide, has not been reported.

4. **Interferon-α** produces responses of in approximately 30% of patients, when used in high doses, greater than 20 mU/m^2 three times/week, but fewer responses at lower doses when used alone, although responses at low doses is improved when combined with protease inhibitors. Interferon-α can result in neutropenia, flu-like symptoms, and depression. Use of pegylated interferon for KS has not yet been reported.

B. **Patients with poor risk KS** should be treated with HAART combined with chemotherapy or investigational agents. Pharmacologic doses of systemic corticosteroids should be avoided, because this can cause dramatic acceleration of KS.

1. **Liposomal anthracyclines** are the most appropriate initial therapy, and either liposomal doxorubicin (Doxil, 20 mg/m^2 IV every 2 to 3 weeks) or daunorubicin (DaunoXome, 40 mg/m^2 IV every 2 to 3 weeks) result in response rates of 25% to 90%. Grade 3 or 4 adverse effects include myelosuppresion (36%), nausea and vomiting (15%), and anemia (10%), and hand-food syndrome. The incidence of extravasation injury, mucositis, nausea, alopecia, and cardiomyopathy with liposomal anthracyclines is lower than that with nonliposomal anthracyclines.

2. **Paclitaxel** 100 mg/m^2 q 2 to 3 weeks is generally considered the most effective and tolerated second-line agent, although some oncologists recommend it as first-line therapy for life-threatening KS. Response rates of 59% to 71% have been reported, with a median duration of response of more than 10 months. Myelosuppression (grade 3 or 4 in 35%), alopecia, neuropathy, and hypersensitivity reaction are the major toxicities. Liposomal paclitaxel (xyotax) has not yet been studied in AIDS-KS.

3. **Oral etoposide** may be useful as a third-line agent, given at a dose of 50 mg/day for 7 days of each 14-day cycle. In a trial of 36 patients, the response rate was 36% with a median duration of response of 25 weeks. This therapy was complicated by grade 3 or 4 neutropenia in 36% of patients.

4. **Vinorelbine** has a 43% response rate in patients with one or more prior systemic therapies for KS, but is associated with myelosuppression.

5. **Alternative chemotherapeutic regimens** that may be considered include bleomycin, taxotere, or a combination of doxorubicin, bleomycin, and vincristine.

6. **Duration of therapy** depends on individual patients. Generally, chemotherapy is given until a plateau in the response has been achieved, and then, doses of therapy can be discontinued or given less frequently. Chronic chemotherapy can be associated with limiting cumulative treatment-related toxicities.

IV. **COMPLICATIONS**

A. **Complications of AIDS-KS.** Although visceral KS, especially GI and pulmonary KS, may prove fatal, AIDS-related immunosuppression and OI remain the major cause of morbidity and mortality inpatients with KS. Superimposed bacterial, fungal, and parasitic infections in ulcerated, weeping lesions are not uncommon. Severe dyspnea from pulmonary KS and hemorrhage from GI involvement of KS also may be seen.

B. **Complication of therapy.** The use of HAART with systemic anti-KS therapy, such as paclitaxel may potentially cause profound toxicity in some patients with AIDS-KS. The metabolism of paclitaxel, docetaxel, and anti-HIV protease inhibitors involves cytochrome P-450.

V. FOLLOWUP. The frequency of followup may vary from every 2 weeks to every 6 months depending on the stage of disease, rate of disease progression or regression, and the type of therapy. During followup visits, **indicator lesions** should be measured, number of KS lesions in indicator regions should be counted, and the character of the lesions described. Repeat photographs and followup chest radiographs should be performed as clinically indicated.

VI. BACKGROUND

  A. KS develops in HIV-negative individuals, including older men primarily of Eastern European, Mediterranean, and/or Jewish descent, individuals undergoing immunosuppression (e.g., associated with bone marrow or organ transplantation), and young males in equatorial Africa, as well as in HIV-infected individuals. AIDS-associated KS occurs in individuals who are homosexual or bisexual and very rarely, if at all, in other HIV risk groups. The incidence of AIDS-KS has decreased dramatically with the use of HAART in the United States. However, in other parts of the world with limited access to HAART, KS incidence continues to increase.

  B. Pathogenesis of KS is thought to involve expression by the spindle cells of cytokines such as interleukin (IL-) 6, basic fibroblast growth factor, vascular endothelial growth factor (VEGF), matrix metalloproteinases, tumor necrosis factor-α, oncostatin-M, platelet-derived growth factor, and interferon-γ.

  C. HHV-8, also designated KS-associated virus, is thought to be the etiologic agent of this disorder, with primarily latently infected cells contributing to the development of this disorder. HHV-8 is present in AIDS-KS, as well as KS developing in HIV-negative populations. Several viral genes implicated in the pathogenesis of KS include those encoding homologs of antiapoptosis proteins Bcl-2 and an inhibitor of Fas-mediated apoptosis, IL-6, cyclin-D, interferon-regulatory factors, chemokines, and G protein-coupled receptors. Serologic tests for HHV-8 are not yet routinely available. The median time for KS development in HHV-8-positive, HIV-1 infected individuals is estimated to be approximately 10 years. HHV-8 is thought to be transmitted sexually, although concentrations of virus in semen appear to be very low. Blood-borne transmission is thought to occur, but inefficiently. Mother-to-child transmission also occurs, but the route of transmission is not defined.

VII. CURRENT FOCUS OF RESEARCH

  A. Antiangiogenic agents have been extensively studies in AIDS-associated KS. This includes thalidomide, as well as several agents studied in phase I and II trials, including fumagillin analogue TNP-470, a VEGF receptor inhibitor SU5416, and antiangiogenic dipeptide IM862. The matrix metalloproteinase inhibitor, COL-3, a tetracycline analog, resulted in a 44% response rate for a median duration of more than 25 weeks in a cohort of 17 patients. This therapy was complicated by headache, photosensitivity, or rash. An inhibitor of collagen synthesis, halofuginone, is also undergoing clinical study in AIDS-KS. IL-12 has also been shown to be a potent inhibitor of angiogenesis, perhaps through induction of inducible protein 10, and clinical trials are underway with this agent. An antisense oligonucleotide to VEGF mRNA will also be studied in AIDS-KS. There is also evidence that antiretroviral protease inhibitors may function as angiogenesis inhibitors. There are no literature reports of the use of bevacizumab for KS.

  B. Inhibitors of growth factor receptor signaling are also being studied, including imatinib, as an inhibitor of platelet-derived growth factor and c-KIT receptors. In a trial of 10 individuals given 600 mg/day, 5 exhibited a partial response, but grade 3 or 4 diarrhea, depression or neutropenia occurred in 8 patients. Larger trials are underway with 400 mg/day imatinib. Other studies based on the mediators of this signaling pathway, including phosphatidyl inositol 3-kinase, serine-threonine kinase Akt, extracellular receptor kinase (Erk), nuclear factor κ B, target of rapamycin (TOR), and cyclin-D may be targets for future therapeutic studies.

  C. Cell differentiating retinoids have also been used systemically in AIDS-KS patients. Oral 9-*cis*-retinoic acid (alitretinoin or Panretin) resulted in a 37% response rate, but almost half of the patients discontinued treatment due to headache or skin toxicity. Hypertriglyceridemia and subclinical pancreatitis have also been reported with retinoids, including alitretinoin. There are no reports of the use of bexarotene for AIDS-KS.

D. Anti-HHV-8 therapy with cidofovir or foscarnet have been reported in anecdotal or retrospective studies. For example, time to KS progression was prolonged in patients treated with foscarnet compared to patients treated with ganciclovir (211 days vs. 22 days). Histone deacetylase inhibitors, such as butyrate and valproic acid, which have been shown to induce lytic gene expression of HHV-8, are now being evaluated in clinical trials.

OTHER ACQUIRED IMMUNODEFICIENCY SYNDROME-ASSOCIATED MALIGNANCIES

I. LUNG CANCERS occur 2.5- to 5-fold more commonly in HIV-positive individuals than in the general population, and are the most frequently diagnosed non-AIDS defining malignancy in this population. Lung cancer risk is unrelated to level of HIV-induced immunosuppression.

II. LIP CANCERS occur 3.1-fold more commonly in HIV-infected patients than the general population. Some of these cancers may be HPV-related.

III. CERVICAL CANCERS occur threefold more commonly in HIV-infected women than the general population. Pap smears are recommended at the time HIV is diagnosed, and if normal, repeated at least once within 6 months. If the initial or followup Pap smear shows severe inflammation, a repeat study should be performed in 3 months. If a Pap smear shows squamous intraepithelial lesions or atypical squamous cells of undetermined significance, colposcopic examination, and if indicated, biopsies should be performed. High risk HPV infections are found more commonly in sexually active HIV-infected women than women not infected with HIV. When cervical cancer presents in an HIV-infected woman with CD4 less than $500/mm^3$, it appears at a younger age and with more advanced disease, and it is associated with a worse outcome than women without HIV infection. The incidence and therapeutic response of cervical cancer, however, appears unchanged by HAART therapy. Standard therapies for preinvasive cervical neoplasia, including cryotherapy, laser therapy, cone biopsy, and loop excision appear less effective in HIV-infected women, and are associated with a higher recurrence rate. The use of radiation therapy combined with chemotherapy may also be less well tolerated in HIV-infected women than women lacking HIV. Thus, treatment planning should take into consideration this information.

IV. PENILE CANCER occurs 3.9-fold more commonly in HIV-positive individuals than in the general population.

V. TESTICULAR SEMINOMAS occur twofold more commonly in HIV-positive individuals than in the general population.

VI. MYELOMA. Gammopathy in the HIV population is frequent, and may be transient or persistent. It does not appear to be related to the stage or severity of HIV infection. In a minority of these cases, there are monoclonal paraproteins that specifically recognize HIV proteins. In addition to benign monoclonal gammopathy, there is a 2.6- to 4.2-fold increase in the incidence of myeloma in the HIV-positive patient population compared to the general population. Moreover, presentations of plasma cell malignancy may be different in HIV-positive patients than the general population, with higher rates of extramedullary or solitary osseous plasmacytomas, and unusual locations for plasmacytomas, such as in the breast or liver.

VII. MULTICENTRIC CASTLEMAN'S DISEASE is characterized by polyclonal hypergammaglobulinemia, plasmacytosis, generalized lymphadenopathy, hepatosplenomegaly, and constitutional symptoms. Characteristic pathologic findings within lymph nodes include perifollicular vascular proliferation and germinal center angiosclerosis. HHV-8 is uniformly present, and viral IL-6 expression is thought to play a critical role in pathogenesis. Reported therapeutic approaches have include HAART alone, rituximab, splenectomy, interferon α, ganciclovir, cidofovir, or combination chemotherapy.

VIII. PLASMABLASTIC LYMPHOMA may occur in the oral cavity or other sites. These lymphomas do not express most B- or T-cell markers, but rather express immoglobulin light chain, EMA, and Ki-67. Some tumors are also positive for CD79a and CD138. These lymphomas are strongly associated with infection by HHV8 and EBV.

IX. CARCINOMA OF THE CONJUNCTIVA is commonly observed among HIV-infected patients in Africa. The spectrum of disease ranges from dysplasia, to carcinoma *in situ*, to invasive disease, originating at the limbus of the eye. HPV infection, exposure to ultraviolet light, male sex, and advanced age are thought to contribute to this disorder. Treatment has included surgical resection, external beam irradiation, and mitomycin.

X. LEIOMYOSARCOMAS occur in children and young adults with AIDS. These are uniformly associated with EBV infection.

XI. OTHER. Higher rates of nonmelanotic and melanotic skin cancer, prostate carcinoma, brain tumors, leukemia, have also been described in HIV-infected individuals compared to the general population.

Suggested Readings

General Care of Patient with HIV and Cancer

Yarchoan R, Tosato G, Little RF. AIDS-related malignancies—the influence of antiviral therapy on pathogenesis and management. *Nat Clin Pract* 2005;2:406–415.

AIDS-NHL

Navarro Kaplan LA. AIDS-related lymphoproliferative disease. *Blood* 2006;107:13–20.

AIDS-HD

Hartmann P, Rehwald U, Salzberger B, et al. Current treatment strategies for patients with Hodgkin's lymphoma and HIV infection. *Expert Rev Anticancer Ther* 2004;4:401–10.

AIDS-Anogenital Carcinomas

Clark MA, Hartley, A, Geh JI. Cancer of the anal canal. *Lancet Oncol* 2004;5:149–57.

AIDS-KS

Antman K, Chang Y. Kaposi's sarcoma. *N Engl J Med* 2000;342:1027–1038.

Other References

Cortes J, Thomas D, Rios A, et al. Hyperfractionated cyclophosphamide, vincristine, doxorubicin, and dexamethasone and highly active antiretroviral therapy for patients with acquired immunodeficiency syndrome-related burkitt lymphoma/leukemia. *Cancer* 2002;94:1492–1499.

Gill P, Wernz J, Scadden D, et al. Randomized phase III trial of liposomal daunorubicin versus doxorubicin, bleomycin, and vincristine in AIDS-related Kaposi's sarcoma. *J Clin Oncol* 1996;14:2353–2364.

Kaplan LD, Lee JY, Ambinder RF, et al. Rituximab does not improve clinical outcome in a randomized phase 3 trial of CHOP with or without rituximab in patients with HIV-associated non-Hodgkin lymphoma: AIDS-malignancies consortium trial 010. *Blood* 2005;106:1538–1543.

Levine AM, Li P, Cheung T, et al. Chemotherapy consisting of doxorubicin, bleomycin, vinblastine, and dacarbazine with granulocyte-colony-stimulating factor in HIV-infected patients with newly diagnosed Hodgkin's disease: A prospective, multi-institutional AIDS clinical trials group study (ACTG 149). *J AIDS* 2000;24:444–450.

Little RF, Pittaluga S, Grant N, et al. Highly effective treatment of acquired immunodeficiency syndrome-related lymphoma with dose-adjusted EPOCH: Impact of antiretroviral therapy suspension and tumor biology. *Blood* 2003;101:4653–4659.

Little RF, Wyvill KM, Pluda JM, et al. Activity of thalidomide in AIDS-related Kaposi's sarcoma. *J Clin Oncol* 2000;18:2593–2602.

Ratner L, Lee J, Tang S, et al. Chemotherapy for human immunodeficiency virus-associated non-Hodgkin's lymphoma in combination with highly active antiretroviral therapy. *J Clin Oncol* 2001;19:2171–2178.

Saville MW, Lietzau J, Pluda JM, et al. Treatment of HIV-associated Kaposi's sarcoma with paclitaxel. *Lancet* 1995;346:26–28.

Spina M, Gabarre J, Rossi G, et al. Stanford V regimen and concomitant HAART in 59 patients with Hodgkin disease and HIV infection. *Blood* 2002;100:1984–1988.

Wang ES, Straus DJ, Teruya-Feldstein J, et al. Intensive chemotherapy with cyclophosphamide, doxorubicin, high-dose methotrexate/ifosfamide, etoposide, and high-dose cytarabine (CODOX-M/IVAC) for human immunodeficiency virus-associated Burkitt lymphoma. *Cancer* 2003;98:1196–1205.

SARCOMA

David Kuperman and Douglas Adkins

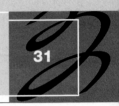

31

I. **APPROACH TO THE SARCOMA PATIENT.** Sarcomas are malignancies of the connective tissue (from the Greek *sarx* for flesh), including fatty tissue, muscle, blood vessels, and bone. Most of these tissues share a common embryologic origin, arising primarily from tissues derived from the mesoderm. There are, however, three notable exceptions (Ewing sarcoma, neurosarcomas, and the peripheral neuroectodermal tumors [PNETs]). The clinical manifestations of sarcomas depend on the anatomic site of origin. The presenting signs and symptoms vary markedly, from a painless lump to debilitating pain. Because of the large number of neoplasms categorized as a sarcoma, the discussion of sarcomas will be divided among the soft tissue neoplasms (extremity, retroperitoneal, and visceral) and the bone sarcomas.

II. **BACKGROUND**

A. **Epidemiology.** In the United States, the incidence of soft tissue sarcomas is approximately 6,000 cases per year, and the incidence of sarcomas of bone is approximately 2,100 cases per year. Sarcomas comprise 1% of adult malignancies and 7% of pediatric malignancies.

B. **Risk factors.** Most cases of sarcoma are sporadic, with no identifiable risk factors. A number of predisposing factors, however, have been recognized.

1. **Radiation.** Sarcomas have been found to originate in or near tissues that have received prior external-beam radiation therapy (RT). These radiation-induced sarcomas generally occur at least 3 years after RT was delivered and often develop decades later. Most of these lesions are high grade, and they are typically osteosarcomas, malignant fibrous histiocytomas (MFHs), and angiosarcomas.

2. **Chemical exposure.** Certain chemicals have also been found to lead to the development of sarcomas. Colloidal thorium dioxide (Thorotrast) has been found to cause hepatic angiosarcomas. Other agents that have been linked to sarcomas include phenoxy herbicides, dioxin, and arsenic. Alkylating chemotherapeutic agents such as cyclophosphamide, melphalan, and the nitrosoureas that are used in childhood cancers have also been associated with the development of sarcomas in adulthood.

3. **Genetic conditions.** Several syndromes are associated with sarcomas. Patients with neurofibromatosis type I have a 10% risk of developing a neurofibrosarcoma. Sarcomas also occur in patients with Li-Fraumeni syndrome. Familial retinoblastoma is linked to the development of osteosarcoma. Gardner's syndrome is a risk for fibrosarcoma. Patients with tuberous sclerosis are at risk for rhabdomyosarcomas.

4. **Other risks associated with sarcomas.** Lymphangiosarcomas have been known to develop in a lymphedematous arm after mastectomy (Stewart-Treves syndrome). Kaposi's sarcoma is associated with human immunodeficiency virus (HIV) disease. Paget's disease of bone is a risk factor for the development of osteosarcoma or fibrosarcoma.

C. **Molecular biology.** Several cytogenetic abnormalities are characteristic of certain sarcomas. The following is a list of selected tumors and their karyotypic mutations.

Peripheral primitive neuroectodermal tumor (PPNET) and Ewing's sarcoma: t(11;22)

Synovial sarcoma: t(X;18)

Clear cell sarcoma: t(12;22)

        Alveolar rhabdomyosarcoma: t(2;13)
        Embryonal rhabdomyosarcoma: trisomy 2q
        Myxoid liposarcoma: t(12;16)
        Uterine leiomyosarcoma: t(12;14)
        Extraskeletal myxoid chondrosarcoma: t(9;22)

III. SOFT TISSUE SARCOMA

A. Overview. Soft tissue sarcomas represent a number of tumor histologies. Pathologic diagnosis is based on the resemblance of these tumors to normal tissues. Despite this diversity, many of the clinical features and treatment decisions are common among various histologies with some notable exceptions.

B. History. The presentation of soft tissue sarcomas varies according to the site of origin. A history should include a search for the risk factors mentioned in the preceding text. An assessment of comorbidities should also be performed.

1. Extremity sarcoma. Approximately half of all soft tissue sarcomas arise in the extremities. The majority are first seen as a painless soft tissue mass. Pain is present in less than one third of patients at the time of presentation. Patients often report an antecedent history of trauma, but the etiologic significance of this is unclear.

2. Retroperitoneal sarcomas. Most patients have an abdominal mass (80%), and approximately half have abdominal pain that is often vague and nonspecific. Weight loss is seen less frequently, with early satiety, nausea, and emesis occurring in fewer than 40% of patients. Neurologic symptoms, particularly paresthesia, occur in up to 30% of patients.

3. Visceral sarcomas. Signs and symptoms relate to the viscus of origin. For example, gastric sarcomas frequently occur with dyspepsia or gastrointestinal bleeding. Rectal bleeding and tenesmus are seen with sarcomas of the rectum. Dysphagia and chest pain are common presenting symptoms of esophageal sarcomas. Painless vaginal bleeding is often seen with uterine leiomyosarcomas.

C. Physical examination. The examination of a patient with sarcoma should include an assessment of the size of the mass and its mobility relative to the underlying soft tissues. A site-specific neurovascular examination should also be performed. An assessment of the patients overall functional status is also important.

D. Diagnosis and staging. In addition to a thorough history and physical examination, the evaluation of patients with soft tissue sarcoma includes a biopsy as well as radiographic imaging.

1. Radiographic imaging. The studies needed for adequate staging vary depending on the site of disease. For soft tissue masses of the extremities and pelvis, magnetic resonance imaging (MRI) is the imaging modality of choice. MRI allows the differentiation of tumor from surrounding muscle and provides a multiplanar view. For retroperitoneal and visceral sarcomas however, computed tomography (CT) scans provide the best anatomic definition of the tumor and provides adequate imaging of the liver, the most common site of metastasis for visceral and retroperitoneal sarcomas.

     Angiography is not usually indicated in the staging of sarcomas because MRI accurately delineates vascular involvement. In addition, nuclear medicine bone scanning has poor specificity and sensitivity in detecting bony invasion and is rarely recommended. Positron electron tomography (PET) has not become routine for most sarcomas but may be helpful for particular sarcomas (high-grade sarcomas and gastrointestinal stromal tumors [GISTs]).

     For patients with sarcoma of the extremities, most metastases (88%) will go to the lung; therefore, chest imaging is necessary. For small, superficial lesions, a preoperative chest radiograph may be sufficient to evaluate for lung metastases, but in patients with high-grade tumors, or tumors larger than 5 cm, a staging CT of the chest should be performed.

2. Pathology

a. Overview. The histologic classification of soft tissue tumors is organized according to the normal tissues they resemble. The ratio of benign to malignant tumors is approximately 100:1. Unlike carcinomas, sarcomas

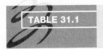

TABLE 31.1	Guidelines to the Histologic Grading of Sarcomas

Low-grade sarcomas	High-grade sarcomas
Good differentiation	Poor differentiation
Hypocellular	Hypercellular
Increased stroma	Minimal stroma
Hypovascular	Hypervascular
Minimal necrosis	Much necrosis
<5 Mitoses/high-power field	>5 Mitoses/high-power field

Adapted from Hajdu SI, Shiu MH, Brennan MF. The role of the pathologist in the management of soft tissue sarcomas. *World J Surg* 1988;12:326–331, with permission.

(malignant soft tissue tumors) do not demonstrate *in situ* changes, nor does it appear that they originate from benign soft tissue tumors (with the exception of malignant peripheral nerve sheath tumors in patients with neurofibromatosis). Clinical behavior is determined more by anatomic site, grade, and size than by a specific histology. Hence most soft tissue sarcomas are treated similarly despite different histologies, with the notable exceptions of GIST and rhabdomyosarcoma.

The histologic grade of a sarcoma is the single best prognostic indicator for the development of recurrent disease. The pathologic features that determine grade include cellularity, differentiation, pleomorphism, necrosis, and number of mitoses (Table 31.1).

The three most common histopathologic subtypes are the MFH, liposarcoma, and leiomyosarcoma. One can often correlate a location of a tumor with its histology. For example, most retroperitoneal sarcomas are liposarcomas or leiomyosarcomas.

b. **Clinical pathologic features of specific tumor types**
   i. **Malignant fibrous histiocytoma (MFH)** is a tumor of later adult life with a peak incidence in the seventh decade. It is usually first seen as a painless mass. The most common site of involvement is the lower extremity, but they also occur in the upper extremity and retroperitoneum.
   ii. **Liposarcoma** is primarily a tumor of adults with a peak incidence between ages 50 and 65 years. It may occur anywhere in the body, but most commonly in the thigh or retroperitoneum. Several types of liposarcoma have been recognized, and they have different clinical outcomes. Well-differentiated liposarcoma is a nonmetastasizing lesion. Sclerosing liposarcoma also is a low-grade lesion. Myxoid and round cell (or lipoblastic) liposarcomas are low- to intermediate-grade lesions and typically have a t(12;16)(q13-14;p11) translocation. Fibroblastic and pleomorphic liposarcomas are higher-grade lesions and typically more aggressive.
   iii. **Leiomyosarcomas** may arise in any location, but more than half are located in the uterus, retroperitoneum, or intraabdominal regions.
   iv. **Kaposi's sarcoma** may occur as raised pigmented lesions on the skin. It classically affects elderly Jewish and Italian men and is fairly indolent. It usually occurs in the lower extremities. An aggressive variant occurs in younger children and is endemic in some areas of Africa. In patients with HIV/acquired immunodeficiency syndrome (AIDS), a disseminated, aggressive form of this disease may develop.

v. **Angiosarcoma** is an aggressive malignant tumor of blood vessels. It may arise in any organ, but is most commonly seen in the head and neck region, the breast, and the liver. The skin is frequently involved. Breast angiosarcomas typically occur in young and middle-aged women, often following radiation for breast cancer. Liver angiosarcomas arise in adults previously exposed to thorium dioxide, insecticides, or polyvinyl chloride. Angiosarcomas are also the most common primary malignant tumor of the myocardium.

vi. **Synovial sarcoma** usually occurs in young adults. The most common site is the knee. Unlike most soft tissue sarcomas, these lesions are usually painful.

vii. **Rhabdomyosarcoma** is a malignant tumor of skeletal muscle. Four categories are recognized: pleomorphic, alveolar, embryonal, and botryoid. Pleomorphic rhabdomyosarcoma usually occurs in the extremities of patients older than 30 years. It is highly anaplastic and may be confused with MFH pathologically. Alveolar rhabdomyosarcoma is a highly aggressive tumor that affects adolescents and young adults. Its histology resembles that of lung alveoli. Embryonal rhabdomyosarcoma arises primarily in the head and neck, especially the orbit. It usually affects infants and children, with a peak incidence at age 4. Botryoid rhabdomyosarcoma has been encompassed in the embryonal category. It has a gross appearance of polypoid masses and has a predilection for the genital and urinary tract. It occurs primarily in children with an average age of 7.

viii. **Gastrointestinal stromal tumor (GIST)** is a sarcoma that can begin anywhere in the gastrointestinal tract but is found most commonly in the stomach (50%) or small bowel (25%). Most GIST tumors have a mutation in c-KIT resulting in constitutive activation of this receptor.

3. **Staging.** The staging system for soft tissue sarcomas incorporates histologic grade (G), size of the primary (T), nodal involvement (N), and distant metastasis (M) (Table 31.2). Grade of the tumor is the predominant feature predicting early metastatic recurrence and death. Beyond 2 years of follow-up, the size of the lesion becomes as important as the histologic grade.

IV. STAGE-DIRECTED APPROACH TO THERAPY
A. Early stage disease (Stage I to III)
1. Extremity soft tissue sarcomas
a. **Surgery.** Surgery is the mainstay of therapy for early-stage soft tissue sarcomas of the extremities. Over the last 20 years, there has been a gradual shift in the surgical management of extremity soft tissue sarcomas away from radical ablative surgery, such as amputation and compartment resection, toward limb-sparing surgery. Currently, limb-sparing surgeries are performed in the vast majority of patients.

When performing a limb-sparing surgery, it is important to obtain adequate margins. In the past, very conservative surgical approaches in which the plane of dissection is immediately adjacent to a pseudocapsule (an area around the tumor that is composed of tumor fimbriae and normal tissue) were associated with a local recurrence rate of 37% to 63%. However, a wide local resection encompassing a rim of normal tissue around the lesion led to improvements in local control, with a local recurrence rate of 30% in the absence of adjuvant therapy. The planned resection should encompass the skin, the subcutaneous tissues, and soft tissue adjacent to the tumor, including the previous biopsy site and any associated drain sites. The tumor should be excised with a minimum of a 1 cm margin of normal surrounding tissue.

There is normally no role for regional lymphadenectomy in most adult patients with sarcoma because of the low (2% to 3%) prevalence of lymph node metastases. Patients with angiosarcoma, embryonal rhabdomyosarcomas, synovial sarcoma, and epithelioid sarcomas, however, have

TABLE 31.1 American Joint Committee on Cancer (AJCC) Staging System for Soft Tissue Sarcoma

Primary tumor (T)	Regional lymph nodes (N)	Distant metastasis (M)	Grade (G)	Stage
TX: primary tumor cannot be assessed	NX: regional lymph node involvement cannot be assessed	MX: presence of metastasis cannot be assessed	G1: low, well differentiated	Stage I: T1a,bN0M0,G1; T2a,bN0M0,G1
T0: no evidence of primary tumor	N0: no regional lymph nodes metastasis	M0: no distant metastasis	G2: intermediate, moderately well differentiated	Stage II: T1a,bN0M0,G2-3; T2aN0M0,G2-3
T1: tumor is <5 cm in greatest dimension	N1: regional lymph node metastasis	M1: distant metastasis	G3: high; poorly differentiated	Stage III: T2bN0M0,G2-3
T1a: tumor is located above and without invasion of the superficial fascia	—	—	—	Stage IV: any T N1 M0, any G; Any T N0 M1, any G
T1b: tumor is located below and/or with invasion of the superficial fascia	—	—	—	—
T2: tumor is >5 cm in greatest dimension	—	—	—	—
T2a: tumor is located above and without invasion of the superficial fascia	—	—	—	—
T2b: tumor is located below and/or with invasion of the superficial fascia	—	—	—	—

Adapted from Greene F, Page D, Fleming I, et al. *AJCC cancer staging manual*, 6th ed. New York: Springer-Verlag, 2002, with permission.

an increased incidence of lymph node involvement and should be examined and imaged for lymphadenopathy.

b. Adjuvant radiation therapy. Wide local excision alone is all that is necessary for small (T1), low-grade, soft tissue sarcomas of the extremities, with local recurrence rate of less than 10%. Adjuvant RT, however, is required in a number of situations: (a) virtually all high-grade extremity sarcomas, (b) lesions larger than 5 cm (T2), and (c) positive or equivocal surgical margins in patients for whom re-excision is impractical. For T2 extremity soft tissue sarcomas or any high-grade sarcomas, limb-sparing surgery plus adjuvant radiation to improve local control has become the standard approach. When adjuvant radiation is planned, metal clips should be placed at margins of resection to facilitate radiation field planning.

c. Adjuvant chemotherapy. The benefit of adjuvant chemotherapy for most extremity soft tissue sarcomas is controversial. A formal meta-analysis of individual data from 1,568 patients who participated in 13 trials was performed by the Sarcoma Meta-analysis Collaboration. The analysis demonstrated a significant reduction in the risk of local or distant recurrence in patients who received adjuvant chemotherapy. There was also a decrease in the risk of distant relapse (metastasis) by 30% in treated patients. Overall survival, however, did not meet criteria for statistical significance between the control group and adjuvant chemotherapy arm, with a hazard ratio of 0.89 (*Lancet* 1997:350:1647). This meta-analysis is limited. Most of the randomized trials examined in this meta-analysis were limited by patient numbers, heterogenous patient and disease characteristics, and varied chemotherapeutic regimens. However, a recent randomized trial of a homogeneous group of patients with high-grade soft tissue sarcomas of the extremities and girdle demonstrated a significant survival advantage of five cycles of adjuvant ifosfamide (1.8 g/m^2 days 1 to 5) and epirubicin (60 mg/m^2 days 1 to 2**)** following definitive local therapy. In this trial, the chemotherapy arm had an overall median survival of 75 months versus 46 months in the observation arm ($p = 0.03$) (*J Clin Oncol* 2001;19:1238). Additional confirmatory randomized trials are required to clarify the role of adjuvant chemotherapy in soft tissue sarcomas. The only exception to this is with rhabdomyosarcomas in which adjuvant chemotherapy is accepted as standard of care.

d. Neoadjuvant therapy. It may be necessary to administer radiation before definitive resection. This is most commonly performed for tumors that are borderline resectable or for tumors located adjacent to the joint capsule. The typical dose is 50 Gy. Sometimes a boost is given postoperatively if margins are not adequate. Neoadjuvant radiation, however, is associated with wound healing difficulties. A phase III National Cancer Institute of Canada (NCIC) trial comparing adjuvant (postoperative) and neoadjuvant (preoperative) radiation demonstrated similar local control rates, metastatic outcome, and overall survival rates between the two arms. However, patients receiving preoperative radiation had a significantly higher incidence of wound complications (35% vs. 17%) (*Lancet* 2002;359:2235).

e. Radiation as definitive therapy. RT alone in the treatment of unresectable or medically inoperable soft tissue sarcoma patients yields a 5-year survival rate of 25% to 40% and a local control rate of 30%. Radiation doses should be at least 65 Gy, if feasible, given the site of the lesion.

f. Brachytherapy. Brachytherapy has also been used in treatment for sarcomas. Iridium 192 is the most commonly used agent. It has comparable local control rates versus adjuvant external-beam RT, although some data suggest a higher rate of wound complications and a delay in healing when the implants are afterloaded before the third postoperative day. The advantages of brachytherapy include a decrease in the patient's entire treatment to 10 to 12 days from 10 to 12 weeks, and the advantage that smaller volumes of tissue can be irradiated, which could improve functional results. However, smaller volumes may not be appropriate, depending on the tumor size and grade.

2. **Retroperitoneal sarcomas**
   a. **Surgery.** As with other soft tissue sarcomas, surgery is the primary treatment of retroperitoneal sarcomas. Tumors that are less than 5 cm in size and not located close to adjacent viscera or critical neurovascular structures are considered resectable. If a tumor has a high clinical suspicion of sarcoma and is resectable, it may not be necessary to perform a preoperative biopsy. One should consider a preoperative biopsy if an incomplete resection is a reasonable possibility to allow neoadjuvant therapy. If a biopsy is performed, it should be a CT-guided core biopsy.

   Unfortunately, only 50% of patients with early-stage retroperitoneal sarcomas are able to undergo complete surgical resection. Of the tumors removed, approximately half will develop a local recurrence. Adjuvant therapy, therefore, plays an important role in the management of retroperitoneal sarcomas.

   b. **Adjuvant and neoadjuvant RT.** Adjuvant RT is most frequently recommended for patients with high-grade tumors or positive margins. The radiation is typically started 3 to 8 weeks following surgery to allow wound healing. Two-year local control rates of 70% have been reported with the addition of postoperative RT.

   Neoadjuvant RT has also been used for patients with retroperitoneal sarcomas. It can be given to patients with marginally resectable tumors and those in whom one would expect to require postoperative radiotherapy. Neoadjuvant RT has a number of advantages over postoperative radiotherapy, including smaller radiation portals and reduction of the extent of the surgical procedure.

   c. **Management of unresectable, locally advanced retroperitoneal sarcomas.** Unresectable retroperitoneal sarcomas can be managed in a number of ways. RT can be given for palliation and with the hope that the tumor could be made resectable. Palliative surgery to reduce local symptoms can be performed. Chemotherapy can also be administered (see Section IV.C.3 for specific regimens). An asymptomatic patient can be observed.

3. **Visceral sarcomas**
   a. **Overview.** Until recently, visceral sarcomas were managed in a similar manner. The discovery of the importance of a mutation in the tyrosine kinase c-KIT in GIST has led to a radical change in therapy for this sarcoma.
   b. **Therapy for visceral sarcomas other than GIST**
      i. **Surgery.** Surgery is the primary treatment of visceral sarcomas.
      ii. **Adjuvant and neoadjuvant radiation.** Adjuvant RT is necessary if the tumor is high grade or if margins are positive. It is usually started 3 to 8 weeks following surgery to allow wound healing. Neoadjuvant radiation can be considered to allow a less radical surgery or make a previously unresectable tumor operable.
      iii. **Management of unresectable, locally advanced visceral sarcomas.** Unresectable intra-abdominal sarcomas can be managed in a number of ways. RT can be given for palliation and with the hope that the tumor could be made resectable. Palliative surgery to reduce local symptoms can be performed. Chemotherapy can also be administered (see Section IV.C.3 for specific regimens). An asymptomatic patient can be observed.
   c. **Therapy for GIST.** Like other sarcomas, surgery is the primary therapy for nonmetastatic GIST tumors. If the tumor is completely removed, there is currently no role for adjuvant therapy. If the tumor cannot be completely removed, treatment with imatinib (Gleevec) should be given. Imatinib is a small molecule tyrosine kinase inhibitor with significant inhibitory activity against c-KIT. Demetri et al. treated 147 patients with metastatic GIST with either imatinib 400 mg/m^2 or 600 mg/m^2 daily. Partial responses were

noted in 54% and stable disease in 28% (*N Engl J Med* 2002;347:472). The initial dose of imatinib is 400 mg p.o. daily, which should be continued until the disease progresses. Upon disease progression, treatment options include higher doses of imatinib (600 or 800 mg/day) or the use of sunitinib, another tyrosine kinase inhibitor, which has shown activity in imatinib resistant GIST.

If a tumor is marginally resectable or the surgery would result in significant morbidity, neoadjuvant therapy with imatinib can be given for 3 to 6 months. Of note, it may take 4 months or more to observe a response to imatinib on CT scan but changes in FDG-PET imaging can be seen very rapidly (within days). The National Comprehensive Cancer Network (NCCN) currently recommends evaluation for response with FDG-PET 2 to 4 weeks following the initiation of therapy with imatinib.

B. Treatment of local recurrence. Local recurrence of soft tissue sarcomas should be treated with surgical resection whenever feasible. Adjuvant radiation is often used. For unresectable recurrence of disease, radiation is preferred.

C. Treatment of metastatic soft tissue sarcomas

1. Overview. Metastatic soft tissue sarcomas can be divided into limited metastasis and extensive metastasis. Limited metastatic disease is defined as resectable metastasis involving one organ system. The prognosis of these two subsets of patients is very different. It is possible to cure limited metastatic disease whereas patients with extensive metastatic disease can only be palliated.

2. Management of limited metastatic disease. For patients with a limited number of pulmonary metastases, metastasectomy has been performed with some improvement in survival when compared with no surgery. Three-year survival rates range from 23% to 42% if a complete resection is performed. In patients with visceral sarcomas and limited liver metastasis, it is sometimes possible to perform a metastasectomy by surgery, chemoembolization, or radio frequency ablation.

3. Management of extensive metastatic disease. The goal of therapy for patients with metastatic sarcoma is palliation and prolongation of survival. Cure is no longer a viable goal. Systemic chemotherapy is the primary modality of treatment. Radiation and surgery may be used with a goal of palliation.

Numerous chemotherapeutic agents have been used as single agents in soft tissue sarcomas. Doxorubicin and ifosfamide are among the most active agents. In the 1980s, a number of drugs including cyclophosphamide, dactinomycin, and vincristine were used as single agents with response rates of 5% to 10%. Doxorubicin was the first significantly active agent against soft tissue sarcomas, with an objective overall response rate of approximately 25%. Continuous infusion of doxorubicin decreases the risk of cardiotoxicity and the severity of nausea while maintaining equivalent antitumor activity when compared with bolus infusion. Dacarbazine (DTIC) has also been found to have activity in soft tissue sarcomas, with a response rate of 17%. It is particularly effective in leiomyosarcomas. Ifosfamide has been found to have significant activity in sarcoma, with a response rate of 24% to 38%. On the basis of evidence of an increasing response rate to higher doses of ifosfamide, trials of "high-dose ifosfamide" ($\sim$12 to 14 g/m^2) showed higher tumor response rates (and toxicities) after an ineffective standard dose (5 to 7 g/m^2) of ifosfamide.

When doxorubicin was combined with DTIC (the AD or ADIC regimen), higher tumor response rates were observed (17% to 40%). To improve the response rate further, several agents were added to the ADIC combination. A phase III trial comparing ADIC, cyclophosphamide plus ADIC (CyADIC), and dactinomycin plus ADIC (DACADIC) resulted in no significant differences in tumor response rates between the three arms. Furthermore, the combination of cyclophosphamide and vincristine with ADIC (the CyVADIC regimen) was no better than doxorubicin alone in a randomized trial.

A combination of [sodium 2-]mercaptoethane sulfonate (MESNA), doxorubicin, ifosfamide, and DTIC (MAID) resulted in a response rate of approximately 47%, with 30% complete responses. A phase III trial comparing MAID with ADIC resulted in a higher overall response rate with MAID (32% to 17%) but significantly more myelosuppression on the MAID arm. Further, overall survival was not significantly different and appeared worse in older patients with MAID. Combination chemotherapy has been compared with single-agent doxorubicin in eight randomized phase III trials. Some of them showed superior response rates with combination chemotherapy, but none of the trials found a significant survival advantage. Kaplan-Meier plots of survival are superimposable within each trial and from trial to trial.

Another combination chemotherapeutic regimen that has had activity in soft tissue sarcomas, in particular leiomyosarcomas, is gemcitabine and docetaxel. Hensley et al. reported the results of a phase II trial in patients with leiomyosarcomas received gemcitabine on days 1 and 8 plus docetaxel on day 8. The patients were given granulocyte colony stimulating factor (G-CSF) support. The overall tumor response rate was 50% (*J Clin Oncol* 2002;20:2824).

Also, in patients with metastatic angiosarcoma, paclitaxel has shown significant antitumor activity.

V. BONE SARCOMA

A. Bone sarcomas may be derived from any of the cells in bone, including cartilage (chondrosarcoma), bone (osteosarcoma, parosteal osteogenic sarcoma), notochord (chordoma), or unknown cells of origin (Ewing's sarcoma, malignant giant cell tumor, and adamantinoma).

B. Presentation. The clinical presentation of bone sarcomas may suggest the pathologic diagnosis before biopsy.

  1. History. Localized pain and swelling are the hallmark clinical features of bone sarcomas. The pain is initially insidious but can become unremitting. Occasionally a pathologic fracture will bring the patient to medical attention. If the tumor arises in the lower extremities, the patient may have a limp. Constitutional symptoms are rare but can be observed in patients with Ewing's sarcoma or patients with metastatic disease. A pertinent history should note how long a lesion has been present and any change in it. Rapid growth or change in a lesion favors a malignant etiology.

  It is also important to inquire about risk factors for development of bone sarcomas. These include any history of RT and chronic bone disease. Paget's disease of bone may give rise to osteosarcoma and giant cell tumors of bone. Sites of chronic osteomyelitis may produce osteosarcomas and squamous cell carcinomas. Fibrous dysplasia may rarely give rise to osteosarcoma. Chondrosarcomas may arise from preexisting benign enchondroma (solitary or multiple in Ollier's disease), or exostoses (hereditary multiple exostoses).

  2. Physical examination. Physical examination may reveal a palpable mass. A joint effusion may be observed, and range of motion of the joint may be limited with stiffness or pain. Neurovascular and lymph node examinations are usually normal.

  3. Diagnosis and staging. Evaluation should include a biopsy and review of appropriate radiographic imaging.

    a. Radiographic imaging should include plain films of the lesion and MRI or CT scan. Biplanar radiographs of the affected bone are helpful in determining the specific site of involvement within the bone, the pattern and extent of bony destruction, periosteal changes, and the presence of matrix mineralization within the tumor.

    Osteolytic (bone-destroying) lesions may be seen in metastatic carcinomas, myeloma, and primary bone tumors. Well-defined (geographic) borders of bone destruction may indicate a slower growing or less aggressive lesion, such as a low-grade chondrosarcoma. As the tumor extends beyond the area of lytic destruction, more aggressive growth may be associated with a "moth-eaten" pattern. Rapid, aggressive growth patterns may be associated with cortical destruction, a soft tissue mass, and a permeative pattern of bone destruction.

Osteoblastic (bone-forming) lesions may be associated with metastatic disease (e.g., prostate, breast, pancreas, and small cell cancer of the lung) or osteosarcoma.

Periosteal reactions may be seen on plain films that give additional clues to the diagnosis. A "sunburst" pattern is associated with classic osteosarcoma. A lamellar or "onion-skin" periosteal reaction is most associated with Ewing's sarcoma. Spiculated periosteal reactions are associated with rapidly growing tumors such as Ewing's sarcoma. A raised periosteal reaction (Codman triangle) may be seen in a number of tumors.

MRI is the imaging study of choice for the evaluation of most bone sarcomas, allowing for visualization of the relation of the tumor to the neurovascular structures, adjacent joints, and the surrounding soft tissues. MRI can also easily demonstrate the intramedullary extent of the tumor and the presence of skip metastases.

CT scan of the primary site may be considered in place of MRI to demonstrate cortical destruction more accurately and for evaluation of pelvic tumors. CT scan of the chest is the preferred imaging of the lungs, which is the most common initial site of metastasis.

Radionuclide technetium Tc 99 bone scan imaging is important for assessing extent of tumor within bone at the primary, and the presence of skip metastases or distant bone metastases.

b. Laboratory features. Anemia or leukocytosis may be present in patients with Ewing's sarcoma. Elevated alkaline phosphatase and lactate dehydrogenase (LDH) levels are observed in patients with osteosarcoma, Ewing's sarcoma, or Paget's disease. An abnormal glucose tolerance test may be seen with chondrosarcoma.

c. Pathology of bone sarcomas. The classification of bone neoplasms is based on the cell of origin. Primary bone sarcomas can exhibit a phenomenon of dedifferentiation, in which these neoplasms exhibit a dimorphic histologic pattern with low-grade and high-grade patterns in the tumor. Treatment is dictated by the high-grade lesion.

i. Osteosarcoma is the most common malignant primary bone tumor, with an annual incidence of three per million. Peaks in incidence occur in adolescents and in the elderly. Most osteosarcomas occur in the metaphyseal region, near the growth plate, of skeletally immature long bones. The distal femur, proximal tibia, and proximal humerus are most common sites.

ii. Ewing's sarcoma represents 10% to 15% of all primary malignant bone tumors. It is the second most common malignant tumor of bone in childhood and adolescence. The peak incidence is the second decade of life. Ewing's sarcoma tends to occur in the diaphysis of long bones. The most common sites are the femur, followed by the pelvis, and then the skin. Ewing's sarcoma and PPNETs share a common genetic origin, a translocation between chromosomes 11 and 22 or 21 and 22. When arising in bone, this tumor is recognized as Ewing's sarcoma and when arising in soft tissue this sarcoma is recognized as a PPNET. Treatment of these tumors is similar, by using a combination of chemotherapy and local measures (surgery and radiation). Ewing's sarcoma is one of the **small round blue cell tumors.** The differential diagnosis of these tumors includes lymphoma, neuroblastoma, retinoblastoma, and rhabdomyosarcoma.

iii. Chondrosarcoma is the second most frequent malignant primary bone tumor, representing approximately 20% of all primary bone malignancies. It usually occurs in patients older than 40 years. It can occur in any bone, but the majority occur in the pelvis (30%), femur (20%), and shoulder girdle (15%).

    iv. Adamantinoma is an indolent, osteolytic tumor that often develops in the upper tibia.

    v. Giant cell tumor of bone or osteoclastoma, represents approximately 5% of all primary bone tumors. The peak incidence is in the third decade of life, with a female predilection. They are typically epiphyseal–metaphyseal tumors, with the majority in the distal femur and proximal tibia.

  d. Staging of bone sarcomas is shown in Table 31.3. Adverse prognostic indicators include an increased LDH, an increased alkaline phosphatase, and an axial primary. Patients with Ewing's sarcoma should have a bone marrow biopsy as part of staging.

C. Treatment of bone sarcomas

  1. General principles of local therapy. Surgical excision is the mainstay of treatment for patients with low-grade bone sarcomas. For high-grade tumors, multimodality therapy is indicated. As an example, for high-grade osteosarcomas, preoperative multiagent chemotherapy is followed by surgical removal of the tumor and then further adjuvant chemotherapy. It is essential to distinguish high-grade osteosarcoma from a low-grade variant, parosteal osteosarcoma, the latter of which has a lower malignant potential and does not require adjuvant chemotherapy. Occasionally, parosteal osteosarcomas will become dedifferentiated (high grade) and their behavior will resemble that of the classic aggressive osteosarcoma.

    a. Limb-sparing surgery. The Musculoskeletal Tumor Society and the NCCN recognizes wide excision, either by amputation or a limb-salvage procedure, as the recommended surgical approach for all high-grade bone sarcomas. Currently, 75% to 80% of patients may be treated with a limb-sparing surgery. This type of resection is predicated on complete tumor removal, effective skeletal reconstruction, and adequate soft tissue coverage. There are three types of limb-sparing procedures.

      i. Osteoarticular resection is an excision of the tumor-bearing bone and the adjacent joint. It is the most common procedure because most bone sarcomas arise in the metaphysis of long bones.

      ii. Intercalary resection is an excision of tumor-bearing bone only.

      iii. Whole bone resection is an excision of the entire bone and adjacent joints. It is used when the tumor extends along or invades the joint. Reconstruction is usually achieved by prosthetic arthroplasty.

  2. Osteosarcoma therapy. The 5-year survival for osteosarcoma with surgery alone is less than 20%. This occurs because microscopic dissemination is likely to be present in 80% of patients at the time of diagnosis. The addition of adjuvant chemotherapy has improved survival for high-grade osteosarcoma, permitting long-term survival as high as 80%.

    a. Neoadjuvant and adjuvant chemotherapy. Neoadjuvant chemotherapy began as a strategy to permit limb-sparing surgery, allowing time for creation of custom-made prosthetics. Since its acceptance, other advantages have been recognized with this approach. It permits earlier treatment of occult micrometastatic disease, preventing emergence of resistant clones, and potentially allowing debulking of the primary to improve chances for limb-sparing surgery.

      Chemotherapeutics active in osteosarcomas include doxorubicin, cisplatin, ifosfamide, and high-dose methotrexate with leucovorin rescue. These agents are typically used in combination to improve response, although the optimal combination and duration of therapy remain controversial. Currently NCCN recommends a combination of at least two of the above for six cycles, with two of the cycles given before surgery.

      Histologic response to preoperative therapy is recognized as a significant prognostic factor. Various systems have been developed for grading histologic response to chemotherapy, but greater than 90% necrosis of tumor cells is associated with the best prognosis. If the tumor has been resected to

TABLE 31.1 American Joint Committee on Cancer (AJCC) Staging System for Bone Sarcoma

Primary tumor (T)	Regional lymph nodes (N)	Distant metastasis (M)	Grade (G)	Stage
TX: primary tumor cannot be assessed	NX: regional lymph node involvement cannot be assessed	MX: presence of metastasis cannot be assessed	G1: low, well differentiated	Stage IA: T1N0M0,G1; T1N0M0,G2
T0: no evidence of primary tumor	N0: no regional lymph nodes metastasis	M0: no distant metastasis	G2: intermediate, moderately well differentiated	Stage IB: T2N0M0,G1; T2N0M0,G2
T1: tumor ≤8 cm in greatest dimension	N1: regional lymph node metastasis	M1: distant metastasis	G3: high; poorly differentiated	Stage IIA: T1N0M0,G3; T1N0M0,G4
T2: tumor is >8 cm in greatest dimension	—	M1a: lung metastasis	G4: undifferentiated (Ewing's sarcoma)	Stage IIB: T2N0M0,G3; T2N0M0,G4
T3: discontinuous tumors in the primary bone site	—	M2b: other sites of metastasis		Stage III: T3N0M0, any G
				Stage IVA: any T N0 M1a, any G
				Stage IVB: any T any N M1b, any G; any T N1 any M, any G

Adapted from Greene F, Page D, Fleming I, et al. *AJCC cancer staging manual*, 6th ed. New York: Springer-Verlag, 2002, with permission.

negative margins and had a good histologic response to chemotherapy, the patient continues on chemotherapy for an additional 2 to 12 cycles. If the tumor was fully resected but has less than 90% necrosis, salvage chemotherapy with agents not used in induction is attempted but the effect of this change in chemotherapy on outcomes is unclear. If the tumor margins are positive, additional local surgery should be attempted.

   b. Radiation therapy. Radiation is not routinely used in the therapy of osteosarcoma, but may prove helpful in patients who refuse definitive resection or palliation of patients with metastatic disease.

   c. Management of metastatic disease. Approximately 10% to 20% of patients with osteosarcoma have evidence of metastatic disease at presentation. Some of these patients may be candidates for surgical resection of pulmonary metastases. For patients with more extensive metastatic disease, chemotherapy is used to provide control of disease and palliation of symptoms.

3. **Therapy for Ewing's sarcoma** and the related PPNETs uses a combined-modality approach.

   a. Treatment of the primary tumor. The optimal treatment for local tumor control is not well defined. Historically, RT has been the mainstay of local therapy, but there has been a recent trend toward surgery. No prospective randomized trials have been performed to compare the two modalities, but retrospective data suggest improvements in local control and survival when surgery is done with a complete resection of the tumor. Patients with unresectable disease or positive margins require RT to improve local control.

   b. Chemotherapy. Before the availability of effective chemotherapeutic agents, fewer than 10% of patients with Ewing's sarcoma survived beyond 5 years, although only 15% to 35% of patients with Ewing's sarcoma/PPNET have evidence of metastatic disease at presentation. This fact suggests that many patients with Ewing's sarcoma had occult microscopic dissemination of the disease at the time of diagnosis. The First Intergroup Ewing's Sarcoma Study demonstrated an improved survival rate for patients receiving systemic therapy with VACA (vincristine, actinomycin D, cyclophosphamide, and doxorubicin). The Second Intergroup Ewing's Sarcoma Study used VACA but on an intermittent schedule and a higher dose and achieved an improved 5-year survival (73%).

   A recent randomized trial demonstrated that the addition of alternating cycles of ifosfamide and etoposide to VAC further improved survival in patients with nonmetastatic Ewing's sarcoma and PPNET. In patients who present with metastatic disease, overall survival was equivalent with these two chemotherapeutic regimens (~20% disease-free survival at 5 years); however, the VAC regimen was less toxic.

   c. Recurrent metastatic Ewing's sarcoma. In this setting, cure is not a realistic goal. Palliation and prolongation of survival are more realistic expectations. Fortunately, aggressive combination chemotherapy (VAC or IE) and RT can still lead to prolonged progression-free survival.

VI. **FUTURE DIRECTIONS** in the treatment of sarcomas include the search for more effective chemotherapeutic agents and combinations, and targeted therapies that will exploit the genetic features of these tumors.

Suggested Readings

Demetri G, von Mehren M, Blanke C, et al. Efficacy and safety of imatinib mesylate in advanced gastrointestinal stromal tumors. *N Engl J Med* 2002; 347: 472.

Frustaci S, et al. Adjuvant chemotherapy for adult soft tissue sarcomas of the extremities and girdles: results of the Italian randomized cooperative trial. *J Clin Oncol* 2001; 19: 1238.

Hensley M, et al. Gemcitabine and docetaxel in patients with unresectable leiomyosarcoma: results of a phase II trial. *J Clin Oncol* 2002; 20: 2824.

O'Sullivan B, et al. Preoperative versus postoperative radiotherapy in soft-tissue sarcoma of the limbs: a randomised trial. *Lancet* 2002; 359: 2235.

Sarcoma Meta-analysis Collaboration. Adjuvant chemotherapy for localized resectable soft-tissue sarcoma of adults: meta-analysis of individual data. *Lancet* 1997; 350: 1647.

32

MALIGNANT MELANOMA AND NONMELANOMA SKIN CANCER
Paul A. Klekotka, Lynn A. Cornelius, and Gerald P. Linette

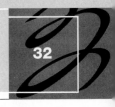

I. MALIGNANT MELANOMA
A. Presentation
1. Subjective
a. Primary cutaneous tumors. Most melanomas arise de novo, although melanoma may also arise in a preexisting nevus, or mole. Patients frequently visit their physician after the appearance of a new skin lesion or change in an existing lesion. Variation in color (variegated, lighter, or darker), a change in size, or a change in border is noted by more than 80% of melanoma patients at the time of diagnosis. Occasionally, patients note associated symptoms such as itching, ulceration, or bleeding that warrant further evaluation of the lesion. Nonpigmented (amelanotic) primary lesions comprise approximately 5% of cutaneous melanomas.

b. Metastatic tumors. Melanoma derives from melanocytes that originate embryonically from the neural crest and are prone to metastasize to multiple sites. Melanoma most commonly metastasizes to the lymph nodes followed by the skin, lungs, liver, brain, and other sites. An uncommon initial presentation of melanoma may be an enlarged lymph node or a pulmonary nodule noted on an incidental chest radiograph without a previously recognized or identifiable primary cutaneous lesion. The symptoms of metastatic melanoma will depend upon the site of the metastasis.

2. Objective.
During the evaluation of the pigmented skin lesion, the ABCDE criteria for evaluating a changing mole are helpful, but not absolute.

a. Asymmetry—one half of the lesion does not match the other.

b. Border irregularity—the lesion has ragged, or blurred, notched edges.

c. Color variegation—pigmentation is a heterogeneous mixture of tan, brown, or black. Red, white, or blue discolorations are particularly of concern.

d. Diameter—lesions that increase in size or are larger than 6 mm in diameter should be carefully evaluated for the presence of melanoma.

e. Evolving—changes in a preexisting lesion over time.

Lesions with one or more of these attributes should be brought to the attention of a physician, preferably a dermatologist, and evaluated for the possibility of melanoma. Other characteristics such as itching, bleeding, and the presence of ulceration should also prompt a careful evaluation for melanoma. In addition to examination and possible biopsy of the lesion in question, a comprehensive skin examination by a dermatologist is also critical in evaluating and monitoring patients with multiple or atypical nevi, a history of excessive sun exposure, nonmelanoma skin cancer or melanoma. Careful examination of axillae, scalp, interdigital webs and soles, genitalia, and oral cavity is essential.

The differential diagnosis of a pigmented skin lesion includes a benign nevus, an atypical ("dysplastic") nevus, hemangioma, seborrheic keratosis, non-melanoma skin cancer (basal cell carcinoma (BCC) and squamous cell carcinoma (SCC), dermatofibroma, and pyogenic granuloma. Benign diagnoses include nevi that are usually well-defined lesions with a smooth surface and uniform pigmentation. Also benign are atypical nevi that can have an irregular shape, color variation, and "smudged" borders. These lesions are characteristically macular, although they may have a papular component, are larger than 5 mm in size, and histologically may display varying degrees of cytologic atypia (graded from mild to severe). Although classified as benign, lesions harboring significant cytologic atypia do require complete surgical excision. Benign hemangiomas are often red to purple to blue-black papules or plaques. A seborrheic keratosis is a verrucous plaque or papule frequently found on the face, neck, or trunk and is of no clinical significance. A benign dermatofibroma is essentially dermal fibrosis that presents as a firm tan to brown papule or nodule. A pyogenic granuloma is a rapidly growing, often ulcerated, nonhealing papule that is often pedunculated. These lesions should always be biopsied, as they are difficult to distinguish clinically from an amelanotic melanoma. With regard to malignant lesions, the nonmelanoma skin cancers, BCC and SCC, may present as erythematous papules with or without scale and characteristically without the pigmentation that occurs on chronically sun-exposed skin.

B. Workup and staging

1. Diagnosis

   a. Excisional biopsy. When the differential diagnosis of a skin lesion includes melanoma, the lesion should not be observed. Full-thickness complete excisional biopsy with 1 to 3 mm margins is optimal. An incisional biopsy or punch biopsy may be performed if the lesion is located in an anatomically or cosmetically compromising area (palm/sole, digit, face, ear). Shave biopsies should be avoided because they compromise the pathologist's ability to stage the cancer adequately. Frozen-section analysis is not recommended for the diagnosis of melanoma.

2. Histologic reporting and classification.
Reporting of Breslow thickness in millimeters, Clarks' level, the presence of ulceration, and peripheral and deep margin status of the biopsy represent minimal elements to be determined and reported by the pathologist. In addition, the presence of satellitosis, as well as lesion location, regression, mitotic rate, tumor-infiltrating lymphocytes, vertical growth phase, angiolymphatic invasion, neurotropism and histologic subtype should be reported. Four major histologic subtypes of melanoma have been described historically. The subtypes include superficial spreading melanoma (SSM), nodular melanoma, lentigo maligna melanoma (LMM) and acral lentiginous melanoma. Desmoplastic melanoma is also a recognized histologic entity and comprises 1% to 2% of all melanomas. The biologic significance of these subtypes is relatively unclear at this time, as the distinction does not predict prognosis independent of other prognostic factors such as Breslow thickness and ulceration.

   Although melanoma can occur in a preexisting nevus (mole), most cases occur de novo. Most melanomas, other than nodular melanoma, are thought to begin as *in situ* lesions that are contained within the epidermis with minimal, if any, ability to metastasize. Nevertheless, melanoma *in situ* should be completely excised with at least a 0.5 cm margin and the patient should be followed closely. Excisional margins for invasive melanomas are determined by Breslow thickness (see subsequent text).

   a. Superficial spreading melanoma (SSM) is the most common type of melanoma. It represents approximately 70% of all cutaneous melanomas. SSM occur most commonly on the trunk in men and the legs in women. SSM often presents as a flat or elevated lesion with an irregular border and variegate color. SSM often spreads horizontally in a "radial growth phase" before penetrating deeper in a "vertical growth phase."

   b. Nodular melanoma (NM) is the second most common type of melanoma. It represents approximately 15% to 30% of cutaneous melanomas. NM occurs most often on the legs and trunk. NM often presents as a brown-black papule that may ulcerate and grow rapidly. NM may also be amelanotic. As NM may not follow the ABCDEs of melanoma diagnosis, they may not be detected early. This may explain why these lesions are often thicker at initial presentation, which leads to a worse prognosis.

   c. Lentigo maligna melanoma (LMM) represents 5% to 15% of cutaneous melanomas. LMM arises in only a small percentage of its precursor lesion, lentigo maligna (LM). LM is characterized as a large, pigmented macule, typically in an elderly patient on sun-exposed areas such as the head, neck, and upper extremities. These lesions are thought to have an extended radial growth phase, and are often present for decades prior to diagnosis. Progression of LM to LMM is usually characterized by changes in pigmentation and/or nodule formation.

    d. Acral lentiginous melanoma (ALM) represents 5% to 10% of melanomas. It occurs most often on the palms, soles, and around the nail. It presents as an irregularly shaped macule with color variation. Although ALM is the most common type of melanoma in patients with pigmented skin, it does not occur more often in those with pigmented skin than in fair-skinned individuals.

3. Current recommendations for clinical and pathologic staging of melanoma. The most commonly used staging system is the American Joint Commission for Cancer (AJCC) Cancer Staging. The revised 2002 AJCC melanoma staging is shown in Table 32.1. Important prognostic factors in the staging of

TABLE 32.1   Revised 2002 American Joint Commission for Cancer (AJCC) Melanoma Staging

Stage	TNM classification	Thick-ness (mm)	Ulceration	Nodes	Metastasis	% 5-yr survival
0	Tis N0 M0	0	–	–	–	100
IA	T1a N0 M0	<1	–	–	–	≥95
IB	T1b N0 M0	<1	+	–	–	89–91
	T2a N0 M0	1.01–2	–	–	–	
IIA	T2b N0 M0	1.01–2	+	–	–	77–79
	T3a N0 M0	2.01–4	–	–	–	
IIB	T3b N0 M0	2.01–4	+	–	–	63–67
	T4a N0 M0	<4	–	–	–	
IIC	T4b N0 M0	<4	+	–	–	45
IIIA	T1–T4a N1a M0	Any	–	1 micro	–	63–69
	T1–T4a N2a M0	Any	–	2–3 micro	–	
IIIB	T1–T4b N1a M0	Any	+	1 micro	–	46–53
	T1–T4b N2a M0	Any	+	2–3 micro	–	
	T1–T4a N1b M0	Any	–	1 macro	–	
	T1–T4a N2b M0	Any	–	2–3 macro	–	
	T1–T4a/b N2c M0	Any	–	In-transit or satellite node	–	30–50
IIIC	T1–T4b N2a M0	Any	+	1 macro	–	24–29
	T1–T4b N2b M0	Any	+	2–3 macro	–	
	Any T N3 M0	Any	Any	>3 macro, In-transit/sat. +node	–	
IV	Any T any N M1a	Any	Any	Any	Distant skin, subcutaneous, or node metastasis, nl LDH	7–19
	Any T any N M1b	Any	Any	Any	Lung metastasis with nl LDH	
	Any T any N M1c	Any	Any	Any	All other visceral metastases with nl LDH Any distant metastasis with Increased LDH	

nl, normal.
Adapted from: Balch CM, Soong SJ, Atkins MB, et al. An evidence-based staging system for cutaneous melanoma. *CA Cancer J Clin* 2004;54(3):131–149.

melanoma are the thickness (Breslow) of the primary lesion measured in millimeters, the presence of histologic ulceration, and regional lymph node involvement. The thickness of the melanoma in millimeters is also known as the *Breslow thickness* and is measured in millimeters from the top of the granular layer in the epidermis to the base of the deepest tumor nest in the dermis. Stage I and II melanoma is localized to the skin only.

Clinical and pathologic evaluation of the lymph nodes will assist the treating physician in assessing the stage of melanoma, prognosis, and treatment options. Regional lymph node involvement (Stage III disease) is determined clinically by physical examination or histologically after a sentinel lymph node biopsy (SLNB), if indicated. Current National Comprehensive Cancer Network (NCCN) recommendations for the performance of an SLNB include intermediate and high-risk primary disease (AJCC clinical stage IB and stage II disease; ≤1 mm thick with ulceration or Clark level IV, V or ≥ 1 mm thick, any characteristic; N0). A sentinel lymph node is the first node that the primary melanoma drains to and therefore is the node with the highest chance of containing metastatic disease. The sentinel lymph node(s) is identified by preoperative injection of technetium 99m radionuclide (lymphoscintigraphy) and perioperative injection of vital blue dye. The node(s) is removed and examined by both histology and immunohistochemistry for the presence of micrometastasis. Sentinel lymph node status is the most powerful predictor of recurrence and survival in patients with metastatic melanoma.

After complete history and physical examination including skin and lymph node evaluations, further workup should include evaluation of lactate dehydrogenase (LDH) level, and a posteroanterior and lateral chest radiograph. In patients with stage 0 (*in situ*) or stage I melanoma, further workup is unnecessary in the absence of symptoms or abnormal laboratory results. In patients with high-risk primary lesions (stage II and III) or suspected distant disease, computed tomographic (CT) scans and possibly, magnetic resonance imaging (MRI), may be helpful, if clinically indicated. The value of fluorodeoxyglucose positron emission tomography (FDG-PET) is undefined and should not replace SLNB for staging most patients with primary cutaneous melanoma. For patients with suspected metastatic (stage IV) melanoma, brain MRI with gadolinium and contrast-enhanced CT of the chest, abdomen, and pelvis is indicated. In certain instances, body FDG-PET imaging (or FDG-PET/CT) can be performed instead of the body CT scan. Head CT with i.v. contrast can be performed in patients unable to undergo MRI; however, the sensitivity of CT is diminished for the detection of small (less than 1 cm) or posterior fossa intracranial metastases.

C. Treatment and prognosis

   1. Primary melanoma. Early diagnosis and excision of cutaneous melanoma may be curative in certain instances. In stage 0 to stage II disease, excision of the primary lesion with NCCN-prescribed margins that are histologically negative for tumor provides the greatest chance of a cure. In all instances, shave excision, curettage, or cryosurgery is contraindicated. Recommendations for excision margin for *in situ* melanoma are 0.5 cm. A margin of 1 cm is adequate for patients with primary melanomas with a Breslow thickness of less than or equal to 1 mm. Surgical margins of 1 to 2 cm are recommended for melanomas with a Breslow thickness of 1.01 to 2 mm. Melanomas greater than 2 mm in Breslow thickness (high-risk primaries) should be removed with at least 2-cm margins.

   2. Lymph node metastases. If the patient has palpable lymph nodes on physical examination at the time of diagnosis, then a complete lymph node dissection should be performed at the time of wide local excision of the primary tumor. As previously described, for patients with melanoma greater than 1 mm in Breslow thickness and no clinical evidence of lymph node metastasis a SLNB should be offered. If micrometastases are found in the sentinel node(s), then a complete lymph node dissection is performed in the involved nodal basin. If the sentinel node is negative, then the patient is spared further lymph node dissection with its additional morbidity. The Multicenter Selective Lymphadenectomy

Trial (*N Engl J Med* 2006;355:1307) provides strong evidence that immediate lymphadenectomy for sentinel node positive patients improves the 5 yr disease-free survival rate (hazard ratio 0.74, 95% CI [0.59–0.93] compared to patients that are spared SLNB at presentation and undergo lymphadenectomy at relapse.

3. **Prognosis.** As stated above, a greater depth of invasion (Breslow thickness), the presence of ulceration, lymph node metastasis, and distant disease all portend a worse prognosis for patients with melanoma (Table 32.1).

D. **Treatment of advanced melanoma**
   1. **Adjuvant therapy.** There is no proven benefit for any adjuvant therapy given to patients with low-risk (stage IA) or intermediate-risk (stage IB, IIA) melanoma. Interferon α 2b was granted U.S. Food and Drug Administration (FDA) approval in 1995 for administration to patients with surgically resected stage IIb, IIc, and III (high-risk) melanoma. The approved schedule is 1 year of adjuvant treatment given intravenously for the initial 4 weeks at 20 MU/m^2 each day (Monday to Friday) followed by subcutaneous administration at 10 MU/m^2 for 48 weeks given three days/week. We routinely hydrate patients with 500 mL saline before each i.v. dose of interferon during weeks 1 to 4. Patients are premedicated with acetaminophen 650 mg p.o.; however, antiemetics are not routinely given. Three randomized controlled clinical trials have been performed using the FDA approved schedule and the results of Eastern Cooperative Oncology Group (ECOG) 1684, ECOG 1690, and ECOG 1694 have been published. A recent update of the three trials (*Clin Cancer Res* 2004;10:1670–1677) confirms the benefit with improved relapse-free survival (RFS) for patients given interferon when compared to the control group. At a median follow-up of 12.6 years, the benefit of adjuvant interferon is durable ($p = 0.02$, hazard ratio [HR] = 1.38) as assessed by RFS. There is no proven benefit for adjuvant cytotoxic chemotherapy or adjuvant high-dose interleukin 2 (IL-2) as treatment of surgically resected melanoma.

      a. **Interferon side effects and toxicities.** The side effects and toxicities of interferon are significant and all patients should be counseled before the initiation of therapy (*Oncologist* 2005;10:739–742). Virtually all patients experience fatigue and many experience fevers, chills, and diaphoresis (70% patients, grade 3 to 4). Myelosuppression, hepatotoxicity, and neurologic symptoms are frequent. Depression can be severe and precautions should be taken with appropriate referral to mental health professionals. Use of selective serotonin reuptake inhibitors (SSRI) is recommended in suitable patients (*N Engl J Med* 2001;344:961–966). Approximately 50% of patients have treatment delay or dose reduction during the initial 4 weeks of induction therapy. In our experience, 75% to 80% of selected patients complete the 1-year course of treatment. Selection criteria used currently in our practice include patients aged 60 or younger with no other significant medical illness, who understand the risks and benefits of treatment. Excellent guidelines to assist in the management of toxicities and side effects have been published (*J Clin Oncol* 2002;20:3703–3718). Finally, there is no role for administration of interferon concurrent with radiation.

   2. **Metastatic disease.** Regional and distant lymph nodes, skin, lung, liver, and brain are the most common distant sites of metastases from cutaneous melanoma. Prognosis depends on the sites of metastases with brain and hepatic metastases having the shortest (3 to 6 months) survival followed by lung metastases; nodal and skin metastases have the most favorable prognosis. Patients with regional nodal disease or a single distant site should be considered for surgical resection (*Ann Surg* 139;961–967). A common example is a late regional recurrence in the draining nodal basin (most often axilla or inguinal areas) considered recurrent stage III melanoma. Complete surgical resection of nodal disease can afford significant long-term survival in many patients (*Cancer J* 2006;12:207–211).

   No systemic treatment has been shown to prolong survival on the basis of any randomized controlled clinical trial. FDA approved systemic therapies for metastatic melanoma include dacarbazine (DTIC) and high-dose IL-2. DTIC is a nonclassic alkylating agent typically used as a single agent as treatment for metastatic melanoma. It is frequently given as a single 30- to 60-min infusion at 850 to 1,000 mg/m2 on day 1 every 21 days; however, many other schedules have been studied and they appear to be equivalent. The objective response rate as reported is between 5% and 15% and responses are generally of short duration (3 to 6 months). Combination chemotherapy has been extensively studied in metastatic melanoma and although response rates are generally higher, there is no survival advantage as compared to DTIC alone. Temozolomide (TMZ) is an oral agent with 100% bioavailability and is frequently used in metastatic melanoma. A randomized clinical trial comparing TMZ versus DTIC showed equivalence; however, TMZ can cross the blood–brain barrier and offers the advantage of convenience and central nervous system (CNS) penetration as treatment for brain metastases. High-dose IL-2 can produce durable complete remission in a small percentage of patients. For example, as reported by Atkins et al., in a series of 270 patients with metastatic melanoma, the overall response rate was 16% (6% CR/10% PR) with a median overall survival of 11.4 months (*J Clin Oncol* 1999;17:2105–2116). However, this regimen is associated with significant toxicities and should be administered at selected centers. Since no therapy has been shown to prolong survival, participation in a clinical trial remains the best option for most patients. For patients ineligible for a clinical trial, initial treatment with single agent DTIC remains the standard of care at most institutions. Patients with brain metastases should be considered for TMZ after definitive treatment with radiotherapy. We do not recommend giving TMZ concurrently with whole-brain radiotherapy in patients with brain metastases pending further study (*J Cancer Res Clin Oncol* 2002;128(4): 214–218).

3. **Investigational therapies.** Clinical investigation is active for the treatment of metastatic melanoma. Various forms of immunotherapy as well as inhibitors of signal transduction and angiogenesis are among the most promising investigational therapies currently under study.

4. **Prognosis.** The median survival of patients with metastatic (stage IV) melanoma is 9 months. Patients with intracranial melanoma metastasis have an especially poor prognosis. Despite definitive treatment with corticosteroids and whole-brain radiotherapy, the median survival is 3 to 4 months. In patients who undergo craniotomy and complete surgical resection of a solitary intracranial metastasis, the median survival is 9 months.

E. **Follow-up.** Patients with a history of melanoma should be followed closely with detailed dermatologic and lymph node examinations. They should be taught skin self-examination, as they are at increased risk for a second primary melanoma, as well as recurrence of disease. In addition, these patients need to be counseled regarding the daily use of a broad-spectrum sunscreen that blocks both UVA and UVB. Patients should also be taught sun avoidance strategies such as avoiding the mid-day sun and wearing protective clothing. Patients diagnosed with melanoma of any stage are not eligible to donate blood, tissue, or solid organs.

Patients with stage 0 melanoma should be followed with periodic skin examinations for life. Current recommendations for stage I to stage II disease are to have a history and physical examination (H&P) every 3 to 6 months for the first 3 years, then every 4 to 12 months for 2 years, and then annual skin examinations for life. These patients should also get an annual chest x-ray (CXR), and LDH levels can be checked every 6 to 12 months. Stage III melanoma warrants clinical examinations every 3 to 4 months for the first 5 years after diagnosis. Patients with stage III melanoma should also be followed up with a CXR, LDH, and complete blood count (CBC) every 3 to 12 months. CT scans should be performed as clinically indicated for patients with surgically resected advanced melanoma. However, there is no accepted role for surveillance imaging (except annual CXR) for patients with stage I/II melanoma. If patients with stage IV melanoma are rendered disease-free, then they should be followed as if they have stage III melanoma according to NCCN guidelines.

F. Special considerations

1. **Melanoma of unknown primary.** Patients may present with metastatic disease without an identifiable primary cutaneous tumor. Cases of melanoma with unknown primary represent less than 5% of melanomas overall. Most patients present with localized lymph node metastasis clinically manifesting as lymphadenopathy. All patients should have a thorough evaluation including examination of the skin, scalp, perineum, eyes, and mucosal membranes, as melanocytes are also present in the eye (conjunctiva and uvea), gut, inner ear, and nasopharynx. Numerous studies have demonstrated that these patients have the same survival as patients with known primaries according to the stage of disease and should be treated accordingly.

2. **Mucosal melanoma.** Mucosal melanoma is rare and represents less than 1% of all melanomas. Melanomas can occur on any mucosal surface including the nasopharynx, oral mucosa, larynx, vulva, and anus. These tumors are generally advanced at the time of presentation and therefore, prognosis is poor. Treatment is wide local excision with negative histologic margins.

3. **Ocular melanoma.** Ocular melanomas also represent less than 5% of the cases of melanoma. Uveal or choroidal melanomas make up most cases, with conjunctival melanomas occurring less frequently. Specialized ultrasonographic evaluation, together with lesional biopsy, is an important tool in initial diagnosis. Treatment for conjunctival melanoma is complete surgical excision. As with cutaneous disease, these tumors tend to metastasize to the regional lymph nodes. For localized uveal or choroidal melanomas, there are multiple treatment options and factors such as size of tumor, pathologic diagnosis, and vision in affected eye and contralateral eye, presence of metastasis, patient age, and performance status should be considered. Treatment options include enucleation, radiation, photocoagulation, and thermotherapy. In contrast to conjunctival melanomas, uveal and choroidal melanomas generally metastasize hematogenously to the liver. There is no effective systemic treatment for metastatic ocular melanoma. For patients with liver dominant metastases, regional therapy should be considered (*Ann Surg Oncol* 2004;11:290–297).

G. Background

1. **Epidemiology of melanoma.** According to 2005 American Cancer Society statistics, melanoma is the fifth most common cancer in men and women, an incidence similar to non-Hodgkin's lymphoma. In addition, the incidence and death rates are rising. The American Cancer Society estimates that in the year 2006 approximately 62,190 cases of melanoma will be diagnosed, and 7,910 individuals will die of melanoma. The lifetime risk of being diagnosed with melanoma in the United States is approximately 1 in 65. Melanoma is approximately twenty times more common in whites than in African Americans.

2. **Risk factors.** In the United States, the risk of developing melanoma is slightly higher in men than in women. Men are more likely to develop melanoma on the trunk, especially the back. Women are more likely to develop melanoma on the extremities, especially the posterior legs. There are multiple risk factors for the development of melanoma and a new or changing mole carries one of the highest relative risks. Less common associated conditions such as the atypical/dysplastic nevus syndrome and the rare genetic disorder xeroderma pigmentosum also have extremely high relative risks. Other reported risk factors include personal history of melanoma; the presence of 50 moles that are more than 2 mm in diameter, 5 moles that are 5 mm in diameter, more than 5 atypical nevi, and large congenital nevi; LM; family history of melanoma; fair skin; exposure to ultraviolet radiation from the sun and/or man-made sources; intermittent sun exposure in fair-skinned individuals; sunburns as a child; immunosuppression; poor suntanning ability; red hair; and higher socioeconomic status.

3. **Pathogenesis.** Melanoma is a cancer of melanocytes, which are melanin (pigment)-producing cells of neural crest origin. A combination of genetic factors

is likely involved in the transformation of a melanocyte to a melanoma. The most important gene involved in development is the CDKN2A or INK4a/ARF gene located on chromosome 9p21. Alternative splicing of this genetic locus produces two proteins. The gene products are the p14 and p16 proteins, both of which are important cell-cycle regulators. Disruption of p16 results in unregulated phosphorylation of the retinoblastoma protein (Rb), which leads to unregulated proliferation. Loss of the p14 protein leads to increased destruction of p53, which leads to enhanced survival and growth of mutated melanocytes. Other pathways implicated in the development of melanoma are the mitogenic pathways such as the Ras/Raf/MAPK pathway that is activated by mutations in N-Ras and B-Raf, and the PI-3 kinase pathway that is activated by PTEN loss and AKT3 amplification in melanomas. Recent studies show that MITF (microphthalmia-associated transcription factor) is a melanocyte-lineage survival oncogene that is often dysregulated by chromosomal amplification.

H. Current focus of research. Effective treatments for stage III and IV melanoma remain elusive. Current strategies focus on early detection, diagnosis, and removal. Current research is focused on elucidating the molecular events involved in transformation of melanocytes to melanoma, in an attempt to translate these findings into new targeted therapies.

II. SQUAMOUS CELL CARCINOMA OF THE SKIN

A. Presentation. SCC generally presents as an enlarging, erythematous, scaly papule or plaque on sun-exposed skin that is persistent and may bleed and be tender. SCC is generally thought to exist on a continuum from precursor lesions known as *actinic keratosis* to squamous cell carcinoma *in situ* (Bowen's Disease) to invasive SCC. Actinic keratoses typically present as keratotic, pink papules on sun-exposed skin of fair-skinned patients.

B. Workup and staging. Although SCC may be suspected clinically, a biopsy is necessary to make a definitive diagnosis. Several biopsy techniques are adequate including shave, punch, incisional, or excisional biopsies. Additionally, a full dermatologic examination and palpation of the draining lymph nodes should be performed. In the absence of evidence of metastatic disease further workup with imaging and laboratory studies is not necessary. Staging of SCCs in the tumor, node, metastasis (TNM) system is based on clinical size in the absence of metastasis.

C. Therapy. Several treatment options exist for the treatment of SCC. Most lesions are removed surgically with 0.4 cm margins for lesions smaller than 2 cm in size and more than 0.6-cm margins for lesions larger than 2 cm. Such margins provide cure rates of 90% to 95%. Mohs micrographic surgery can be employed for lesions that are at high risk for recurrence and metastasis such as SCC on the central face, ears, eyelids, lips, recurrent SCCs, SCCs larger than 2 cm, SCCs with aggressive histologic subtypes, and SCCs that develop in scars. Mohs micrographic surgery involves the use of frozen or permanent sections to evaluate as close to 100% of the surgical margin as possible by cutting the tissue horizontally instead of vertically. Additional therapies for SCCs include cryosurgery, curettage and electrodesiccation, radiation, and rarely, intralesional chemo- or immunotherapy. Radiation therapy is generally reserved for patients who are poor surgical candidates or are infirm. Radiation is used as adjunct therapy in patients with metastatic disease and high-risk SCCs. Chemotherapy is not routinely used, but patients with advanced disease may benefit from platinum-based combination chemotherapy.

There has been some attempt to employ chemoprevention in patients with a high risk of developing cutaneous SCC, particularly solid organ transplant patients. These modalities range from the use of topical immunomodulators, such as imiquimod, to topical and oral retinoids and topical 5-fluorouracil (Efudex). The use of these topical agents results in irritation that is typically well tolerated. Oral retinoid therapy, however, may be associated with serum lipid abnormalities that may already be problematic in this patient population. In addition, the discontinuation of oral retinoids may be associated with a rebound in the number of SCCs.

D. Prognosis. The vast majority of SCCs can be cured surgically. However, the incidence of recurrence is 1% to 10% depending on the method used and can be approximately 20% for high-risk lesions in high-risk locations such as the ear. The incidence of metastasis from cutaneous SCC is 2% to 6%. When SCCs metastasize they typically go to the first draining lymph node. Certain SCCs have a more aggressive course and are designated as high-risk. High-risk SCCs carry a metastatic risk greater than 10% and include lesions on the lips and ears, lesions larger than 2 cm, deeper lesions, SCCs in scars, recurrent SCCs, SCCs with perineural invasion, and SCCs in immunosuppressed patients.

E. Follow-up and prevention. Low-risk SCCs are followed up with full–body skin examinations every 3 months for the first year, every 6 months for the next year, and annually thereafter. High-risk SCCs should be followed up with skin examinations and lymph node examinations every 3 months for the first 2 years, with progressive lengthening of the interval thereafter. Sun protection and sun avoidance need to be stressed in these patients.

F. Background
  1. **Epidemiology.** SCC is the second most common type of skin cancer in the United States. The overwhelming majority of SCCs occur on chronic sun-exposed skin in older individuals. Men are twice as likely to develop SCC, and its incidence is more than 20 times higher in fair-skinned individuals than in patients with pigmented skin.
  2. **Risk factors.** The major risk factor for development of SCC is exposure to ultraviolet (UV) radiation or the sun. Therapeutic sources of UV radiation such as psoralen plus ultraviolet A (PUVA) also increase the risk for SCC. Other risk factors include immunosuppression (especially in solid organ transplant patients), fair skin, exposure to ionizing radiation, infection with certain human papillomavirus subtypes, burn scars, nonhealing ulcers, increased age, and hereditary disorders such as xeroderma pigmentosum.
  3. **Pathogenesis.** Multiple factors play a role in the development of SCC. Exposure of epidermal keratinocytes to UV light induces DNA damage, some of which may inactivate the p53 tumor suppressor gene. Exposure to UV radiation also induces local and systemic immunosuppression that likely plays a role in the development of SCC. Immunosuppression in solid organ transplant recipients also markedly increases their risk of developing SCCs, indicating the importance of an intact immune system in SCC prevention.

G. Current research. Areas of current research include developing immune modulators and other nonsurgical methods for treating SCCs.

III. BASAL CELL CARCINOMA

A. Presentation. (BCC) typically presents as a pink, pearly papule with a rolled border on sun-exposed skin. Patients may report that the lesion bleeds easily, does not heal, and is tender.

B. Workup and staging. As with SCC, a biopsy is critical for making a diagnosis of BCC. Any one of several biopsy techniques is acceptable including shave, punch, incisional, or excisional biopsies. BCCs rarely metastasize and further workup, beyond a full skin examination, is generally not necessary.

C. Therapy. BCCs are typically treated with destructive or surgical measures. Curettage and electrodessication provides a rapid and effective method to destroy BCCs with a cure rate of approximately 90%. Surgical excision of BCCs with at least a 4-mm margin provides a cure rate of approximately 95%. Similar to SCCs, BCCs in high-risk locations, BCCs near vital structures, and recurrent BCCs can be treated with Mohs micrographic surgery. Cryotherapy and radiation therapy are also options for patients with low-risk BCCs who are poor surgical candidates.

  Topical therapy is also available for certain subtypes of BCC, such as superficial spreading BCCs on the trunk. Topical 5-fluorouracil can effect cure rates of more than 90%, whereas imiquimod has been shown to clear approximately 80% of such BCCs.

D. Prognosis. The prognosis for patients with BCC is excellent. Most patients are cured by the aforementioned modalities. If left untreated, BCCs continue to enlarge and are locally destructive. Metastases occur in less than 0.1% of patients and common sites are the lymph nodes, lungs, and bones. Death from BCCs is extremely rare.

E. Follow-up and prevention. Patients with a history of BCC have a 50% chance of developing a second BCC within 5 years. Therefore, similar to patients with SCC, close follow-up is recommended. Avoidance of precipitating factors such as sun exposure, tanning beds, ionizing radiation, and arsenic exposure needs to be stressed in these patients.

F. Background

1. **Epidemiology.** BCC is the most common cancer in the United States. It is more common in men then in women and typically presents on sun-exposed areas of fair-skinned individuals.

2. **Risk factors.** Risk factors for the development of BCC include UV light exposure from the sun and/or tanning beds, exposure to ionizing radiation, fair skin, immunosuppression, exposure to arsenic, history of a nonmelanoma skin cancer, increased age, and hereditary disorders such as xeroderma pigmentosum and basal cell nevus syndrome.

3. **Pathogenesis.** BCCs are thought to arise from the pluripotent cells of the pilosebaceous unit that are capable of producing sebaceous glands, apocrine glands, and hair. Mutations in the p53 gene from UV radiation have been implicated in some cases. Studies on patients with basal cell nevus syndrome demonstrated the roles of the PATCHED gene and dysregulation of the SONIC HEDGEHOG pathway in BCC formation.

IV. MERKEL CELL CARCINOMA

A. Presentation. Merkel cell carcinoma (MCC) typically presents as an asymptomatic, pink to red, dome-shaped papule on the head or neck. Patients may present with metastatic disease and constitutional symptoms or symptoms related to the site of the metastasis.

B. Workup and staging. Biopsy and histologic examination is required to make the diagnosis of MCC. Following diagnosis, MCC patients should have a complete history and physical examination, including a CBC and liver function tests. The physical examination should include a full dermatologic and lymph node examination. Patients should also have a staging CT or MRI to screen for both regional lymph nodes and distant metastases.

C. Therapy. Wide local excision with 3-cm margins is recommended. There is some evidence that wide local excision combined with complete lymph node dissection and radiation therapy may provide a survival benefit. Sentinel lymph node biopsies are often performed; however, the therapeutic benefit is unproven. Patients with recurrent MCC may be treated with wide local excision, radiation and rarely chemotherapy. Chemotherapy is generally reserved for patients with metastatic disease. Chemotherapy and radiation may decrease tumor size, but neither is curative.

D. Prognosis. The overall 5-year survival rate for MCC is approximately 50%. About half of the patients with MCC develop lymph node metastases and about one third metastasize to distant organs. Common sites of metastases are the liver, bone, brain, lung, and skin. Poor prognostic factors include large tumor size, high number of mitotic cells, and small cell size.

E. Follow-up and prevention. Given the high rates of local recurrence and metastatic disease, patients should be followed up closely. As with other cutaneous cancers, prevention focuses on sun and UV radiation avoidance.

F. Background

1. **Epidemiology.** MCC is the least common of all cutaneous cancers. In the United States, approximately 400 cases are diagnosed a year. MCC is more common in fair-skinned, elderly individuals and generally presents on the head and neck followed by the extremities.

2. **Risk factors.** Risk factors for the development of MCC include exposure to the sun and man-made sources of UV radiation, immunosuppression, a history of skin cancer, fair skin, and age more than 70.

3. **Pathogenesis.** MCC is thought to arise from the Merkel cell in the skin. The Merkel cell is of neural crest origin and its function is unclear. Several chromosomal abnormalities have been described in MCC with the most common one on the short arm of chromosome 1.

Suggested Readings

Balch CM, Buzaid AC, Soong SJ, et al. Final version of the American Joint Committee on Cancer staging system for cutaneous melanoma. *J Clin Oncol* 2001;19(16):3635–3648.

Balch CM, Soong SJ, Gershenwald JE, et al. Prognostic factors analysis of 17,600 melanoma patients: validation of the American Joint Committee on Cancer melanoma staging system. *J Clin Oncol* 2001;19(16):3622–3634.

Johnson TM, Bradford CR, Gruber SB, et al. Staging workup, sentinel node biopsy, and follow-up tests for melanoma: update of current concepts. *Arch Dermatol* 2004;140(1):107–113.

McMasters KM, Reintgen DS, Ross MI, et al. Sentinel lymph node biopsy for melanoma: controversy despite widespread agreement. *J Clin Oncol* 2001;19(11):2851–2855.

Miller AJ, Mihm MC Jr. Melanoma. *New Engl J Med* 2006;355:51–65.

National Comprehensive Cancer Care Network. *Clinical practice guidelines in oncology— v.2.2006: melanoma.* http://www.nccn.org/professionals/physician_gls/PDF/melanoma .pdf, 2006.

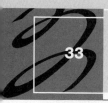

33 | CANCER OF UNKNOWN PRIMARY SITE
Daniel Morgensztern

I. DEFINITION. Carcinoma of unknown primary (CUP) is defined as a biopsy-proven metastatic malignant tumor whose primary site cannot be identified during pretreatment evaluation including a thorough history and physical examination, laboratory and radiographic studies, and a detailed histologic investigation.

II. PRESENTATION

    A. Subjective. Although CUPs comprise a heterogeneous group of tumors with different natural histories, there are still some typical characteristics. Some of the clinical features include a short history of local symptoms related to the metastatic sites (pain, swelling, and cough) and constitutional symptoms (weight loss, fatigue, and fever).

    B. Objective. The physical examination is frequently abnormal with findings such as effusions, lymphadenopathy, and hepatomegaly, indicating the site of metastatic involvement. Patients should undergo a thorough examination of the skin to rule out the presence of melanoma or nonmelanoma tumors, breast, rectum, pelvis, and genitals. The most common sites involved are lymph nodes, liver, bone, lungs, and pleura. Most patients present with multiple metastatic sites because of early dissemination and, unlike known primary tumors, the pattern is usually unpredictable.

III. DIAGNOSIS. The diagnosis is made by biopsy. Since several studies may need to be performed, it is important to consult with the pathologist to determine whether the specimen is sufficient, as the commonly used fine needle aspiration contains limited tissue and does not provide information on tissue architecture.

IV. WORKUP

    A. Initial assessment. With the histologically proven diagnosis of malignancy, patients should undergo a limited clinical investigation to identify the primary site and favorable subsets. This evaluation should include a complete history physical examination including pelvic and rectal examination, complete blood count (CBC), chemistry profile, urinalysis, occult blood stool testing, chest radiography, computer tomography (CT) of the abdomen and pelvis, and symptom-oriented endoscopy. Subsequent diagnostic tests are based on the clinical presentation, gender, and histopathologic findings. Comprehensive and exhaustive radiographic and endoscopic tests should not be performed because even with extensive workup, the primary site becomes evident in less than 25% of the patients. Up to 80% of primaries can be found in autopsy series, most commonly in the lungs and pancreas.

    B. Imaging. The initial radiological evaluation may be limited to chest radiographs and CT scans of the abdomen and pelvis. Chest radiograph is usually performed during the initial evaluation, even in the absence of respiratory symptoms, since a large number of patients will eventually have the diagnosis of lung cancer. However, chest radiograph cannot reliably distinguish primary lung tumors from metastatic disease to the lungs, particularly in malignancies that may metastasize to endobronchial sites such as carcinomas of the breast, colon, and kidney. Contrast radiographic studies have a low yield and should be reserved for patients with findings related to the organ to be examined. The role of CT scan of the chest has not been defined, although it may help determine the extent of metastatic disease. CT scan of the abdomen and pelvis may detect the primary site in approximately one third of patients. It can also be particularly useful in the detection of occult pancreatic carcinomas. Mammogram is indicated in the diagnostic investigation of all women with CUP, particularly in the cases of adenocarcinoma metastatic to axillary lymph nodes. Breast magnetic resonance imaging (MRI) may be indicated in cases where the suspicion for primary breast remains high despite a negative mammogram.

The experience with fluorodeoxyglucose positron emission tomography (FDG-PET) scan in CUP has been limited so far and larger prospective series are needed before its routine use. Some of the problems associated with the use of PET include the high cost, elevated false positive rate, and lack of improved survival after the identification of the primary tumor. Nevertheless, PET may be particularly useful in patients with squamous cell carcinoma in the cervical lymph nodes, where it may allow the detection of a primary site in the head and neck area in approximately one third of the cases, and in patients with single metastatic site, where additional metastases may influence the treatment.

C. Endoscopy. Endoscopy cannot be recommended during the routine workup for patients with CUP in asymptomatic patients. Instead, it should be used according to the clinical presentation Therefore, ENT endoscopy should be performed in patients with isolated cervical lymph node involvement by squamous cell carcinoma, bronchoscopy in patients with pulmonary symptoms, gastrointestinal endoscopies in patients with abdominal symptoms or occult fecal blood, and proctoscopy or colposcopy in patients with inguinal lymph node involvement.

D. Pathology

1. Light microscopy. Routine light microscopy of the tissue specimen after staining with hematoxylin and eosin may identify the four main histologic subtypes of CUP; adenocarcinoma (50% to 60%), poorly differentiated carcinomas or adenocarcinomas (30%), squamous cell carcinomas (5% to 15%), and undifferentiated malignant neoplasms (5%).

2. Immunohistochemistry. Immunohistochemistry (IHC) represents the most widely available specialized technique for the classification of neoplasms and may help identify the tumor lineage by the use of peroxidase-labeled antibodies against specific tissue antigens. Immunoperoxidase (IP) can be used on formalin-fixed specimens, which usually makes repeated biopsy unnecessary and may identify several cell components, resulting in the narrowing of diagnostic possibilities (Table 33.1). Cytokeratins (CKs) are a family of intermediate filaments characteristic of carcinomas. The CK profile may be useful in the identification of the primary tumor site and the ones most commonly used in patients with CUP are the CK7 and CK20. CK7 is found in tumors of the lung, ovary, endometrium, and breast, and is absent in lower gastrointestinal tumors. CK20 is expressed in the gastrointestinal and urothelial cells. Therefore, the CK7/CK20 phenotype can be very useful in the diagnosis of CUP, particularly for adenocarcinomas (Table 33.2).

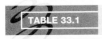 **TABLE 33.1**   **Immunoperoxidase Staining**

Tumor type	Immunohistochemistry
Carcinoma	CK, EMA
Lymphoma	CLA
Melanoma	S-100, vimentin, HMB-45
Sarcoma	Vimentin, desmin, factor VIII antigen (angiosarcoma)
Breast cancer	ER, PR, CK, EMA
Germ cell tumor	β-HCG, AFP, PLAP, CK, EMA
Neuroendocrine tumor	Chromogranin, synaptosyn, NSE, CK, EMA
Prostate cancer	PSA, CK, EMA
Thyroid	Thyroglobulin, TTF-1, calcitonin (MTC), CK, EMA

AFP, α-fetoprotein; CK, cytokeratin; CLA, common leukocyte antigen; EMA, epithelial membrane antigen; ER, estrogen receptor; β-HCG, beta-human chorionic gonadotropin; HMB, human melanoma black; MTC, medullary thyroid carcinoma; NSE, neuron-specific enolase; PLAP, placental alkaline phosphatase; PR, progesterone receptor; PSA, prostate-specific antigen; TTF-1, thyroid transcription factor 1.

TABLE 33.2	Cytokeratin Phenotype

CK phenotype	Tumors
CK7−/CK20−	Head and neck, liver, lung (squamous and small cell), prostate, renal
CK7+/CK20−	Biliary tract and pancreas, breast, cervical, endometrial, lung (adenocarcinoma), ovarian (nonmucinous), thyroid
CK7−/CK20+	Colon, Merkel cell carcinoma
CK7+/CK20+	Biliary tract and pancreas, ovarian (mucinous), urothelial

3. **Electron microscopy.** Electron microscopy (EM) allows the visualization of the ultrastructural features of the tumors such as cellular organelles, granules, and cell junctions. It may be useful in the identification of neuroendocrine tumors (neurosecretory granules), melanoma (premelanosomes), and poorly differentiated sarcomas. It may also help in differentiating between lymphoma and carcinoma or adenocarcinoma and squamous cell carcinoma although it does not localize the primary site of the malignancy. Since EM is expensive, time consuming, and not widely available, its use should be reserved for the cases with unclear lineage after light microscopy and IHC.

4. **Tumor markers.** Commonly used serum tumor markers such as (CEA), CA 19-9, and CA 125 are of limited value in the diagnosis of patients with CUP. Thyroglobulin may be increased in patients with bone metastases, suggesting an occult thyroid primary. CA 125 may be helpful in women with peritoneal papillary adenocarcinomatosis. Male patients should have serum beta-human chorionic gonadotropin (β-HCG), alpha fetoprotein (AFP), and prostate-specific antigen (PSA) tested to exclude testicular and prostate cancer respectively.

5. **Genetics.** Genetic analyses of the biopsy specimen may provide further characterization regarding the origin of the malignancy since a large number of tumors display characteristic cytogenetic abnormalities (Table 33.3).

V. THERAPY AND PROGNOSIS

A. **Favorable subsets.** Following the exclusion of lymphoma and sarcoma by a careful pathologic evaluation, the vast majority of the patients will have the diagnosis of carcinoma. The next step in the investigation is to determine whether they belong to one of the several subsets of CUP patients that require specific treatment approaches that may lead to improved outcomes and possibly cure (Table 33.4).

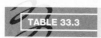

TABLE 33.3	Selected Cytogenetic Abnormalities

Tumor	Abnormality
Lymphomas	
Anaplastic large cell lymphoma	t(2;5)
Burkitt's lymphoma	t(8;14)
Follicular lymphoma/diffuse large B-cell lymphoma	t(14;18)
Mantle cell lymphoma	(11;14)
Sarcomas	
Alveolar rhabdomyosarcoma	t(2;13)
Uterine leiomyoma	t(12;14)
Synovial sarcoma	t(X;18)
Germ cell tumors	i(12p)
Retinoblastoma	del(13)
Wilm's tumor	del(11)

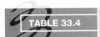

TABLE 33.4	Favorable Subsets and Treatment

Subset	Treatment
Women with adenocarcinoma involving only axillary lymph nodes	Treat as stage IIA (T0 N1) or IIIA (T0 N2) breast cancer
Women with papillary serous adenocarcinoma in the peritoneal cavity	Treat for stage III ovarian carcinoma
Men with blastic bone metastases and elevated PSA	Treat for prostate cancer with hormonal therapy
Men with poorly differentiated carcinoma with midline distribution	Treat as extragonadal germ cell tumors
Squamous cell carcinoma of the cervical lymph nodes	Treat as locally advanced head and neck cancer
Isolated inguinal lymphadenopathy by squamous cell carcinoma	Inguinal node dissection with or without adjuvant radiation therapy
Poorly differentiated neuroendocrine carcinoma	Platinum-based chemotherapy
Single metastasis	Local treatment with surgery or radiation therapy

PSA, Prostate-specific antigen.

1. **Women with isolated axillary adenopathy.** Patients with CUP and isolated axillary adenopathy are usually females and the diagnosis is most likely breast cancer. The lymph node specimen should be tested for ER, PR, and HER2/neu. In case of a negative mammogram, the occult breast primary may be seen on MRI. The primary tumor can be identified after mastectomy in 40% to 80% of cases. Patients with mobile axillary lymph nodes (N1) should be treated as stage IIA breast cancer, whereas patients with fixed nodes (N2) should be treated as stage IIIA disease.

2. **Women with papillary serous adenocarcinoma of the peritoneal cavity.** The presence of ascites and peritoneal adenocarcinoma in women is typical of ovarian carcinoma although this pattern of spread may also occur in tumors of the lung, breast, and gastrointestinal tract. However, a primary tumor is not found in a large number of these patients. Although the origin of these cells is unknown, histologic features such as papillary configuration or psammoma bodies are typical of ovarian carcinoma. Patients should be considered to have as stage III ovarian carcinoma and treated with cytoreductive surgery followed by platinum-based chemotherapy.

3. **Men with blastic bone metastases and elevated PSA.** Elderly men with adenocarcinoma of unknown primary and metastatic disease involving predominantly the bones and those with increased serum PSA or positive PSA staining in the biopsy specimen should be treated for metastatic prostate cancer.

4. **Men with poorly differentiated carcinoma of midline distribution.** Young men with predominant midline tumor distribution (mediastinum and retroperitoneum) of uncertain histogenesis should be treated as extragonadal germ cell tumors even in the absence of elevated serum levels of AFP or β-HCG. The presence of isochromosome 12p in some tumors allows their classification as germ cell tumors.

5. **Squamous cell carcinoma of the cervical lymph nodes.** Patients with mid or upper cervical lymph nodes are usually middle aged or elderly, with frequent history of tobacco and alcohol abuse. The main suspicion in these patients is of a primary head and neck tumor, and the workup should involve the complete evaluation of the upper airways. In the absence of an identifiable primary site, patients should be considered to have locally advanced head and

neck cancer. Patients with lower cervical lymph or supraclavicular lymph nodes may have lung cancer and should undergo fiberoptic bronchoscopy during the workup, particularly in the case of unrevealing head and neck examination and nondiagnostic chest radiograph. If no primary site is found, the prognosis for this subset of patients is usually poor.

6. **Isolated inguinal lymphadenopathy from squamous cell carcinoma.** Most patients with inguinal lymph nodes have a detectable primary tumor either in the genital or in the anorectal area. Therefore, both the genitalia and rectum should be evaluated during the initial workup. If the primary cancer cannot be identified, long-term survival may be achieved with inguinal lymphadenectomy with or without adjuvant radiation therapy. Some patients may also benefit from the addition of chemotherapy, either in the neoadjuvant or adjuvant settings.

7. **Poorly differentiated neuroendocrine carcinoma.** These are usually very poorly differentiated tumors but with positive IHC stains for chromogranin or neuron-specific enolase (NSE). The origin for this heterogeneous group of tumors is unclear and some may represent undifferentiated variants of known neuroendocrine tumors or small cell carcinomas. Patients usually present with diffuse hepatic or bone metastases and usually respond to cisplatin-based chemotherapy.

8. **Single metastasis.** In a small number of patients, only a single metastatic lesion is identified despite a complete clinical and radiologic evaluation. Although other metastatic sites may become evident within a short period of time, some patients may achieve prolonged disease-free interval with local therapies such as surgery or radiation therapy. Despite the uncertain role, adjuvant chemotherapy may be considered for patients with good performance status.

B. **Unselected patients.** With the exception of patients in the favorable subsets, most patients with CUP remain relatively resistant to chemotherapy indicating a very poor prognosis. Although the median survival for patients enrolled into clinical trials ranges between 6 and 10 months, population data from tumor registries report median survivals of 2 to 3 months in unselected patients. A prognostic model proposed by the French study group was based on ECOG (Eastern Cooperative Oncology Group) performance status higher than 1 and abnormal lactate dehydrogenase (LDH). Patients with none, one, or two risk factors had median survivals of 10.8, 6.0, and 2.4 months respectively (*J Clin Oncol* 2002;20:4679–4683). Patients with good performance status may benefit from chemotherapy. No single chemotherapeutic regimen has emerged as the treatment of choice and the most commonly used include a combination of platinum and a taxane (Table 33.5). The role for a third agent such as gemcitabine or etoposide remains unclear.

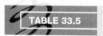

TABLE 33.5 Selected Chemotherapeutic Regimens for Cancer of Unknown Primary

Regimen	Assessable patients	Response rate (%)	Median survival (mo)
PCb[a]	70	39	13
PCbE[b]	66	48	11
PCbG[c]	113	25	9
DCb[d]	40	22	8
DCp[d]	23	26	8

[a] Briasoulis E, Pavlidis N. Cancer of unknown primary origin. *J Clin Oncol* 2000;18:3101–3117.
[b] Greco FA, Burris HA III, Erland JB, et al. Carcinoma of unknown primary site: long-term follow-up after treatment with paclitaxel, carboplatin, and etoposide. *Cancer* 2000;89:2655–2660.
[c] Greco FA, Burris HA, Litchy S, et al. Gemcitabine, carboplatin, and paclitaxel for patients with carcinoma of unknown primary site: a Minnie Pearl Cancer Research Network study. *J Clin Oncol* 2002;20:1651–1656.
[d] Greco FA, Erland JB, Morrissey LH, et al. Carcinoma of unknown primary site: phase II trials with docetaxel plus cisplatin or carboplatin. *Ann Oncol* 2000;11:211–215.
Cb, carboplatin; Cp, cisplatin; E, etoposide; D, docetaxel; G, gemcitabine; P, paclitaxel.

VI. BACKGROUND. Metastatic CUP is a common entity, accounting for 2.3% of all cancers reported to the Surveillance, Epidemiology, and End Results (SEER) database between 1973 and 1987. It represents the seventh to eight most common type of cancer and the fourth commonest cause of death in both men and women. The median age at presentation is approximately 60 years and it is slightly more prevalent in men.

The characteristic of CUP is the development of metastases before the primary tumor becomes detectable. These tumors are characterized by early dissemination, unpredictable metastatic spread, and very aggressive behavior.

Suggested Readings

Briasiykus E, Tolis C, Bergh J, et al. ESMO minimum clinical recommendations for diagnosis, treatment and follow-up of cancers of unknown primary site (CUP). *Ann Oncol* 2005;16(Suppl 1):75–76.

Culine S, Kramar A, Saghatchian M, et al. Development and validation of a prognistic model to predict the length of survival in patients with carcinoma of an unknown primary site. *J Clin Oncol* 2002;20:4679–4683.

Dowel JE. Cancer from an unknown primary site. *Am J Med Sci* 2003;326:35–46.

Hillen HPF. Unknown primary tumours. *Postgrad Med J* 2000;76:690–693.

Pavlidis N, Briasoulis E, Hainsworth J, et al. Diagnostic and therapeutic management of cancer of unknown primary. *Eur J Cancer* 2003;39:1990–2005.

Pavlidis N, Fizazi K. Cancer of unknown primary. *Crit Rev Onc Hematol* 2005;54:243–250.

Rubin BP, Skarin AT, Pisick E, et al. Use of cytokeratins 7 and 20 in determining the origin of metastatic carcinoma of unknown primary, with special emphasis on lung cancer. *Eur J Cancer Prev* 2001;10:77–82.

Van De Wouw AJ, Jansen RLH, Speel EJM, et al. The unknown biology of the unknown primary tumor: a literature review. *Ann Oncol* 2003;14:191–196.

Varadhachary R, Abbruzzese JL, Lenzi R. Diagnostic strategies of unknown primary cancer. *Cancer* 2004;100:1776–1785.

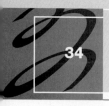

34 CANCER AND THROMBOSIS
Charles Eby

I. INTRODUCTION. Oncologists deal with the sequelae of numerous interactions between malignant diseases and the hemostatic systems of their patients: venous thrombosis, accompanying or preceding the discovery of cancer; thrombotic and hemorrhagic complications of cancer management; and the challenges of thromboembolism prophylaxis and treatment. Malignancy-associated venous thromboembolic events (VTEs) account for approximately 20% of all VTEs, affecting approximately 25% of cancer patients at some point during the course of their illness. In addition, patients with a VTE have poorer survival rates compared to thrombosis-free patients with similar types and stages of cancer (*Medicine* 1999;78:285–291). Finally, chronic oral anticoagulation therapy is less effective and more dangerous in cancer patients, with higher rates of bleeding and clotting complications, compared to patients without malignancies.

II. PATHOPHYSIOLOGY. A clearer understanding of the complex pathophysiology of cancer-associated thrombosis is beginning to emerge. Expression of tissue factor (TF) or cancer procoagulant on the surface of cancer cells, as well as aberrant expression of TF on the surface of monocytes and endothelial cells in response to cancer-induced production of inflammatory cytokines, play a central role in promoting a hypercoagulable state, angiogenesis, and tumor metastasis (*Semin Thromb Hemost* 2005;31:104–110). In addition to tumor–host hypercoaguable interactions, decreased activity due to disease or therapy leads to increased venous stasis, and vascular injury from surgery, chemotherapy, radiation, and central venous catheters (CVCs) are major risk factors for symptomatic VTE, completing Vichow's triad.

Results from recent, prospective trials confirm anticoagulant prophylaxis is not necessary for most cancer patients with CVC, and low molecular weight heparin (LMWH) is more effective in preventing recurrent VTE than oral vitamin K antagonists. Areas of ongoing clinical investigation include the optimal form and duration of VTE prophylaxis in certain perioperative and chemotherapy situations. In addition, preliminary studies suggest that LMWH therapy may improve survival in some cancer patients independent of VTE prevention.

III. VENOUS THROMBOSES AND OCCULT CANCER. Patients who present with idiopathic venous thromboses may harbor an undiagnosed malignancy. In the landmark study of Prandoni et al., (*N Engl J Med* 1992;327:1128–1133) 250 consecutive outpatients with an objectively diagnosed deep vein thrombosis (DVT) were periodically monitored for signs or symptoms of subsequent cancers. Initial findings on routine history, physical examination, and screening laboratory studies led to cancer diagnoses in 5 out of 153 patients with an idiopathic DVT and in none of 107 patients. During a 2-year follow-up period, symptomatic malignancies were diagnosed in 13 (5.2%) patients, 11 (7.6%) patients with an idiopathic DVT, and 2 (1.9%) patients with a secondary DVT. There were 35 recurrent VTEs in the idiopathic group, and 6 (17%) subsequently developed cancer. Gastrointestinal (GI), gynecologic, or urologic adenocarcinomas (*n* = 8) were most common, two were glioblastomas, and the remaining three were adenocarcinomas of the lung and breast, and a leiomyoscarcoma.

Retrospective surveys of large population databases linking hospital discharge diagnoses of unprovoked VTE and subsequent cancer diagnoses (Sorensen, White) confirm an increased risk of future cancer diagnosis particularly involving malignancies of the pancreas, brain, ovary, lung, kidney, and liver, acute myelogenous leukemia, and non-Hodgkin's lymphomas (*N Engl J Med* 1998;338;1169–1173; *Arch Intern Med* 2005;165;1782–1787). Most malignancies are diagnosed within 4 to 6 months of a VTE, and approximately 40% will have metastasized. On the basis of a retrospective cohort study, it is estimated that approximately 2.5% of adults presenting with an idiopathic VTE harbor an occult malignancy, and most cancers will become clinically apparent within 4 to 6 months of the VTE and will already be metastatic (*Arch Intern Med* 2005;165;1782–1787).

Owing to the general awareness of an association between VTE and malignancies, oncologists may be asked to evaluate patients with idiopathic VTE for occult cancer. Limited prospective data are available for guidance. The screening for occult malignancy in patients with symptomatic idiopathic venous thromboembolism (SOMIT) trial (*J Thromb Hemost* 2004;2:884–889) randomized 201 patients with idiopathic VTEs to either aggressive cancer screening (abdominal/pelvic ultrasonography, abdominal/pelvic computed tomography [CT]) scan, upper endoscopy, colonoscopy, hemoccult testing, sputum cytology, carcinoembryonic antigen [CEA], α-fetalprotein [αFP], CA-125, mammogram and pelvic examination with PAP smear for women, and prostate-specific antigen [PSA] plus prostate ultrasonography for men), or routine follow up after deferring 32 patients in whom cancers were diagnosed based on initial history, physical, and routine laboratory studies (Piccioli). An additional 13 of 99 cancers were identified in the aggressive screening arm. During the 2-year follow-up, one cancer was diagnosed in the screening arm compared to 10 out of 102 in the control arm. Although there was no significant difference in mortality at 2 years (2.0% screening, 3.9% control), the study did not meet its enrollment target of 1,000 due to poor accrual. A subsequent analysis of the SOMIT data (*J Thromb Hemost* 2005;3:2391–2396) concluded that abdominal/pelvic CT scanning was the most cost-effective cancer screening test, and that tumor markers were associated with high false-positive rates that generated additional unnecessary testing.

In a larger, prospective cohort study (*J Thromb Hemost* 2004;2:876–881), investigators used a two-step approach to cancer screening in idiopathic VTE patients. Step 1: a thorough history, physical examination, including rectal examination, and pelvic and breast exams in women, complete blood count (CBC), erythrocyte sedimentation rate (ESR), serum protein electrophoresis (SPEP), urine analysis (UA), comprehensive metabolic panel (CMP), and chest x-ray (CXR). Abnormalities suggestive of cancer were pursued with additional diagnostic procedures and biopsies to confirm the presence of a malignancy. Patients who did not have a cancer diagnosed in step 1 ($n = 830$) underwent Step 2: a "limited" work-up consisting of an abdominal/pelvic ultrasonography, CEA and PSA in men and CA-125 in women. Abnormalities suggestive of cancer were pursued with additional diagnostic steps and biopsies to confirm the presence of a malignancy. Patients who were cancer-free after steps 1 and 2 were followed for 12 months for the occurrence of symptomatic cancer. Step 1 evaluation identified 167 out of 864 patients for further cancer screening, primarily due to histories of weight loss, change in bowel habits, abdominal pain, and bleeding, and 34 out of 167 (20%) were diagnosed with cancers. Fifty-four patients were suspected of cancer based on findings during step 2 screening, and **13** out of 54 (24%) additional cancers were detected. Finally, **14** cancers were diagnosed during a 12-month follow-up. The results of this study suggest that in adults with idiopathic VTE, a cancer screening strategy employing a heightened scrutiny of information obtained from a careful history and physical examination, and general hematology, chemistry, and urine laboratory tests, combined with additional diagnostic tests in patients with abnormal finding will lead to diagnosis of approximately 50% of occult malignancies. In addition, it would be reasonable to perform age- and gender-appropriate general cancer screening procedures if they are not up to date. Although additional imaging, endoscopy, and currently available tumor marker tests may diagnose additional occult cancers, evidence that earlier detection will improve survival is lacking. **Therefore, aggressive searching for occult cancers in asymptomatic patients with idiopathic VTEs is not recommended.**

IV. PREVENTION OF VTE IN PATIENTS WITH CANCER

A. Prophylaxis against VTE in patients with cancer in the perioperative setting.

Cancer patients have a sevenfold increased risk of VTE compared to persons without a malignancy, and the risk is 54-fold higher in the first 3 months after cancer diagnosis, based on a recent case–control study (*JAMA* 2005;293:715–722). A considerable portion of the marked increase in cancer-associated VTE risk shortly after diagnosis is likely due to surgical, chemotherapy, and hormonal interventions, and can be reduced by employing appropriate prevention strategies. The incidence of VTE after cancer surgery may be as high as 50% without prophylaxis. Although mechanical prophylaxis methods can reduce postoperative VTE rates by approximately 50%, they are inferior to anticoagulant prophylaxis. Prospective studies comparing LMWH (qd.), and unfractionated heparin (UFH) (5,000U t.i.d.) postoperative prophylaxis, typically for 7 to 10 days, in cancer patients have consistently shown equivalent efficacy and safety with VTE rates of approximately 15% (primarily asymptomatic calf DVTs) and major bleeding incidents of approximately 4% (*N Engl J Med* 2002;249:146–153). Prospective studies comparing the synthetic pentasaccharide fondaparinux to UFH or LMWH specifically for VTE prophylaxis in cancer surgery have not been completed. However, cancer surgery patients who received fondaparinux in the PEGASUS trial, a prospective, randomized study comparing fondaparinux (2.5 mg/day) to daltaparin (5,000 U/day) in high-risk abdominal surgery patients, had significantly fewer DVTs (7.7%) compared to cancer patients in the dalteparin arm (7.7%) and equivalent low risk of bleeding complications (*Blood* 2003;102: Abstract 40).

There are compelling data to support extended DVT prophylaxis following some types of cancer surgery. In the ENOXACAN II study, patients were randomized to receive enoxaparin, 40 mg/day for 6 to 10 or 25 to 31 days after planned curative open surgery for abdominal or pelvic malignancies (*N Engl J Med* 2002;346:975–980). The endpoints were DVT, and major bleeding complications. The incidence of DVT was significantly different: 12% for routine and 4% for extended DVT prophylaxis, while bleeding complications were comparable (3.6% and 4.7% respectively). However, most thrombi were asymptomatic distal DVTs. A smaller prospective trial comparing routine to extended DVT prophylaxis with daltaparin 5,000 U/day reported similar results, and the 2004 American College of Chest Physicians (ACCP) guidelines recommend extended DVT prophylaxis with LMWH for patients undergoing abdominal/pelvic open cancer surgery (*Chest* 2004;126:338S–400S). Although there is no consensus regarding DVT prophylaxis following laparoscopic cholecystectomy in patients without additional VTE risk factors, patients undergoing laparoscopic colorectal, urologic, and gynecologic cancer surgeries are also at high risk for VTE complications (*Chest* 2004;126:338S–400S). Seven to ten days of postoperative DVT prophylaxis with UFH or LMWH would be reasonable until future studies determine the ideal prophylaxis schedule for this population (*J Thromb Hemost* 2005;3:210–214).

Patients who undergo surgery for central nervous system neoplasms have one of the highest rates of postoperative VTE and lowest tolerance for bleeding complications. However, several prospective randomized trials have validated the safety and efficacy of anticoagulant VTE prophylaxis with UFH and LMWH starting approximately 24 hours after surgery (*Br J Hematol* 2004;128:291–302).

B. Prophylaxis against VTE in patients with cancer and acute medical illness.

All oncology patients admitted to hospital for management of acute medical conditions or cancer therapy should be considered for mechanical or anticoagulant VTE prophylaxis. Several prospective, randomized VTE prevention studies have confirmed the efficacy and safety of LMWH and UFH prophylaxis in acutely ill medical patients, but cancer patients have comprised only 5% to 14% of these populations. Subset analysis of cancer patients in the MEDENOX (*N Engl J Med* 1999;341:793–800) study detected a 50% reduction in VTE risk in patients receiving enoxaparin versus placebo, and the 2004 ACCP guidelines recommend UFH or LMWH for VTE prophylaxis in hospitalized cancer patients (*Chest* 2004;126:338S–400S). Temporary risk factors for bleeding complications, including invasive procedures or thrombocytopenia, may require interruption of anticoagulant prophylaxis and substitution of mechanical devices until the bleeding risk is resolved, and should not lead to complete avoidance of UFH or LMWH. Ambulation should also be conscientiously encouraged during hospitalization.

It should be assumed that all patients receiving chemotherapy or hormonal therapy are at increased risk of VTE, although estimates of the absolute risks are available for only selected malignancies and treatment modalities. Plausible pro-thrombotic mechanisms include decreased activity of physiologic anticoagulants, release of procoagulants from apoptotic cancer cells, and drug-induced injury to endothelial cells. A prospective multicenter observational study of ambulatory cancer patients beginning chemotherapy reported a VTE incidence of 0.8% per month. Independent risk factors associated with treatment-related VTE included baseline platelet count greater than 350,000, primary site (lung, upper GI, and lymphoma), and anemia (hemoglobin less than 10, or use of erythropoietin (EPO)). Treatment-association risk of VTE has been most thoroughly examined in women with, or at risk for, breast cancer. Tamoxifen approximately doubles the VTE incidence in both the primary prevention and adjuvant therapy setting (Cuzick). The VTE risk is similar with raloxifene, a selective estrogen receptor modulator, and lower with aromatase inhibitors. One prospective, double blind trial, ran-domizing women with metastatic breast cancer receiving multidrug chemotherapy to warfarin 1 mg/day for 6 weeks followed by dose adjustment to an interna-tional normalized ratio (INR) target of 1.3 to 1.9, versus placebo, showed an 85% reduction of symptomatic VTE in the treatment arm (incidence 0.16% per month compared to a 0.7% per month in the control group) without a significant increase in major bleeding complications (*Lancet* 1994;343:886–889). Despite the efficacy and safety of primary VTE prophylaxis in this population, confirmatory studies have not been reported, and, with rare exceptions, routine primary VTE prophylaxis with warfarin or parenteral anticoagulants during chemotherapy has not been adopted by medical oncologists.

The increased incidence of VTE complications in multiple myeloma patients treated with thalidomide when combined with dexamethasone or doxorubicin has focused attention on the need for routine VTE prophylaxis during treatment of this cancer population. Studies comparing different VTE prophylaxis approaches in patients with multiple myeloma receiving thalidomide have not been reported to date, and there is no consensus regarding the optimal VTE strategy. Oral anticoagulation targeted to an INR of two to three, and prophylactic dosing of LMWH appear to be effective, but low-intensity oral anticoagulation is not effec-tive (*Br J Haematol* 2004;126:715–721). In a single institution study of liposomal doxorubicin, vincristine, dexamethasone, and thalidomide for newly diagnosed or relapsed multiple myeloma, VTE occurred in 10 of the first 35 patients. Hemosta-sis tests showed an increase in von Willebrand factor levels postchemotherapy, suggesting a pathologic role for platelet–endothelial interaction, and leading to the addition of low dose aspirin (81 mg/day) prophylaxis for subsequent subjects. The VTE incidence in patients who never took aspirin was 58% compared to 19% for patients who took aspirin from the start of chemotherapy (*Mayo Clin Proc* 2005;80:1568–1574). Until more data comparing different prophylactic strategies in multiple myeloma patients receiving thalidomide combination chemother-apy are available, clinicians must use their clinical judgment and select the approach they deem appropriate for each patient (*Mayo Clin Proc* 2005;80:1549–1551).

Although the interactions between the malignant plasma cells, dexametha-sone, doxorubicin, and thalidomide that produce a hypercoagulable state are incompletely understood at this time, there may be a class effect for antiangiogen-esis drugs because thrombotic complications have been reported for thalidomide treatment of systemic lupus erythematosus (SLE) and renal cell cancer, as well as for levolidomide and bortezomib treatment of multiple myeloma.

V. CVC AND THROMBOSIS. Percutaneous inserted central catheters and port-a-caths provide reliable venous access for administration of chemotherapy, medications, nutrition, and blood components to cancer patients, as well as for collection of blood for diagnostic tests. However, complications associated with CVC include insertion-related trauma (bleeding and pneumothorax), infection (cellulitis, bacteremia, sepsis), and thrombosis (occluded catheter lumen, external catheter fibrin sheath, partial or occlusive venous thrombus). The reported frequencies of symptomatic upper extremity DVT associated with CVC in cancer patients not using prophylactic anticoagulants decreased from 33% to 38% (*Ann Intern Med* 1990;112:423–428) from 38% (*J Thromb Haemost* 1996;2:876–881) in the 1990s to 3% to 4% in the last 5 years (*J Clin Oncol* 2005;23:4057–4062), most likely reflecting refinements in catheter materials and insertion techniques. Although earlier randomized control trials (RCTs) previously demonstrated a significant reduction in venography-confirmed upper extremity DVTs with either warfarin 1.0 mg/day or dalteparin 2,500 IU/day , recent, RCTs have failed to show a significant reduction of asymptomatic or symptomatic CVC-associated DVTs for 1.0 mg/day warfarin, 40 mg/day enoxaparin, or 5,000 IU/day dalteparin compared to placebo. On the basis of the results of these contemporary studies, the 2004 "Chest" (American College of Chest Physicians) guidelines no longer recommend routine DVT prophylaxis with the currently available anticoagulants for cancer patients with CVCs. However, selected cancer patients may benefit from DVT prophylaxis if they have had a previous CVC-associated thrombosis, or a spontaneous VTE. Patients with hematologic malignancies treated with intensive chemotherapeutic regimens appear to have a two to fourfold higher risk of CVC-associated symptomatic DVTs compared to patients receiving out-patient chemotherapy for solid tumors. However, studies evaluating the risks and benefits of DVT prophylaxis in the hematologic malignancy population have not been published, and routine anticoagulation is not indicated. Although several cohort studies have shown an increased relative risk of CVC-associated DVT in cancer patients who are also heterozygous for factor V Leiden (FVL) or prothrombin gene G20210A mutation, routine screening of cancer patients who have no VTE history for these inherited thrombophila risk factors is not recommended.

Management of symptomatic CVC-associated DVTs is controversial. Although the risk of symptomatic pulmonary embolism (PE) appears to be low in this situation, it remains a potentially serious complication. Typically, the catheter is removed, even when the lumens are still patent, therapeutic anticoagulation with UFH or LMWH is started, and chronic anticoagulation is continued with either warfarin or LMWH for a limited period. However, clinical circumstances may support anticoagulation without removing the catheter, or deferral of anticoagulation therapy if symptoms are mild and bleeding risk unacceptable.

VI. DIAGNOSIS AND TREATMENT OF VTE IN CANCER PATIENTS

A. Diagnosis of VTE. Although the combination of a low clinical assessment score and a negative quantitative D-dimer result has been validated for ruling out VTE in patient populations with a low prevalence of thrombosis, this strategy should be used with great caution in cancer patients suspected of having an acute DVT or PE in whom a higher underlying prevalence of VTE may produce an unacceptably high false negative D-dimer rate, and low negative predictive value. In addition, D-dimer concentration is typically elevated in cancer patients in the absence of an underlying VTE, producing a high false-positive rate and very low positive predictive value for thrombosis. A clinical suspicion for VTE in cancer patients requires sensitive imaging studies, guided by the presenting signs and symptoms, to assess for venous thrombus in the affected limb and emboli in pulmonary arteries. The noninvasive imaging techniques: lower extremity color duplex ultrasonography, spiral chest CT, and ventilation–perfusion scan, are likely to have similar sensitivities for detection of DVT and PE in cancer patients as have been reported in symptomatic patients without underlying malignancies. However, CVC-associated upper extremity DVTs tend to be more centrally located, and published sensitivities of ultrasonographic techniques range from 56% to 94% whereas specificities are consistently 100%. Therefore, although a positive upper extremity duplex color ultrasonographic study confirms a suspected CVC-associated DVT, a negative study requires more sensitive imaging techniques such as venography or possibly CT or magnetic resonance imaging (MRI), to rule out a thrombus. Periodic use of CT scans to assess treatment response or disease progression in solid cancers can lead to the discovery of asymptomatic partial or occlusive thrombi. Management of these "incidental" clots of indeterminant age is problematic and must be individualized.

B. Therapy of VTE in Patients with Cancer

1. Special issues in patients with cancer. Three important issues related to treatment of cancer-associated VTE are the safety, type, and duration of anticoagulation therapy. The only absolute contraindication to therapeutic anticoagulation is major active bleeding that cannot be rapidly and reliably controlled. However, the bleeding risk associated with some relative contraindications can be difficult to assess in a quantitative manner for individual patients. Treatment of VTEs in patients with primary and metastatic brain tumors is particularly challenging, due to the potentially devastating complications of intracranial hemorrhage (ICH) associated with anticoagulation therapy, the risk of recurrent VTE, and the inadequacy of high quality evidence to guide management (Fig. 34.1). Therapeutic anticoagulation is considered by some oncologists and neurosurgeons to be an absolute contraindication in VTE patients with highly vascular brain metastases or recent craniotomies. For patients in whom the benefit of anticoagulation therapy is judged to outweigh the risk, one approach involves cautious initiation of a continuous infusion of UFH, and if tolerated, followed by long-term anticoagulation therapy.

Thrombocytopenia, either cancer-related, or secondary to marrow suppression from chemotherapy, frequently complicates anticoagulation therapy. While data to define an evidence-based safe, minimal platelet count are not available, expert opinions and anecdotal clinical experience support initiation of therapeutic anticoagulation when the platelet count is greater than $50,000/\mu L$, and lower intensity, or interruption, of chronic anticoagulation when the platelet count drops below this level.

2. Role of inferior vena cava (IVC) filters. Placement of an IVC filter is an option in cancer patients with acute VTE and unacceptable bleeding risk or major bleeding complications during anticoagulation therapy. However, IVC filters are thrombogenic, and it would be appropriate to initiate or resume anticoagulation therapy if the acute bleeding risk factor resolves. Removable IVC filters are now FDA-approved medical devices. However, an endovascular procedure is required to remove them, and attempts to do so are not always successful. It is reasonable to speculate that the potential ability to remove an IVC filter will lower the threshold to insert one, and that once inserted, most will become permanent.

3. Role of thrombolytic therapy. Indications for thrombolytic therapy in cancer patients with VTE are limited due to the increased risk of bleeding, especially in patients with brain tumors, but should be considered for a PE causing severe hemodynamic instability, a DVT causing arterial insufficiency in the affected limb due to severe venous congestion, clinically significant extension of a thrombus despite therapeutic anticoagulation, and an occluded CVC that must be kept patent.

4. Initial treatment of VTE—role of heparin. Following objective confirmation of a DVT or PE in a cancer patient, the traditional approach to treatment was initial anticoagulation with UFH, using the activated partial thromboplastin time (aPTT) for therapeutic monitoring, and concurrent oral anticoagulation with warfarin until two therapeutic INRs (2–3) were obtained ≥ 24 hours apart at which time heparin was stopped. Meta-analysis of prospective, randomized studies confirms LMWHs are more effective and safe compared to UFH for initial anticoagulation in medical patients. Results of subset analyses of cancer patients with acute VTEs from several large prospective studies indicate that initial anticoagulation with LMWH and UFH have equivalent VTE recurrence rates at 3 months. However, LMWH is the preferred initial anticoagulant in cancer patients due to the ease of administration, elimination of therapeutic monitoring due to dependable weight-based pharmacokinetics, and lower risk of heparin-induced thrombocytopenia. Dosing of different LMWHs in cancer patients is the same as for medical patients, with similar caveats for patients with severe renal insufficiency (CrCl [creatinine clearance] <30 mL/minute), extremely high or low weight, and women who are pregnant. In a study comparing twice-daily (1 mg/kg), and once-daily (1.5 mg/kg) dosing of enoxaparin for treatment of acute VTE, the cancer patient subgroup had a nonsignificant higher VTE recurrence rate with once-daily dosing (12.2%) compared to twice daily (6.4%) (*Ann Int Med* 2001;134:191–202). It is unclear at the moment whether twice-daily dosing of enoxaparin is more efficacious than once-daily dosing in cancer patients. Owing to the study design, once daily dosing of enoxaparin is only approved for in-hospital treatment of acute VTE.

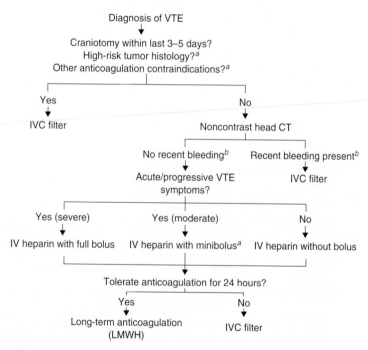

Figure 34.1. Proposed approach to the initial treatment of venous thromboembolism (VTE) in patients with brain tumors. IVC, inferior vena cava; IV, intravenous; LMWH, low molecular weight heparin. [a]Melanoma, renal cell carcinoma, choriocarcinoma, and thyroid cancers are considered relative contraindictions depending on clinical circumstances. [b]Acute bleeding appears hyperdense on computed tomography (CT) scan for approximately 10 days; in postoperative patients, blood in the surgical cavity is a common radiographic finding and does not preclude anticoagulation. (Garber DE. Management of venous thromboembolism in patients with primary and metastatic brain tumors. *J Clin Oncol* 24:1310–1318. Reprinted with permission from the American Society of Clinical Oncology.)

5. **Long-term anticoagulation for VTE in patients with cancer.** Cancer patients who receive anticoagulant therapy for a VTE have more thrombotic recurrences and bleeding complications than patients without malignancies during both the initial period of parenteral heparin therapy and long-term oral anticoagulation. The VTE recurrence and major bleeding rates are approximately four times and two times higher respectively in cancer patients compared to patients without a malignancy, which translates into cumulative recurrent VTE and bleeding incidences of 20% and 12% respectively after 1 year of anticoagulation therapy (*Blood* 2002;100:3484–3488). Among cancer patients, both thrombotic and bleeding complications are more likely with more extensive cancer.

In addition to the higher morbidity associated with chronic oral anticoagulation therapy in cancer patients, treatment is complicated by the requirement for frequent INR monitoring and dose adjustments due to the impact of cancer treatments, disease progression, and other comorbidities on the pharmacokinetics and pharmacodyamics of warfarin, and the delay in reversal and onset of anticoagulant effect when warfarin is stopped or restarted.

Two prospective, randomized, open-label studies have confirmed that chronic anticoagulation with LMWH is superior to oral anticoagulation in cancer patients. In the comparison of low molecular weight heparin versus oral anticoagulant therapy (CLOT) study Lee, 2002 cancer patients with acute VTEs were randomized to 6 months of treatment with a coumarin anticoagulant or dalteparin after initial therapy with dalteparin (200 IU/kg/day). Dosing for patients randomized to dalteparin was continued at 200 IU/kg/day for 1 month, then reduced to 75% to 80% for the remaining 5 months. Symptomatic VTE recurrences were reduced by 52% in the dalteparin arm (17% vs 9%), and there was no significant difference in major bleeding rates between the two arms. The LITE trial (Long-term Innovations in TreatmEnt program) randomized 200 cancer patients with acute VTEs to standard treatment (initial UFH then warfarin, INR two to three) or initial and chronic anticoagulation with tinzaparin (175 IU/kg/day Hull). After 3 months, warfarin anticoagulation therapy was continued (standard treatment arm) or initiated (LMWH arm) for patients considered to be at continued risk for recurrent VTE. After 1 year, 16% of patients randomized to standard treatment experienced a recurrent VTE compared to 7% in the LMWH arm ($p = 0.044$). There was no significant difference in bleeding complications between the two groups. Two small prospective randomized trials comparing chronic anticoagulation with enoxaparin to warfarin detected an insignificant trend toward fewer VTE recurrences in the enoxaparin arms, and a meta-analysis of these four studies favors LMWHs compared to oral vitamin K antagonists for a reduction of VTE recurrence (risk ratio 0.50 [95% confidence interval [CI] 0.35 to 0.72]) and noninferiority in terms of bleeding complications.

The seventh ACCP conference guidelines recommend both initial and chronic anticoagulation with either dalteparin or tinzaparin, as dosed in the studies of Lee and Hull, for treatment of acute VTE in cancer patients. Although generalizing these guidelines to include other brands of LMWH is not currently supported by adequately powered randomized controlled studies, in some situations, LMWH choices may be limited due to formulary restrictions, necessitating substitution.

The duration of anticoagulation therapy following a VTE in cancer patients must be individualized. In general, if treatment leads to cure or a durable remission, 3 to 6 months of anticoagulation therapy is appropriate. If the malignancy is locally or diffusely advanced at the time of VTE occurrence, the risk of recurrence is higher, and continued anticoagulation therapy is appropriate, whether or not ongoing cancer treatment is planned. However, the mortality rate for patients with VTEs was 40% at 6 months in the CLOT study and 47% at 12 months in the LITE study due to cancer progression, and the risk/benefit assessment of anticoagulation therapy during palliative care of cancer patients has not been adequately examined.

Although similar mortality rates have been observed for cancer patients with VTEs in randomized prospective trials comparing chronic anticoagulation with LMWH and vitamin K antagonists, subset analyses of patients with lower tumor burdens have consistently shown a survival benefit associated with LMWH treatment.

Suggested Readings

Agnelli G, Bergqvist D, Cohen A, et al. A randomized double-blind study to compare the efficacy and safety of postoperative fondaparinux (Arixtra) and preoperative dalteparin in the prevention of venous thromboembolism after high-risk abdominal surgery: the PEGASUS study [abstract 40]. *Blood* 2003;102(11 pt 1):15a.

Baz R, Li L, Kottke-Marchant K, et al. The role of aspirin in the prevention of thrombotic complications of thalidomide and anthracycline-based chemotherapy for multiple myeloma. *Mayo Clin Proc* 2005;80:1568–1574.

Bergzvist D, Agnelli G, Cohen AT, et al. Duration of prophylaxis against venous thromboembolism with enoxaparin after surgery for cancer. *N Engl J Med* 2002;346:975–980.

Bern M, Lokich JJ, Wallach SR, et al. Very low doses of warfarin can prevent thrombosis in central venous catheters. A randomized prospective trial. *Ann Intern Med* 1990;112:423–428.

Blom J, Doggen C, O Santo S, et al. Malignancies, prothrombotic mutations, and the risk of venous thrombosis. *J Am Med Assoc* 2005;293:715–722.

Buller H, Agnelli G, Hull RD, et al. Antithrombotic therapy for venous thromboembolic disease. *Chest* 2004;126(Suppl 3):401S–428S.

Couban S, Goodyear M, Burnell M, et al. Randomized placebo-controlled study of low dose warfarin for the prevention of venous catheter-associated thrombosis in patients with cancer. *J Clin Oncol* 2005;23:4063–4067.

Cuzick J, Powles T, Veronesi U, et al. Overview of the main outcomes in breast-cancer prevention trials. *Lancet* 2003;361:296–300.

Di Nisio M, Otten H, Piccioti A, et al. Decision analysis for cancer screening in idiopathic venous thromboembolism. *J Thromb Haemost* 2005;3:2391–2396.

Di Nisio M, Rutjes W, Büller HR, Combined use of clinical pretest probability and D-dimer test in cancer patients with clinically suspected deep venous thrombosis. *J Thromb Haemost* 2005;4:52–57.

Falanga A. Thrombophilia in cancer. *Semin Thromb Hemost* 2005;31:104–110.

Geber D, Grossman S, Streiff MB, Management of venous thromboembolism in patients with primary and metastatic brain tumors. *J Clin Oncol* 2006;24:1310–1317.

Geerts W, Pineo G, Heit JA, et al. Prevention of venous thromboembolism. *Chest* 2004;126:338S–400S.

Group EBCTC. Tamoxifen for early breast cancer: an overview of the randomized trials. *Lancet* 1998;351:1451–1467.

Huisman M. Is antithrombotic prophylaxis required in cancer patients with central venous catheters? Yes for special patient groups. *J Thromb Haemost* 2006;4:10–13.

Hull R, Pineo G, Brant RF, et al. Long-term low-molecular-weight-heparin versus usual care in proximal-vein thrombosis patients with cancer. *Am J Med* 2006;119:1062–1072.

Lee A. Management of thrombosis in cancer: primary prevention and secondary prophylaxis. *Br J Haematol* 2004;128:291–302.

Lee A, Levine M, Baker RI, et al. Low-molecular weight heparin versus a coumarin for the prevention of recurrent venous thromboembolism in patients with cancer. *N Engl J Med* 2002;249:146–153.

Levine M, Hirsh J, Gent M, et al. Double-blind randomized trial of a very-low-dose warfarin for prevention of thromboembolism in stage IV breast cancer. *Lancet* 1994;343:886–889.

Levitan N, Dowlas A, Remick S, et al. Rates on initial and recurrent thromboembolic disease among patients with malignancy versus those without malignancy. Risk analysis using Medicare claims data. *Medicine* 1999;78:285–291.

Merli G, Spiro T, Olsson CG, et al. Subcutaneous enoxaparin once or twice daily compared with intravenous unfractionated heparin for treatment of venous thromboembolic disease. *Ann Intern Med* 2001;134:191–202.

Monreal M, Alastrue A, Rull M, et al. Upper extremity deep venous thrombosis in cancer patients with venous access devices-prophylaxis with a low molecular weight heparin (Fragmin). *Thromb Haemost* 1996;75:251–253.

Monreal M, Lensing A, Prins MJ, et al. Screening for occult cancer in patients with acute deep vein thrombosis or pulmonary embolism. *J Thromb Haemost* 2004;2:876–881.

Piccioli A, Lensing A, Büller HR, et al. Extensive screening for occult malignant disease in idiopathic venous thromboembolism: a prospective randomized clinical trial. *J Thromb Haemost* 2004;2:884–889.

Prandoni P, Lensing A, Piccoli A, et al. Deep-vein thrombosis and the incidence of subsequent symptomatic cancer. *N Engl J Med* 1992;327:1128–1133.

Prandoni P, Lensing A, et al. Recurrent venous thromboembolism and bleeding complications during anticoagulant treatment in patients with cancer and venous thrombosis. *Blood* 2002;100:3484–3488.

Rajkumar S. Thalidomide therapy and deep venous thrombosis in multiple myeloma. *Mayo Clin Proc* 2005;80:1549–1551.

Rasmussen M. Preventing thromboembolic complications in cancer patients after surgery: a role for prolonged thromboprophrophylaxis. *Cancer Treat Rev* 2002;28:141–144.

Rasmussen M. Is there a need for antithrombotic prophylaxis during laparascopic surgery? Always. *J Thromb Haemost* 2005;3:210–211.

Reichardt P, Kretzschmar A, Blakhov M, A phase III double-blind, placebo-controlled study evaluating the efficacy and safety of daily low-molecular-weight heparin (dalta-perin sodium, fragmin) in preventing catheter-related complications in cancer patients with central venous catheters [abstract 1474]. *Proc Annu Meet Am Soc Clin Oncol* 2002;21:396a.

Samama M, Cohen A, Darmon JY, et al. A comparison of enoxaparin with palcebo for the prevention of venous thromboembolism in acutely ill medical patients. Prophylaxis in Medical Patients with Enoxaparin Study Group. *N Engl J Med* 1999;341:793–800.

Sorensen H, Mellemkjaer L, Steffensen FH, et al. The risk of a diagnosis of cancer after primary deep venous thrombosis or pulmonary embolism. *N Engl J Med* 1998;338:1169–1173.

Van Rooden C, Tesselaar M, O Santo S, et al. Deep vein thrombosis associated with central venous catheters-a review. *J Thromb Haemost* 2005;3:2409–2419.

Verso M, Agnelli G, Bertoglio S, et al. Enoxaparin for the prevention of venous thromboembolism associated with central vein catheter: a double-blind, placebo-controlled, randomized study in cancer patients. *J Clin Oncol* 2005;23:4057–4062.

White R, Chew H, Zhev H, et al. Incidence of thromboembolism in the year before diagnosis of cancer in 528,693 adults. *Arch Intern Med* 2005;165:1782–1787.

Zangari M, Barlogie B, Angissis E, et al. Deep vein thrombosis in patients with multiple myeloma treated with thalidomide and chemotherapy: effects of prophylactic and therapeutic anticoagulation. *Br J Haematol* 2004;126:715–721.

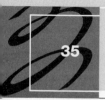

35 ONCOLOGIC EMERGENCIES
Vamsidhar Velcheti and Ramaswamy Govindan

I. METABOLIC EMERGENCIES
A. Hypercalcemia

1. **Signs and symptoms.** Symptoms generally develop at total calcium levels greater than 12 mg/dL. Symptoms are dependent on the rapidity of increase as well as on the absolute level. Serum calcium of 14 mg/dL or higher developing over days may render a patient comatose, whereas the same level developing over months may be relatively asymptomatic. Patients with severe hypercalcemia usually present with nausea, vomiting, anorexia, abdominal pain, constipation, altered mental status, and seizures. Patients usually have some renal impairment, with dehydration, elevated creatinine, polyuria, and polydipsia. Nephrolithiasis is relatively uncommon in hypercalcemia due to malignancy as opposed to other metabolic causes of hypercalcemia. Long-standing hypercalcemia can result in demineralization and frequent fractures of the long bones. Physical examination may reveal altered mental status, distended abdomen from ileus, and signs of dehydration. In the absence of prompt recognition and treatment, hypercalcemia can progress to renal failure, coma, and death.

2. **Workup.** The normal range for total serum calcium is 8.6 to 10.3 mg/dL (2.15 to 2.57 mM). About half the amount of the circulating calcium is bound by albumin, and the remaining unbound ionized calcium (normal range, 4.5 to 5.1 mg/dL) is responsible for the biologic functions. A low albumin level results in a higher fraction of ionized calcium. The effective total calcium should be calculated with the formula: corrected Ca (mg/dL) = measured Ca (mg/dL) − albumin (g/dL) + 4.

   In patients with hypercalcemia without a previous history of malignancy, other causes of hypercalcemia should be considered. Chief among these is hyperparathyroidism. Because the immunoassay for parathyroid hormone (PTH) does not detect parathyroid hormone-related protein (PTH-rp), patients with elevated PTH are more likely to have hyperparathyroidism than malignant hypercalcemia. The other causes of hypercalcemia includes thyrotoxicosis, adrenal insufficiency, 1,25(OH)$_2$ vitamin D toxicity (through ingestion or granulomatous conversion), and inherited disorders of calcium metabolism.

3. **Treatment.** The treatment of hypercalcemia depends on the serum calcium level and the symptoms. The main goals of treatment are increasing renal excretion of calcium and inhibiting bone reabsorption.

   a. **Volume expansion.** Patients with symptomatic hypercalcemia are often dehydrated. Dehydration decreases the renal glomerular perfusion, thereby reducing the ability of the kidney to excrete excess serum calcium. Such patients should be rehydrated with normal saline at an initial rate of 200 to 300 mL/hour up to 2 to 3 L and later maintained on oral fluids to maintain the urine output at 100 to 150 mL/hour. If the patients appear to be fluid overloaded due to a decrease in renal ability to excrete the administered salt, loop diuretics can be used. Loop diuretics not only reduce the volume load but also decrease calcium reabsorption in the loop of Henle. Electrolytes should be carefully monitored and potassium and magnesium repletion achieved as necessary. Hypophosphatemia is common in hypercalcemia but should not be replete unless symptomatic, because an increase in the calcium × phosphorus product to 70 or more can cause precipitation of calcium salts in the kidney and other soft tissues.

b. **Intravenous bisphosphonates.** The bisphosphonates are nonhydrolyzable analogs of inorganic pyrophosphate that are selectively concentrated in the bone and that adsorb to the surface of bone hydroxyapatite. They inhibit calcium reabsorption by reducing the activity of the osteoclasts. These drugs have become the agents of choice for malignancy-associated hypercalcemia, and can successfully control serum calcium in 80% to 90% of patients. Zoledronate is a third-generation bisphosphonate, approved for treatment of hypercalcemia. It is administered typically at a dose of 4 mg i.v. over 15 minutes. The main side effect is hypocalcemia, which is often asymptomatic. Serum calcium will generally normalize 3 to 4 days after administration, and the nadir is reached around day 10. Serum calcium levels should be monitored, and patients with recurrent hypercalcemia may require repeated dosing every 3 to 4 weeks. Pamidronate, another bisphosphonate, is used less often these days for this indication. Oral bisphosphonates have not been shown to be as effective and are not recommended.

c. **Calcitonin.** Salmon calcitonin is a peptide sequence similar to human calcitonin; it functionally antagonizes the effects of PTH. Salmon calcitonin (4 to 8 IU/kg) is usually administered intramuscularly or subcutaneously every 12 hours. The administration of calcitonin with saline should reduce the serum calcium concentrations within 12 to 48 hours. The efficacy of calcitonin is limited to the first 48 hours, after which there appears to be a receptor downregulation resulting in tachyphylaxis, thereby limiting the use of calcitonin in the long-term management of hypercalcemia. However, calcitonin is safe and rapidly acting, and may be used to manage severe hypercalcemia before bisphosphonates reach full effect.

In patients with malignancies producing $1,25(OH)_2$ vitamin D such as myeloma or lymphomas, corticosteroids may be effective in controlling hypercalcemia. A dose of 60 mg prednisone p.o. or its equivalents given intravenously can be used alone or in combination with bisphosphonates in patients with hematologic malignancies before definitive therapy of the underlying malignancy. Steroids are not effective in the treatment of hypercalcemia in patients with solid tumors.

Several new inhibitors of bone resorption such as osteoprotegerin (an antagonist of RANKL receptor), monoclonal antibodies directed against RANKL, monoclonal antibodies neutralizing PTHrP, and 22-oxacalcitriol are being studied currently.

4. **Pathophysiology.** Hypercalcemia of malignancy results from three main mechanisms, namely, secretion of a PTHrP, local osteolytic activity and, abnormal $1,25(OH)_2$ vitamin D production. Malignant hypercalcemia due to osteolytic activity usually develops in patients with extensive skeletal metastases (e.g., breast cancer, lung cancer, prostate cancer, or multiple myeloma). Humoral secretion of PTHrP is seen in a variety of cancers such as squamous cell cancer, (e.g., of head and neck, esophagus, cervix, or lung), renal cancer, ovarian cancer, endometrial cancer, and breast cancer. Some lymphomas secrete the active form of vitamin D, 1, 25-dihydroxycholecalciferol, resulting in increased osteoclastic bone resorption and intestinal absorption of calcium resulting in hypercalcemia.

B. **Tumor lysis syndrome**

1. **Signs and symptoms.** The onset of TLS can be before initiation of cytotoxic therapy but is often within 12 to 72 hours after administration of cytotoxic therapy and/or radiation therapy. A high level of suspicion is required because TLS symptoms can be very nonspecific. Symptoms are often a result of ensuing electrolyte imbalances. The patients may present with nausea, vomiting, fluid overload, congestive heart failure, cardiac arrhythmias, seizures, tetany, syncope, and possibly sudden death ,often due to cardiac arrest.

The most worrisome metabolic consequences of TLS are hyperkalemia, hypercalcemia and renal failure. Acute renal failure results from precipitation of phosphate and urate salts in the renal tubules, which creates a vicious cycle thereby resulting in further deterioration of renal function. Patients at risk for TLS are those with elevated levels of uric acid, phosphorus, and lactate dehydrogenase (LDH) before treatment.

Laboratory TLS is diagnosed with the presence of two or more of the following parameters: (a) uric acid less than or equal to 8 mg/dL or 25% increase from baseline (b) potassium less than or equal to 6.0 mEq/L or 25% increase from baseline (c) phosphate level 4.5 mg/dL or 25% increase from baseline (d) calcium 7 mg/dL or 25% decrease from baseline. *Clinical TLS* is defined (Cairo-Bishop definition) as the presence of laboratory TLS plus renal failure and/or cardiac arrhythmias and/or seizures and/or sudden death.

2. **Management.** The best approach to managing the problem of TLS is prevention. Patients at risk need to be identified and have prophylactic measures instituted before and during initial treatment. Blood chemistries (electrolytes, creatinine, phosphorus, calcium, and LDH) need to be checked in patients at risk every 8 to 12 hours during the first 2 to 3 days of treatment. Patients with high risk should be pretreated for at least 2 days with allopurinol (600 mg/day) plus isotonic saline to maintain high urine output (greater than 2.5 L/day). The dose of allopurinol should be decreased for preexisting renal insufficiency and as tumor bulk decreases. Brisk hydration helps eliminate the cellular breakdown products and also preserve the function. Furosemide may be given to maintain urine output and also to decrease the hyperkalemia. Urine alkalinization with either one ampoule of $NaHCO_3$ in 0.5 N saline or two to three ampoules in D5W may be needed to maintain the urine solutes (calcium, uric acid, oxalates) in ionic form and thereby prevent crystallization and also to help correct metabolic acidosis accompanying TLS. Management of TLS involves treatment of the underlying electrolyte abnormalities along with any coexisting renal failure or cardiac arrhythmias.

Hyperkalemia may develop rapidly, and patients at risk should have serum electrolytes checked at least every 12 hours, and more frequently if TLS develops. Mild hyperkalemia (5.5 to 6.0 mEq/L) may be treated with sodium polystyrene sulfonate (Kayexalate resin) and hydration as described earlier. More serious hyperkalemia (greater than 6 mEq/L or with electrocardiogram [EKG] changes) may be treated immediately with 50 mL of 50% glucose solution with 15 units of regular insulin, i.v. piggyback over an hour. Indications for hemodialysis include volume overload, serum uric acid greater than 10 mg/dL, or rapidly increasing phosphorus levels and uncontrolled hyperkalemia. Renal failure caused by TLS is usually reversible, and even patients requiring hemodialysis often regain normal kidney function as the TLS subsides.

Rasburicase, a newer recombinant form of urate oxidase was recently approved for prophylaxis and treatment of TLS in pediatric patients. Rasburicase appears to decrease the uric acid levels much more rapidly than allopurinol. However, the safety and efficacy of rasburicase needs to be further evaluated for use in adults and geriatric patients.

3. **Pathophysiology.** The tumor lysis syndrome (TLS) results from excessive tumor breakdown either spontaneously or during therapy, leading to a variety of metabolic abnormalities. There is a sudden release of potassium, phosphates, and purine metabolites from tumor cells undergoing cell death. The TLS occurs most frequently in patients with tumors having high growth fraction and substantial systemic tumor burden that are very sensitive to chemotherapy and radiotherapy such as leukemias with high leukocyte counts and lymphomas. TLS is rarely encountered in patients with epithelial malignancies.

C. **Syndrome of inappropriate antidiuretic hormone (SIADH)**

1. **Signs and symptoms.** Patients initially present with headache and fatigue and if left uncorrected may rapidly progress to confusion, seizure, coma, and death. A low plasma osmolality with elevated urine osmolality (more than 100 mosmol/kg), urine Na more than 40 meq/L, low blood urea nitrogen (BUN) and serum uric acid level, and normal acid–base and potassium balance are all suggestive of SIADH.

2. **Management.** Fluid restriction is the initial step of management for patients with mild to moderate SIADH. In patients with acute (less than 48 hours)

and symptomatic hyponatremia, a more rapid correction of Na may be needed with 3% saline. Very rapid correction of the hyponatremia is complicated by central pontine myelinosis and fluid overload, particularly in patients who were euvolemic. The rate of correction should be maintained at less than 1 mEq/L/hour and less than 20 mEq/L of total daily correction. When the serum Na levels reach 120 mEq/L then the 3% saline should be stopped and fluid restriction instituted. For chronic SIADH demeclocycline (inhibits the renal action of antidiuretic hormone (ADH)) at a daily dose of 600 to 1200 mg/day is effective and usually returns the serum Na levels to normal within 2 weeks.

3. **Pathophysiology.** SIADH is a syndrome of excessive secretion of ADH resulting in hyponatremia. Excessive secretion of ADH leads to increased sodium loss and increased urine osmolality. Small cell lung cancer (SCLC) is the most common cancer causing SIADH, with over 15% patients with SCLC developing SIADH at some point during the course of the illness.

II. NEUROLOGIC EMERGENCIES

A. Spinal cord compression

1. **Signs and symptoms.** The symptoms of cord compression may occur abruptly or progress gradually. Back pain occurs in almost all patients with spinal cord compression. The pain may be localized to the back or may radiate either unilaterally or bilaterally in the distribution of spinal roots. Back pain may be exacerbated by flexion of the back, Valsalva manoeuvre, and coughing. Unlike back pain resulting from degenerative disc disease, the back pain due to spinal cord compression is not relieved by recumbency and may even be exacerbated. Initially there may be weakness and sensory paresthesias along the dermatome of the corresponding spinal roots involved in the compression. More general signs of spinal cord dysfunction such as weakness and sensory disturbances, along with bowel and bladder disorders soon follow the radicular pain.

Patients with thoracic cord compression develop weakness and sensory paresthesias and/or loss of sensation in the legs that is usually ascending. Gait disorders are usually prominent and may be a result of the sensory ataxia due to posterior column compression. Motor symptoms and sphincter disturbances such as urinary/fecal incontinence or retention usually develop late and are associated with poor prognosis. With lumbar (L1-2) spinal compression, sphincter disturbances may occur early.

New onset of back pain in a patient at risk mandates a careful neurologic examination. In cases of gradual cord compression, patients may be unaware of sensory deficits that may be detectable by neurologic examination. Regions distal to the cord compression may be weak and hyper-reflexic with upgoing (extensor plantar) reflexes in the toe, whereas reflexes at the level of a lesion are decreased. Urinary retention should be determined by obtaining a postvoid bladder residual value. Anal sphincter function is usually preserved until late in cord compression; early deficits in sphincter tone or sensation may be due to involvement of the cauda equina. Acute, severe cord compression can cause spinal shock, with hyporeflexia and flaccid paralysis of all regions below the lesion.

2. **Workup.** The clinical neurologic examination may prompt further evaluation of the spine but is not precise enough to be used to plan treatment. All patients with suspected cord compression should undergo imaging of the spine. Magnetic resonance imaging (MRI) is the modality of choice when available. Contrast computed tomography (CT) is recommended if MRI cannot be performed. It is important to image the entire spine, as some patients may have more than one region of compression. Plain films and bone scans have a limited role because they may miss soft tissue components of tumors. If the nature of the compressing mass is uncertain, surgical or image-guided biopsy for tissue diagnosis is essential. When cord compression is the initial presentation of cancer, further evaluation may reveal a lesion such as a lymph node, on which it may be easier to perform a biopsy.

3. **Management.** Spinal cord compression requires prompt recognition because delay in treatment usually results in reduced recovery of function and poor outcome. Corticosteroids should be started as soon as spinal cord compression is suspected. Steroids decrease edema associated with spinal cord compression and improve symptoms transiently. We recommend that dexamethasone be used, with a 10-mg loading dose i.v. or p.o., followed by 4 mg every 6 hours. Dexamethasone should be tapered off over a few weeks.

External-beam radiation is the treatment of choice and should begin as soon as the diagnosis is confirmed. Standard radiation doses range from 2,500 to 4,000 cGy delivered in 10 to 20 fractions. Traditional indications for surgical intervention include the need for a tissue diagnosis, resection of "radioresistant" tumors and tumors primarily treated by surgery (such as sarcomas), and cord compression in a previously irradiated spine. A very rapid onset of symptoms suggests the possibility of vertebral burst fracture causing bony impingement on the cord. This is an indication for urgent surgical intervention to remove bone fragments from the spinal canal. Patients with extensive bony destruction by tumor and vertebral instability may be at risk for further compression fracture and symptom recurrence after completing x-ray therapy (XRT); these patients should be considered for vertebral stabilization. Surgical patients usually require 7 to 10 days for wound healing before beginning radiation. In select group of patients addition of decompressive surgery to radiation therapy improved neurologic outcomes as compared with radiotherapy alone (Patchel: *Lancet* 2005;366(9486):643–648).

Systemic therapy using hormonal and/or chemotherapeutic agents should be included when appropriate (e.g., in patients with lymphoma). An additional treatment option available (apart from radiation) for patients with hormone-sensitive prostate cancer is androgen blockade in patients who are not hormone-resistant. High-dose ketoconazole (400 mg p.o. every 8 hours) rapidly reduces testosterone levels into the castrate range and should be considered in patients with cord compression known or suspected to be caused by prostate cancer. Patients receiving high-dose ketoconazole should be given replacement doses of corticosteroids (prednisone, 5 mg p.o. in the morning and 2.5 mg p.o. at bedtime), as ketoconazole may cause adrenal insufficiency. One strategy is to initiate treatment with ketoconazole and flutamide (a peripheral androgen blocker) on presentation, and then a few days later discontinue ketoconazole and administer a gonadotropin hormone–releasing hormone (GnRH) agonist (e.g., leuprolide). Flutamide must be continued for 3 to 4 weeks when starting a GnRH agonist to prevent tumor flare.

4. **Course of the disease.** An estimated 1% of cancer patients develop spinal cord compression, and this number is expected to increase as improvements in systemic therapy allow these patients to live longer. Metastatic breast, lung, and prostate cancers account for most malignant cord compressions. Although cord compression is usually not life-threatening, patients with neurologic impairment secondary to cord compression have a markedly reduced quality of life and a significantly shortened overall survival. Exophytic metastases to a vertebral body account for 80% to 90% of cases, with the remaining due to epidural metastases and vertebral fractures. Other less common causes of cord compression include metastases to the posterior vertebral elements, benign and malignant tumors primary to the spine, vascular malformations, and infections. It is critical to begin therapy as soon as possible.

5. **Pathophysiology.** Spinal cord compression is most commonly due to extradural metastases involving the thoracic spine (70%), the lumbosacral spine (20%), and the cervical spine (10%). Intramedullary, intradural, or leptomeningeal metastases are rarely encountered. Spinal cord compression is seen most commonly in patients with lung and breast cancer. The main mechanisms involved in spinal cord compression are direct extension of the soft tissue epidural disease, direct neural compression due to vasogenic cord edema and venous hemorrhage, and loss of myelin and ischemia resulting from an

increase in the synthesis of prostaglandin E2, interleukin (IL)-1 and IL-6, and serotonin.

III. HEMATOLOGIC EMERGENCIES

A. Leukostasis

1. **Signs and symptoms.** Leukostasis is a clinical diagnosis; symptoms are nonspecific and may be attributed to infection or heart failure. Patients in leukostasis are usually hypoxemic, although live blasts in an arterial blood sample obtained for arterial blood gas (ABG) estimation may lower the Po_2 content spuriously if the specimen is not processed in a timely manner. A nonspecific diffuse infiltrate is often present on chest radiograph (CXR). There may be impairment of other end organs, including the eye, kidney, and liver. Lactic acidosis may be a late event. Symptoms may be fulminant, leading to death in a matter of days or even hours. These patients have a propensity for central nervous system (CNS) bleeds after chemotherapy is begun, often in the absence of disseminated intravascular coagulation (DIC) or thrombocytopenia.

2. **Management.** Leukapheresis is often a lifesaving intervention and needs to be instituted before the differential diagnoses are ruled out. Patients who receive leukapheresis have a lower incidence of intracerebral bleeds after starting chemotherapy and also decrease the incidence of TLS. Leukapheresis should be considered in all patients with a total white count greater than 100,000/dL. Hydroxyurea might be considered as an adjunct to leukapheresis to decrease cell proliferation before definitive treatment. Red blood cell transfusion should be avoided since it can worsen the symptoms associated with leukostasis. Thrombocytopenia and coagulation factors need to be corrected to minimize the risk of CNS bleeding. Patients with signs of sepsis need to have blood drawn for culture and treated empirically with broad-spectrum antibiotics. The underlying malignancy needs to be treated appropriately.

3. **Pathophysiology.** It is a syndrome commonly seen in acute leukemias and comprises of respiratory distress, abnormal CXR, confusion, and CNS bleeding. High and rapidly increasing blast counts are characteristic of leukostasis, with white counts often greater than 100,000/dL. Despite the very high blast counts that can occur in lymphoid leukemias, leukostasis is not very common in acute lymphoblastic leukemia (ALL). The classic pathologic finding in leukostasis is occlusive intravascular aggregates of blasts blocking the circulation in multiple organs, especially the lungs and brain.

IV. CARDIAC EMERGENCIES

A. Cardiac tamponade

1. **Signs and symptoms.** Dyspnea is the most common presentation of pericardial tamponade. Cough, chest pain, and generalized weakness are often present. Hypotension is a common feature due to the decline in cardiac output. Severe hypotension and pulseless electrical activity are the final consequences of untreated tamponade. More often cardiac tamponade manifests in a less dramatic way with increased filling pressures and decreased cardiac output. Features of right-heart failure, such as peripheral edema, hypotension, and elevated jugular venous pressure (JVP) may be seen. Pulsus paradoxus (a decrease in systolic blood pressure of 10 mm Hg or more on inspiration) is classically associated with pericardial effusion.

2. **Workup.** The clinical diagnosis of cardiac tamponade is usually confirmed by the physical findings supplemented by echocardiography. The EKG in tamponade shows sinus tachycardia. The characteristic findings on EKG in patients with pericardial effusion include low voltage and possibly electrical alternans as the heart swings within the distended pericardium. Electrical alternans has a high specificity but is lacking in sensitivity for tamponade. CXR may reveal an enlarged cardiac silhouette (water-bottle heart) with clear lung fields. At least 200 mL of fluid must accumulate before the cardiac silhouette is enlarged on chest x-ray and hence this is often absent in acute tamponade. CT or MRI images of the heart may reveal the presence of a pericardial effusion but cannot determine hemodynamic significance. Echocardiography is the most frequently

obtained study and can demonstrate both the effusion and diastolic collapse of the right atrium and right ventricle. Collapse of the right atrium occurs when the extrinsic compression by the effusion overcomes venous pressure and prevents right heart filling. Right atrial collapse for more than one third of the cardiac cycle, is highly sensitive and specific for cardiac tamponade. Examination of pericardial fluid is often required in cancer patients to ascertain the diagnosis of malignant effusion and to rule out other causes. In malignant pericardial effusion, cytology will be positive in only 65% to 85% of cases. A positive cytology may be predictive of a poorer outcome in patients with neoplastic pericardial disease. Pericardial biopsy is the gold standard for establishing malignant involvement.

Other causes of pericardial effusion include inflammatory disorders, infections, radiation, uremia, and hypothyroidism. Acute cardiac tamponade presenting with signs of right heart failure must be differentiated from a right-sided acute myocardial infarction and an aortic dissection.

3. **Management.** Asymptomatic patients with mild effusion do not require treatment unless the etiology is unclear. The rapid onset of dyspnea, chest pain, and fatigue should prompt therapeutic intervention. The initial goal in treating tamponade is to drain the fluid. Pericardial fluid can be drained by catheter pericardiocentesis or surgical pericardiectomy. Pericardiocentesis is done after local anesthesia; the needle is inserted to the right of the xiphoid and advanced toward the tip of the left scapula, with constant aspiration during the procedure. A large syringe or a catheter with a stopcock should be available to allow removal of 50 to 60 mL of fluid. This results in rapid improvement in symptoms. Despite dramatic improvement in the symptoms, reaccumulation of fluid occurs in as many as 60% of patients. In this situation, a surgical pericardial window will usually prevent repeated accumulation and is the treatment of choice, even if the effusion cannot be confirmed to be malignant by cytology. Balloon pericardiotomy is an alternative to surgical creation of a pericardial window. In this procedure an un-inflated balloon catheter is placed in the pericardial space using a subxiphoid approach under guidance. The balloon is then inflated and pulled out of pericardium to create a "window," thereby allowing drainage of fluid into the pleural or peritoneal space. This technique has shown a decrease in the reaccumulation in 80% to 100% of cases. This approach may be a reasonable alternative to surgery in patients with malignant tamponade, especially in those who are poor surgical candidates.

4. **Pathophysiology.** Over 10% of patients dying of cancer are found to have pericardial involvement at autopsy. However, only a small proportion of these patients actually develop clinical symptoms in real life. Thoracic malignancies are the most common cause of malignant pericardial effusion and tamponade.

B. **Superior vena cava syndrome**
1. **Signs and symptoms.** Patients with superior vena cava (SVC) syndrome commonly complain of dyspnea, swelling of the face, neck, and upper extremities, and pain (chest pain or headaches). Symptoms may develop rapidly or gradually and may vary in severity by position. Bending forward or lying flat may worsen symptoms as a result of increased venous pressure proximal to the obstruction. Even in the presence of severe symptoms, patients are rarely critically ill as a result of SVC syndrome alone. Dilated neck veins are usually present along with collateral veins which develop as a result of longstanding occlusion.
2. **Workup.** The CXR may show mediastinal widening and pleural effusion. Contrast-enhanced CT is extremely helpful in delineating the location and extent of venous blockage and presence of collateral venous drainage. It also provides very useful information regarding the adjacent structures, including the presence or absence of compressive mass lesions, and is useful in planning subsequent biopsy or therapeutic intervention. MRI may be useful for

patients who are unable to undergo a contrast CT. A histologic diagnosis is essential in the management of SVC syndrome, as specific treatment may be influenced by the tumor type. Patients without a tissue diagnosis or in whom the diagnosis is uncertain should undergo surgical or percutaneous biopsy of an accessible site. Sputum cytology, pleural fluid cytology, and biopsy of enlarged thoracic lymph nodes may be diagnostic in most cases. Bronchoscopy, mediastinoscopy, or thoracotomy may be required if the diagnosis is in doubt.

3. **Treatment.** Treatment of the underlying disease is the mainstay in the treatment of SVC syndrome. Endovascular therapy (i.e., intraluminal stenting) may be considered in some patients with very severe symptoms and in patients with advanced cancers not responsive to chemotherapy or radiation. The role of steroids in managing SVC syndrome is questionable.

Accurate histologic diagnosis of the underlying etiology is essential before the initiation of any form of therapy. Pre-biopsy empirical treatment may obscure the histologic diagnosis and make further management of the underlying disease complicated. SVC syndrome is rarely a medical emergency unless it presents with central airway obstruction or severe laryngeal edema with stridor, in which case it needs to be managed emergently. Several thoracic malignancies mainly lymphomas, germ cell neoplasms and limited-stage SCLC are responsive to chemotherapy with or without radiation therapy. These patients are often relieved of the symptoms from SVC obstruction within weeks of initiation of therapy.

SVC obstruction resulting from indwelling central venous catheters and pacemakers can be managed effectively by thrombolytic therapy (unless contraindicated) especially if the patient's symptoms were for less than 5 days. The central catheter should be left in place and used to administer lytics, and patients should be given anticoagulation therapy afterward, as with any deep vein thrombosis (DVT).

4. **Mechanism.** SVC syndrome results from obstruction of blood flow in the SVC caused by invasion or external compression of the SVC. Thoracic malignancies are the most common cause of SVC syndrome. Other causes of compression of the SVC include indwelling central venous devices that result in SVC thrombosis, aortic aneurysms, and fibrosing mediastinitis.

Suggested Readings

Ahmann FR. A reassessment of the clinical implications of the superior vena cava syndrome. *J Clin Oncol* 1984;2:961–969.

Arrambide K, Toto RD. Tumor lysis syndrome. *Semin Nephrol* 1993;13:273–280.

Body JJ, Bartl R, Burckhardt P, et al. Current use of bisphosphonates in oncology. *J Clin Oncol* 1998;16:3890–3899.

Dempke W, Firusian N. Treatment of malignant pericardial effusion with ^{32}P-colloid. *Br J Cancer* 1999;80:1955–1957.

List AF, Hainsworth JD, Davis BW, et al. The syndrome of inappropriate secretion of antidiuretic hormone (SIADH) in small-cell lung cancer. *J Clin Oncol* 1986;4:1191–1198.

Loblaw DA, Laperriere NJ. Emergency treatment of malignant extradural spinal cord compression: an evidence based guideline. *J Clin Oncol* 1998;16:1613–1624.

Mundy GR, Guise TA. Hypercalcemia of malignancy. *Am J Med* 1997;103:134–145.

Shepherd FA. Malignant pericardial effusion. *Curr Opin Oncol* 1997;9:170–174.

Silverman P, Distelhorst CW. Metabolic emergencies in clinical oncology. *Semin Oncol* 1989;16:504–515.

Spinazze S, Caraceni A, Schrijvers D. Epidural spinal cord compression. *Crit Rev Oncol Hematol* 2005;56:397–406.

Spinazze S, Schrijvers D. Metabolic emergencies. *Crit Rev Oncol Hematol* 2006;58:79–89.

Stewart AF. Hypercalcemia associated with cancer. *N Engl J Med* 2005;352:373–379.

Tanigawa N, Sawada S, Mishima K, et al. Clinical outcome of stenting in superior vena cava syndrome associated with malignant tumors. *Acta Radiol* 1998;39:669–674.

Wuthner JU, Kohler G, Behringer D, et al. Leukostasis followed by hemorrhage complicating the initiation of chemotherapy in patients with acute myeloid leukemia and hyperleukocytosis. *Cancer* 1999;85:368–374.

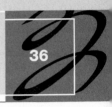

MANAGEMENT OF COMPLICATIONS OF CHEMOTHERAPY – A NURSING PERSPECTIVE

36

Eve Gilstrap and Beth Zubal

I. INTRODUCTION. Great strides have been made in the treatment of cancer patients, even since the first edition of The Washington Manual of Oncology in 2002. As health care providers in the area of oncology, we have the opportunity to help our patients live longer and with better quality of life. With the addition of biologically targeted therapies, new cytotoxic agents, and novel ways of administering these agents, our patients will benefit from a well informed nursing staff with strong working knowledge of the management of cytotoxic and biological treatment-related symptoms. This is the focus of this chapter.

II. EXTRAVASATION AND HYPERSENSITIVITY, ANAPHYLAXIS

    A. Hypersensitivity. Although hypersensitivity reactions to chemotherapy and targeted drugs are rare, they can be life threatening and are predominant with the intravenous route. Most of the clinical reactions are immediate (type 1) immunoglobulin E (IgE) mediated that manifest with target organ signs and symptoms including fever, myalgias, arthralgias, nausea/vomiting, dyspnea, pruritus, urticaria, angioedema, headache, and often a feeling of impending doom. Skin testing on patients with a history of drug reactions is common with agents including L-asparaginase that requires close observation with a test dose.

        Chemotherapy and targeted drugs most associated with an anaphylactic reaction are the platinum agents, taxanes, epipodophyllotoxins, asparaginases, and intravenous monoclonal antibodies. Premedication with histamine 1 (H_1) antagonists, H_2 blockers, antipyretics, and corticosteroids can reduce the incidence of reaction; however, there is no standard regimen that has been developed. In the event of a type 1 reaction, the drug flow should be halted immediately while maintaining patent intravenous access, resuscitation airway, breathing and circulation (ABCs) assessed and first-line treatment administered including adrenaline, oxygen, and crystalloid intravenous solutions. Based on client assessment, desensitization may be warranted with slow, escalating doses.

        Type 2 hypersensitivity may present as hemolysis with an antibody-mediated reaction causing inflammation. Type 3 reactions activate in circulation and manifest as vasculitis, arthritis, and nephritis. Type 4 delayed reactions are seen as graft rejections and cutaneous reactions.

    B. Chemotherapy vesicants and irritants. Intravenous chemotherapeutic agents are classified as *irritants*, causing irritation or redness at the site without tissue necrosis or *vesicants*, causing tissue necrosis or ulceration if there is leakage of the agent into the local tissue (extravasation). Should extravasation be suspected or detected, the intravenous (IV) chemotherapy flow should be stopped, any residual medication aspirated, IV antidote (if recommended) administered, needle removed, and supportive measures administered such as heat or cold compress and extremity elevation if peripheral IV (Table 36.1).

III. CARDIAC COMPLICATIONS. Systemic therapy for the treatment of cancer can result in cardiac complications, which may be transient to dose-dependent. Cardiovascular manifestations may be exacerbated in patients with a heart disease history, prior anthracycline exposure and ionizing radiation to the mediastinum. The anthracyclines, particularly doxorubicin, may manifest cardiotoxicity from acute arrhythmias to mitochondrial damage leading to congestive cardiomyopathy. As the anthracyclines play a significant role in treating various forms of liquid and

TABLE 36.1	Irritant and Vesicant Chemotherapeutic Drugs

Irritants	Vesicants
Bleomycin	Cisplatin (>20mL of 0.5 mg/mL concentration)
Carboplatin	Dactinomycin-D
Carmustine	Daunorubicin HCL
Cisplatin	Doxorubicin HCL
Cyclophosphamide	Epirubicin HCL
Dacarbazine	5-Fluorouracil
DaunoXome	Idarubicin
Doxil	Mechlorethamine HCL
Etoposide	Mitomycin-C
5-Fluorouracil	Mitoxantrone HCL
Ifosfamide	Paclitaxel
Irinotecan	Vinblastine
Melphalan	Vincristine
Oxaliplatin	Vinorelbine
Pentostatin	—
Plicamycin	—
Streptozocin	—
Teniposide	—
Topotecan HCL	

solid tumors, dose limitations, scheduling, and close patient monitoring is essential. Doxorubicin should be limited to a cumulative dose of 450 mg/m^2 to avoid chronic cardiomyopathy with radionuclide ventriculograms obtained pretherapy, serially and postadministration.

Nonanthracycline therapy including antibody agents are associated with cardiac complications, including hypotension, hypertension, arrhythmias, ischemia, cardiomyopathy, and myocardial infarction (Table 36.2). Undergoing intense single and combination drug therapy in compromised cancer patients may lead to the development of sepsis and the need for antibiotic and antifungal therapy which often results in hypotension or ultimately heart failure. Most of the cardiac side effects are reversible and irreversible cardiotoxicity is well managed with diuretics, selective β-blockers and angiotensin-converting enzyme inhibitors.

IV. CAPILLARY LEAK SYNDROME. Capillary leak syndrome is a rare disorder of chemotherapeutic agents and primarily a manifestation of biological (i.e., interleukin-2 [IL-2], and sargramostim) resulting in a capillary permeability shift of intravascular to interstitial fluid. Peripheral and pulmonary edema is normally reversible with the administration of diuretics, vasopressors, and intravenous fluids.

V. CUTANEOUS. Alopecia is the most commonly seen cutaneous direct or indirect side effect of single and combination antineoplastic agents. Anagen effluvium is complete hair loss or thinning induced by direct alteration of mitotic activity of the hair cell; therefore, occurring within 7 to 10 days of the affecting agent. Hair growth gradually returns after cessation of the agent(s) and often with new color or texture. In addition, alopecia can be exacerbated by the underlying severe biological and psychological stress of the disease. Treatments such as scalp hypothermia to manage hair loss with chemotherapeutic regimens have demonstrated a slowing, not prevention, of the process. A multitarget tyrosine kinase inhibitor (TKI), sunitinib, orally results in a benign, reversible hair depigmentation (graying) predominantly found in scalp and facial hair. Table 36.3 lists the chemotherapeutic regimens associated with alopecia.

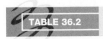

TABLE 36.2	Chemotherapy and Targeted Agent-Induced Cardiotoxicity
Agent	**Cardiovascular risk**
Alemtuzamab	Arrhythmias, hypotension
Amsacrine	Left ventricular dysfunction/heart failure
Anthracyclines	Left ventricular dysfunction/heart failure
Daunorubicin	—
Doxorubicin	—
Epirubicin	—
Idarubicin	—
Arsenic trioxide	Arrhythmias
Bevacizumab	Heart Failure/hypertension/thromboembolism
Busulfan	Endomyocardial fibrosis/tamponade
Capecitabine	Coronary artery spasm
Cetuximab	Hypotension
Cisplatin	Heart Failure/hypertension
Cyclophosphamide	Hemorrhagic myopericarditis/heart failure
Denileukin	Hypotension
Etoposide	Hypotension
Fluorouracil	Coronary artery spasm
Homoharringtonine	Hypotension
Ifosfamide	Heart failure/arrhythmias
Interferon-α	Hypotension/hypertension
Interleukin-2	Ventricular arrhythmias/hypotension
Imatinib	Heart failure/pericardial effusion
Mitomycin	Heart failure
Mitoxantrone	Left ventricular dysfunction/heart failure
Paclitaxel	Heart failure/arrhythmias
Rituximab	Arrhythmias/hypotension
Thalidomide	Bradycardia/edema/thromboembolism
Trastuzumab	Left ventricular dysfunction/heart failure
Tretinoin	Heart failure/edema/hypotension
Vinblastine, vincristine, vinorelbine	Myocardial infarction

Taxane therapy results in nail discoloration and on occasion, oncholysis. Transient erythema (especially at an irritated intravenous site of infusion), pruritus, telangiectasis, nail pitting or ridging, and photosensitivity are common manifestations of chemotherapy.

Painful paronychial inflammation most often seen in the great toe can develop following infusion of cetuximab, an epidermal growth factor receptor (EGFR) inhibitor, requiring dose interruption or discontinuation. Hyperpigmentation is commonly seen with capecitabine, doxorubicin, etoposide, and bleomycin.

A common site of darkening appears over the phalanges but can also be seen in nails, hair, and mucous membranes. The discoloration, which normally decreases after treatment, is more predominant in the African-American population and those of Mediterranean descent.

Radiation recall is defined as an inflammatory condition to tissue that has been previously irradiated such as the skin, gastrointestinal (GI) tract, lungs, and heart. The dose-dependent recall effect is brought on by such agents as doxorubicin, bleomycin, methotrexate (MTX), etoposide, vinca alkaloids, and hydroxurea. These agents, in addition to the anthracyclines, exacerbate tissue inflammation if received within 1 week of irradiation or even much later. The common dermatologic side

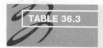

TABLE 36.3	Single and Combination Chemotherapeutic Regimens Causing Alopecia

Aminocamptothecin	Ifosfamide
Amsacrine	Irinotecan
Bleomycin	Irinotecan/5-FU/leucovorin
Busulfan	Mechlorethamine
Carmustine	Melphalan
Chlorambucil	Methotrexate
Cisplatin	Mithramycin
Cisplatin/etoposide	Mitomycin
Cyclophosphamide	Mitoxantrone
Cytarabine	Paclitaxel
Dacarbazine	Pacilitaxel/carboplatin
Dactinomycin	Taxotere
Daunorubicin	Teniposide
Doxorubicin (>50 mg)	Topotecan
Epirubicin HCL	Vincristine
Etoposide	Vinblastine
5-Fluorouracil (5-FU)	Vindesine
Hydroxyurea	Vinorelbine
Idarubicin	—
FAC (fluorouracil, doxorubicin, cyclophosphamide)	—
MOPP/ABVD (MOPP+doxorubicin, bleomycin, vincristine, dactinomycin, 5FU)	—
MOPP (Nitrogen mustard, vincristine, procarbazine, prednisone)	—

effects range from minor skin irritation to erythematous macules but can exacerbate to toxic epidermal necrolysis.

Capecitabine, a prodrug of 5-Fluorouracil (5-FU), can produce a hand–foot syndrome (palmar–plantar erythrodysesthia [PPE]) that can quickly progress from tingling to a painful burning sensation. Cracking of the skin, desquamation, and papules to the palms and/or soles result in a discontinuation or break from therapy.

The most common dermatologic reaction of skin rash is seen with EGFR targeted agents. The acneform or erythematous rash predominantly presents on the face, chest, and back (upper torso). Topical steroids (hydrocortisone) and antibiotics (clindamycin gel/lotion) are useful for mild, grade 1 macular/papular rashes with the addition of oral antibiotics such as minocycline 100 mg/b.i.d. or triethoprim/sulfamethoxazole b.i.d. for grade 2 eruptions (rash covering less than 50% of body surface area). Severe grade 3 rash, defined as covering more than 50% with associated signs and symptoms including pain, require reassessment to continue the drug and/or treat with oral steroids in addition to the oral antibiotic and/or topical lotions.

Patients should be educated to use lotions that are alcohol-, perfume- and dyefree, minimize sun exposure and wear sunscreen to exposed skin when outdoors. Although most of these rashes are non–life threatening, careful attention to the patient's psychological well-being should be considered.

VI. FLULIKE SYMPTOMS (FLS). In the oncology setting, fever most often presents in either the immunocompromised, neutropenic patient or during a blood product transfusion. The problem of febrile neutropenia is addressed in section IX.

Biotherapy and chemotherapeutic agents can induce FLS of "drug fever," chill/rigors, myalgias, arthralgias, headache, nasal congestion, and malaise in combination or separately. Biological substances and cytokines are found naturally in the body and the immune system is accelerated when these agents are administered. Therefore, when these agents are discontinued, the symptomatology normally resolves. Etiology of FLS is unknown but believed to be related to endogenous and exogenous pyrogens, also known as cytokines, released as the body's inflammatory response following biological and chemotherapeutic treatment.

Treatment choices for FLS, whether by medication or nonpharmacologic intervention, are usually based on the subjective description given by the patient. Although non–life threatening, these symptoms significantly impact the patient's quality of life.

VII. FATIGUE. Fatigue is one of the most common problems in treatment with cytotoxic agents, biologic response modifiers, bone marrow transplantation and radiation therapy affecting more than 75% of cancer patients during and after treatment. It can be cyclic and worsen during the period of nadir. However, fatigue due to radiation treatment may increase toward the end of treatment. It is more prevalent with multimodality or dose-intense treatment protocols, and in the setting of metastatic disease. Although consistently underreported, oncology patients identify fatigue as the most distressing symptom and the most common problem. Patients often fear that fatigue is the symptom of recurrent disease. Fatigue is often overlooked by the health care provider and the patients themselves, as a treatable cause of treatment-related morbidity and therefore, must be assessed thoroughly and reevaluated with every encounter with our patients. Fatigue has gained widespread acceptance in medical literature as a persistent sense of tiredness or exhaustion. The term fatigue is preferentially used to cover fatigue, asthenia, and malaise as one entity during the treatment of cancer.

Owing to success with many cancer treatments, all health care professionals will likely encounter patients presenting with prolonged states of fatigue related to the effect of treatment. As health care professionals, we can be advocates for our patients in the areas of work environment, private insurance, and disability benefits. Each of the problems that may contribute to fatigue may also contribute to the maintenance of other symptoms. For example, untreated cancer pain can increase or cause depression and anxiety that can further exacerbate insomnia, which may further exacerbate fatigue symptoms (Table 36.4 and 36.5).

Proposed mechanisms of pathophysiologic causes include the following:

- Loss of muscle mass, defective muscle energy metabolism, and/or abnormalities in the generation or use of adenosine triphosphate (ATP)
- Neurophysiologic skeletal muscle changes
- Chronic stress response, possibly mediated through the hypothalamic pituitary axis
- Systemic inflammatory response
- Immune activation associated with production of proinflammatory cytokines.
- Disrupted sleep or circadian rhythms
- Hormonal changes
- Direct central nervous system (CNS) toxicity
- Deficiency of L-carnitine may reduce energy production through fatty acid oxidation

When sleep disruption is suspected as an underlying cause of fatigue, zaleplon or zolpidem are two commonly recommended hypnotics that do not usually cause oversedation. Triazolam, oxazepam, temazepam, lorazepam, estazolam, clonazepam, quazepam, and flurazepam all represent commonly prescribed benzodiazepine hypnotics. Antidepressants with sedative effects to consider include

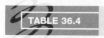

TABLE 36.4 Primary Evaluation of Fatigue

Primary evaluation (during and following treatment)	Interventions	Patient education
Focused history to assess for disease recurrence or progression; review of systems; onset, pattern, duration, change over time, associated factors, interference with ability to function	Interventions should begin at the time of initial diagnosis	Teach daily self-assessment and interventions focused on the underlying cause of fatigue
—	Education and strategies for management; reassessment with each encounter	Reassurance that treatment-related fatigue is not necessarily an indicator of disease progression
Quality of life assessment and/or numeric scale	Energy conservation	—
Assess performance status	—	Massage and healing touch; relaxation; optimize sleep quality; energy conservation and activity management
Assessment of psychosocial support systems	Set priorities, pace, delegate, schedule activities at times of peak energy, labor-saving devices, postpone nonessential activities, naps that do not interrupt night-time sleep, structured daily routine, attend to one activity at a time; distraction	Acupuncture
Review current medications	Titrate opioid analgesics to avoid excessive sedation.	Educate patients in self assessment
—	Consider psychostimulants after ruling out other causes of fatigue	—
—	Treat anemia as indicated	—
—	Continued reassessment	—
—	Consider trial of low-dose corticosteroids (administered in the morning)	—
—	NSAIDs found to reduce tumor stimulated cytokines	—

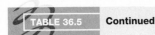

| TABLE 36.5 | Continued |

Primary evaluation (during and following treatment)	Interventions	Patient education
—	Methylphenidate trial, may however, exacerbate insomnia; limited data on use of SSRIs tricyclics, and bupropion in depressed and nondepressed cancer patients	—
Assessment of contributing factors that are treatable including pain, emotional distress (depression or anxiety), sleep disturbance, anemia, nutritional assessment (weight/caloric intake and fluid/electrolyte imbalance; activity level; comorbidities) infection; cardiac, pulmonary, renal, hepatic, neurologic or endocrine dysfunction (hypothyroidism)	See Table 36.5	See Table 36.5

NSAID, nonsteroidal anti-inflammatory drug; SSRI, selective serotonin reuptake inhibitors.

trazodone, amitriptyline, doxepin, mirtazapine, and olanzapine. This group of antidepressants may provide help with correction of sleep patterns as well as treat depression that is associated with the disruption. Mirtazapine may also provide some stimulation of appetite. One must be cautious of oversedation, especially in the elderly or compromised patient.

The drugs associated with fatigue include the opioids used for pain control and most of all the traditional chemotherapeutic agents and biological agents. In addition, several anticancer drugs such as interferon (IFN), IL-2, and asparaginase can cause hypothyroidism, which may indirectly contribute to fatigue. Many of the medications used to treat the underlying cause of fatigue may also have the common side effect of fatigue.

In the United States there are more than 9 million people living with cancer. Improvements in survival have led to efforts to enhance quality of life. Fatigue can be a long-term or late effect of disease or treatment. More research needs to be dedicated to studying these groups as we have limited knowledge of fatigue in these survivors.

VIII. GI side effects

A. Nausea and/or vomiting. The incidence of chemotherapy induced emesis (CIE) has declined dramatically over the past two decades. There are three distinct types of CIE that have been defined—acute, delayed, and anticipatory.

TABLE 36.6 **Treatable Causes of Fatigue**

Treatable cause of fatigue	Assessment	Pharmacologic	Nonpharmacologic
Pain	Current and past history with pain; pain assessment scale, visual analog, or happy/sad faces scale; educate patients on how to quantify their pain both before and after interventions	See Chapter 14, Pain Management	Guided imagery
—	—	NSAIDs, then weak opioids, then strong opioid drugs and adjuvant drugs added at any step	Meditation
—	—	—	Massage
—	—	—	Exercise
—	—	—	Education of patient and caregivers
Emotional distress (depression or anxiety)	DSM diagnostic criteria for major depression: (>2 weeks) depressed mood or diminished interest in activities AND four or more of the following: changes in appetite or weight, insomnia or hypersomnia, psychomotor agitation or retardation, fatigue, feeling worthless or guilty, inability to concentrate, suicidal ideation	Antidepressants, antianxiety agents; selective serotonin reuptake inhibitors such as fluoxetine may exacerbate insomnia	—
—	Physician psychiatric evaluation recommended to formulate plan of care and identify high-risk patients	Patient may also require specific hypnotic medication	Counseling individual, family, and support groups

Anemia	Assess acute vs. nonacute; Classify mild (Hgb 10–11 g/dL), moderate (Hgb 8–10 g/dL), or severe (Hgb <8 g/dL);	See Chapter 37, 'Growth Factor Support in Oncology'	Use of erythropoietic therapy requires close assessment of blood pressure; seizures reported in CRF patients receiving erythropoietic drugs; titrate hgb to 11–12 g/dL to decrease risk of thromboembolic events
—	Review of systems	Symptomatic Hgb 10–11 (consider starting erythropoietic therapy)	—
—	Assess comorbidities and perform reproducible functional assessment	Hgb <10 (strongly consider starting erythropoietic therapy) and consider iron studies	—
—	—	Consider iron supplementation if ferritin <100; transferrin saturation <20%)	—
—	—	Hgb < 8 consider transfusion	—
Sleep disturbance	Review diagnostic criteria; consider predisposing, precipitating, and perpetuating factors (maladaptive behaviors and cognitions)	Nonbenzodiazepine hypnotic agents (zaleplon, polpidem) have less residual side effects	Sleep hygiene
—	Review medications for potential side effects	If secondary to depression, consider treating the underlying psychiatric disturbance with trazodone, amitriptyline, doxepin (caution with oversedation)	Cognitive behavioral intervention
—	Identify if transient (<2 weeks), short-term (2–4 weeks) or chronic (>4 weeks); evaluate for delayed sleep onset, impaired sleep continuity or early-morning awakening	See commonly prescribed medications	Relaxation training; stimulus control therapy (going to bed only when sleepy; sleep consolidation (reduce nap time); consistent bedtime and awakening time
—	Consider sleep apnea	—	Biofeedback
—	—	—	Progressive muscle relaxation and guided imagery

(continued)

TABLE 36.5 Treatable Causes of Fatigue

Treatable cause of fatigue	Assessment	Pharmacologic	Nonpharmacologic
Nutrition	—	—	Exercise
	Assess electrolytes, calcium, phosphorus, magnesium; hemoglobin/hematocrit, serum albumin, creatinine clearance, blood sugar	Correct abnormalities	Dietitian referral
	Food diary	Anorexia/cachexia consider megestrol acetate; dronabinol; metoclopramide	Oral supplements (Instant Breakfast, Forta Shakes, NutraShakes, Lactose free Ensure: Boost); PEG for additional calories; calorie dense for tube feedings – Ensure or Sustacal Plus, Jevity, Osmolite
	Assess barriers to intake such as alterations in GI function: nausea, vomiting, anorexia, stomatitis, esophagitis	Consider intermittent IV hydration with correction of electrolyte abnormalities.	
	Assess for psychosocial influence due to depression, anxiety	—	—
	Assess height/weight: gain or loss; muscle loss; poor wound healing; condition of skin, nails, mucous membranes	—	—
	Consider candida, pain or tumor effects	—	—
Activity level	(Re) Assessment of performance status through Karnofsky and/or ECOG scale	Consider referral to physical therapy	Exercise physical therapy

NSAID, nonsteroidal anti-inflammatory drug; DSM, Diagnostic and Statistical Manual of Mental Disorders; CRF, chronic renal failure patients; PEG, percutaneous endoscopic gastrostomy; ECOG, European Cooperative Oncology Group

Acute CIE occurs within the first 24 hours and peaks at 5 to 6 hours. **Delayed-onset emesis** develops after 24 hours of chemotherapy administration. **Anticipatory nausea** is a conditioned response that patients experience after prior cycles of chemotherapy have induced nausea and vomiting. The most effective way to prevent this type of nausea and vomiting is to have aggressive control of acute and delayed onset emesis. The objective of antiemetic therapy is the complete absence of chemotherapy-induced nausea and vomiting.

Biotherapy such as IFN or IL-2 may cause nausea and vomiting as part of an FLS. Monoclonal antibodies may induce nausea and vomiting during the infusion due to the infusion process, not the antibodies.

The health care provider should always keep in mind that emesis in cancer can also be caused by partial or complete bowel obstruction, vestibular dysfunction, brain metastases, electrolyte imbalance, uremia, concomitant drug treatments, including opiates, gastroparesis induced by tumor, chemotherapy or underlying diabetes, and psychophysiologic factors such as anxiety and anticipatory nausea and vomiting.

The known pathophysiologic basis of CIE are as follows:

1. Emetic center. The emetic center is an anatomically indistinct collection of receptor and effector nuclei predominantly localized in the nucleus *tractus solitarius*. It appears to coordinate the efferent respiratory, GI, and autonomic activity associated with nausea and vomiting. The emetic center functions as the final effector pathway through which a variety of afferent stimuli can activate emesis.

2. Chemoreceptor trigger zone (CTZ). The CTZ is located in the area postrema in the floor of the fourth ventricle. Since it lies outside of the blood–brain barrier, it is accessible to emetic stimuli borne either in the blood or cerebrospinal fluid. The CTZ appears to be an important source of afferent input to the emetic center and is an important site for muscarinic (M_1), dopamine (D_2), serotonin (5-HT_3), neurokinin-1(NK_1), and histamine (H_1) receptors.

3. Two other sources of afferent input to the emetic center with CIE include higher brain stem and cortical structures, which may play a role in anticipatory emesis, and input from the GI tract, which is conveyed by the vagus and splanchnic nerves.

4. Although more than 30 neurotransmitters have been associated with the peripheral and CNS sites involved in CIE, the three most important neurotransmitters, namely dopamine, serotonin, and substance P, appear to have the most clinical relevance. Several therapeutic agents are designed to antagonize the action of these neurotransmitters and all have shown clinical benefit as antiemetics.

Considerable progress has been made over the last two decades in the development of more effective and better-tolerated methods of controlling nausea and vomiting induced by cytotoxic chemotherapy and radiation. Studies of the neurotransmitter serotonin (5-HT) led to the introduction of the type 3, 5-hydroxytryptamine receptor (5-HT_3) antagonists into clinical practice during the early 1990s. These drugs have become the mainstay of current antiemetic therapy for CIE and include dolasetron, granisetron, ondansetron, palonosetron, and tropesitron.

1. **Management of chemotherapy-related nausea**

    High risk (level 5). For patients receiving high-dose cisplatin and other highly emetogenic (level 5) agents, the optimal regimen to prevent both acute and delayed emesis appear to be a 5-HT_3 receptor antagonist, dexamethasone, and aprepitant. The rates of complete protection from acute emesis using this combination are between 83% and 89%, while complete emesis protection for 5 days following chemotherapy can be expected in 63% to 73% in such patients.

Moderate risk (level 3, 4). For patients receiving moderately emetogenic chemotherapy, the current regimen of choice is a combination of an effective dose of a 5-HT$_3$ receptor antagonist and IV dexamethasone given immediately before chemotherapy. For patients receiving cyclophosphamide combined with an anthracycline or carboplatin with another agent, the addition of aprepitant to a 5-HT$_3$ receptor antagonist and dexamethasone should be considered as a reasonable option.

Low risk (level 2). Low-risk chemotherapeutic drugs are associated with 10% to 30% incidence of acute emesis. Common clinical situations in which this level of risk is encountered include the administration of topotecan or gemcitabine. Please refer to Table 36.6 for emetogenic potential for the specific agent.

When using **combination** chemotherapy, the following algorithm is helpful in determining the level of emetogenicity: (Table 36.7 and 36.8)

- Identify the most emetogenic agent of the chemotherapeutic agents being prescribed.
- Level 1 agents do not contribute to the total emetogenicity.
- As one or more level 2 agents are added, the level of emetogenicity increases by one level.
- Adding a level 3 agent to the combination increases the level by one level per agent.

2. **Radiation-induced nausea** caused by high-risk total body irradiation can be effectively controlled with a 5-HT$_3$ receptor antagonist, such as ondansetron, which currently has the largest clinical evidence of its effectiveness, with or without a corticosteroid before each fraction and for at least 24 hours afterwards. There is limited evidence of the effectiveness of corticosteroids with medium and low emetic risk radiation, but a 5-HT$_3$ receptor antagonist can be recommended in this setting.

3. **Nonpharmacologic treatment options and education**
   - Use optimal antiemetic therapy during **every** cycle of treatment.
   - We recommend telephone calls to patients and families within 24 to 48 hours of treatment to reassess for symptoms due to treatment.
   - One should not wait until the next cycle to reassess tolerance.
   - Behavioral therapy may include relaxation and systematic desensitization, hypnosis/guided imagery, music therapy, acupuncture or acupressure.

B. **Diarrhea.** GI toxicity is a common problem for cancer patients receiving cyto-toxic and biological therapy. Chemotherapy-induced diarrhea (CID) is the most common dose-limiting toxicity (Table 36.9). When evaluating a patient with diarrhea, one should also consider an intestinal infection such as *Clostridium difficile*, radiation effects, and a history of prior intestinal resection as an under-lying cause. The presence of fever, dizziness, or abdominal pain should raise the possibility of a complication such as sepsis or bowel obstruction and may often require hospitalization for the proper assessment and treatment of diarrhea. The clinician should grade the diarrhea, assess for blood, incontinence, and conduct a thorough history and physical examination.

Both 5-FU and irinotecan cause exudative diarrhea which results in acute damage to the intestinal mucosa, leading to loss of epithelium. 5-FU causes mitotic arrest of crypt cells, which increases the ratio of immature secretory crypt cells to mature villous enterocytes. This causes an increased volume of fluid that leaves the small bowel leading to clinically significant diarrhea. Irinotecan and 5-FU have overlapping toxicity profiles; therefore, the risk of GI toxicity may be even higher. These drugs are commonly used together for the treatment of colorectal cancer.

Irinotecan and topotecan can cause cholinergically-mediated early-onset diarrhea, which occurs during, or within several hours of drug infusion in 45% to 50% of patients. This effect is thought to be due to its structural similarity to

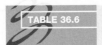

	Emesis Risk Level for Specific Cytotoxic and Biological Agents

Risk level	Drug
5 (High)	Carmustine
—	Cisplatin
—	Cyclophosphamide
—	Dacarbazine
—	Mechlorethamine
—	Streptozocin
—	Lomustine
—	Pentostatin
—	Dactinomycin
4/3 (Moderate)	Cyclophosphamide
—	Carmustine (<250 mg/m^2)
—	Doxorubicin
—	Cisplatin (<50 mg/m^2)
—	Epirubicin
—	Cytarabine (>1 g/m^2)
—	Idarubicin
—	Mitoxantrone (>12 mg/m^2)
—	Hexamethylmelamine
—	Ifosfamide
—	Carboplatin
—	Irinotecan
—	Melphalan
—	Procarbazine
—	Mitoxantrone (>12 mg/m^2)
—	Cytarabine (>1 g/m^2)
2 (Low)	methotrexate (>100 mg/m^2)
—	Fluorouracil (<1 mg/m^2)
—	Doxorubicin (<20 mg/m^2)
—	Docetaxel
—	Mitoxantrone (<12 mg/m^2)
—	Topotecan
—	Cytarabine (<1 mg/m^2)
—	Thiotepa
—	Temozolomide
—	Paclitaxel
—	Etoposide
—	Mitomycin
—	Asparaginase
—	Gemcitabine
1 (Minimal)	capecitabine
—	Methotrexate
—	Vincristine
—	Trastuzumab
—	Vincristine
—	Rituximab
—	Vinblastine
—	Bleomycin
—	Vinorelbine (IV)
—	Etoposide (IV)
—	Teniposide (IV)

TABLE 36.7   CIE Prevention and Treatment Guidelines

Chemotherapy risk level	Drug	Day 1	Day 2	Day 3	Day 4	As needed
High	Dexamethasone	X	X	X	If needed	—
—	Aprepitant	X	X	X	—	—
—	5-HT$_3$ antagonist	X (palo)[a]	—	—	—	If needed
—	Lorazepam	PRN	PRN	PRN	If needed	—
—	Metoclopramide, H1 blockers, or phenothiazines	Oral or IV p.r.n	Oral p.r.n	Oral p.r.n	Oral p.r.n	Oral p.r.n
Moderate	Dexamethasone	X	X	X	If needed	—
—	—	And (palo)	Or	Or	Or	—
—	5-HT$_3$ antagonist		X	X	X	—
—	Lorazepam	PRN	PRN	PRN	PRN	—
—	Aprepitant	X	X	X	—	—
—	Metoclopramide, H1 blockers, or phenothiazines	Oral/IV p.r.n	Oral p.r.n	Oral p.r.n	Oral p.r.n	Oral p.r.n
Low	Dexamethasone	X (IV)	—	—	—	—
—	Phenothiazine, Metoclopramide	PRN	PRN	PRN	PRN	PRN

[a]Palonosetron (has longer half-life).

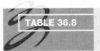

TABLE 36.8	Consider the Following Recommendations for Management of Breakthrough or Refractory Nausea and Vomiting:

- Addition of other dopamine antagonists such as metoclopramide, thiethylperazine, or butyrophenones such as haloperidol. Metoclopramide given on a schedule for this purpose has been found to be effective in preventing nausea and vomiting
- Consider switching to a different 5-HT$_3$, although limited investigational trial data suggest it may sometimes be efficacious
- Consider the addition of an anxiolytic agent in combination with the antiemetic agents
- If the patient has dyspepsia, consider antacid therapy such as an H$_2$ blocker or proton pump inhibitor
- Consider adding oral or intravenous corticosteroids
- Consider cannabinoid such as dronabinol

the drug acetylcholine. Other symptoms include abdominal cramping, rhinitis, lacrimation, and salivation. These symptoms usually last approximately 30 minutes and are usually well controlled by atropine during the administration of the drug. In contrast, late irinotecan-associated diarrhea is not cholinergically mediated. It is more common when given at doses exceeding 350 mg/m^2 and less common when given as an every 3-week cycle. Irinotecan can produce mucosal changes that result in the accumulation of the active metabolite of irinotecan, SN-38, in the intestinal mucosa which itself does not appear to cause diarrhea but it can be deconjugated in the intestines, resulting in diarrhea.

Studies have demonstrated that 10% of the population has the common genetic polymorphisms of the UDP-glucuronyltransferase 1A1 (UGT1A1) gene which can predict the increased risk of severe side effects, including neutropenia and diarrhea related to the use of irinotecan. The UGT1A1 molecular assay for irinotecan toxicity is a test that is now U.S. Food and Drug Administration (FDA) approved. Patients who are at risk for this polymorphism should have their initial dose of irinotecan lowered.

TABLE 36.9	Agents Causing Diarrhea

Cytotoxic agents causing diarrhea	Biotherapy agents causing diarrhea
Irinotecan	Interleukin 2
Topotecan	Interferons
5-FU, UFT	Monoclonal antibodies
Fludarabine	—
Cytarabine	—
Idarubicin	—
Plicamycin	—
Mitoxantrone	—
Pentostatin	—
Floxuridine	—
Capecitabine	—
Cisplatin	—
Oxaliplatin	—
Docetaxel	—
Pemetrexed	—
UFT	—

Dihydropyrimidine dehydrogenase (DPD) deficiency or partial DPD deficiency may result in a severe form of life-threatening diarrhea, mucositis, nausea, vomiting, rectal bleeding, and pancytopenia with the administration of 5-FU. Recently, a breath test was developed to evaluate the entire pyrimidine catabolic pathway. This test is being examined and is not yet FDA approved for use in the standard clinical setting.

Capecitabine is an oral fluoropyrimidine that is converted to 5-FU. UFT is a combination of ftorafur, a 5-FU prodrug, and uracil that has been in widespread use in Japan for more than 20 years and has been introduced in the United States. Uracil competitively inhibits DPD, leading to higher intratumoral concentrations of 5-FU. Grade 3 to 4 diarrhea can occur in 10% to 20% of patients. Prompt discontinuation of UFT usually prevents severe GI toxicity.

The molecularly targeted agents including the EGFR, TKIs, and the vascular endothelial growth factor (VEGF) inhibitors may cause diarrhea. Dose-limiting toxicities can typically be easily managed by the use of loperamide. In some cases, diarrhea necessitates dose reduction or treatment interruptions. Erlotinib and gefitnib may cause diarrhea in up to 60% of patients. Sorafenib and imatinib cause diarrhea in 30% to 45% of patients and severe diarrhea occurs in less than 5%. Diarrhea is seen in as many as half the patients treated with bortezomib, a proteasome inhibitor used in the treatment of multiple myeloma. Eight percent of the events were graded as level 3 or 4 toxicities.

Pharmacologic and nonpharmacologic interventions. Mucosal injury may lead to a temporary lactase deficiency, and therefore, the ingestion of milk-containing foods may need to be avoided. The mainstay of drug therapy of CID is the opiates. Loperamide (Imodium) and diphenoxylate (Lomotil) are the most commonly used and both are FDA-approved for this indication. Loperamide appears to be more effective and has been recommended in treatment guidelines. The standard dose of loperamide is not usually effective. A more aggressive regimen (4 mg initially, then 2 mg every 2 hours or 4 mg every 4 hours until diarrhea-free for 12 hours) is often required, particularly for irinotecan-induced diarrhea.

Octreotide is a synthetic long-acting somatostatin analog that works by decreasing the secretion of a number of hormones, such as vasoactive intestinal peptide (VIP), prolongation of intestinal transit time, and reduced secretion and increased absorption of fluid and electrolytes. Octreotide is used for the treatment of diarrhea related to VIP-secreting tumors, symptoms due to carcinoid syndrome, and is also beneficial in patients with CID from fluoropyrimidines and irinotecan, although the optimal dose has not been determined. Octreotide is generally reserved as a second-line therapy for patients who do not respond to high-dose loperamide because of its high cost and general effectiveness of loperamide. The side effects of octreotide are generally mild, including bloating, cramping, flatulence, and fat malabsorption. Hypersensitivity-like reactions and hypoglycemia can occur at higher doses.

C. **Mucositis.** Mucositis is a general term referring to all mucosal inflammation. Stomatitis is oral mucositis. Disruption in the integrity of the oral mucosa is a common problem in patients receiving cytotoxic therapy and radiation therapy. It occurs in 30% to 40% of cytotoxic therapy, 80% of stem cell transplant recipients and 100% of head and neck radiation treatment patients. Xerostomia or dry mouth occurs less frequently. The alteration in taste is termed *dysgeusia* or the absence of taste is called *ageusia*.

The initial clinical manifestation is soft tissue erythema of the buccal mucosa or soft palate with a burning sensation in the mouth and may begin just 7 days after the first dose of chemotherapy. Cytotoxic therapy or radiation therapy damage DNA resulting in cell, tissue, and blood vessel damage. DNA damage results in the upregulation of messenger signals, releasing proinflammatory cytokines such as tumor necrosis factor (TNF), IL-1β and IL-6. This is what results in the appearance of solitary, elevated, white desquamative patches that are slightly painful. With further progression, epithelial sloughing results in multiple shallow ulcerations with a pseudomembranous appearance, which coalesce to form large painful lesions and may cause dysphagia and reduced oral intake. Oral or gingival bleeding can occur if the patient becomes thrombocytopenia with platelet counts less than $15,000/\mu L$. Poor oral hygiene can worsen this condition.

Severe pseudomembranous or erosive mucositis can lead to secondary infection with *Candida albicans* or even bacterial sepsis, particularly in the presence of neutropenia, and can necessitate the use of parenteral nutrition and/or opiates. A topical application of morphine sulfate has been used; however, most oral preparations of morphine contain glycerin or ethanol or both. These are not suitable for topical application because alcohol and glycerin can directly injure the mucosa. The pain may be severe enough to require systemic parenteral opiates. Morphine is recommended as the opioid of first choice for patient-controlled analgesia. Efforts to limit mucositis progression by blocking the mechanism of chemotherapy-induced toxicity have had a relatively limited role. Lesions spontaneously begin to resolve within several days, and are usually completely healed within 10 to 14 days of chemotherapy. Severe symptoms may necessitate dose reduction during subsequent chemotherapy cycles.

The cytotoxic drugs most commonly associated with mucositis are in the class of antimetabolities, antitumor antibiotics, alkylating agents, and plant alkaloids. Biotherapeutic agents such as IL-2, lymphokine-activated killers (LAKs), TNF and IFN have been associated with mucositis. Local radiation of structures around the head or neck can also cause stomatitis by also altering supportive structures such as salivary glands and bone. Uncomplicated mucositis is a self-limiting condition. Prophylactic administration of nystatin suspension is not effective and is not recommended but useful for active Candida infections.

The oral cavity can also be secondarily infected by viral pathogens. The most common is reactivation of herpes simplex virus (HSV) type 1 infection, which occurs in up to 65% to 90% of seropositive patients receiving high-dose chemotherapy. HSV-associated mucositis tends to be more severe and of longer duration than non–HSV-associated mucositis. The typical vesicular lesions may not be evident in the presence of chemotherapy-induced mucositis. A swab of one of the lesions can be sent for viral culture; HSV is usually isolated within 72 hours. Empiric antiviral therapy with parenteral or oral acyclovir oral valacyclovir can be initiated while awaiting culture results. Because of high reactivation rates, HSV-seropositive patients who are undergoing either induction chemotherapy for acute leukemia or receiving high dose "conditioning" regimens followed by high-dose chemotherapy should receive acyclovir antiviral prophylaxis.

The treatment of mucositis is supportive and aimed at symptom control. It consists of a combination of oral care, mucosal protectants, and either topical or systemic analgesia. The clinician should include an initial thorough oral examination to identify patients who might be at higher risk of mucositis due to periodontal disease, which should be treated before starting chemotherapy. Following the administration of chemotherapy, routine mouth care including removal of dentures, atraumatic cleansing, and oral rinses with a weak solution of salt and baking soda (one half teaspoonful of salt and one teaspoonful of baking soda in a quart of water) should be performed every 4 hours. The oral cavity should be rinsed and wiped after meals, and dentures cleaned and brushed often to remove plaque. A soft toothbrush cleans teeth effectively but may be too harsh for patients with moderate to severe stomatitis. Hydrogen peroxide (diluted 1:1 with saline or water) may be used for gentle debridement. Use of hydrogen peroxide should be limited, as chronic therapy may delay healing. The diet should be limited to foods that do not require significant chewing; acidic, salty, or dry foods should be avoided.

A variety of mucosal coating agents have been used, including topical kaolin/pectin, diphenhydramine, oral antacids, and maltodextrin. These agents provide an adherent barrier over mucosal surfaces, thereby shielding oral lesions from the effect of food, liquids, and saliva. Topical Lidocaine solutions provide pain relief but require frequent administration. Topical Lidocaine is frequently combined with coating agents, a mixture that is often referred to as *magic mouthwash*. One example consists of equal parts of viscous Lidocaine, diphenhydramine, antacids such as Maalox, and nystatin with instructions to swish and swallow every 2 hours as needed. Although the optimal dose and method of administration has yet to be clarified, amifostine data suggest significant reductions in mucositis compared to placebo.

D. Xerostomia. Although more commonly attributed to radiation therapy exposure, changes in salivary gland function can also be attributable to chemotherapy. Reduced salivary flow can also result from anticholinergic medications given for therapy-induced nausea or diarrhea. Clinical presentation can vary, with some patients presenting with dry mucous membranes of varying severity, whereas others complain of excessive saliva with drooling as a result of dysphagia or odynophagia. The major symptoms associated with xerostomia are dry, uncomfortable mucosal tissues and thick ropy saliva, which may impair speech and swallowing. Therapy is symptomatic such as rinsing with saline or the use of commercially available saliva substitutes. Dry cracked lips can be treated with petroleum-based lubricants.

E. Constipation. Constipation occurs in approximately one third of cancer patients and can be defined as a decreased frequency of defecation (usually less than three bowel movements per week) accompanied by discomfort or difficulty. It is usually because of a combination of poor oral intake and drugs, such as opioid analgesics or antiemetic agents, that slow intestinal transit time.

Constipation is rarely a dose-limiting toxicity for chemotherapeutic agents except for the vinca alkaloids, such as vincristine, vinblastine, and vinorelbine. These drugs have pronounced neuropathic effects and reduce GI transit time. The constipating effect of vinca alkaloid therapy is usually apparent after the first dose and is typically not cumulative. It is most prominent 3 to 10 days after chemotherapy and then resolves in most cases after a few days. Thalidomide has shown promise in the treatment of refractory multiple myeloma and other disorders. Constipation occurs approximately one third to one half of the time it is administered.

The most frequently used laxatives are docusate, senna or bisacodyl. If these agents are not effective, magnesium salts, lactulose, or sorbitol are often useful. Patients and their families require frequent reassessment of this problem accompanied by specific written directions for the use of medications and dietary changes.

F. Colitis. Neutropenic enterocolitis (a form of necrotizing enterocolitis or typhlitis) is one of the most common GI complication in leukemic patients who are undergoing induction therapy and following stem cell–supported high-dose chemotherapy. This type of colitis is caused by primary mucosal injury due to chemotherapy followed by a secondary infection. The most common invoked pathogens are opportunistic pathogens, pseudomonas, clostridial species, and fungal infections, which are often documented postmortem.

Neutropenic enterocolitis typically develops when the ANC falls below 500. Patients usually present with fever, abdominal pain, nausea, vomiting, diarrhea, and not uncommonly, sepsis. Patients with abdominal pain can be masked by steroid therapy. The diagnosis is based on signs and symptoms, as well as imaging studies, mainly computed tomography. The optimal therapy of neutropenic enterocolitis remains controversial, as both conservative medical management (bowel rest, decompression, nutrition, supportive measures, and broad-spectrum antibiotics) and surgery have been proposed.

A small number of cases of ischemic colitis have been reported with docetaxel-containing regimens in patients. The clinical manifestations are similar to neutropenic enterocolitis, but not all patients are neutropenic at presentation.

C. difficile colitis is a common problem in patients with cancer, mostly due to oral antibiotic use and hospitalization; however, it has been described in patients without any prior antibiotic use following chemotherapy. The proposed mechanism is chemotherapy-induced intestinal damage which facilitates the proliferation of *C. difficile*. Frequent occurrences of *C. difficile*-related diarrheal episodes have been reported in patients treated with dose-dense paclitaxel-containing regimens. Stool specimens for *C. difficile* can identify the organism but are not always required before initiating standard treatment.

G. Intestinal Perforation. Bevacizumab, a monoclonal antibody that binds VEGF, has occasionally been associated with intestinal perforation and hemorrhage. Perforation can occur at sites of residual cancer, surgical anastomoses, or uninvolved sites where it can cause GI ulcers or nasal septal perforations. These complications may be severe or fatal. Management may include observation, antibiotics, and/or surgery, depending upon the site and extent of perforation and requires discontinuation of bevacizumab.

Sunitinib, an inhibitor of multiple enzymes in the tyrosine kinase pathway, is used in patients with gastrointestinal stromal tumors (GISTs) refractory to imatinib and in renal cell carcinoma. In rare cases, necrosis of large GISTs involving the intestines results in perforation, the development of fistulas, and/or bleeding. If the initial event can be managed and other masses potentially at risk for perforation removed, continued treatment may be warranted, because the tumor necrosis is a predictor of continued control of the disease.

H. Perirectal cellulitis. Perirectal cellulitis is an inflammation and edema of the perineal and rectal area caused by tears of the anorectal mucosa, allowing for infection. The most common pathogens include gram-negative aerobic bacilli, enterococci, and bowel anaerobes. Patients who are at risk for this include patients with neutropenia or thrombocytopenia, especially if more chronic. Other risk factors include constipation, diarrhea, radiation therapy, hemorrhoids, anal fissures or any rectal trauma, including enemas and rectal thermometers, which should be avoided in these patients.

Antibiotics can be used for antianaerobic coverage, including clindamycin or metronidazole in addition to broad spectrum aerobic coverage. An effective bowel regimen should be established and patients and their families must be educated in perineal hygiene and the use of appropriate barrier creams.

IX. MYELOSUPPRESSION

A. Neutropenia. Neutropenia is the most common hematologic toxicity. White blood cell (WBC) nadirs generally occur 5 to 14 days following the administration of chemotherapy and recover by days 7 to 21. Agents such as docetaxel can result in an early, short-lasting type of neutropenia at a dose of more than 100 mg/m^2 when infused over 1 hour every 3 weeks.

The ANC is the objective clinical indicator. It is equal to the product of the WBC count and the fraction of polymorphonuclear cells (PMNs) and band forms noted on the differential analysis: ANC = WBC (cells/microL) × ([PMNs + bands] ÷ 100).

Mild (grade 1) neutropenia is defined as ANC between the lower limit of normal and 1,500/mm^3. Moderate (grade 2) is ANC of 1,000 to 1,500/m^3. Severe is ANC between 500 and 1,000/mm^3 and grade 4 (life threatening) is ANC less than 500/mm^3.

Fever associated with neutropenia is treated with intravenous antibiotics that are effective against gram negative bacteria. Available data does suggest that regimens with a greater than 40% chance of risk of febrile neutropenia, may justify the use of colony-stimulating factors (CSFs). Other high-risk group patients include patients with preexisting neutropenia, more advanced cancer, poor performance status, tumor involvement in the bone marrow, history of prior neutropenia with treatment, hepatic or renal dysfunction, protein–calorie malnutrition, concurrent therapy with antibiotics, antifungals, sulfas, allopurinol, and steroids.

Patients and their families can be taught preventive methods such as hand washing, dietary precautions with preparation and proper washing of foods. Prevention of trauma to the skin and mucous membranes, good oral hygiene, use of an electric razor instead of a blade razor, and use of a water-soluble lubricant during intercourse are simple things patients can do to prevent infections. Patients should not receive live vaccines during treatment, which includes oral vaccination for polio, varicella, smallpox, and nasal flu vaccine. Patients and families should be taught to monitor their temperature and should call for fever higher than 100.6F (38C).

One should avoid the use of CSFs with concomitant chemotherapy and radiation due to the increased risk of myelosuppression CSF has not been proved to reduce morbidity or mortality in this group. Dose reduction of the chemotherapy agent should be considered as the primary therapeutic option after an episode of severe neutropenia, except in the setting of a curable tumor. CSFs are NOT recommended as adjunctive treatment for febrile neutropenic patients. However, if an individual patient is at high risk of poor outcome, the use of adjuvant CSF may be considered, but the specific benefit has not been determined. CSF should be not given with concurrent chemotherapy, but must be given at least 24 hours after chemotherapy and stopped several days before the next chemotherapy administration.

B. Anemia. Anemia can occur in up to 40% to 50% of cancer patients, even before they have started cancer treatment. After the initiation of chemotherapy and/or radiation therapy, the incidence of anemia may climb to 90%; therefore, patients should be screened carefully before starting any particular regimen. Cancer and treatment-related anemia is caused by multiple factors, including bleeding, hemolysis, bone marrow infiltration, nutritional deficiencies, and anemia of chronic disease (ACD). Serum ferritin levels can be elevated in patients with cancer as a result of inflammation; therefore, this will not accurately reflect a patient's iron stores. A thorough iron workup is usually recommended and many patients benefit from iron replacement, either orally or intravenously.

Erythropoietic (EPO) therapy is usually initiated when the hemoglobin is less than 10 g/dL but may be considered at 10 to 11 g/dL if the patient is symptomatic. Several dosing schedules for epoetin alfa and darbepoetin alfa are available. Darbepoetin alfa has a half-life of 33 to 48 hours when given subcutaneously, compared to 16 to 19 hours for epoetin alfa. Therefore, darbepoetin alfa may be given at 2- or 3-week intervals instead of weekly. Side effects of both epoetin alfa and darbepoetin alfa include nausea, dyspnea, cough, weakness, constipation, fever, and vomiting. Thrombotic events were reported in 6.2% of patients on darbepoetin compared to 4.1% of patients on placebo. The goal of treatment, supported by quality of life evidence, is an Hgb of 11 to 12 g/dL (see Chapter).

EPO stimulates the production of red blood cells (RBCs) by increasing the number of stem cells, and shortening the time stem cell takes to become a mature RBC. EPO receptors have been identified on endothelial, renal, neuronal, and cardiac cells *in vitro*, which may explain why many patients also experience neuropathic toxicities with anemia.

Drugs that cause decreased RBC production related to either bone marrow suppression or impaired EPO response include platinum drugs, combination therapy with cyclophosphamide, MTX, and 5-FU, biotherapy, and ifosfamide. The clinician should perform a thorough history and physical before proceeding with therapy.

C. Thrombocytopenia. Thrombocytopenia occurs due to bone marrow suppression and usually occurs with neutropenia. It is common practice to hold chemotherapy if the platelet count is less than 100,000. Cytotoxic drugs commonly associated with thrombocytopenia include platinums, dacarbazine, daunorubicin, docetaxel, doxorubicin, gemcitabine, lomustine, mitomycin, thiotepa, trimetrexate, and the taxanes. A delayed-onset type of thrombocytopenia has been reported with carmustine, dactinomycin, fludarabine, lomustine, mitomycin, paclitaxel, streptozocin, thiotepa, and 6-thioguanine.

Risk factors for thrombocytopenia include the use of myelosuppressive chemotherapy, concurrent therapy or radiation therapy alone. Other risks include bone marrow infiltration, disseminated intravascular coagulation, and elevated temperature leading to the destruction of platelets. The existence of other cormorbidities such as liver impairment, diabetes, infection, sepsis, HIV, connective tissue disorders, or aplastic anemia put patients at even more risk for thrombocytopenia. Numerous drugs can also decrease platelet production including antibiotics, anticoagulants, antidepressants, aspirin, codeine, ethanol, indomethacin, nonsteroidal anti-inflammatory drugs (NSAIDs), and sulfa drugs.

Platelet counts less than 50,000/mm^3 create moderate risk for bleeding for patients. A platelet count less than 15,000/mm^3 usually indicates severe risk and a transfusion is usually indicated. Patients and their families can be taught bleeding precautions which includes the following:

- Avoidance of high-risk activities
- Maintenance of good skin and mucous membrane integrity
- Effective and safe oral hygiene
- Avoiding intercourse if platelets are less than 50,000/mm^3
- Avoid dental care
- Avoidance of enemas or suppositories
- Maintenance of optimal nutrition
- Avoidance of medications that can induce bleeding

Consider using IL-11, approved as a megakaryocyte growth factor in nonmyeloid malignancies and nonmyeloblative chemotherapeutic regimens.

X. NEUROTOXICITY. Neurologic toxicities that develop from antineoplastic compounds result from direct agent toxicity, which is usually reversible and/or dose limited, or indirect toxicity that results in metabolic disturbances or cerebral changes. The platinum agents and taxanes along with thalidomide, MTX, and vincristine are the most neurotoxic. Of the platinum compounds, cisplatin is primarily associated with sensorineural ototoxicity and peripheral neuropathy, affecting the dorsal root ganglion and peripheral nerves. Carboplatin, given at standard dosages, is less likely to manifest neurotoxicity. When administered, oxaliplatin (third-generation platinum) results in a transient, day's long, cold sensitivity leading to painful parasthesias and dysesthesias. Oxaliplatin neurotoxicity is cumulative, acute, or chronic, and, in most of the patients, slowly reverses over time. On occasion, neurotoxicity presents weeks to months following completion of therapy referred to as a *coasting phenomenon.*

Taxanes, docetaxel, and paclitaxel, affect the sensory nerves leading to a dose-dependent, cumulative neurotoxicity exhibited primarily with sensory neuropathy. Docetaxel produces a "glove and stocking" paraesthesia, which is accelerated in patients with prior neuropathies or those receiving combination therapies with cisplatin.

Thalidomide, an antiangiogenic treatment, produces somnolence in patients that usually decreases over weeks of therapy. With lengthy, cumulative thalidomide therapy (more than 12 months), neuropathies present with the most frequent symptom of parasthesias.

MTX, given intrathecally, exhibits a self-limiting neurotoxicity of aseptic meningitis and is; therefore, best administered with a corticosteroid to prevent the toxicity. Rarely, a delayed toxicity of leukoencephalopathy is exhibited in patients receiving MTX alone or potentiated in patients with a previous or concurrent cranial irradiation. CNS effects of malaise and blurred vision have also been reported in moderate dosages.

Biologic response modifiers (BRMs) and monoclonal antibody neurotoxicity are primarily dose dependent. Higher doses of BRMs, IFN, and IL, tend to trigger neuropsychiatric disturbances such as confusion, depression, irritability and insomnia. Neurotoxicities with BRMs, such as motor weakness, are rare with the exception of intrathecal IFN which can result in an acute (within 24 hours) or later onset of encephalopathy (Table 36.10).

XI. PULMONARY TOXICITY. Pulmonary toxicities occur with a myriad of chemotherapeutic agents and range from direct drug-induced pulmonary disease to immune suppression resulting in infectious and noninfectious states. Pulmonary infections can

TABLE 36.10	Cytotoxic Agents Causing Neurotoxicity

Asparaginase	Ifosfamide
5-Azacytidine	Interferons
Busulfan	Interleukins
Carboplatin	Levimisole
Carmofur	Methotrexate
Cisplatin	Mitomycin C
Cytarabine	Nitrogen mustard
Cytosine arabinoside	Paclitaxel
Dacarbazine	Pentostatin
Doxorubicin	Procarbazine
Etoposide	Suramin
Extramustine	Tamoxifen
Fludarabine	Teniposide
5-fluorououracil (5-FU)	Thiotepa (high dose)
Gemcitabine	Vinca alkaloids
	Vincristine

occur in any compromised patient but are found primarily in neutropenic patients with nonhematopoietic cancers resulting in the number one reason for hospitalization. Conventional bacteria are responsible for most pneumonitis states. Viruses, fungi, and uncommon organisms are also known to cause pulmonary infections with or without dual bacteria.

Careful consideration must be taken in treating patients who are elderly, have preexisting pulmonary compromise, and/or receiving concomitant therapies with similar pulmonary and cardiac toxicity (i.e., anthracyclines, dexamethasone, MTX, and cyclophosphamide). Of the cytotoxic agents, bleomycin (more than 400 U total dose) causes the greatest direct insult to the pulmonary system (Table 36.11).

XII. CYSTITIS. Patients receiving chemotherapy and those with primary bladder or cancers adjacent are at risk of developing cystitis. The most serious cystitis is hemorrhagic and more common in the autologous bone marrow transplant patient receiving higher doses of cytotoxic agents. Aside from hematuria, clinical manifestations include urinary frequency, dysuria, oliguria, or nocturia. As microscopic hematuria is possible without associated symptoms, a baseline and sequential urinalysis is obtained with cytotoxic agents posing the greatest risk.

The two chemotherapeutic agents primarily responsible for hemorrhagic cystitis are ifosamide and cyclophophosphamide (intravenous with greatest risk). Conventional doses may result in trace hematuria with or without symptomatology or high doses resulting in frank hematuria. Mesna, a bladder protectant, is administered with higher doses of cyclophosphamide and standard with ifosfamide infusion with the addition of vigorous hydration. Amifostine, an aminothiol, has also shown potential as a cytoprotective in renal tissue. Hemorrhagic cystitis management includes discontinuation of the offending drug, continuous bladder irrigation, administration of an antifibrinolytic agent, and a urologic consultation.

Preventative measures to be included to monitor for hemorrhagic cystitis, in addition to subjective patient information, are baseline and sequential blood urea nitrogen (BUN), creatinine, and urine cultures as warranted.

Immunocompromised patients are at risk of developing infectious renal symptoms, which may be exacerbated by irradiation to the renal field. Common pathogens responsible for the infectious state include, *Escherichia coli*, *Staphylococcus saprophyticus*, Proteus and Klebsiella. Therefore, antibiotic choice should be prescribed according to pathogen taking into account any concomitant cytotoxic agent.

TABLE 36.11 | Chemotherapy Agents Causing Drug-Induced Pulmonary Toxicity

Agent	Characteristic pulmonary effects
Alemtuzumab	Bronchospasm, shortness of breath
Arsenic trioxide	Mild to moderate reversible cough, dyspnea, pleural effusion
Bleomycin	Interstitial pneumonitis and fibrosis
Busulfan	Rare but serious bronchopulmonary dysplasia and fibrosis
	Onset of complications can be months or years
Carmustine	Interstitial pneumonitis, delayed pulmonary fibrosis
Capecitabine	Mild toxicity of dyspnea
	Manageable with symptom treatment and dose adjustment
Chlorambucil	Interstitial pneumonitis
Cyclophosphamide	Pulmonary edema
Cytarabine	Interstitial pneumonitis
Docetaxel	Pleural effusion, pulmonary infiltrates
Doxorubicin	Hypersensitivity infusion-related pulmonary reactions
Etoposide	Hypersensitivity infusion-related pulmonary reactions
Fludarabine	Dyspnea, cough and rare interstitial pulmonary infiltrations
Gefitinib	Interstitial lung disease
Gemcitabine	Dyspnea and rare parenchymal lung disease
Gemtuzumab ozogamicin	Hypersensitivity infusion-related pulmonary reactions
Imatinib mesylate	Fluid retention leading to pleural effusion, edema and ascites
Interleukin 2	Pulmonary edema
Melphalan	Interstitial pneumonitis
Methotrexate	Interstitial pneumonitis
Mitomycin	Interstitial pneumonitis
Mitoxantrone	Interstitial pneumonitis
Oprelvekin (Interleukin 11)	Edema, resolves within days of drug cessation with diuretics
Oxaliplatin	Hypersensitivity infusion-related pulmonary reactions
Paclitaxel	Hypersensitivity pneumonitis
Rituximab	Hypersensitivity infusion-related pulmonary reactions
Thiotepa	Interstitial pneumonitis
Trastuzumab	Hypersensitivity infusion-related pulmonary reactions
Vinorelbine tartrate	Rare but serious acute dyspnea and bronchospasm

XIII. SYNDROME OF INAPPROPRIATE ANTIDIURETIC HORMONE SECRETION (SIADH). SIADH is a manifestation of water intoxication, which, in some circumstances, can escalate to a critical situation if sodium level drops (below 105 mEq/L). The syndrome results in decreased water excretion, hyponatremia, hypervolemia, and hypoosmolality due to an inappropriate antidiuretic secretion. Treatment includes fluid restriction, diuresis, and hypertonic saline infusion. Most common cytotoxic agents that pose a threat are bortezomib, cisplatin, cyclophosphamide, ifosfamide, melphalan, and the vinca alkaloids.

XIV. NEPHROTOXICITY. Patients receiving IFN and bevacizumab are screened for proteinuria. With IL-2 infusions, monitoring for hypotension, cardiac, and intravascular volume is crucial to prevent nephrotoxicity and subsequently prerenal azotemia.

Renal dysfunction (creatinine clearance less than 60 mL/minute) poses a need for dose reduction in the following cytotoxic agents:
- MTX
- Cisplatin
- Carboplatin
- Bleomycin
- Etoposide
- Hydroxyurea
- Deoxycoformycin
- Fludarabine
- Cladribine
- Topotecan

Common chemotherapeutic and targeted agents causing nephrotoxicity:
- Carmustine (with cumulative doses)
- Cisplatin
- IL-2
- Lomustine (with cumulative doses)
- MTX (with high-dose therapy)

XV. HEPATOTOXICITY. Hepatic function must be assessed before and during chemotherapeutic administration as most of these agents are metabolized by the liver. Preexisting liver disease disrupts metabolism of the toxic agents resulting in extrahepatic toxicity to other organs and to the hematopoietic system. Not all toxicities are dose dependent but rather cause a hypersensitivity or metabolic response. A distinction must be analyzed in the symptomatic patient and when liver enzymes are elevated to discern causes including liver disease, hypersensitivity, concurrent medications, and alcohol intake. Elevation of particular liver enzymes may assist in diagnosis but a true distinction is sometimes difficult. For patients undergoing cytotoxic treatment, although there are few available guidelines to follow, there are standardized criteria developed by the National Cancer Institute to assist in grading liver function test (LFT) abnormalities. In addition to LFTs, complete blood chemistry, complete blood count, and prothrombin time should be monitored. Hepatotoxicity with cytotoxic therapy varies based on intrinsic and extrinsic factors and therefore should be monitored regardless of agent utilized in treatment.

Risk factors for developing hepatic dysfunction include the following:
- History of alcohol abuse with or without cirrhosis or concomitant alcohol use during cytotoxic treatment
- Elderly
- Prior irradiation to the liver or right upper abdominal quadrant
- Use of illicit drugs before or during treatment
- Current or prior liver tumor involvement
- Prior or current liver infection
- Prior hepatic damage
- History of transplant (peripheral blood stem cell or marrow, liver, kidney)
- Concurrent use of medications metabolized by the liver including narcotics and noncytotoxic medications

Clinical presentation of hepatic dysfunction with preexisting disease or during cytotoxic treatment include the following:

- Hepatosplenomegaly
- Portal hypertension
- Anorexia or developing weight loss
- Onset of right upper quadrant pain
- Nausea and/or emesis
- Ascites
- Pruritus
- Encephalopathy
- Bruising and/or active bleeding
- Fatigue
- Elevated transaminases
- Prolonged prothrombin times
- Diarrhea, dehydration
- Dyspepsia
- Clay-colored stools, darkened urine

Chemotherapeutic agents requiring dose modification with liver disease:

Amasacrine	5-Flouracil
Cytarabine	Ifosfamide
Cyclophosphamide	Irinotecan
Daunorubicin	Mitoxantrone
Dactinomycin	Paclitaxel
Docetaxel	Procarbazine
Doxorubicin	Vincristine
Etoposide	Vinorelbine

XVI. SEXUAL DYSFUNCTION. Alterations occur in sexual well-being, function and reproduction in men and women receiving both chemotherapeutic and hormonal treatments. Careful counseling should not only precede treatment with comprehensive education of possible and known side effects with each agent to be administered, but also, an ongoing open communication with subsequent visits should ensue.

Chemotherapy and hormonal agents can affect gonadal function leading to temporary or permanent dysfunction. In women, ovarian suppression results in side effects of hot flashes, vaginal dryness, dyspareunia, vaginal infections, and irregular menses. Permanent menopause brought on by particular agents (alkylating regimens) can result in short-term hot flashes, depression, and ultimately result in urogenital atrophy from estrogen deficiency. Urogenital atrophy in women, erectile dysfunction in men and overall loss of sexual libido can affect sexual desire. Estrogen deficiency in the vaginal vault results in urogenital atrophy, dryness, and subsequent pain during sexual activity. Vaginal dryness and resulting pain can be eased with the use of a water-based lubricant. Hormonal therapy received by men may result in gynecomastia.

Infertility risk increases with particular agents for males and females; therefore, ovum and sperm banking should be discussed before receiving treatment. However, birth control options and consequences of birth defects should be addressed with both genders as the reproductive ability may exist throughout treatment and afterwards.

Sexuality for both genders is not only affected by the drugs given and the disease itself, but also the psychological impact of the diagnosis and the self-image consequences. A referral to a gynecologist or counselor should be offered to patients to address their sexual feelings and treatment available (Table 36.12).

XVII. OCULAR TOXICITY. Cytotoxic agents are indirectly and directly related to ocular toxicities. Loss of eyelashes with particular agents poses an infection risk to the neutropenic patient by removing a barrier to the eye. Cytotoxic agents are secreted

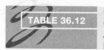

| TABLE 36.12 | Common Hormonal and Chemotherapeutic Treatments Affecting Sexual and Reproductive Functioning | |

Treatment	Effect
Hormonal treatments	
Androgens	Masculine traits
Antiandrogens	Impotence, decreased sexual desire
Estrogens	Gynecomastia
Antiestrogens	Gynecomastia
Alkylating agents and antimetabolites	Amenorrhea, azoospermia, oligospermia
Vinblastine	Decreased libido, erectile dysfunction, ovarian dysfunction
Vincristine	Erectile dysfunction

in fluids including tears, causing irritation and excessive tearing. Also, the vasculature to the eye can be affected by cytotoxic and targeted agents affecting vision.

Chemotherapeutic and targeted Agents associated with ocular toxicities.

- Alkylating agents
- Antimetabolites
- Biologics
  Granulocyte-colony and macrophage stimulating factors (G-CSF/GM-CSF) IFNs, IL-2, retinoids
- Cytotoxic antibiotics
- Taxanes
- Tamoxifen
- Vinca alkaloids

XVIII. SECOND PRIMARY MALIGNANCIES. Chemotherapeutic (or combined, i.e., irradiation) modalities used to treat primary malignancies can induce liquid and solid secondary malignancies months to years later. Debate ensues whether the secondary malignancy is manifested from the primary treatment received or from the initial (treated) diagnosis. The alkylating agents, anthracyclines, and epipodophyllotoxins are associated with the development of secondary leukemias with the most common diagnosis of acute nonlymphocytic leukemia. Therefore, patients with a primary diagnosis receiving these agents are at risk.

Common **primary diagnosis receiving chemotherapeutic agents developing second primary malignancies:**

- Bone marrow transplant patients receiving chemotherapy with total body irradiation
- Hodgkin's disease
- Lymphoma
- Testicular cancer
- Pediatric cancers due to length of expected survival

Suggested Readings

Hicklin DJ, Ellis LM. Rose of the vascular endothelial growth factor pathway in tumor growth and angiogenesis. *J Clin Oncol* 2005;23:1011.

Homes Gobel B. Chemotherapy-induced hypersensitivity reactions. *Oncol Nurs Forum* 2005;32(5):1027–1042.

Itano JK, Taoka KN. *Core curriculum for oncology nursing*, 4th ed. St. Louis: Elsevier Science, WB Saunders, 2005.

Lynch MP. *Essentials of oncology care*. NewYork: Professional Publishing Group, Ltd, 2005.

Saltz LB. Understanding and managing chemotherapy-induced diarrhea. *Support Oncol* 2003;1(1):35–47.

Schrijvers DL. Extravasation: a dreaded complication of chemotherapy. *Ann Oncol* 2003;14(*Suppl 3*):iii26–iii30.

Smith RJ, Khatcheressian J, Lyman GH, et al. 2006 update of recommendations for the use of white blood cell growth factors: an evidence – based clinical practice guideline. *J Clin Oncol* 2006;24:1–19.

Sykes NP. The pathogenesis of constipation. *Support Oncol* 2006;4(5):213–218.

Wilkes GM, Barton-Burke M, eds. *2006 oncology nursing drug handbook*. Boston: Jones and Bartlett Publishers, 2006.

Yarbro CH, Frogge MH, Goodman M, eds. *Cancer symptom management*, 3rd ed. Boston: Jones and Bartlett Publishers, 2004.

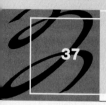

GROWTH FACTOR SUPPORT IN ONCOLOGY
37
Rama Suresh

I. INTRODUCTION. Hematopoiesis is the process of production of circulating blood cells in the bone marrow. The proliferation and differentiation of the pluripotent stem cell to the myeloid and the lymphoid progenitors and the further differentiation of those to the mature circulating blood cells involves complex interaction of the stem cells, bone marrow stromal cells, and cytokines. The cytokines also activate the mature hematopoietic cells. The action, affected cell lines, and chromosomal location of these cytokines, otherwise called hematopoietic growth factors, have been identified to some extent and comprise a field of ongoing research.

II. MYELOID GROWTH FACTORS

A. Granulocyte colony-stimulating factor (G-CSF)

1. **Endogenous G-CSF.** This is a lineage-specific growth factor located on chromosome 17 that promotes the maturation of granulocyte colony-forming unit to polymorphonuclear leukocyte and also enhances neutrophil function. It is a 174–amino acid glycoprotein and is produced by monocytes, fibroblasts, and endothelial cells. Mice that lack G-CSF have chronic neutropenia, reduced bone marrow myeloid precursors and have impaired ability to increase neutrophil count in response to infections (*Blood* 1994;84(6):1737–1746). The serum G-CSF level normally ranges from 20 to 100 pg/mL. Fever, neutropenia, gram-negative and fungal infections, and impaired kidney function and liver function lead to increase in G-CSF levels.

2. **Recombinant preparations (rHuG-CSF).** Three formulations of recombinant G-CSF are available. Filgrastim (Neupogen) and pegfilgrastim (Neulasta) are 175–amino acid glycoproteins, synthesized in *E. coli* expression system and available in the United States. Lenograstim synthesized from Chinese hamster ovary cells is analogous to the 174–amino acid glycoprotein but is not available in the United States. Pegfilgrastim (Neulasta), which is a covalent conjugate of filgrastim and monomethoxypolyethylene glycol, has a prolonged half life. The half life of filgrastim is 3.5 hours and that of pegfilgrastim is 15 to 80 hours. Filgrastim and pegfilgrastim have a similar mechanism of action in that they stimulate the production of neutrophils and activate the mature neutrophils.

3. **Recommended dose.** The recommended dose of filgrastim is 5 μg/kg/day administered subcutaneously for all situations except peripheral blood stem cell (PBSC) mobilization where the dose of 10 μg/kg/day is preferable. It can be started only 24 hours after administering chemotherapy and is discontinued once the absolute neutrophil count (ANC) exceeds 10,000/mm³following the chemotherapy-induced nadir. It should not be administered in the period 24 hours before chemotherapy. In the setting of high-dose therapy and autologous stem cell rescue, G-CSF can be given between 24 and 120 hours after administration of high-dose therapy. G-CSF should be continued till reaching an ANC of 2 × 10^9 to 3 × 10^9/dL.

Pegfilgrastim should be given once subcutaneously, at a dose of 6 mg, 24 hours after the completion of chemotherapy and 14 days before the next dose of chemotherapy. The safety and efficacy of this drug in a dose-dense chemotherapy setting is not yet fully established. Pegfilgrastim is currently not indicated for stem cell mobilization (*J Clin Oncol* 2006;24(19):4451). Dosage does not have to be adjusted for kidney dysfunction.

4. **Adverse effects.** Generally adverse effects are mild, consisting primarily of bone pain, myalgias, and arthralgias. In patients with sickle cell disease, it can trigger sickle cell crisis and multiorgan failure (*Blood* 2001;97:3998–3999). A flare of metastatic bone lesions and increased tracer uptake in the axial skeleton could be seen in bone scans after administration of recombinant G-CSF. There could be transient neutropenia with intravenous injections and transient dyspnea with pulmonary infiltrates on chest radiograph (CXR). In patients receiving chronic treatment with G-CSF, benign splenomegaly may arise, secondary to extramedullary hematopoiesis. Cases of splenic rupture and adult respiratory distress syndrome (ARDS) have been reported with the use of pegfilgrastim. Allergic reaction and injection-site rash can occur with either drug.

B. **Granulocyte–macrophage colony-stimulating factor (GM-CSF)**

1. **Endogenous GM-CSF.** This is a growth factor that broadly stimulates hemato-poiesis as it increases the production of all types of leukocytes including neutrophils, lymphocytes, eosinophils, and monocytes and acts directly on mega-karyocyte development. It also enhances neutrophil and monocyte/macrophage function. It plays a greater role in the local inflammatory response than inducing proliferation and differentiation of cell lines. GM-CSF knock-out mice are not neutropenic but they develop pulmonary alveolar proteinosis and pneumonia. GM-CSF is not detected in the serum of humans even in infected states. It is a 127–amino acid glycoprotein and is secreted by a variety of cells including T lymphocytes, macrophages, monocytes, endothelial cells, smooth muscle cells, and fibroblast cells. The gene is located on chromosome 5.

2. **Recombinant granulocyte–macrophage colony-stimulating factor (rHuGM-CSF).** Among the three preparations of rHuGM-CSF that have been devised (Sargramostim, Regramostim and Molgramostim), sargramostim produced using yeast is available in the United States as Leukine. Administration of rHuGM-CSF resulted in an increase in peripheral blood neutrophils, eosinophils, monocytes, and macrophages. It also stimulated the functional activity of these cells. The half life is 2 hours. Sargramostim is a 127–amino acid glycoprotein that differs from natural GM-CSF by substitution of leucine at position 23, and the carbohydrate moiety may be different.

3. **Recommended dose.** A dose of 250 μg/m^2/day of GM-CSF should be used for all settings. Subcutaneous dosing is preferred, although intravenous dosing is safe if required. GM-CSF may be administered 24 to 72 hours after chemotherapy and discontinued once the ANC has recovered to 10,000/mm^3 or the ANC is more than 1,500/mm^3 for 3 days.

4. **Adverse effects.** When administered intravenously, immediate but transient neutropenia may occur. The common adverse effects include dyspnea, headache, diarrhea, fever, myalgias, arthralgias and injection-site reactions. Some patients may develop tachycardia, hypotension, flushing, and syncope with the first dose. With higher doses, rarely, weight gain, pericarditis, pleuritis, and capillary leak syndrome have been reported. Higher incidence of fever has been reported with GM-CSF as compared to G-CSF and combination of G-CSF/GM-CSF in bone marrow transplant settings (*J Clin Oncol* 2000;18:3558–3585). Rare patients may have anaphylaxis and arrhythmias.

C. **Clinical applications of myeloid growth factors.** The following recommendations are based on the 2005 American Society of Clinical Oncology (ASCO) clinical practice guidelines for the use of colony-stimulating factors (CSFs) (*J Clin Oncol* 2006:4451).

1. **Primary prophylaxis is** recommended for the prevention of febrile neutropenia (FN) in patients with high risk (20% or more) of FN on the basis of age, medical history, disease characteristics, and myelotoxicity of the chemothera-peutic regimen. For dose-dense regimens, CSFs are required and recommended. In deciding on the use of prophylactic CSF, one should consider not only the optimal chemotherapeutic regimen but also the individual patient risk factors and intention of treatment (curative vs. palliative). It is appropriate to use this in patients who are undergoing treatment for cure to prevent dose reduction

and delays. In patients with a high risk for chemotherapy-induced infectious complications, such as age above 65 years, poor performance status, extensive previous treatment, bone marrow involvement by cancer, poor nutritional status, open wounds, and other serious comorbidities, primary prophylaxis can be used even with regimens where the risk for FN is less than 20%.

2. **Secondary prophylaxis.** For patients who experienced a neutropenic complication from an earlier cycle of chemotherapy (for which primary prophylaxis was not received), in which a reduced dose may have compromised disease-free or overall survival or treatment outcome, secondary prophylaxis is recommended. In other patients it is appropriate to consider dose delay and dose reduction.

3. **Afebrile neutropenia.** CSFs should not be used for afebrile patients with neutropenia routinely.

4. **Febrile neutropenia.** CSFs should not be routinely used as adjunctive treatment for patients with fever and neutropenia. However, in FN patients with a high risk for infection associated complications such as prolonged neutropenia, uncontrolled primary disease, pneumonia, hypotension, multiorgan dysfunction, invasive fungal infection, and in patients older than 65, use of CSFs is recommended.

5. **To allow dose-dense/dose-intense regimens.** Dose-dense/dose-intense regimens have been shown to increase survival in some situations such as node-positive breast cancer, non-Hodgkin's lymphoma, and small cell lung cancer. In those situations, it is appropriate to use CSFs to enable giving dose-dense/dose-intense chemotherapy.

6. **Bone marrow transplant.** As per the current standard of care, CSFs can be used to mobilize PBSCs often in conjunction with chemotherapy and after autologous but not allogenic PBSC transplant.

7. **Acute myeloid leukemia.** Several studies have shown that CSF administration can produce a modest decrease in the duration of neutropenia when begun shortly after completion of the initial induction chemotherapy. Beneficial effects on the endpoints such as duration of hospitalization and incidence of severe infections have been variable. No unfavorable impact has been reported on remission rate, remission duration, or survival. Patients older than 55 are likely to be benefited. Use of CSF for priming effects is not recommended. CSFs can be recommended after the completion of consolidation chemotherapy because of the potential to decrease the incidence of infection. CSFs should be used judiciously or not at all in patients with refractory or relapsed myeloid leukemia.

8. **Acute lymphoid leukemia.** The use of G-CSF for children with acute lymphoid leukemia (ALL) was associated with small benefits in days of antibiotics or in-hospital days, although with small additional costs. For adults, cost estimates have not been reported. G-CSF can be given with continued steroid/antimetabolite therapy without increasing the risk of myelosuppression.

9. **Myelodysplastic syndromes.** Although CSFs can increase ANC, there is no data supporting long-term continuous use. Intermittent administration may be considered in the subset of patients with severe neutropenia and recurrent infection.

10. **Concomitant chemoradiotherapy.** CSFs should be avoided in patients receiving concomitant chemotherapy and radiation therapy, particularly involving the mediastinum. It can be considered in patients receiving radiation therapy alone if prolonged delays secondary to neutropenia are expected.

III. ERYTHROID GROWTH FACTORS

A. Erythropoietin (EPO)

1. **Endogenous erythropoietin (EPO).** This is a lineage-specific growth factor located on chromosome 7 and it stimulates the proliferation and maturation of erythroid colony-forming units (CFU-E) and is essential for the terminal maturation of the erythroid cells. Knock-out mice form erythroid blast-forming unit (BFU-E) and CFU-E but fail to produce mature erythrocytes. Several factors including Steel factor, IL-3, GM-CSF, and activin work synergistically with EPO in stimulating erythropoiesis. It is a 193–amino acid protein produced in the kidney. The level of oxyhemoglobin and the rate of delivery of oxygen to

the tissues are the main regulators of erythropoiesis. Normally EPO levels in the serum range from 4 to 30 U/L. In anemic patients with hematocrit (Hct) levels less than 35%, levels of EPO increase up to 1,000 folds.

2. **Recombinant erythropoietin (rHuEPO).** There are three preparations of recombinant EPO, produced in Chinese hamster ovary cells—epoetin alpha, darbepoetin alpha and epoetin beta. Only epoetin alfa (Epogen and Procrit) and darbepoetin alfa (Aranesp) are available in the United States. Darbepoetin alpha is closely related to EPO and is a 165–amino acid protein that differs from recombinant human EPO in containing five N-linked oligosaccharide chains, whereas recombinant human EPO contains three chains. The two additional N-glycosylation sites result from amino acid substitutions in the EPO peptide backbone. These drugs stimulate the division and differentiation of committed progenitor cells. There is a dose–response relationship with this effect. The half life of epoetin alfa is 4 to 13 hours in patients with renal failure and 20% shorter in healthy volunteers. The half life of darbepoetin is longer (49 hours) when given subcutaneously.

3. **Recommended dose.** Subcutaneous route is preferred over intravenous route because of the less amount of drug required. It is important to use the lowest dose of these drugs that will gradually increase the hemoglobin concentration to the lowest level sufficient to avoid the need for RBC transfusion and not to exceed 12 g/dl.

   The recommended starting dose of epoetin is 150 U/kg thrice weekly for 8 weeks with possible increase in dose level to 300U/kg thrice weekly for an additional 4 to 8 weeks in those who do not respond to the initial dose. An alternative weekly dosing regimen (40,000 U/week) based on common clinical practice may be considered, although it is not supported well by clinical data. Dose escalation to 60,000 U/week may also be considered in patients who do not respond to the initial dose.

   As with epoetin, the preferred route is subcutaneous for darbepoetin. The recommended starting dose for darbepoetin alpha administered weekly is 2.25 μg/kg and in those who do not respond adequately, the dose should be increased to 4.5 μg/kg. For the every 2-week regimen, the initial dose is 200 μg and if there is inadequate response, the dose can be increased to 300 μg every 2 weeks. For the every 3 week regimen, the dose is 500 μg/week given every 3 weeks.

   If the rate of hemoglobin increase is more than 1 g/dl in 2 week period the dose of epoetin should be decreased by 25% and the dose of darboepoetin should be decreased by 40%.

   If the rise in hemoglobin is less than 1 g/dL at 6 to 8 weeks of treatment, evaluation for iron deficiency and tumor progression should be done and the discontinuation of EPO should be considered.

   Once the hemoglobin level is ≥ 12 g/dl, the dose of EPO should be withheld and then restarted when the hemoglobin falls to 11 g/dl.

   Darbepoetin alfa every 2 weeks has been compared to epoetin alfa every week in patients with chemotherapy-induced anemia and found to have comparable efficacy. Darbepoetin alfa dosage schedule allows the convenience of synchronizing the administration of the drug while the patient is in the clinic to receive chemotherapy.

4. **Clinical indications.** In cancer patients with non-myeloid malignancies EPO is indicated for the treatment of anemia due to the effect of concomitantly administered chemotherapy. It is currently not FDA approved to be used in the treatment of anemia due to cancer and myelodysplastic syndrome. The use of these drugs in anemia due to cancer and myelodysplastic syndrome is under debate.

5. **Adverse effects.** A rare but serious adverse event is antibody-mediated pure red cell aplasia (PRCA) and severe anemia with epoetin alfa and darbepoetin. Patients who have a loss of response should be evaluated for this and these drugs should not be given to patients with PRCA. The more likely adverse effects include edema, high blood pressure, fever, headache, insomnia, rash, nausea, vomiting,

injection-site reaction, arthralgia, myalgias, fatigue, cough, and dyspnea. Chest pain, arrhythmia, diarrhea, seizure, and thromboembolic events are less likely. Very rarely allergic reactions and flu-like syndrome are noticed. Iron deficiency is quite common because of the consumption of available stores and decline in transfusion rate.

As of March 2007, there are new black box warnings with erythropoiesis stimulating agents. They can increase the risk of thromboembolic events, serious cardiovascular events and death when administered to target hemoglobin greater than 12 g/dl. In cancer patient use of ESAs shortened time to tumor progression in patients with advanced head and neck cancer receiving radiation therapy and shortened overall survival in patients with metastatic breast cancer receiving chemotherapy, when administered to target hemoglobin greater than 12 g/dl. Antithrombotic prophylaxis should strongly be considered when Epogen/Procrit is used pre-operatively to reduce allogeneic red blood cell transfusions. Aranesp is not approved for this indication.

IV. PLATELET AND MEGAKARYOCYTIC GROWTH FACTORS

A. Thrombopoietin (TPO)

1. **Endogenous TPO.** This is a lineage-specific growth factor that amplifies the basal production of megakaryocytes and platelets and the gene is located in chromosome 3. Knock-out mice model shows that the megakaryocyte and platelet levels are reduced by more than 80% but the animals are healthy and do not bleed (*J Exp Med* 1996;182:651–656). It was discovered in 1994 and is otherwise called c-Mpl ligand, megakaryocyte growth and development factor, and megapoietin. The receptor for TPO is called *c-Mpl*. TPO is mainly produced in the liver and to some extent is also produced in the kidney and bone marrow. TPO is a polypeptide of 353 amino acids, with an amino terminal end responsible for receptor binding, and has 46% sequence similarity to the EPO protein and a carboxyl end, which increases the bioavailability of the protein, with no homology to any known proteins. Data from several studies suggest that plasma levels of TPO are regulated through circulating platelet numbers by binding to platelet TPO receptors (*Transfusion* 2002;42:321–327). Intermittent platelet transfusions in the thrombocytopenic patient may actually blunt the TPO response (*N Engl J Med* 1998;339:746–754).

2. **Recombinant thrombopoietin (rHuTPO).** Two forms of recombinant human TPO are currently under clinical trials. One is a full-length glycosylated molecule developed in CHO cells. The second is a nonglycosylated, 163–amino acid recombinant human TPO developed in *Escherichia coli* and conjugated to polyethylene glycol (PEG-rHuMGDF). Both are yet to be approved by the U.S. Food and Drug Administration (FDA) and made available for commercial use.

B. Oprelvekin (Neumega).
Interleukin (IL)-11 is a thrombopoietic growth factor that directly stimulates the proliferation of hematopoietic stem cells and the megakaryocyte progenitor cells and induces megakaryocyte maturation resulting in increased platelet production. Oprelvekin, the active ingredient in Neumega is produced in *E. coli*. The polypeptide is 177 amino acids in length and differs from the native one in lacking proline. It is FDA approved for use in chemotherapy-induced thrombocytopenia. The dose is 50 µg/kg/day given subcutaneously starting 24 hours after chemotherapy, until the post nadir platelet count is more than 50,000/µL. The most common side effects associated with Oprelvekin treatment included peripheral edema, dyspnea, tachycardia, atrial arrhythmia, papilledema and conjunctival redness.

V. FUTURE DIRECTIONS.
There are other hematopoietic growth factors in development. EPO is also being studied for its nonhematologic activity on brain and heart tissue. A better understanding of the stem cell trafficking will help in the manipulation of these events. Small molecules/peptides with greater affinity to the specific receptors are being developed.

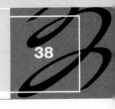

TRANSFUSION MEDICINE

Joshua Field, Douglas Lublin, and George Despotis

38

I. RED BLOOD CELLS (RBCs). The therapeutic goal of a blood transfusion is to increase oxygen delivery according to the physiologic need of the recipient. It is difficult to determine an appropriate transfusion threshold, however, because the benefits of blood are hard to define and measure. In a multi-institutional Canadian study by Hebert et al., 418 critical care patients were to receive red cell transfusions when the hemoglobin (Hgb) level decreased to less than 7 g/dL, with Hgb maintenance in the range of 7 to 9 g/dL, and 420 patients were to receive transfusions when the Hgb was less than 10 g/dL, with Hgb levels maintained in the range of 10 to 12 g/dL. The 30-day mortality rates were not different between the two groups (18.7% vs. 23.3%; $p = 0.11$), indicating that a transfusion threshold as low as 7 g/dL is as safe as a higher transfusion threshold of 10 g/dL in critical care patients without active end-organ ischemia. An important confounding factor in the efficacy of red cell transfusions involves the variable capacity of red cell units to enhance or provide tissue oxygenation based on 2,3-diphosphoglycerate (DPG) levels, which vary with the age of the red cell units. Clearly, more data are needed to determine when transfusion in this setting is beneficial.

Data on morbidity also are unclear. Silent perioperative myocardial ischemia has been observed in patients undergoing noncardiac as well as cardiac surgery. Hemoglobin levels in the range of 6 to 10 g/dL as well as clinical signs or indicators of end-organ ischemia other than [Hgb] may identify patients who may benefit from blood transfusion. Accordingly, elderly patients undergoing elective, noncardiac surgery have been shown to be at risk for intraoperative or postoperative myocardial ischemia with hematocrits less than 28%, particularly in the presence of tachycardia. In the absence of a physiologic need (i.e., no evidence of end-organ ischemia) in a stable, nonbleeding patient, correction of anemia may not be indicated and may, in fact, predispose patients to adverse outcomes.

Guidelines for blood transfusion have been issued by several organizations including a National Institutes of Health consensus conference on perioperative transfusion of red cells, the American College of Physicians, the American Society of Anesthesiologists, and the Canadian Medical Association. These guidelines consistently recommend that blood should not be transfused on a prophylactic basis and suggest that in patients who are not critically ill, a Hgb level of 6 to 8 g/dL is well tolerated and acceptable. Adherence to these guidelines has raised questions about whether transfusion is now underused. A Hgb level of 8 g/dL seems an appropriate threshold for transfusion in surgical patients with no risk factors for critical or target end-organ) ischemia, whereas a threshold of 10 g/dL may be more appropriate for patients who are considered at risk. However, prophylactic transfusion of blood (i.e., in anticipation of blood loss) cannot be endorsed, particularly because studies have found an association between transfusion and less favorable outcomes in critically ill patients. It is unlikely that one specific hemoglobin value can be used as a universal threshold for transfusion.

II. TRANSFUSION THERAPY

A. General considerations. The transfusion of blood or blood components has inherent risks, summarized in Table 38.1. Informed consent (a clear explanation of relative benefits, risks, and alternatives regarding the transfusion to the patient) is mandatory, and is accompanied in many institutions by a consent form that documents the conversation and patient acceptance. In the elective transfusion setting, alternatives to blood transfusion may include autologous or directed (from a donor known to and selected by the patient) blood. In addition, patients should

445

TABLE 38.1   **Risks with Blood Transfusion**

Risk factor	Frequency/unit transfused
Infection	
Hepatitis A	1/1,000,000
Hepatitis B	1/30,000 to 1/250,000
Hepatitis C[a]	1/1,600,000
HIV[a]	1/2,100,000
HTLV types I and II	1/250,000 to 1/2,000,000
Parvovirus	1/10,000
Bacterial Contamination	
Platelets	1/12,000
Red cells	1/500,000
Acute hemolytic reaction	1/250,000 to 1/1,000,000
Delayed hemolytic reaction	1/1,000
Transfusion-related acute lung injury	1/5,000

Modified from Goodnough LT, Brecher ME, Kanter MH, et al. Transfusion medicine, part I: blood transfusion. *N Engl J Med* 1999;340:438–447, with permission. HIV, human immunodeficiency virus; HTLV, human T-cell leukemia virus.
[a]Data from Busch MP, Kleinman SH, Nemo GJ, et al. Current and emerging infectious risks of blood transfusions. *JAMA* 2003;289:959–962.

be evaluated with respect to uncovering treatable anemias (e.g., iron, folate, B$_{12}$, erythropoietin) before initiating blood transfusion.

Risks, side effects, and indications of blood and blood products are available in the Circular of Information for Blood and Blood Products, issued jointly by the American Red Cross, America's Blood Centers, and the American Association of Blood Banks (AABB) under the direction of the U.S. Food and Drug Administration (FDA), and can be obtained from hospital transfusion services. Administration of blood must be preceded by confirmation that three different and specific identifiers (such as name, birth date, and hospital number or social security number), match between the patient and the blood-unit label, immediately before initiating infusion of the blood unit. The blood must be infused through a dedicated intravenous line with no other concurrent drugs or fluids, except 0.9% NaCl (normal saline). Vital signs are recorded immediately before transfusion and within 5 to 10 minutes after starting; the patient is also carefully monitored, and at regular intervals (e.g., hourly) thereafter. Each blood unit should be administered within 4 hours. A standard macroaggregate filter (170 to 260 μm) is used to prevent infusion of fibrin, cell clumps, and debris.

An order for blood type and screen involves testing the patient's RBCs for the A, B, and D (Rh) antigens whereas the antibody screen involves testing the serum for the presence of alloantibody against other (minor) RBC antigens. The frequency of detecting such alloantibodies varies between patient populations (e.g., 0.5% of the general population vs. 2% of hospitalized patients vs. 8% of hospitalized surgical patients), and is related to previous exposure from pregnancy or transfusion. A cross-match order leads to *in vitro* testing of the patient's serum against donor RBCs to confirm compatibility between the blood unit selected and the patient.

B. Complications of transfusion

1. **The Transfusion Medicine Service provides distinct criteria with respect to transfusion reactions** to alert medical personnel regarding potential problems with the transfusion. These criteria include a temperature elevation of greater than 1°C; the appearance of symptoms (e.g., shortness of breath, nausea/vomiting, pruritus, pain at infusion site, back pain, palpitations); or signs (changes in vital signs, rash, hives, edema, or stridor) indicating a change in the

patient's clinical status. When a transfusion reaction is considered, the transfusion is stopped immediately, and a physician is notified to assess the patient's status. The transfusion is terminated if there is a significant change in the patient's clinical status during the transfusion. At that time, the blood bag, patient blood samples, and urine are sent to the blood bank, where patient and blood-unit identification are reverified; blood group and antibody screen are repeated; serum and urine are inspected for signs of hemolysis; and the residual contents of the blood bag are cultured. The patient's blood should be drawn for blood culture if fever or blood pressure changes occurred during the transfusion.

2. **Nonhemolytic febrile-associated transfusion reactions (FATRs)** are characterized by fever and accompanied variably by chills, pruritus, rash, or hives. They occur in 0.5% to 2% of RBC transfusions and in 8% to 30% of platelet transfusions. Within certain populations such as multiparous women and frequently (or chronically) transfused patients, the prevalence can be higher. These reactions are generally mild and occur during the latter part of the transfusion. The potential mechanisms involve either antibodies against donor leukocyte antigens and/or donor plasma proteins, soluble cytokines, (interleukins, tumor necrosis factor), or both. Symptoms are treated with acetaminophen (650 mg) for fever and diphenhydramine (25 to 75 mg), p.o. or i.v. for more significant allergic reactions or when the patient is NPO. Occasionally, rigors and chills may require meperidine (25 to 50 mg i.v.). Epinephrine and glucocorticoids are utilized infrequently for severe allergic reactions (e.g., 1:300 to 1:1,000). The transfusion may be continued at the discretion of the physician, particularly in patients with prolonged transfusions with mild reactions. Some patients may benefit from prophylactic treatment shortly before transfusion, to prevent or attenuate reactions. Bedside leukodepletion filters can be utilized for patients with a history of two or more febrile reactions but prevent only 50% of reactions, because they affect only those due to antibodies against leukocytes. However, severe hypotension can occur in susceptible patients (e.g., patients on angiotensin-converting enzyme [ACE] inhibitors) and is secondary to the hemodynamic effects of bradykinin, which is released due to the filtration process and sustained because of reduced clearance (i.e., as related to use of ACE inhibitors). The clinical manifestations include vital sign instability, particularly, hypotension. Bedside leukodepletion filters should therefore be avoided in patients with cardiovascular compromise and in those treated with ACE inhibitors.

   Severe anaphylactic reactions have been observed (i.e., generally with the first or second transfusion) in patients with immunoglobulin A (IgA) deficiency who have anti-IgA antibodies and receive blood products (all of which contain IgA).

3. **Acute hemolytic transfusion reactions are caused** by preformed antibodies (IgM or IgG antibodies against A or B antigens, or complement-fixing IgG antibodies against minor RBC antigens, such as Kidd) in the patient and are characterized by complement-mediated intravascular hemolysis subsequent to initiation of the transfusion. Hypotension, fever, nausea/vomiting, and back and/or chest pain may develop, along with hemoglobinuria, renal failure, and disseminated intravascular coagulation (DIC). If such a reaction is suspected, the transfusion should be immediately terminated. Treatment includes resuscitative measures, support of intravascular volume, and preservation of renal function with i.v. hydration, along with alkalinization of urine (i.e. sodium bicarbonate therapy).

4. **Delayed transfusion reactions** are usually detected 7 to 21 days after RBC transfusion. They are related to a primary or anamnestic IgG response on exposure to minor RBC antigens, the latter seen particularly in patients previously exposed to such antigens through pregnancy or previous blood transfusion. Clinical manifestations may include icterus or jaundice (due to accelerated intravascular RBC destruction), a failure to increase Hgb (1 g/dL/unit) levels after RBC transfusion, or most commonly through serologic evidence (i.e., the appearance of a new alloantibody on antibody screen before subsequent

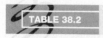

TABLE 38.2	Indications for Leukocyte-Reduced Blood Components

Established indications
    Prevention of recurrent nonhemolytic febrile transfusion reactions to red blood cell transfusions
    Prevention or delay of alloimmunization to leukocyte antigens in select patients who are candidates for transplantation or transfusion on a long-term basis
Indications under review
    Prevention of the platelet-refractory state caused by alloimmunization
    Prevention of recurrent febrile reactions during platelet transfusions
    Prevention of cytomegalovirus transmission by cellular blood components
Not indicated for
    Prevention of transfusion-associated graft-versus-host disease
    Prevention of transfusion-related acute lung injury due to the passive administration of anti-leukocyte antibody
    Patients who are expected to have only limited transfusion exposure
    Acellular blood components (fresh frozen plasma, cryoprecipitate)

From Lane TA, Anderson KC, Goodnough LT, et al. Leukocyte reduction in blood component therapy. *Ann Intern Med* 1992;117:151–162, with permission.

transfusion). Occasionally the reactions can be clinically severe, with renal impairment and even reported deaths (Table 38.2). Treatment in these cases is the same as for acute reactions. Patients should be informed that they have an allergy (e.g., antibody to non-ABO antigens) to prevent subsequent delayed hemolytic transfusion reactions since many of these antibodies (50%) fade within 3 to 6 months.

5. **Transfusion-related acute lung injury (TRALI)** is an under-recognized and serious reaction to transfusion often due to an anti–human leukocyte antigen (HLA) or antineutrophil antibody from a donor (usually a multiparous woman) that reacts to the corresponding antigen on recipient leukocytes. Alternatively, accumulation of lipids or cytokines in the plasma of stored blood products has also been implicated as a cause of TRALI, especially from platelet units. TRALI is now the leading cause of transfusion-related mortality in the United States, exceeding the number of deaths due to transfusion of ABO-incompatible or bacterially contaminated units. Most studies have indicated that plasma is associated with roughly 50% of TRALI cases, whereas apheresis or whole blood platelets are the next most common precipitant, and packed red cells and cryoprecipitate are rare causes of TRALI. Other publications, however, have indicated the highest incidence with platelets (1:400 platelet units). Clinical manifestations of TRALI include fever, hypotension, tachycardia, and noncardiogenic pulmonary edema that can lead to profound hypoxemia and respiratory distress. Chest radiographs demonstrate bilateral infiltrates without cardiomegaly consistent with acute respiratory distress syndrome. Typically, signs and symptoms of TRALI occur within 2 hours of receipt of the blood product, but can occur up to 6 hours following transfusion. Treatment is supportive, and more than 70% of patients require mechanical ventilation; however, most patients are extubated within 24 to 72 hours.

    Confirmation of TRALI first requires the identification of potentially involved blood products and their respective donors. Other blood products from the donor(s) suspected in a TRALI case must be quarantined during evaluation. To implicate a donor in a case of TRALI, the presence of an anti-HLA or antineutrophil antibody with specificity to an antigen expressed by the recipient is required. Implicated donors are typically permanently deferred from further donation.

To date, measures to prevent TRALI have focused on the identification and deferral of donors at high risk to form anti-HLA or antineutrophil antibodies. The United Kingdom adopted a policy to manufacture and import male donor plasma only, whereas centers in Spain screen previously pregnant donors for anti-HLA antibodies and, if positive, do not manufacture plasma products from these donors. In multiparous donors from the United States, the incidence of anti-HLA antibodies is approximately 25% and, therefore, policies to exclude high-risk donors can potentially adversely affect the supply of blood products. Insuza et al., reported a 6% loss of apheresis platelets and an 8% loss of fresh frozen plasma (FFP) following the implementation of the Spanish policy. It is currently unclear if these preventative measures can definitively decrease the incidence of TRALI.

6. **Volume overload** with symptoms and signs of congestive heart failure can be seen in patients with cardiopulmonary compromise, particularly in elderly patients with substantial anemia who already have expanded plasma volume. Diuretic therapy should be used prophylactically in such patients to minimize this complication. The distinction between volume overload and TRALI can be difficult. Recently, a small study involving 19 patients suspected to have transfusion-associated circulatory overload (TACO) found beta natriuretic peptide (BNP) to be 81% sensitive and 89% specific in the diagnosis of volume overload following a transfusion. BNP may be a helpful marker to distinguish TACO from TRALI, although future studies are needed.

7. **Transfusion-associated graft-versus-host disease (GVHD)** is a syndrome in which donor lymphocytes that share an HLA haplotype with the patient's lymphocytes successfully engraft and attack the host (patient) with clinical manifestations of rash, pancytopenia, and liver and gastrointestinal damage (diarrhea). This appears to be unique to immunocompromised patients such as solid organ or bone marrow transplantation patients, and patients with certain malignancies (Hodgkin's disease, non-Hodgkin's lymphoma, leukemia, multiple myeloma), particularly in those undergoing intensive chemotherapy (e.g., fludarabine or myeloablative therapy). Interestingly, a patient with human immunodeficiency virus (HIV) infection has not yet been reported to have this complication, probably because of the suppressive effect of HIV infection on donor lymphocytes. Mortality is in excess of 80% and is usually secondary to bone marrow failure. This complication can be prevented by irradiation of blood products (see later) for patients at risk. On the basis of the pathogenesis, directed blood transfusions from any blood relative of the transfusion recipient also must be irradiated.

8. **Posttransfusion purpura (PTP)** is a rare complication, which is manifested by a profound immune-mediated thrombocytopenia that is observed 7 to 10 days after blood transfusion. Platelet alloantibodies within the recipient initiate the destruction of allogeneic platelets and are thought to trigger a complement-mediated consumption of the patient's own platelets. Most commonly, recipients lack human platelet antigen (HPA)-1a, which is present in approximately 99% of whites. Although controversial, additional platelet transfusions with HPA-1a–positive units may increase complement generation, so further transfusions are often withheld unless an HPA-1–negative donor is identified. The treatment for PTP is intravenous IgG (IVIG) and, if this fails, plasma exchange may be initiated.

C. **Infections**

1. **Human immunodeficiency virus infection.** Since the recognition that HIV infection is transmissible by blood, major advances in blood safety have been made. With the implementation of nucleic acid testing (NAT) for direct detection of viral (HIV and hepatitis C) contamination, the window period (time from infection to detectability by testing) is 11 days for HIV and 8 to 10 days for hepatitis C. Following the institution of NAT testing, the estimated risk for HIV and hepatitis C transmission is $1:1.8 \times 10^6$ and $1:1.6 \times 10^6$, respectively. **The risk of fatality from acute hemolytic transfusion reaction (usually due to**

ABO incompatibility secondary to patient or blood-unit misidentification) approximates $1:1.5 \times 10^6$ which now exceed the estimated death risk from viral transmission. Nevertheless, prudent utilization of transfusion support is important because blood is a scarce resource and because of possible, unknown future blood risks.

2. **West Nile Virus (WNV).** Queens, New York was the epicenter of a WNV epidemic in 1999, which thereafter spread to numerous states throughout the country. The first of the cases of transfusion-transmitted WNV was reported in 2002, when Pealer et al. identified 23 transfusion recipients who developed symptoms of a viral illness within 4 weeks of transfusion and then had laboratory confirmation of WNV. The cases were linked to 16 donors who were viremic at the time of collection. NAT testing of blood donors was started in 2003 and data from the American Red Cross reported 540 positive donations in 2003 and 2004. It is not clear if NAT testing for WNV in blood donors will need to continue as the number of WNV cases throughout the country has declined since 2002.

3. **Cytomegalovirus (CMV) infection.** CMV infection has been a substantial cause of morbidity and mortality for immunocompromised oncology patients. Patients who receive allogeneic bone marrow/stem cell transplantation are at risk because of cytotoxic preparative regimens, immunosuppressive therapy (cyclosporine and corticosteroid), and/or GVHD. Up to 60% of this patient population will experience CMV infection, with half of them developing CMV disease. Even with the use of CMV-negative blood products, CMV seroconversion has been reported in 1% to 4% of CMV-negative donor–recipient transplantation patients.

   CMV infection and CMV disease are much less common in patients undergoing conventional chemotherapy or autologous bone marrow/stem cell transplantation, and are not thought to be a significant clinical problem.

   A randomized, controlled clinical trial in allogeneic bone marrow transplantation patients compared the value of CMV-seronegative blood products with unscreened blood products that were subjected to bedside leukofiltration. Four (1.3%) of 252 patients in the CMV-seronegative cohort developed CMV infection, with no CMV disease or fatalities; 6 (2.4%) of 250 patients in the leukoreduced cohort developed CMV disease, of whom 5 died. A much larger study would have to be performed to eliminate a type II statistical error with the insignificant rise in CMV infection of 40%. The filtered cohort had an increased probability of developing CMV disease by day 100 (2.4% vs. none; $p = 0.03$). Even when the investigators eliminated CMV infections that occurred within 21 days of transplantation, two cases of fatal CMV disease occurred in the filtered arm as compared with none in the leukoreduced arm. The conclusion by the authors of this study that leukoreduced blood products are "CMV safe," remains controversial. In a consensus conference held by the Canadian Blood Service, 7 of 10 panelists concluded that patients considered at risk for CMV disease should receive CMV-seronegative products, even when blood components are leukoreduced.

4. **Bacterial Contamination.** The risk of platelet-related sepsis is estimated to be 1:12,000 for apheresis platelets but is greater with transfusions of pooled platelet concentrates from multiple donors (e.g., 1:2,000 after receiving six concentrates). Transfusion-related sepsis was the second leading cause of transfusion-associated fatalities from 1990 to 1998. In descending order, the organisms most commonly implicated in fatalities (as reported to the FDA) are *Staphylococcus aureus, Klebsiella pneumoniae, Serratia marcescens,* and *Staphylococcus epidermidis.* Platelets are prone to bacterial contamination because they are stored at 20°C to 24°C (room temperature). There is an increasing risk of bacterial overgrowth with time and, consequently, the shelf life of platelets is limited to 5 days. However, with new procedures this may be extended to 7 days. In 2004, AABB implemented standards that require blood banks to perform bacterial testing of platelets. The bacterial testing systems are inoculated 24 hours after collection (to allow for bactrerial growth) and then incubate for an additional 24 hours.

Approximately 1:2,000 platelet units is found to be bacterially contaminated and often bacteria are detected after the 24-hour incubation and subsequent transfusion. Late positive tests likely indicate a reduced bacterial load and a smaller risk of sepsis. When platelets are released from bacterial testing, only 3 days remain of the 5-day shelf life, which challenges blood banks to maintain an adequate platelet inventory without substantial wastage. Recently, the FDA has approved a bacterial testing system that prolongs the shelf life of platelets to 7 days, which is currently being utilized in some centers.

Another method to reduce the risk of transfusion-associated sepsis is photochemical treatment of platelet products. Photochemical treatments utilize ultraviolet (UV) light and psoralen to inactivate a broad range of gram-negative and gram-positive organisms, as well as viruses. Treatment of platelet concentrates with amotosalen (a synthetic psoralen) and UVA light will result in a >4.5-log reduction in bacterial pathogens. Two randomized, controlled trials have evaluated the safety and efficacy of platelet concentrates treated with psoralen and UVA and both concluded that platelet products treated with photochemical inactivation were as efficacious as conventional platelets in achieving hemostasis with a comparable safety profile. Further studies are needed to better elucidate the role of pathogen inactivation in platelet products to reduce transfusion-associated sepsis and the risk reduction, if any, these methods provide in addition to the AABB-mandated bacterial cultures.

The clinical presentation of bacterially contaminated platelet infection can range from mild fever (which may be indistinguishable from febrile, nonhemolytic transfusion reactions) to acute sepsis, hypotension, and death. Sepsis caused by transfusion of contaminated platelets is under-recognized in part because the organisms found in platelet contamination are frequently the same as those implicated in "catheter" or "line" sepsis. The overall mortality rate of identified platelet-associated sepsis is 26%.

In the clinical setting, any patient in whom fever develops within 6 hours of platelet infusion should be evaluated for possible bacterial contamination of the component, and initiation of empiric antibiotic therapy should be considered. Because of their storage at room temperature, platelets are more prone to bacterial infection than are other blood products. FATRs occur in only 0.5% of red cell transfusions; of these, 18% and 8% of patients experience a second and third FATR, respectively. Approximately 18% of platelet transfusions are associated with FATR, although the prevalence of platelet-associated FATR can be as high as 30% in frequently transfused populations such as oncology patients. Reactions characterized as severe occur in only 2% of platelet transfusions, and bedside leukofiltration has not been found to reduce the overall prevalence of FATR. Risks of transfusion-transmitted diseases are the same as those for red cells and are summarized in Table 38.1.

D. Plasma therapy. Plasma therapy should be administered to patients who have abnormal prothrombin time (PT) or partial thromboplastin time (PTT) assays in the setting of correction with a mixing study and clinically significant hemorrhage. The most common setting is in patients with liver disease who have multiple coagulation deficiencies, along with ongoing consumption due to impaired reticuloendothelial system (RES) clearance of substances activating the coagulation system. Another setting is in vitamin K deficiency. Vitamin K is derived from dietary sources and from intestinal bacteria, so that deficiency is caused by poor dietary intake and/or with antibiotic therapy (e.g., intubated or cachectic patients treated with prolonged and multiple antibiotic therapy). Patients who have had Coumadin overdose or who are sensitive to this agent can also have markedly elevated international normalized ratio (INR) values. Parenteral vitamin K (5 to 10 mg s.q. or i.v. daily) administration should be considered in both patients with liver disease (impaired enterohepatic circulation of bile salts leading to deficiency of vitamin K and the vitamin K–dependent coagulation factors II, VII, IX, and X) and patients with Coumadin overdose. For patients with life-threatening hemorrhage, 15 mL/kg of plasma will increase factor levels by 20% to 30%.

E. Platelet transfusions

1. Platelet-transfusion practices

a. Threshold for transfusion. Several studies have evaluated prophylactic platelet-transfusion practices and thresholds for patients who are thrombocytopenic due to myelosuppressive therapy. One study found that most patients undergoing stem cell transplantation were transfused prophylactically with platelets when their platelet counts were between 10×10^9/L and 20×10^9/L, indicating that a threshold of 20×10^9/L was most common. Only 9% of hemorrhagic events reported in this study occurred when platelet counts were less than 10×10^9/L.

Two prospective, randomized studies evaluated the relative merits of platelet-transfusion thresholds of 10×10^9/L versus 20×10^9/L for leukemia patients undergoing chemotherapy. One found that the lower transfusion threshold was associated with 22% fewer platelet transfusions. No differences between the two patient cohorts were seen with respect to hemorrhagic complications, number of red cell transfusions, duration of hospital stay, or mortality. In a second study, a platelet threshold of 10×10^9/L was safe and effective when compared with a threshold of 20×10^9/L. Two (1.9%) of the 105 patients in this study died of hemorrhagic complications; each patient had a platelet count greater than 30×10^9/L at the time of death. However, these studies were not adequately powered to detect a difference in fairly infrequent but catastrophic complications (e.g., subarachnoid bleeds). Nevertheless, it seems that other patient-related factors (i.e., qualitative platelet abnormalities, von Willebrand disease, or other hemostatic system defects) may play a role with respect to bleeding complications in the setting of thrombocytopenia.

b. Platelet dose. Standards of the AABB require that 75% of single-donor platelet (SDP) or apheresis products contain more than 3×10^{11} platelets and that 75% of platelet concentrates (i.e., six pack is equivalent to a SDP) contain more than 5.5×10^{10} platelets. However, there is a broad range of platelet doses in several clinical trials, indicating that there is no consensus for a standardized platelet-transfusion dose.

High-dose platelet therapy was investigated in a clinical trial that randomized patients with hematologic malignancies to prophylactic platelet transfusions with standard, high, and very high platelet doses (4.6×10^{11}, 6.5×10^{11}, and 8.9×10^{11} platelets, respectively) to maintain a platelet count of 15×10^9 to 20×10^9/L. The high and very high platelet dose cohorts had greater platelet-count incremental increases and prolonged time to next transfusion when compared with the standard platelet dose cohort. However, as the platelet dose increased, the ratio of median number of platelets transfused/median transfusion interval decreased, suggesting that lower platelet doses may decrease the overall number of platelets required to maintain a platelet count of 15×10^9 to 20×10^9/L.

Mathematical modelling of platelet survival predicts that lower doses of prophylactic platelet therapy (approximately 2×10^9 vs. 4×10^9) transfused to maintain a platelet count of 10×10^9/L would decrease platelet usage by 22%. To evaluate the effects of low-dose platelet therapy on platelet utilization and risk of hemorrhage, Tinmouth et al. randomized thrombocytopenic patients receiving high-dose chemotherapy or a stem cell transplant to low dose (approximately 2×10^{11}) versus standard-dose (approximately 4×10^{11}) platelet therapy. Over the course of their hospitalization, patients in the low-dose arm required 25% fewer platelet units and had a comparable number of bleeding events to the standard-dose group. Further studies of platelet-transfusion dosage strategies are needed to determine an optimal dose.

2. Platelet refractoriness. Infusion of an SDP generally results in a platelet count rise of 30,000 to 60,000/μL. *Platelet refractoriness* is defined as a reduced or absent rise in platelet count, especially when measured within 1 hour of transfusion. The differential diagnosis of platelet refractoriness in oncology patients include infection, disseminated intravascular coagulation (DIC), thrombotic thrombocytopenia purpura (TTP), splenomegaly, drugs, or antibody-mediated mechanisms. The first step in managing patients who respond poorly to platelet transfusions is to identify the specific cause of platelet refractoriness, which first requires the measurement of a corrected count increment (CCI), which accounts for the dose of platelets and the recipient size. Platelet refractoriness is typically defined as a CCI of less than 5,000 to 7,500 on two occasions when the patient receives ABO-compatible platelets.

$$CCI = \frac{\text{Platelet count increment/mm}^3 \times \text{Body surface area (m}^2)}{\text{Number of platelets transfused } (\times 10^{11})}$$

Upon diagnosis of platelet refractoriness, the causative factor must be sought. In multiply transfused patients, a poor response to transfusion may be commonly due to anti-HLA-related antibodies. Antibody-mediated accelerated clearance of platelets is supported by a poor increment when the count is obtained within 30 to 60 minutes posttransfusion. The formation of antibodies to HLA antigens occurs when there is exposure to foreign HLA molecules through pregnancy or transfusion. As platelets express HLA class I antigens, the presence of these antibodies may result in platelet refractoriness. Leukocytes present in transfused products have been implicated in the formation of HLA antibodies and, therefore, a large, randomized trial was conducted to examine the benefit of leukoreduced blood products in the reduction of platelet alloantibodies. The TRAP study (Trial to Reduce Immunization to Platelets) found that clinical platelet refractoriness associated with HLA antibody seropositivity was reduced from 13% of patients transfused with unprocessed platelet concentrates to 3% to 5% of patients receiving leukoreduced apheresis platelets, leukoreduced platelet concentrates, or psoralen/UVB–treated platelets. Notably, there was no difference in the rate of hemorrhage or overall mortality between the groups. The authors concluded that leukoreduced blood helped prevent the formation of alloantibodies.

Alloantibodies to HLA antigens can be detected by methods of lymphocytotoxicity, enzyme-linked immunosorbent assay (ELISA), or flow cytometry. If HLA alloantibodies are found, providing matched platelets at the A and B loci can improve platelet increments. Alternatively, if specificity of the HLA antibody can be determined, antigen-negative platelets may be effective. In fact, some centers utilize cross-match procedures to identify platelet units that will improve responsiveness to platelet transfusion. The largest obstacle to providing HLA-matched platelets is a limited donor pool, which can be mitigated through single antigen mismatches with cross-reactive groups (CREGs). CREGs are structurally similar HLA antigens that react with common antisera. Transfusing alloimmunized patients with selectively HLA-mismatched platelets can increase the number of potential donors while improving platelet increments.

Persistent refractoriness to platelet transfusions despite HLA-matched platelets is not uncommon in heavily alloimmunized patients. Although many immunosuppressive medications have been tried in this circumstance, the only therapy that has demonstrated some success is IVIG. Case reports and small series comprise most of this literature and the efficacy of IVIG in the treatment of alloimmunized patients is variable between reports. IVIG should not be used as a first-line therapy for alloimmunized patients; however, it has a role in patients who are persistently refractory to well-matched platelets or who are refractory and have active bleeding.

Although alloantibodies are an important cause of platelet refractoriness, in some cases patient-specific factors can also influence the response to transfusion. In patients undergoing stem cell transplantation, the type of therapy administered and extent of disease are important predictors of platelet increment following a transfusion. A study of stem cell transplant recipients noted that factors usually associated with patient response to platelets (history of previous transfusion, pregnancy, the presence of HLA or platelet-specific antibodies) did not significantly correlate with CCI. Rather, patient-specific variables such as disease status (advanced rather than early), conditioning regimen (including total body irradiation or not), progenitor cell source (bone marrow rather than peripheral stem cell), and type of transplant (allogeneic vs. autologous) are significant predictors of platelet refractoriness in patients undergoing stem cell transplantation.

F. Special blood products

1. **Washed RBCs** are rarely indicated, except in patients with severe reactions to plasma or platelets, such as patients with IgA deficiency or in patients who cannot tolerate potassium loads (e.g., end-stage renal disease).

2. **Irradiation of blood products** eliminates engraftment by immunologically competent donor lymphocytes and is recommended for immunocompromised patients (high-dose chemotherapeutic regimens, immunosuppressive therapy in allogeneic transplantation, or fludarabine therapy), and any patient receiving directed transfusions from a blood relative.

3. **Leukoreduced blood products** (i.e., defined as 99.9% of white blood cells [WBCs] removed) have been recommended for the following patients: (a) patients with previous febrile transfusion reactions not prevented by acetaminophen and diphenhydramine therapy; (b) patients undergoing red cell exchange transfusions; (c) patients for whom cross-match compatible blood is difficult to obtain; (d) patients who are candidates for solid organ (kidney, heart, lung) or stem cell (aplastic anemia) transplantation; and (e) patients who should receive CMV-negative blood (e.g., platelets) when CMV-seronegative products are unavailable (Table 38.2).

III. APHERESIS. Apheresis is a procedure that removes a specified component of whole blood. It can be broadly classified into plasmapheresis (removal of plasma) and cytapheresis (removal of cells). Whole blood is continuously (i.e., 50 to 100 mL/min) removed from the patient either through a central venous catheter or a peripheral vein with a large bore needle and enters the pheresis machine through an extracorporeal circuit. Within the machine, the components of blood are separated by centrifugation, the desired portion (plasma, platelets, white cells, or red cells) is removed, and the remainder is then returned to the patient along with replacement solutions (e.g. plasma, albumin, or hetastarch). In the case of plasmapheresis, filtration instead of centrifugation can be used and similarly a replacement fluid is necessary, which may be albumin, plasma, or a combination.

A. Plasmapheresis. In general, plasmapheresis is used to remove disease-inducing antibodies and the amount of antibody removed per procedure depends on the vascular distribution of the pathologic antibody. IgG is 45% intravascular and approximately five procedures (1.5-blood volume exchange) are necessary to remove 90% of the antibody; in contrast, IgM is 80% to 90% intravascular and requires roughly two to three procedures to remove 90% of the antibody. Plasmapheresis is used to treat many disease states in patients with cancer diagnoses. The frequency of required maintenance procedures also depends on the half-life of the specific immunoglobulin class (i.e., 21 days for IgG vs. 10 days for IgM and IgA).

Waldenstrom's macroglobulinemia (WM) is a low-grade lymphoma often associated with hyperviscosity symptoms due to excess IgM. If patients with WM present with symptoms of hyperviscosity (dizziness, shortness of breath, bleeding, confusion, visual changes) emergent plasmapheresis can markedly improve symptoms. Additionally, patients with WM who cannot tolerate other therapies may be maintained on a chronic program of plasmapheresis to control symptoms. Plasma-pheresis is also effective in the treatment of hyperviscosity associated with multiple myeloma; however, IgG or IgA paraproteins may require more than one procedure for symptom resolution. Recently, a randomized, controlled trial investigated the role of plasmapheresis in acute renal failure of multiple myeloma. Patients were randomized to conventional therapy (supportive care plus treatment of multiple myeloma) or to conventional therapy plus five to seven plasma exchange procedures. No significant differences in dialysis dependence, glomerular filtration rate, or death were noted between the plasmapheresis and standard therapy cohorts. Finally, plasmapheresis can be utilized in stem cell transplantation patients who receive a transplant from an ABO-incompatible donor. In the case of a major incompatibility (A donor→O recipient), recipient isohemagglutinins (anti-A) may persist until erythroid engraftment (A cells) occurs, with resultant potentially life-threatening hemolysis. This incompatibility may also lead to a protracted red cell engraftment period. Alternatively, if the donor is of O and the recipient of A groups, a minor incompatibility is present. Donor lymphocytes (which produce anti-A) are delivered along with stem cells, and after approximately 10 days synthesize anti-A in quantities sufficient to cause clinically significant hemolysis. This phenomenon is referred to as *passenger lymphocyte syndrome*. Monitoring forward/reverse blood types, blood counts, lactate dehydrogenase (LDH), and direct antigen test results in susceptible patients (e.g., those with anti-A or anti-B titers >1:8) can allow early identification of patients who might require apheresis management for these hemolytic processes. In major or minor incompatibilities, plasmapheresis can effectively remove the isohemagglutinins and help abate hemolysis. However, if hemolysis is related to IgG (anti-A or anti-B), then plasmapheresis may not be immediately effective (i.e., since five procedures are required for a log reduction in IgG levels). In the case of a minor incompatibility, red cell exchange with O units may be indicated to reduce hemolytic related sequelae.

B. Cytapheresis is used to collect peripheral blood stem cells for transplantation as discussed in Chapter 5. Outlined in the Chapter 35 is leukoreduction for hyperviscosity of acute leukemia.

Suggested Readings

Bernstein SH, Nademanee AP, Vose JM, et al. A multicenter study of platelet recovery and utilization in patients after myeloablative therapy and hematopoietic stem cell transplantation. *Blood* 1998;91:3509–3517.

Bowden RA, Slichter SJ, Sayers M, et al. A comparison of filtered leukocyte-reduced and cytomegalovirus (CMV) seronegative blood products for the prevention of transfusion-associated CMV infection after marrow transplant. *Blood* 1995;86:3598–3603.

Finch CA, Lenfant C. Oxygen transport in man. *N Engl J Med* 1972;286:407–415.

Goodnough LT, Brecher ME, Kanter MH, et al. Transfusion medicine, part I: blood transfusion. *N Engl J Med* 1999;340:438–447.

Hebert PC, Wells G, Blajchman MA, et al. A multicenter, randomized, controlled clinical trial of transfusion requirements in critical care. *N Engl J Med* 1999;340:409–417.

Lane TA, Anderson KC, Goodnough LT, et al. Leukocyte reduction in blood component therapy. *Ann Intern Med* 1992;117:151–162.

Norol F, Bierling P, Roudot-Thoraval F, et al. Platelet transfusion: a dose-response study. *Blood* 1998;92:1448–1453.

Pealer LN, Marfin AA, Petersen LR, et al. Transmission of west nile virus through blood transfusion in the United States in 2002. *N Engl J Med* 2003;349:1236–1245.

Stramer SL, Fang CT, Foster GA, et al. West nile virus among blood donors in the United States, 2003 and 2004. *N Engl J Med* 2005;353:451–459.

Stramer SL, Glynn SA, Kleinman SH, et al. Detection of HIV-1 and HCV infections among antibody-negative blood donors by nucleic acid-amplification testing. *N Engl J Med* 2004;351:760–768.

The Trial to Reduce Alloimmunization to Platelets Study Group. Leukocyte reduction and ultraviolet B irradiation of platelets to prevent alloimmunization and refractoriness to platelet transfusions. *N Engl J Med* 1997;337:1861–1869.

Wandt H, Frank M, Ehninger G, et al. Safety and cost effectiveness of a 10 × 10(9)/L trigger for prophylactic platelet transfusions compared with the traditional 20 × 10(9)/L trigger: a prospective comparative trial in 105 patients with acute myeloid leukemia. *Blood* 1998;91:3601–3606.

Welch HG, Mehan KR, Goodnough LT. Prudent strategies for elective red blood cell transfusion. *Ann Intern Med* 1992;116:393–402.

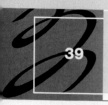

39

NUTRITIONAL SUPPORT
Carolina C. Javier

I. IDENTIFICATION AND ASSESSMENT OF PATIENTS AT NUTRITIONAL RISK. Nutrition plays a supportive role in the care of the patient with cancer, whether the goal of therapy is curative or palliative. Nutritional interventions will maintain and preserve body composition and lean body mass, support functional status, and enhance the quality of life. Proactive assessments of nutritional status are essential to assure success in intervention and to improve patient outcome. Treatment modalities could have an impact on the nutritional status of the patient and could increase the risk for weight loss and malnutrition. Oncology dietitians play a key role in optimizing nutrition for the cancer patient through counseling and education of patients and their families, and other members of the health care team. The assessment and nutritional surveillance of the patient with cancer can help meet therapeutic goals.

II. NUTRITIONAL ASSESSMENT. Nutritional assessment is an essential component in the nutritional care of the patient with cancer, because it will provide an estimate of body composition, such as fat, skeletal muscle protein, and visceral protein. It will likewise identify patients who are at risk of cancer-induced malnutrition and determine the magnitude of nutritional depletion in patients who are already malnourished.

A. Patient history and examination. Information that pertains to the patient's medical history and physical examination will reveal usual body weight, any recent weight change, or inclusion of new or special diets. Unintentional weight loss of 10% or more of body weight within the previous 6 months could mean a significant nutritional deficit and is a good indicator of clinical outcome. Signs of malnutrition such as muscle wasting, loss of muscle strength, and depletion of fat stores may be revealed by a physical examination. However, body weight alone is insufficient as a nutritional assessment tool and will fail to show important changes in disease or therapy-related caloric intake or metabolic rate.

In addition, detailed information should be obtained regarding change in appetite, food intake, gastrointestinal problems, and concomitant disease.

B. Anthropometric assessment. Anthropometric measurements are often used in the assessment of nutritional status, particularly when a chronic imbalance occurs between protein and energy intake. Such disturbances change the patterns of physical growth and the relative proportions of body tissues such as fat, muscle, and total body water. The measurement of the triceps skinfold is used to calculate an estimation of fat stores, whereas the midarm muscle circumference (includes the basic anthropometrics of weight and height) assesses lean body mass.

$$MMC\ (cm) = Arm\ circumference\ (cm) - 0.314 \times TSF\ (mm)$$

where MMC is the midarm muscle circumference, and TSF is the triceps skinfold thickness.

Standards for age and gender have been established; however, there are wide variations among individuals, and interobserver measurement variability is considerable.

Anthropometric measurements may be markedly affected by non-nutritional factors and are rarely performed in the routine clinical setting.

C. Assessment of protein status. Serum protein concentrations such as retinol-binding protein, transferrin, prealbumin, and albumin can be used to assess the degree of visceral protein depletion.

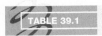

Protein	Half-life	Body pool size (g/kg body weight)
Serum albumin	14–20 d	3–5
Serum transferrin	8–10 d	<0.1 g
Serum thyroxine–binding prealbumin (TBPA)	2–3 d	0.01
Serum retinol–binding protein (RBP)	12 h	0.002

The relation between malnutrition and serum protein levels is related to the patient's hydration status and the half-life of the individual protein. Visceral protein status is frequently assessed by the measurement of one or more of the serum proteins (Table 39.1). One of the first organs to be affected by protein malnutrition is the liver, which is the main site of synthesis for most of these serum proteins.

The synthesis of serum proteins is impaired by the limited supply of protein substrates, resulting in a decline in serum protein concentrations. Many non-nutritional factors influence the concentration of serum proteins (Table 39.2) and reduce their specificity and sensitivity. Total serum protein is easily measured and has been used as an index of visceral protein status in several national nutrition surveys; however, it is a rather insensitive index of protein status. For example, normal limits of total serum protein concentration are maintained initially despite a restricted protein intake, with significant depletion when clinical signs of protein malnutrition become apparent. This marked decrease in the serum albumin concentrations, which represents 50% to 60% of the total serum protein, is the cause of this decline.

Serum albumin reflects changes within the intravascular space and not the total visceral protein pool. Serum albumin is not very sensitive to short-term changes in protein status; it has a long half-life of 14 to 20 days (Table 39.1). Reduced catabolism largely compensates for reductions in hepatic synthesis of serum albumin.

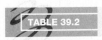 **Factors Affecting Serum Protein Concentrations**

Inadequate protein intake resulting from low dietary intakes, anorexia, unbalanced diets, hypocaloric intravenous infusions

Altered metabolism generated by trauma, stress, sepsis, and hypoxia

Specific deficiency of plasma proteins caused by protein-losing enteropathy and liver disease

Reduced protein synthesis resulting from inadequate energy intake, electrolyte deficiency, trace element deficiencies (e.g., iron and zinc), vitamin deficiency (e.g., vitamin A)

Pregnancy induces changes in the amount and distribution of body fluids

Capillary permeability changes

Drugs (e.g., oral contraceptive agents)

Strenuous exercise

(Adapted with permission from Jeejeebhoy KN. Protein nutrition in clinical practice *Br Med Bull* 1981;37:11–17.)

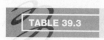

TABLE 39.3	Factors Considered in Subjective Global Assessment (SGA)[a], of Nutritional Status

A. History
   Weight change (loss in 1, 3, 6 mo, change in the past 2 wk)
   Dietary intake change (relative to normal, type of diet)
   GI symptoms (persisting >2 wk)
   Functional capacity (ECOG 0–4)
   Disease and relation to nutritional requirements (primary diagnosis, stage, metabolic stress)
B. Physical
   Subcutaneous fat, muscle wasting, edema, ascites
C. SGA rating
   A, Well nourished
   B, Moderately malnourished
   C, Severely malnourished

GI, gastrointestinal; ECOG, Eastern Cooperative Oncology Group; SGA, subjective global assessment.
[a]Modified SGA used at Fox Chase Cancer Center (short version).

Each transferrin molecule binds with two molecules of iron, and thereby serves as an iron-transport protein. Transferrin responds more rapidly to changes in protein status because of its shorter half-life and smaller body pool than albumin. Like serum albumin concentrations, serum transferrin concentrations are affected by a variety of factors, including gastrointestinal, renal, and liver disease.

The nutritional status of the patient also can be defined by using objective data. The Prognostic Nutritional Index (PNI) has been shown to predict clinical outcome in cancer patients. The PNI is based on serum albumin level, serum transferrin level, delayed cutaneous hypersensitivity, and triceps skinfold thickness.

D. Immune function. Tests of immunocompetence are sometimes used as functional indices of protein status; however, their sensitivity and specificity are low. Nutritional deficiencies can impair nearly all aspects of the immune system, and no single measurement can assess adequacy of the immune response. Examples of immunologic tests include lymphocyte count, measurement of thymus-dependent lymphocytes, and delayed cutaneous hypersensitivity.

E. Subjective global assessment (SGA). SGA of nutritional status includes relevant history data (dynamic weight loss, dietary intake, specific symptoms, performance status, primary disease, and metabolic demand) as well as clinical data (subjective estimate of fat/protein stores.) The use of a standardized, simple, and validated assessment method such as Detsky's SGA is recommended (Table 39.3) for further specific studies. The nutritional assessment tools used for clinical routine are summarized in Table 39.4.

III. INTERVENTIONS AND NUTRITIONAL THERAPY. An estimate of current energy and protein balance is useful in providing nutritional intervention.

Nitrogen metabolism. The measurement of the nitrogen balance can document the effectiveness of nutritional therapy; nitrogen balance is calculated by the formula:

$$\text{Nitrogen balance} = \frac{\text{protein intake}}{6.25} - (\text{urinary urea nitrogen} + 4)$$

The apparent net protein utilization is generated by using the relationship. The obligatory nitrogen loss is roughly equal to 0.1 g/kg of body weight.

Calorie expenditure. The calculation of basal energy expenditure (BEE) is performed by using the following formula:

For men: BEE = $66 + (13.7 \times W) + (5 \times H) - (6.8 \times A)$;
For women: BEE = $655 + (9.6 \times W) + (1.7 \times H) - (4.7 \times A)$,

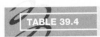

TABLE 39.4   **Synopsis of Nutritional Assessment Parameters**

Minimal screening assessment
  Present weight in relation to ideal weight (weight/height index)
  Weight change (percentage weight change/time interval)
  Serum albumin
Complete assessment
  History
    Dietary data (food records, recall methods)
    Concomitant disease
  Physical examination
    Body fat, muscle wasting
    Specific nutritional deficiencies
  Anthropometrics
    Triceps skin fold (caliper method)
    Midarm muscle circumference
  Laboratory tests
    Creatinine/height index
    Serum transferrin or albumin
  Immune function
    Total lymphocyte count
    Delayed hypersensitivity skin tests
  Subjective global assessment, clinical experience
Apparative assessment
  Bioelectrical impedance analysis

where W is the actual weight in kilograms; H is the height in centimeters; and A is the age in years. By using the value for BEE, the caloric intakes can be expressed as a multiple of BEE:

$$\text{Kilocalorie intake as percentage of BEE} = \frac{\text{Caloric intake}}{\text{Basal energy expenditure}} \times 100$$

Caloric-intake evaluation. Table 39.5 provides the figures for a rough estimation of protein and calorie requirements for all hospitalized patients. An evaluation of caloric intake also can be determined by using Table 39.6. Guidelines for making decisions for nutritional therapy based on energy and protein balance are given in Table 39.7.

A. Oral nutrition. The preferred method for providing nutrition for patients who are able to eat is by oral diet, which can be modified according to the physiologic and anatomic constraints of their illness. Nutritional support considerations for

TABLE 39.5   **Rapid Estimation of Protein and Calorie Requirements of Adult Patients**

Degree of stress	Caloric requirements (kcal/kg[a]/d)	Protein requirements (g/kg[a]/d)
None	25	0.8
Mild metabolic stress	35	1.0
Moderate–severe metabolic stress	45	1.5

[a] Desired body weight.

TABLE 39.6	**Nutrition Planning for Patients with Moderate to Severe Protein–Calorie Malnutrition**
Protein and calorie balance	**Nutrition plan**
Negative	
Long period of support anticipated	Increase intake now
Short period of support anticipated	Delay intensive therapy; minimize losses until acute illness subsides; reevaluate frequently
Zero	Delay intensive therapy; minimize losses until acute illness subsides; reevaluate frequently
Positive	Try to maintain 500–1,000 kcal and 15–30 g protein/d over requirement

individuals with daily energy deficits (e.g., patients with anorexia and resulting weight loss, dysphagia), are given in Tables 39.8 and 39.9.

B. Dietary supplements. Nutrients, vitamins, and minerals that are essential for human health as well as a variety of nonessential nutrients such as phytochemicals, hormones, and herbs are used as dietary supplements; however, these should never replace whole foods. The American Cancer Society (ACS) warns against massive doses of any dietary supplement, recommends supplements that are close to the daily percentage value for most vitamins and minerals, and states that there is no substitute for a well-balanced diet that follows the United States Department of Agriculture (USDA) Food Pyramid. The daily percentage value (DV) on food labels, formerly known as the recommended daily allowance is the average daily dietary intake level that is adequate to meet the nutrient requirements of nearly all (97% to 98%) individuals in a specific life stage and gender group. To account for differences in need and ability for absorption, the DV is set considerably higher

TABLE 39.7	**Nutritional Therapy**	
A. Energy requirements		**Kilocalories required (kcal/24 h)**
Type of therapy		
Parenteral anabolic		$1.75 \times$ BEE
Oral anabolic		$1.50 \times$ BEE
Oral maintenance		$1.20 \times$ BEE
B. Prescriptions for anabolism[a]	**Protein (g/d)**	**Kilocalories (kcal/d)**
Type of therapy		
Oral protein sparing	$1.5 \times$ weight[b]	
Total parenteral nutrition	$(1.2–1.5) \times$ weight	$40 \times$ weight
Oral hyperalimentation	$(1.2–1.5) \times$ weight	$35 \times$ weight

BEE, basal energy expenditure.
[a]Levels of protein intake are to be adjusted according to blood urea nitrogen values and nitrogen balance.
[b]Weight, actual weight in kilograms.
(Reprinted with permission from Blackburn GL, Bistrian BR, Maini BS, et al. Nutritional and metabolic assessment of the hospitalized patient. *J Parenter Nutr* 1977;1:11.)

TABLE 39.8	Nutritional Support Considerations for Individuals with Daily Energy Deficits

Potential problem	Intervention
Anorexia	Small frequent meals seasoned according to individual taste
	Snacks of nutrient-dense liquids such as instant breakfast, milk shakes, or commercial supplements can provide significant protein and calories and are easily consumed. (See Table 39.9)
Dry mouth/thick saliva	Encourage good oral hygiene
	Artificial saliva and use of a straw may facilitate swallowing
	Petroleum jelly applied to the lips may help prevent drying
	Avoid coarse foods; some patients may require a liquid diet
Dysphagia	Encourage a soft, more liquid diet and easy-to-swallow foods
	Small frequent meals
	Use liquid nutritional formulas
	Determine the appropriate consistency of food and fluids or any special swallowing techniques given by the speech therapist
Radiation esophagitis	Soft bland diet, using creamy, lukewarm, or cool foods
	Avoid coarse, dry, or scratchy textured foods
	Avoid tart and acidic fruits and juices, alcohol, and irritating spices

than the estimated average requirement. Any recommendations for nutritional supplementation at doses higher than twice the DV should be individualized and are dependent on each individual's dietary and disease status. The American Dietetic Association recommends getting all the nutrients needed from the diet first and then considering supplementation only if it is adequately researched.

C. Enteral feeding. Enteral feeding refers to the provision of nutrients, either to supplement oral intake, or as the sole source of nutrition, delivered through a catheter or a tube to the gastrointestinal tract for absorption. Enteral feeding is preferred to parenteral feeding because it preserves the gastrointestinal architecture and prevents bacterial translocation from the gut. Enteral feeding has the advantage of delivering nutrients beyond areas of obstruction, at rates that can maximize nutrient absorption. Nutrients should be administered distal to the ligament of Treitz to avoid complications of aspiration pneumonia and gastric ileus. For short-term feeding, a nasoduodenal tube may be used. If there is a need for long-term enteral support, the preferred method is either a gastrostomy or jejunostomy tube, which can be placed either surgically or endoscopically. Nutritionally complete enteral-feeding formulas as well as specialized modular products to meet specific disease-related nutrient requirements are commercially available.

D. Total parenteral nutrition (TPN). Providing nutritional support by the parenteral route is an important option for patients for whom oral or enteral nutrition is unsuitable. The hyperosmolar TPN solutions require central venous access to reduce complications of venous thrombosis and phlebitis. Inherent complications such as pneumothorax occur infrequently. Parenteral nutrition is more expensive than enteral or oral nutrition, and adherence to specific guidelines is of utmost importance to minimize complications. Some studies on the use of TPN in cancer patients demonstrated improvement in body weight and total body fat content. Specific minerals, trace elements, and vitamins can be provided with TPN, but TPN does not stop the catabolic process of cancer cachexia, as nitrogen losses continue for patients receiving TPN, or alter the increased protein turnover and the process of lipolysis. When appropriately selected, certain cancer patients receiving

TABLE 39.9 Examples of Commonly Used Nutritional Products

Product	Serving size	Calories	Protein (g)	Fat (g)	Remarks
Boost High Protein (Mead Johnson)	8 oz	240	15.0	6.0	Use as oral or tube feeding Ready to serve
Boost Plus (Mead Johnson)	8 oz	360	14.0	14.0	Use proper dilution for tube feeding Use as oral or tube feeding Ready to serve
Nestle Carnation Instant Breakfast	1 packing with 1 cup whole milk	315	12.0	10.0	Use proper dilution for tube feeding High protein, high calories
Ensure (Ross)	8 oz	250	8.8	6.1	Use as oral or tube feeding Complete balanced nutrition
Ensure Plus (Ross)	8 oz	355	13.0	11.4	Use as oral or tube feeding Complete balanced nutrition
Ensure Fiber with FOS (Ross)	8 oz	250	8.8	6.1	For oral or tube feeding With fructo-oligosaccharides
Equate Plus (Wal Mart)	8 oz	360	13.0	13.0	High calories, high protein Lower cost
2 Cal HN (Ross)	8 oz	475	19.9	21.5	Calorie dense (2 cal/cc) High protein For oral or tube feeding
Isocal HN Plus (Mead Johnson)	8 oz	280	12.8	9.5	Tube-feeding product Contains MCT
Ultra Slim Fast	11 oz	200–220	7–10	1.5–3.0	Lower calorie, low fat
Sweet Success (Nestle)	11 oz	200	11.0	3.0	For oral use
Scandi–Shake (Scandipharm)	3 oz Powder with 1 cup whole milk	600	12.0	30.0	Very high calorie, high protein and fat Lactose-free available For oral use
Nutritional Supplement (Walgreens)	8 oz	355	13.0	12.6	Lower cost For oral use

FOS, fractooligo saccharides; MCT, medium-chain triglyceride.
Prices and local availability for these products may vary greatly. Products may be purchased in drug stores, grocery stores, and department stores.
Modular components that can be added for extra calories: Polycose or Sumacal, 23 cal/tbsp.; Lipomul, 6 cal/cc (90 cal/tbsp.); MCT Oil, 8 cal/cc (116 cal/tbsp.).

TPN have shown significant decreases in morbidity and mortality. This includes patients with severe malnutrition receiving perioperative TPN and bone marrow transplant recipients. The American Society of Parenteral and Enteral Nutrition has recommended TPN supplementation in patients expected to have inadequate oral or enteral nutritional intake for more than 10 to 14 days.

Suggested Readings

Alpers DH, Stenson WF, et al. *Manual of nutritional therapeutics,* 3rd ed. Boston: Little, Brown and Company, 1995.

American Cancer Society. *Alternative methods: dietary and herbal remedies, dietary supplements.* Atlanta: American Cancer Society, 1997.

American Dietetics Association. American Dietetics Association Position of the American Dietetics Association: vitamin and mineral supplementation. *J Am Diet Assoc* 1996;96:73–77.

Am J Pub Health 1973;63:1.

Blackburn GL, Bistrian BR, Maini BS, et al. Nutritional and metabolic assessment of the hospitalized patient. *J Parenter Nutr* 1977;1:11.

Buzby GP, Mullen JL, Matthews DC, et al. Prognostic nutritional index in gastrointestinal surgery. *Am J Surg* 1980;139:160–167.

Calabresi P, Schein PS, eds. *Medical oncology: basic principles and clinical management of cancer,* 2nd ed. New York: McGraw-Hill, 1993:1151–1172.

Delmore G. Assessment of nutritional status in cancer patients: widely neglected? *Support Care Cancer* 1997;5:376–380.

Dempsey DT, Mullen JL. Prognostic value of nutritional indices. *J Parenter Nutr* 1987;11:109S.

Detsky AS, McLaughlin JR, Baker JP, et al. What is subjective global assessment of nutritional status? *J Parenter Enteral Nutr* 1987;11(1):8–13.

Food and Nutrition Board, Institute of Medicine. *Recommended daily allowances,* 10th ed. Washington, DC: National Academy Press, 1989.

Gibson RS. *Principles of nutritional assessment.* New York: Oxford University Press, 1990.

Golden MH. Transport proteins as indices of protein status. *Am J Clin Nutr* 1982;35:1159–1165.

Hirsch S, de Obaldia N, Petermann M, et al. *Nutrition* 1991;7:35–38.

Jeejeebhoy KN. Protein nutrition in clinical practice. *Br Med Bull* 1981;37:11–17.

J Parenter Enter Nutr 1980;10:441–445.

Klein S, Koretz RL. Nutrition support in patients with cancer: what do the data really show? *Nutr Clin Pract* 1994;9:91–100.

Koretz RL. Parenteral nutrition: is it oncologically logical? *J Clin Oncol* 1984;2:534–538.

Monsen ER. Dietary reference intakes for the antioxidant nutrients: Vitamin C, vitamin E, selenium, and carotenoids. *J Am Diet Assoc* 2000;100:637–640.

National Cancer Institute. *Eating hints for cancer patients.* 1998.

Ottery FD. Rethinking nutritional support of the cancer patient: the new field of nutritional oncology. *Semin Oncol* 1994;21:770–778.

Rivadeneira DE, Evoy D, Fahey TJ III, et al.. Nutritional support of the cancer patient. *CA Cancer J Clin* 1998;48:69–80.

Shils ME, Olson JA, Shike M, eds. *Modern nutrition in health and disease,* 8th ed. Philadelphia: Lea & Febiger, 1994:182–183.

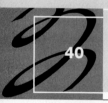

40 SMOKING CESSATION AND COUNSELING
Megan E. Wren

I. CIGARETTE SMOKING AFTER A DIAGNOSIS OF CANCER. Cigarette smoking is an important contributor to many malignancies. In addition, continuing to smoke after diagnosis may reduce the effectiveness of treatment, reduce survival rates, increase the side effects of treatment and increase the likelihood of a second malignancy. As one example, in a study of breast cancer survivors, smoking was a significant risk factor for the later development of lung cancer (odds ratio [OR] 6.0). A history of thoracic radiotherapy was not a risk factor for lung cancer in nonsmokers (OR 0.5) but was synergistic with smoking (OR 9.0).

After the publication of the first Surgeon General's Report on Smoking and Health in 1965, the rate of smoking among adult Americans gradually decreased from 42% down to 20.9% in 2004. Among current smokers, 70% report they want to quit. Although individual quit attempts have a low success rate, many people can be successful with repeated attempts. In fact, *of all Americans who have smoked, half have successfully quit*. The clinician should recognize tobacco dependence as a chronic disease, subject to periods of remission and relapse, and requiring ongoing counseling. Fortunately, effective interventions are now available that may be able to increase long-term quit rates from 15% to 30%.

II. SMOKING CESSATION PRACTICE GUIDELINES. A consensus guideline from the US Public Health Service ("the PHS Guideline") provides practical advice on treating tobacco addiction. This evidence-based guideline was sponsored and supported by many organizations, including the National Cancer Institute (NCI). The full guideline is available for free at www.surgeongeneral.gov/tobacco, as well as a Quick Reference Guide and a Clinician's Packet. Key recommendations include the following:
- Tobacco dependence is a chronic condition that often requires repeated intervention.
- Effective treatments exist that can produce long-term or even permanent abstinence; every patient who uses tobacco should be offered at least one of these treatments.
- There is a strong dose–response relation between the intensity of tobacco dependence counseling and its effectiveness. Treatments involving person-to-person contact (through individual, group, or proactive telephone counseling) are consistently effective, and their effectiveness increases with treatment intensity (e.g., minutes of contact).
- Numerous effective pharmacotherapies for smoking cessation now exist. Except in the presence of contraindications, these should be used with all patients attempting to quit smoking.

III. SMOKING CESSATION COUNSELING
- **A. The "Five A's"** technique for brief office counseling of smokers is familiar to many clinicians. A brief summary is provided in the subsequent text; more detail is available in the PHS Guideline.
  - **1. Ask** about smoking... every patient, every visit. Make it one of the vital signs so it is not forgotten.
  - **2. Advise** smokers to quit. Be empathetic, not confrontational. Use a clear, strong message such as, "Quitting smoking is the most important thing you can do to protect your health now and in the future. I can help you." Personalize the message by stressing the relevance to the patient's cancer diagnosis and treatment. Smoking cessation may increase the chance of remission, permit better wound healing, may decrease the toxicity of treatments, and reduce the chances of developing new cancers in the future.

3. **Assess** willingness to make a serious quit attempt in the next 30 days. Many clinicians use Prochaska's Transtheoretical Model of "Stages of Change" to help categorize a patient's readiness for change.
   a. Precontemplation—The patient has no plan to quit smoking. He is unaware or underaware of the consequences of smoking, or is demoralized by previous failures. The clinician's aim is to get the patient to *think about* quitting.
   b. Contemplation—The patient is thinking about quitting in the next 6 months. He is ambivalent about the pros and cons of quitting. The clinician's goal is to help the patient emphasize the factors in favor of quitting, and address any misconceptions.
   c. Preparation—The patient is intending to take action in the next month. The clinician should invest time to help the patient quit (see Section 4).
   d. Action—The patient has quit smoking; provide practical advice and moral support.
   e. Maintenance—The patient is working to prevent relapse and becomes increasingly confident over time.
4. **Assist** in the quit attempt. If the patient is ready to make a serious attempt to quit, then make smoking cessation the focus of the visit:
   a. Help the patient set a specific "quit date" in the next couple of weeks. Write it in the chart and on a prescription blank to make it official.
   b. Discuss anticipated triggers and challenges and strategies to cope with them.
   c. Provide educational materials. Offer referrals to classes, websites such as www.smokefree.gov, or a telephone Quitline (1-800-QUITNOW) for additional counseling.
   d. Recommend pharmacotherapy, except in special circumstances
5. **Arrange** follow-up. Follow-up in person or by phone within the first week and again within the first month.

IV. MEDICATIONS TO AID SMOKING CESSATION

A. **Pharmacotherapy is effective.** The PHS Guideline recommends that pharmacotherapy be offered to all patients attempting to quit smoking, except in the presence of contraindications. Although not a guarantee of success, all forms of pharmacotherapy can approximately double the abstinence rate as compared with the placebo group in randomized controlled trials. The PHS Guideline recognizes five first-line medications: bupropion sustained release (SR), nicotine gum, nicotine inhaler, nicotine nasal spray, and the nicotine patch. Two second-line drugs may also be considered: clonidine, and nortriptyline.

B. **Nicotine replacement therapy (NRT).** NRT provides an alternative source of nicotine to ease withdrawal symptoms while the patient learns new nonsmoking behaviors.
   1. **Effectiveness.** Many studies have documented that the use of NRT can double the long-term success rate. NRT is even more effective when combined with counseling. The effectiveness of counseling increases with the intensity of treatment, but even brief interventions are of benefit.
   2. **Health effects.** Nicotine is addictive but the adverse health effects of smoking are from other constituents in tobacco and its smoke. Cigarette smoke contains more than 4,000 chemical compounds, ranging from carbon monoxide to hydrogen cyanide and 69 known carcinogens, including arsenic, benzene, and radon. Essentially all the carcinogenic activity of cigarettes is attributable to the smoke, not the nicotine itself; therefore, a cigarette is a contaminated drug delivery device. Many in the public falsely believe that NRT is just as harmful as cigarettes and they think that NRT can cause heart attacks, lung cancer, and asthma.
   3. **Safety**
      a. The most common side effect of nicotine is local irritation, such as a rash under a nicotine patch or throat irritation from inhaled nicotine.
      b. Although nicotine does cause sympathetic neural stimulation, NRT provides lower nicotine doses and slower delivery as compared with cigarette smoking. Also, the dose–response relation for nicotine is flat so the effects of

smoking plus NRT are similar to smoking alone. Numerous studies have documented the safety of NRT, especially as compared with continued smoking.

c. The American Heart Association supports the use of NRT to aid in smoking cessation.

d. NRT does not increase cardiovascular deaths or hospitalizations, even in patients who smoked while using NRT and/or used NRT for more than a year.

e. Stress testing in smokers with coronary artery disease showed that addition of a nicotine patch improved exercise tolerance and decreased perfusion defect size, despite continued smoking and increased serum nicotine levels. The reduction in ischemia correlated with reduced exhaled carbon monoxide levels, as the subjects spontaneously reduced their smoking while wearing the nicotine patches.

4. Specific NRT products and patient instructions. Some products are available over-the-counter (OTC) and others by prescription only (Rx).

a. Nicotine polacrilex gum (OTC)

i. The nicotine is absorbed only through the lining of the mouth. Rapid chewing, eating, or drinking will cause the nicotine to be swallowed and it will cause heartburn, hiccups, or stomach upset.

ii. It takes several minutes for the nicotine to reach the bloodstream, so there will not be the immediate "satisfaction" of smoking.

iii. Chew slowly and intermittently, just enough to release the peppery flavor and then park the gum between cheek and gum to let the nicotine be absorbed. Alternate slow chewing and parking for 15 to 30 minutes.

iv. Use the gum on a fixed schedule, one piece every 1 to 2 hours. Try to use at least nine pieces per day for the first month; using less increases the chance of relapse. Additional pieces may be used as needed up to a maximum of 24 pieces per day.

v. After a month or 2 of abstinence, start to slowly taper the number of pieces per day (one piece per day every 4 to 7 days).

b. Nicotine lozenges (OTC) have been marketed since the PHS Guideline was published. Like the gum, the nicotine is absorbed through the buccal mucosa.

c. Nicotine transdermal patches (OTC and Rx)

i. Apply a fresh patch each morning to a relatively hairless area on the upper chest, back, or outer arm (body hair may be shaved, but do not apply the patch on broken skin).

ii. Wash hands after handling patches. The used patch should be folded in half and thrown away out of reach of children and pets.

iii. To minimize skin irritation, apply the patch in a different place each day. It is common to feel tingling under the patch for the first hour.

iv. Any brand of patch may be used for either 16 or 24 hours. Leaving the patch on overnight will ensure adequate blood levels of nicotine on awakening, to help deal with early morning cravings. Taking the patch off at night may reduce sleep disturbances.

d. Varenicline is the newest smoking cessation medication, a partial nicotine agonist. It binds to the $\alpha4b2$ nicotinic acetylcholine receptors, stimulating dopamine release to reduce craving and withdrawal symptoms while also blocking binding of nicotine to reduce the reinforcing effects of smoking ("satisfaction") (*JAMA.* 2006;296:47–55 and *JAMA.* 2006;296:56–63).

i. Effectiveness. Varenicline has been shown to more than double the placebo quit rate.

ii. Dosage. Varenicline should be started 1 week prior to the patient's quit date at 0.5 mg once daily for 3 days, then 0.5 mg twice daily for 4 days then 1 mg twice daily for 12–24 weeks.

iii. Safety. The most common adverse effects of varenciline were nausea (in more than ¼ patients), headache, vomiting, flatulence, insomnia, abnormal dreams, and dysgeusia.

e. Nicotine inhaler (Rx)

   i. The vapor is absorbed in the mouth and throat. The inhaler is puffed frequently for 20 minutes (much more frequently than a cigarette).

   ii. Use at least six cartridges a day to reduce withdrawal symptoms and relapse. The maximum number of cartridges per day is 16.

   iii. The side effects of mouth and throat irritation, cough, or upset stomach usually subside over time.

f. Nicotine nasal spray (Rx)

   i. Spray once into each nostril. *Do not sniff or inhale while spraying.* Wait 2 to 3 minutes before blowing nose.

   ii. Avoid contact with skin, eyes, or mouth.

   iii. Do not use more than 5 times an hour or 40 times in 24 hours.

   iv. The side effects of irritation in the nose and throat, sneezing, coughing, watery eyes, or runny nose usually subside over time.

g. Combination therapy. It is appropriate to use transdermal nicotine for "basal" delivery and one of the other forms of NRT for "breakthrough" cravings.

C. Bupropion sustained release (SR) is the only non-nicotine medication approved by the FDA for use in smoking cessation; sold under the brand name Zyban, it is identical to Wellbutrin SR. It is thought to work by enhancing dopaminergic activity in the central nervous system.

   1. Effectiveness

   a. In randomized controlled trials, subjects treated with bupropion SR had abstinence rates of about twice that in the placebo group.

   b. Efficacy is independent of a history of depression.

   c. In direct comparison studies bupropion SR was more effective than nicotine patches and the combination of bupropion plus nicotine patch was slightly more effective than either alone.

   d. There is some evidence that bupropion SR, with or without NRT, may attenuate the weight gain associated with smoking cessation.

   2. Dosage. Bupropion SR should be started 1 week prior to the patient's quit date, at 150 mg once daily for 3 days, then 150 mg twice daily; late evening dosing may lead to insomnia. Duration of treatment should be 7 to 12 weeks or longer.

   3. Safety. The most common side effects are insomnia, dry mouth, and nausea. Because of a 1 in 1000 risk of seizures, bupropion SR should not be used in patients with a history of seizure, head trauma, brain tumor, or in those with anorexia/bulimia, hepatic failure, or those using drugs that may increase the risk of seizures (theophylline, systemic steroids, antipsychotics, antidepressants, hypoglycemics/insulin; or abuse of alcohol or stimulants).

D. Other medications. Nortriptyline and clonidine are considered second-line agents.

   1. The tricyclic antidepressant nortriptyline is not FDA approved for smoking cessation, but there have been several published reports that demonstrate that its efficacy in smoking cessation is better than placebo but less than bupropion SR. As with other tricyclic antidepressants, nortriptyline can cause dry mouth, constipation, and sedation. An advantage of nortriptyline is its affordability.

   2. Clonidine can approximately double the quit rate and is inexpensive, but it is rarely used for smoking cessation due to troublesome side effects including dry mouth, sedation, and orthostatic hypotension. Abrupt cessation of high-dose clonidine can cause rebound hypertension. It may be used at 0.1 to 0.2 mg twice daily.

   3. Benzodiazepines and selective serotonin reuptake inhibitors (SSRIs) are *not* effective for smoking cessation.

V. CONCLUSIONS. Smoking cessation remains an important goal, even after the diagnosis of cancer. Tobacco dependence is a chronic condition that often requires repeated intervention. However, effective treatments exist that can produce long-term or even permanent abstinence. All patients should be offered at least brief counseling, and essentially all patients attempting to quit should be offered pharmacotherapy. NRT, bupropion, and perhaps nortriptyline approximately double the abstinence rate. With patience and persistence, many smokers can eventually achieve long-term abstinence.

Suggested Readings

Cigarette smoking among adults—United States, 2000. *MMWR* 2002;51(29):642–645.

Cigarette smoking among adults—United States, 2004. *MMWR* 2005;54(44);1121–1112.

Fiore MC, Bailey WC, Cohen SJ, et al. *Treating Tobacco Use and Dependence: Clinical Practice Guidelines*. Rockville: U.S. Department of Health and Human Services, Public Health Service, 2000.

Gold PB, Rubey RN, Harvey RT. Naturalistic, self-assignment comparative trial of bupropion SR, a nicotine patch, or both for smoking cessation treatment in primary care. *Am J Addict* 2002;11(4):315–331.

Gritz ER, Fingeret MC, Vidrine DJ, et al. Successes and failures of the teachable moment: smoking cessation in cancer patients. *Cancer* 2006;106(1):17–27.

Hughes JR, Stead LF, Lancaster T. Antidepressants for smoking cessation (Cochrane Review). *Cochrane Libr* 2003;2, Oxford: Update Software.

Hughes JR, Stead LF, Lancaster T. Nortriptyline for smoking cessation: a review. *Nicotine Tob Res* 2005;7(4):491–499.

Hurt RD, Sachs DP, Glover ED, et al. A comparison of sustained-release bupropion and placebo for smoking cessation. *N Engl J Med* 1997;337(17):1195–1202.

Jorenby DE, Leischow SJ, Nides MA, et al. A controlled trial of sustained-release bupropion, a nicotine patch, or both for smoking cessation. *N Engl J Med* 1999;340:685–691.

Mahmarian JJ, Moye LA, Nasser GA, et al. Nicotine patch therapy in smoking cessation reduces the extent of exercise-induced myocardial ischemia. *J Am Coll Card* 1997;30(1):125–130.

Murin S, Inciardi J. Cigarette smoking and the risk of pulmonary metastasis from breast cancer. *Chest* 2001;119:1635–1640.

Murray RP, Bailey WC, Daniels K, et al. Safety of nicotine polacrilex gum used by 3,094 participants in the Lung Health Study. *Chest* 1996;109(2):438–445.

Ockene IS, Miller NH. Cigarette smoking, cardiovascular disease, and stroke; a statement for healthcare professionals from the American Heart Association. *Circulation* 1997;96:3243–3247.

Prochaska JO, Goldstein MG. Process of smoking cessation. Implications for clinicians. *Clin Chest Med* 1991;12(4):727–35.

Silagy C, Lancaster T, Stead L, et al. Nicotine replacement therapy for smoking cessation (Cochrane Review). *Cochrane Libr* 2002;4, Oxford: Update Software.

U.S. Department of Health and Human Services, Centers for Disease Control and Prevention. *The Health Consequences of Involuntary Exposure to Tobacco Smoke: A Report of the Surgeon General*. U.S. Department of Health and Human Services, Centers for Disease Control and Prevention, National Center for Chronic Disease Prevention and Health Promotion, Office on Smoking and Health, 2006.

UK National Smoking Cessation Conference. www.uknscc.org/2005_UKNSCC/speakers/alex_bobak.html. 2005.

41

PAIN MANAGEMENT
Robert A. Swarm, Rahul Rastogi, and Daniel G. Morris

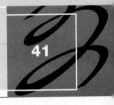

I. **INTRODUCTION TO CANCER PAIN MANAGEMENT.** Pain is a common problem in oncology practice, although the vast majority of patients could receive good cancer pain control with regular use of standard analgesic therapies. Unfortunately, standard therapies are inconsistently applied. In developed countries, up to 30% of people at initial cancer diagnosis, 50% to 70% of those receiving active antitumor therapy, and up to 80% of those with advanced malignant disease suffer from inadequately controlled pain. Improving cancer pain management will require health care professionals to have better knowledge of pain pathophysiology, epidemiology, and therapy; patients to be more effective self-advocates and better-informed health care consumers; and a health care delivery system that requires aggressive symptom control as part of individualized, patient-centered goals of therapy for cancer care. Because pain control not only improves quality of life for cancer patients but may also impact survival, optimized pain control is an integral component of comprehensive cancer care.

A. **Barriers to cancer pain management (Table 41.1).** To have pain due to cancer consistently well controlled, each practitioner must insure that each cancer patient under his/her care receives optimized pain control. Factors known to limit optimal cancer pain management must be identified in clinical practice and appropriately managed.

II. **COMPREHENSIVE PAIN ASSESSMENT.** The starting point for good pain control requires a thorough pain history and physical examination. Consider repeating diagnostic evaluations because tumor progression or metastasis is the most common cause of increasing pain in patients with cancer. When feasible, antitumor therapies may be the most effective pain management therapy.

A. **Pain assessment scales** are used to facilitate measurement of pain intensity and establish a baseline from which to judge the success of pain treatments. A numeric pain scale ("0 = No pain" up to "10 = Worst pain imaginable") is easily used by most adults, but the face scale (happy to sad faces) may be more easily used by young children. Measuring pain intensity is only the starting point in understanding the severity and consequence of a patient's pain.

B. **The comprehensive pain evaluation** includes "PQRST" factors: P = Provocative factors and palliative factors; Q = Quality(characteristics) of pain; R = Region, radiation, and referred distribution of pain; S = Severity of pain intensity; T = Temporal factors including onset, duration, time of maximum intensity, frequency, and daily variation. Patients should be queried about a previous history of pain and what drugs were effective or ineffective in his or her management.

C. **Consider comorbid conditions** that may greatly influence analgesic therapy, especially in elderly or those with advanced disease. Renal and/or hepatic insufficiency will significantly impact choice of analgesics. Intractable coagulopathy may preclude use of interventional pain therapies. Advanced medical illness may increase risk of opioid adverse effects (gastrointestinal disease: constipation or ileus; respiratory disease: respiratory depression).

D. **Assess components of pain.** Nociceptive, neuropathic, affective, behavioral, cognitive, social. Neuropathic pain may respond best to treatments including anticonvulsant and/or antidepressant therapy. Affect, cognition, and social context may markedly influence selection and/or efficacy of analgesic therapies.

E. **Believe the patient' own report of pain.** It is the most reliable indicator of pain. Malingering is rare in cancer pain management. If you do not (or conclude that you cannot) trust the patient' description of pain, pain will not be controlled.

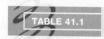

| TABLE 41.1 | Barriers to Optimal Cancer Pain Management |

Patient-related barriers	Physician-related barriers
1. Poor communication with physicians 2. Reluctance to report pain 3. Misconceptions about pain and available treatments 4. Reluctance to take medications 5. Fear of opioid addiction 6. Fear of medication adverse effects 7. Inability to access therapy, follow plan	1. Inadequate pain assessment of patient 2. Inadequate knowledge, underuse of available techniques 3. Bias limits opioid prescribing specially for female, elderly, minorities, well-functioning patients 4. Reluctance to prescribe opioids
Health care system–related barriers	**Disease- and treatment-related barriers**
1. Reimbursement encourages curative interventions over symptom control 2. Cost of analgesic therapies 3. Excessive state opioid regulations 4. Insufficient pain education, training among health care professionals 5. Poor availability, underutilization of advanced modalities for pain 6. Multiple specialists, fragmented care	1. Progressive disease increasing tissue damage and pain 2. Injury, inflammation, nerve damage, opioid tolerance facilitate pain signal processing, increasing pain 3. Coexisting/comorbid diseases may limit use of analgesic therapies 4. Incomplete efficacy of available pain therapies, including opioids

III. SYSTEMIC ANALGESICS

A. The World Health Organization (WHO) ladder (Fig. 41.1), the most widely used and validated protocol for cancer pain management, is a stepwise approach based on pain intensity Opioids are the cornerstone of pharmacotherapy for moderate to severe cancer pain, but adjuvant analgesics (nonopioid analgesics, antidepressants, and anticonvulsants) are used to enhance pain relief when needed. Analgesics should be given *"by the mouth"* (or the simplest, most effective route of administration); *"by the clock"* (regular dosing schedule rather than sporadic "as-needed" dosing); *"by the ladder;"* and *"for the individual"* (titrate analgesic to effect, monitor for adverse effects). Unrelieved pain can almost always be controlled by reevaluating the patient and reapplying the principles of the WHO ladder. For pain refractory to systemic analgesics, advanced pain therapies (beyond the WHO ladder) should be utilized.

B. Nonopioid analgesics (Table 41.2) are used as the principal analgesics for mild pain. In more severe pain, nonopioids are used as adjuvant analgesics (in addition to opioid) to improve pain control and reduce opioid dose (to reduce opioid-related adverse effects and the risk of opioid tolerance).

1. Aspirin and the nonacetylated salicylates are modestly potent analgesics and antipyretics. Aspirin is a uniquely potent inhibitor of platelet function but the nonacetylated salicylates have no impact on platelet function. The risk of gastrointestinal ulceration, somewhat greater with aspirin than other salicylates, significantly limits the analgesic utility of these agents, especially in medically ill or elderly patients. Salicylate is metabolized in the liver with renal excretion of salicylate and inactive metabolites.

2. Acetaminophen is a modestly potent but effective analgesic and antipyretic. Typical doses (650 mg to 1,000 mg q.i.d., maximum 4,000 mg/day) are well tolerated, but excessive doses may result in potentially fatal hepatotoxicity. Acetaminophen is available for oral and rectal administration, but rectal absorption is poor.

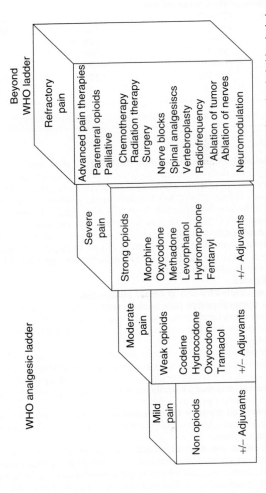

Figure 41.1. The continuum of therapies for cancer pain, based on the World Health Organization (WHO) analgesic ladder, includes a wide range of system analgesics, interventional pain therapies, and adjuvant therapies.

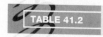

| TABLE 41.2 | Nonopioid Analgesics | | |

	Single oral dose (mg)	Maximum daily dose (mg)	Half-life (h)
Acetaminophen	650–1,000	4,000	2–3
Aspirin	650–1,000	5,000	0.3–0.5[a]
Salsalate	500–1,000	3,000	1[a]
Nonsteroidal anti-inflammatory drugs (NSAIDs)			
Ibuprofen	200–800	3,200	3–4
Celecoxib	100–200	800	10–12
Diclofenac	50	225	1–2
Ketoprofen	50–75	300	2.1
Nabumetone	500–750	2,000	24
Naproxen	220–500	1,500	10–20
Piroxicam	10–20	20	50

[a]Metabolized to salicylic acid which has a half-life of 20–30 hours with repeated dosing.

C. Nonsteroidal anti-inflammatory drugs (NSAIDs) are most useful in pain from inflammatory processes and/or boney metastases. NSAIDs limit facilitation of pain signal transmission by inhibiting prostaglandin synthesis in peripheral tissues and central nervous system (CNS). Renal insufficiency, gastrointestinal intolerance, and coagulopathy limit NSAID utility, especially in medically ill patients. Selective cyclooxygenase 2 (COX-2) inhibitors (celecoxib 200 mg daily or b.i.d.) have lower risk of gastrointestinal ulceration and no platelet dysfunction, but risk of thromboembolic events limits use. Ketorolac (15 to 30 mg i.v./i.m., q.i.d.) is the only parenteral NSAID available in United States, but therapy is limited to 5 days due to risk of gastrointestinal ulceration.

D. Opioid analgesics

1. General principles for use of opioid analgesics

a. Use a comprehensive pain assessment (outlined in the preceding text) to gather information upon which to base decisions for prescribing opioids. Repeat/review assessment at each patient contact and whenever pain is not controlled.

b. Teach patients and their families to assess pain by using a numeric score to facilitate communication. Documentation of pain intensity rating as the fifth vital sign is standard practice for outpatient and inpatient care.

c. Administer analgesics orally or through the least invasive route that provides effective pain control.

d. Document all narcotic prescriptions in the medical record to aid in the monitoring and adjustment of pain therapy (and to comply with federal and state regulations).

e. Individualize the dose of opioid. The correct dose is the one that adequately controls pain while minimizing adverse effects. Depending on pain severity, degree of opioid tolerance, and comorbid factors, the required daily dose of opioid can range over two to three orders of magnitude.

f. Avoid use of combination analgesic preparations, which contain opioid together with an NSAID or acetaminophen, unless that specific combination of medications is indicated for the specific patient. Separate preparations of opioid and nonopioid compounds will often allow more flexible dosing than combination analgesic preparations.

g. Anticipate opioid-related adverse effects and treat promptly (Table 41.3). Almost everyone taking opioid on a daily basis will need daily treatment for constipation.

TABLE 41.3 Managing Common Opioid Side Effects

Side effects	Comments and management	
Constipation	Most common side effect No tolerance Use agents regularly and prophylactically Educate patients Combine agents	Stool softeners (docusate) Stimulants (senna, bisacodyl) Bulk laxatives (psyllium) Osmotic agents (lactulose, polyethylene glycol) Enemas Opioid antagonist (oral naloxone)
Sedation	Avoid confounding medications Lower opioid dose by 25% Use stimulants Opioid substitution Add adjuvant to reduce opioid dose Use neuroaxial route of delivery	Dextroamphetamine Methylphenidate Modafinil Donepezil
Nausea and vomiting	Manage constipation Treat with antiemetics Correct metabolic factors Switch to another opioid Tolerance develops slowly	Promethazine Prochlorperazine Olanzapine Ondansetron, dolasetron Scopolamine Hydroxyzine Dexamethasone
Myoclonus	Usually with high dosages Switch to another opioid Lower dose of opioid Avoid meperidine	Lorazepam Clonazepam Diazepam
Pruritus	Treat with antihistamines Consider a different opioid	Diphenhydramine Hydroxyzine Ondansetron Nalbuphine
Withdrawal symptoms	Taper dose by half every other day when discontinuing	Clonidine
Opioid toxicity syndrome (OTS)	Risk factors: rapidly increasing, high-dose opioid; dehydration; renal failure Severe myoclonus may mimic seizures.	Opioid rotation, adequate hydration, opioid dose reduction

Seizures rarely have been reported with high-dose opioid infusion, typically associated with preservative agents. If using high-dose infusion, use preservative-free opioid preparations.

h. **Use regularly scheduled, long-acting analgesic preparations** (extended-release preparations of morphine, oxycodone, oxymorphone; fentanyl transdermal patch; methadone) to improve compliance and provide more consistent pain relief than repeated dosing of short-acting opioid preparations. Extended release oral opioid tablets should be swallowed whole and not cut or crushed.

i. **Prescribe supplemental doses of opioid for "breakthrough pain"** not controlled by the regularly scheduled doses. For this purpose, it is best to use short-acting, immediate-release preparations of opioid (morphine; oxycodone, hydromorphone). Doses of pain medication for breakthrough pain are typically 10% to 15% of the total daily opioid dose.

j. **Be flexible but aggressive in treating severe, uncontrolled pain.** Hospital admission for parenteral opioids and frequent reassessment of analgesic efficacy may be required. In a pain emergency, opioid should be given intravenously (e.g., morphine 1 to 4 mg i.v., every 10 minutes) and titrated to effect. Once pain is improved, a patient-controlled analgesia (PCA) device may facilitate access to, and documentation of, needed opioid for subsequent conversion to oral dosing.

k. **Be aware of equipotent doses of various opioid analgesics** to facilitate changes between agents or routes of administration (Table 41.4).

l. **Use naloxone to treat severe respiratory depression related to opioid overdose**. Give naloxone 0.1 to 0.2 mg i.v./i.m. every 1 to 5 minutes as needed; however, opioid antagonism with naloxone may cause extreme pain and other opioid withdrawal symptoms, and use should be carefully considered.

2. **Specific opioid analgesics (Table 41.4)**

   a. **Morphine** is hepatically metabolized to active metabolites which may account for components of morphine analgesic effect and toxicity. Morphine and metabolites undergo combined fecal and urinary excretion: morphine should be used with caution in renal insufficiency as metabolites may accumulate and cause toxicity. Although oral administration is preferred for most patients, morphine can be administered through intravenous, intramuscular, subcutaneous, sublingual, rectal, topical (for painful skin ulceration), epidural, and intrathecal routes.

   b. **Hydromorphone**, and its active hepatic metabolites, are cleared by the kidneys and can accumulate in renal failure to precipitate opioid toxicity. In some individuals, common opioid adverse effects may be less with hydromorphone than with morphine. Hydromorphone can be administered through intravenous, intramuscular, subcutaneous, sublingual, rectal, epidural, and intrathecal routes.

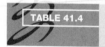 **TABLE 41.4**   Opioid Analgesics for Chronic Pain, with Estimates of Equivalent Doses Used at the Washington University Pain Management Center

	Elimination (t$\frac{1}{2}$) in hours	Dose by injection equivalent to morphine injection 10 mg (single dose)	Dose by mouth equivalent to morphine injection 10 mg (single dose)
Morphine	2–4	10 mg	20–60 mg
Codeine	3	120 mg	200 mg
Fentanyl[a]	4	100 μg	N/A
Hydrocodone	4	N/A	30–40 mg
Hydromorphone	3	2 mg	10 mg
Levorphanol	14	2 mg	4 mg
Meperidine[b]	3	100 mg	300 mg
Methadone[c]	30	10 mg	10–20 mg
Oxycodone	3	N/A	20–30 mg
Oxymorphone	2	1 mg	10 mg
Propoxyphene[b]	14	N/A	400 mg
Tramadol	6	Only the oral formulation of this is available in the United States; limit to 50–100 mg/dose and 400 mg/d due to seizure risk with higher doses	

[a] Transdermal fentanyl patch 100 μg/h = morphine 300 mg/day p.o.
[b] CNS toxicity of active metabolites limits use in chronic pain management.
[c] Very long elimination half-life causes methadone to accumulate over many days. Because methadone is eliminated ten times more slowly than morphine, with repeated dosing methadone is ten times more potent than morphine and must be dosed with caution.

c. **Fentanyl** has high lipid solubility and is metabolized by the liver to inactive metabolites which are enterally cleared. Fentanyl is given through intravenous, intramuscular, subcutaneous, transdermal, transoral mucosal, epidural, and intrathecal routes. Fentanyl transdermal patches may provide an attractive option for patients unable to swallow pills. Typically changed every 72 hours, some patients will require patch replacement every 48 hours. Patients who are cachectic or are experiencing night sweats may have poor absorption of transdermal fentanyl. Fentanyl transmucosal preparations, oralet (Actiq—initial dose 200 μg) and buccal tablet (Fentora—initial dose 100 μg), are partially absorbed through the oral mucosa and may be used for breakthrough pain.

d. **Oxycodone** is hepatically metabolized to active (oxymorphone) and non-active metabolites. Oxycodone should be used cautiously in patients with renal and hepatic insufficiency. It is only available for oral administration.

e. **Methadone** has a remarkably long elimination half-life (30 $\pm$ 19 hours). Although equianalgesic to morphine with single-dose administration, methadone accumulates with repeated dosing so that, at steady state, it is fully ten times more potent that morphine. Methadone must be increased slowly (every 5 to 10 days) and supplemented with as-needed doses of short-acting opioid (morphine, oxycodone) to avoid overdose. Metabolized in the liver by cytochrome P-450 enzymes to inactive metabolites, methadone metabolism is markedly affected by medications that induce or impede P-450 activity. Methadone and metabolites are enterally excreted and do not accumulate in renal failure. Methadone should be avoided in hepatic insufficiency because prolongation of normally long elimination half-life may preclude timely dose titration. Methadone also had nonopioid analgesic effects, through N-methyl D-aspartate (NMDA) receptors which may add to analgesic effect, especially in neuropathic pain. Methadone, especially at high doses (greater than 100 mg/day), has been associated with prolongation of QT interval and cardiac arrhythmia. Methadone can be given through oral, rectal, or intravenous routes (local tissue reaction may complicate repeated subcutaneous or intramuscular administration) with high bioavailability.

f. **Oxymorphone** is a potent, semisynthetic opioid. For parenteral administration it is approximately ten times more potent than morphine, but due to modest oral bioavailability, oral oxymorphone is only three times more potent than morphine. Elimination half-life of oxymorphone is 1.3 $\pm$ 0.7 hours with active and inactive oxymorphone metabolites excreted in the urine. Hepatic and/or renal insufficiency greatly influences oxymorphone pharmacokinetics. Oxymorphone is available for oral, parenteral, and rectal administration. Drinking alcohol significantly increases peak oxymorphone absorption from the extended release oral formulation (Opana ER).

g. **Codeine** provides almost no pain relief directly; rather, its active hepatic metabolites (morphine and morphine-6-glucuronide) provide codeine-derived analgesic effect. It may have higher risk of nausea than hydrocodone or oxycodone. Codeine is available for oral, intramuscular, or subcutaneous administration (intravenous administration should be avoided due to the risk of histamine release and subsequent cardiovascular instability).

h. **Hydrocodone,** a derivative of codeine, is metabolized by cytochrome P-450 into hydromorphone, which may mediate some of the pharmacologic effects of hydrocodone. It is only available for oral administration in preparations combined with nonopioid analgesics.

i. **Tramadol** (50 to 100 mg p.o. q.i.d., maximum 400 mg/day) has modest analgesic efficacy due to weak affinity for μ-opioid receptors. Dose is limited to a maximum of 400 mg/day, due to increased risk of seizures with higher doses. Tramadol also has effect as a norepinephrine and selective serotonin reuptake inhibitor, similar to some antidepressant medications, which may result in advantageous nonopioid effects. It should not be used in individuals receiving full doses of antidepressants, because overlapping effects of these medications could result in excess toxicity. Tramadol undergoes hepatic metabolism by the cytochrome P-450 system. In the United States, it is only available for oral administration.

j. **Meperidine** has almost no utility in cancer pain. It is metabolized to normeperidine, which accumulates due to a long half-life, and is associated with excitatory effects including tremulousness and seizures. Severe reactions, after even a single dose of meperidine, may occur in patients being treated with monoamine oxidase (MAO) inhibitors, including excitation, delirium, hyperpyrexia, convulsions, and death.

k. **Propoxyphene** is a low potency congener of methadone with almost no utility in cancer pain. It may cause severe drug interactions with carbamazepine, warfarin, or alcohol. It is metabolized to norpropoxyphene, which accumulates due to a long half-life, and is associated with excitatory effects including tremulousness and anxiety/depression, as well as prolongation of QT interval may lead to cardiac arrhythmias.

3. **Opioid rotation** involves intentionally switching from one opioid analgesic to another, using appropriate guidelines for equianalgesic dosing. Consider opioid rotation when an analgesic regimen proves inadequate despite attempts at opioid dose adjustment. Although individuals tolerant to one opioid will have cross-tolerance to other opioids, the cross-tolerance may be incomplete. In other words, the effective analgesic dose of the new opioid may be 50% (or less), the anticipated equianalgesic dose based on the prior opioid requirement. The dose-sparing effect often seen with opioid rotation may allow better pain control with fewer analgesic-related adverse effects. Opioid rotation must be undertaken with caution to avoid overdosing or underdosing, potentially resulting in excess adverse effects, inadequate pain control, or other problems. Although the data is limited to case reports and case series, opioid rotation is widely utilized in clinical practice. Special caution is required when switching to methadone from another systemic opioid, due to the long elimination half-life of methadone (see preceding text).

E. **Adjuvant analgesics (Table 41.5)**

1. **Anticonvulsants** are effective analgesics in neuropathic pain. Gabapentin (300 to 1200 mg/p.o., three times daily) is the most widely used anticonvulsant for pain control, with analgesic efficacy for acute postoperative pain, as well as neuropathic pain. Other anticonvulsants (i.e., topiramate, levetiracetam, lamotrigine, pregabalin, oxcarbazepine) should be considered upon failure/intolerance to gabapentin. Dosing of anticonvulsants must be adjusted in renal and/or hepatic insufficiency. They are only available for oral administration.

2. **Antidepressants**, especially tricyclic antidepressants (TCAs), have analgesic efficacy in chronic neuropathic pain and as recommended as adjuvant analgesics. Newer antidepressants (e.g., citalopram, duloxetine, venlafaxine, fluoxetine) may be less effective analgesics than TCAs but are generally better tolerated. If one antidepressant is poorly tolerated or provides ineffective analgesia, a different antidepressant should be tried. Antidepressants are only available for oral administration.

3. **Miscellaneous agents**

a. **Muscle relaxants** have not been studied in cancer pain, but are commonly used for musculoskeletal pain. Sedation is a common adverse effect. **Baclofen** (10 to 20 mg p.o., three times daily) is widely used for control of spasticity, but also has analgesic efficacy in neuropathic pain. To avoid potentially serious withdrawal, chronic baclofen therapy must be slowly tapered over several days, rather than abruptly discontinued. **Tizanidine** (2 to 8 mg p.o., three to four times daily) is an effective agent for spasticity with limited efficacy in chronic pain. Potential adverse effects include hypotension and hepatotoxicity. Renally cleared, tizanidine dosing must be reduced in renal insufficiency. Other muscle relaxants (carisoprodol,

TABLE 41.5	Adjuvant Analgesics		
	Usual, single oral dose (mg)	Maximum daily dose (mg)	Half-life (h)
Anticonvulsants			
Gabapentin	100–1,200	3,600	5–9
Lamotrigine	50–250	500	15–30
Levetiracetam	250–1,000	3,000	6–8
Pregabalin	50–300	600	10–12
Topiramate	25–200	400	20–30
Valproate	100–500	2,000	6–15
Antidepressants			
Amitriptyline	25–300	300	16–30
Bupropion	50–150	450	14
Citalopram	10–40	40	30–36
Doxepin	25–300	300	16–30
Duloxetine	30–120	60–120	10–14
Fluoxetine	10–80	80	100
Sertraline	50–200	200	24–60
Trazodone	25–400	400	8
Venlafaxine	25–100	375	5–11

cyclobenzaprine, metaxalone) have only a limited role in management of cancer-related musculoskeletal pain.

b. **Local anesthetics**, especially **lidocaine**, given systemically (intravenous infusion or oral administration) are effective analgesics. A lidocaine infusion (1 to 2 mg i.v./minute, after a 25- to 50-mg loading dose) may be especially effective for intractable neuropathic pain which has proven ineffective to systemic opioid. For long-term use, intravenous lidocaine infusion is difficult to maintain and serum level must be checked regularly to avoid toxicity. Unfortunately oral **mexiletine** (10 mg/kg/day, divided into three doses daily) has only modest analgesic efficacy. Lidocaine 5% patch provides pain relief through topical anesthetic action, and is especially indicated where neuropathic pain is associated with markedly increased skin sensitivity (cutaneous mechanoallodynia). With little systemic absorption, lidocaine patch has negligible systemic effects, but the water-based adhesive may cause dermatitis if left in place for more than 12 hours daily.

c. **Systemic corticosteroids** are used in cancer patients to provide analgesia, improve appetite, prevent nausea and malaise, and improve quality of life. Corticosteroids may be particularly useful in acute pain due to boney metastases, infiltration or compression of neural structures, increased intracranial pressure (headache), obstruction of a hollow viscus or organ capsule distention, or spinal cord compression. Long-term use of steroids may lead to gastrointestinal ulceration, so use of gastroprotective agents is advised.

IV. **SPECIAL TECHNIQUES FOR MANAGEMENT OF RESISTANT CANCER PAIN**

A. **Psychological and behavior medicine techniques**. Multidisciplinary cancer care would be incomplete without including care for the psyche. Cancer pain is a complex emotional experience. Cancer patients with pain undergo emotional distress, especially anxiety and depression, which increase pain and suffering. Pharmacologic and nonpharmacologic therapies for treatment of psychological and psychiatric comorbidities are essential to the overall management of cancer pain. **Cognitive behavioral therapies (CBT)** are the most frequently used psychological modalities in chronic pain management. Through CBT, patients learn to control the thoughts, emotions, and behaviors that modulate pain experience. CBT includes hypnosis, relaxation techniques (including progressive muscle relaxation, meditation, and guided imagery), biofeedback, coping skills training, music therapy, cognitive restructuring, supportive and group therapy, and stress management techniques.

B. Physical and occupational therapies are essential to optimize functional status after prolonged medical illness or surgical intervention. Therapeutic and conditioning exercise programs are essential components to the successful long-term management of chronic pain. Specific therapies such as orthotic bracing and assistive devices, may greatly aid pain control and/or patient functional status.

C. Complementary and alternative therapies are widely used, alone or in conjunction with conventional therapies, for pain control by persons with cancer. Patients should be routinely asked about complementary and alternative (CAM) therapies, if only to allow screening for potential adverse interactions between CAM and conventional therapies. Alternative therapies such as acupuncture, massage, healing touch, and many herbal therapies have shown benefits in controlling pain and other symptoms, but comparative trials with other analgesic therapies are lacking.

D. Interventional techniques for severe cancer pain are important components of comprehensive care for severe cancer pain and should not be relegated to treatments of last resort. Interventional pain therapies should be considered if pain is not adequately controlled with systemic analgesics, or if use of such analgesics is associated with adverse effect (e.g., sedation, constipation, and/or nausea). Interventional pain therapies can potentially improve quality of life by (a) providing more effective pain control and (b) allowing reduction in analgesic dose, with reduced analgesic adverse effects. Improved pain control and reduced adverse effects through appropriate use of interventional pain therapies may improve life expectancy in patients with terminal disease.

1. **Spinal administration of analgesics** delivers medication more potently to the spinal cord to enhance analgesic efficacy and minimize systemic (brain) adverse effects of analgesics, especially sedation. Spinal analgesics (opioids, local anesthetics, clonidine, and/or baclofen) are used singly or in combination for either intrathecal or epidural administration. The spinal administration of combined opioid, local anesthetic, and clonidine is an especially potent analgesic therapy. Spinal analgesics may be administered by epidural or intrathecal (subarachnoid) systems, but an implanted pump (for intrathecal infusion) is most commonly used.

   a. **Spinal opioids** (especially morphine, hydromorphone) have significantly increased potency: 100 mg/day parenteral morphine is roughly equivalent to 10 mg/day epidural morphine, which is roughly equivalent to 1 mg/day intrathecal morphine; however, actual doses must be titrated to effect. Fentanyl, because of its high lipid solubility, has rapid systemic absorption after spinal administration; therefore spinal administration of fentanyl may have little advantage over systemic administration. Potential adverse effects include sedation, respiratory depression (onset may be delayed for several hours), constipation, nausea, pruritus, peripheral edema, and urinary retention. Exceptionally high doses of spinal opioids may result in myoclonic jerks or even diffuse muscle rigidity.

   b. **Spinal local anesthetics** (bupivacaine, lidocaine) may markedly decrease pain without sedation or some other of the potential adverse effects associated with opioid analgesics. After spinal administration of low doses of local anesthetic, pain relief may be obtained without significant motor blockade or extremity numbness. Potential adverse effects include hypotension (especially orthostatic hypotension), extremity weakness, and urinary retention.

   c. **Spinal clonidine** has analgesic efficacy after epidural or intrathecal administration, through action at spinal α_2-adrenergic receptors. Potential adverse effects include hypotension (especially orthostatic hypotension), bradycardia, congestive heart failure, and sedation.

2. **Vertebroplasty and kyphoplasty** are procedures for the percutaneous injection of bone cement (methyl methacrylate) into vertebral bodies affected by compression fractures due to metastatic tumor, destructive vertebral hemangiomas, or osteoporosis. Kyphoplasty differs from vertebroplasty in that bone cement is injected after a balloon has been used to create a cavity in the vertebral body, in an attempt to restore vertebral body height. Vertebroplasty/kyphoplasty can be highly effective in control of pain from vertebral compression fractures due to osteoporosis and/or tumor. Thorough radiographic evaluation is essential before vertebroplasty/kyphoplasty. Potential adverse effects include spread of unhardened cement beyond the vertebral body, through direct spread to the spinal canal or through vascular embolization. Vertebroplasty/kyphoplasty need not delay treatment of spinal metastases with radiation therapy, but may provide rapid onset of pain relief, which may facilitate the use of appropriate antitumor therapies.

3. **Neurolytic neural blockade** should be considered for patients with terminal disease in whom pain is poorly controlled with less-invasive therapies and pain is localized to a particular region of the body. If pain recurs after several months, neurolytic blockade may be repeated, but repeated blockade is generally not necessary.

   a. **Neurolytic celiac plexus block**, the most commonly performed neurolytic technique for cancer pain, is indicated for upper abdominal visceral pain from pancreatic or other upper abdominal malignancy. Up to 85% of appropriately selected patients report good-to-excellent pain relief after neurolytic celiac plexus block. The side effects of orthostatic hypertension and increased frequency of bowel movements (diarrhea) transiently affect most persons after neurolytic celiac plexus block, but only 1% to 2% requires long-term medical management of these symptoms. Significant neural damage or paralysis is a rare but devastating complication of celiac plexus block that generally precludes the use of this technique in nonterminal illness. The risk of paralysis may cause some patients to decide against celiac plexus block, but to others, the potential for good-to-excellent pain relief (75% to 85%) that may be associated with improvements in constipation, nausea, and general sense of well-being outweighs the risk of paralysis (0.1% to 0.2%).

   b. **Neurolytic hypogastric plexus block** may be an effective technique for management of visceral pain from pelvic malignancy. Its use is not significantly associated with extremity weakness, but ejaculatory failure/inorgasmia is a potential adverse effect. Neurolytic hypogastric plexus block is not likely to provide good pain control if there is tumor invasion of somatic or neural structures.

E. **Neurosurgical techniques** for pain control are rarely used, but are potentially powerful tools in the management of resistant pain. Spinal cord procedures (e.g., cordotomy) and even brain surgeries (e.g., cingulotomy) may be of real benefit in management of intractable pain. Especially for unilateral lower body or lower extremity pain, in the setting of terminal illness, cordotomy (percutaneous or open surgical approach) may provide remarkable control of previously intractable pain.

F. **Management of refractory pain and/or other symptoms of terminal illness.** In the last hours to days of life, some people who are dying develop severe symptoms such as intractable pain, dyspnea, delirium, and/or emesis (e.g., fecal emesis due to distal bowel obstruction beyond surgical intervention). If such symptoms are intolerable to the dying patient, but would be refractory to further acceptable efforts at palliative intervention, consideration should be given to alleviation of distress through administration of sedatives. Terminal, palliative sedation should be considered only for those who have requested not to be resuscitated ("no code") in the event of cardiac/respiratory arrest. Midazolam is the most commonly used drug for palliative sedation (1 to 2 mg i.v., i.m., or subcutaneously q1h, p.r.n.; or loading dose of 1 to 2 mg i.v. with infusion 0.5 to 2 mg/hour) but other benzodiazepines (diazepam, 5 to 10 mg p.o., 2 mg i.v. q2h, p.r.n.) can be used instead. Benzodiazepines may worsen agitation in some persons, and they may be better treated with barbiturates (thiopental infusion, 0.5 mg/kg i.v. loading dose, followed by 0.25 to 0.5 mg/kg/hour i.v. infusion), or neuroleptic sedatives (haloperidol, 1 to 4 mg i.v./p.o. q1h, p.r.n.) titrated to good effect to ease suffering from otherwise intractable symptoms. These drugs generally have long elimination half-lives and will accumulate to steady-state level over a few days. The use of palliative terminal sedation to provide a dying person relief from intractable, intolerable suffering is firmly within the realm of good, supportive palliative care and should not be confused with euthanasia.

V. SPECIFIC PAIN SYNDROMES

A. **Mucositis** is one of the most debilitating, refractory adverse effects following chemotherapy and/or radiotherapy damage to tissues of the alimentary canal. Mucositis is associated with pain and increased risk of infection and can lead to impaired nutritional status and dehydration. Traditional management of oral mucositis has involved patient education for avoidance of dehydration, oral rinses (saline, chlorhexidine), topical and systemic analgesics, nutritional support, and prevention/management of infection. Palifermin, a recombinant keratinocyte growth factor, helps in prevention and faster healing of oral mucositis.

B. **Bone pain** or skeletal pain from cancer is a frequent problem and is especially common with boney metastasis. Bone pain can be managed by various modalities including NSAIDs, opioids, corticosteroids, bisphosphonates, radiation therapy, radioisotopes, hormonal and/or chemotherapy, and orthopedic surgery.

1. **Bisphosphonates** inhibit osteoclast-mediated bone resorption and are an important component in the treatment of painful bone metastasis. Zoledronic acid 4 to 8 mg every 3 to 4 weeks, Pamidronate 90 mg i.v. over 1 to 2 hours every 3 to 4 weeks, and Ibandronate 3 mg every 3 months, have been shown to relieve pain, reduce the number of metastases, prevent osteolysis, and decrease the frequency of fractures. All bisphosphonates can induce gastrointestinal upset, renal damage, and mandibular osteonecrosis. Dose should be adjusted based on renal function.

2. **Radioisotopes,** through parenteral administration, provide systemic radiation to diminish multifocal painful skeletal metastasis. Strontium-89 and Samarium-153 have shown selectivity for bone metastasis and found to be effective in reducing pain. High cost, delayed pain relief, and severe hematologic toxicity result in limited use of these agents.

3. **External-beam radiation** is used in relieving local tumor-related bone pain. Focal lesion can be managed by localized external-beam irradiation (also known as *involved-field irradiation*). Multiple painful sites can be managed by wide-field external-beam irradiation (e.g., hemibody irradiation). Side effects include bone marrow suppression and radiation tissue damage.

C. **Neuropathic pain from tumor invasion of major nerve plexus.** Neuropathic pain may be relatively less responsive to opioid analgesics than more typical tissue-injury (nociceptive) pain, especially when tumor directly invades a major nerve or plexus. Clinical situations such as tumor invasion of brachial plexus (Pancoast tumor), or retroperitoneal sarcoma invading the lumbosacral plexus, require aggressive pain therapies early in the course of disease. Adjuvant, nonopioid analgesics (anticonvulsants, antidepressant) therapies should be optimized. Although rarely needed, severe neuropathic pain not responding to systemic analgesics is a relatively common indication for spinal administration of analgesics, typically through an implanted spinal infusion pump.

D. **Tumor treatment–related neuropathic pain syndromes**

1. **Chemotherapy-induced peripheral neuropathy (CIPN)** can present as a pure motor disturbance, a pure sensory disturbance or as a mixed sensory-motor disturbance. Typically, paresthesias or dysesthetic sensations follow chemotherapy including: paclitaxel and related compounds, vincristine, platinum compounds, ifosfamide, antiganglioside-G-D2 monoclonal antibody, bortezomib, and cytarabine. Agents that have been used in an attempt to prevent CIPN include: amifostine, Org-2766, Leukemia inhibitory factor, lithium,

α-lipoic acid, folinic acid, glutathione, pyridoxine, IGF-1, nimodipine, glutamate and calcium–magnesium solution. There is no specific treatment for CIPN but antineuropathic pain medications (gabapentin, pregabalin, levetiracetam, and topiramate) may be of benefit.

2. **Radiation neuropathy** presents in patients who have undergone radiation therapy. The incidence is variable and appears to be dose dependent. The most common injuries occur to the brachial plexus (after radiation therapy for breast cancer, lung cancer or Hodgkin' lymphoma) and the lumbosacral nerves (after radiation for pelvic and abdominal malignancies). Peripheral neuropathy is also seen, but usually is self-limited and less symptomatic. Injury can occur to any nerve in the beam of the radiation therapy device. The common complaints include paresthesias, dysesthesias, allodynia, hyperalgesia, and hyperpathia in the area of nerve injury. Most of these neuropathies present weeks after radiation therapy. Treatment includes anticonvulsants, opioids, NSAIDs, TCAs, and local and topical anesthetics. In very severe cases, consideration of intrathecal therapy should be undertaken. Psychological and physical therapy modalities should be entertained as a part of a multidisciplinary program.

3. **Postsurgical pain syndromes**
   a. **Postmastectomy pain syndrome,** involving persistent pain in the anterior chest, axilla, and medial and posterior portions of the arm, occurs after surgical procedures involving the breast. It has a prevalence of 4% to 30% and occurs between 2 weeks and 6 months following surgery. The pain is quite variable between somatic and neuropathic, but is usually a combination of the two (tight, constricting, paresthesias, hyperpathia, burning, electric shock, or stabbing). Treatment includes opioids, anticonvulsants, topical agents (lidocaine patch), physical therapy, and cognitive behavioral therapy.
   b. **Postradical neck dissection pain syndrome** is a combination neuropathic and myofascial pain condition that occurs in as many as 50% of postsurgical patients. It is a persistent, neuropathic pain involving one or more branches of the superficial cervical plexus (SCP). It is usually described as spontaneous, continuous burning pain, shooting pain, or allodynia. Treatment is similar to other postsurgical neuropathic pain syndromes, but additional consideration should be given to myofascial trigger point injections using local anesthetic and/or botulinum toxin.
   c. **Postthoracotomy pain syndrome (PTPS)** is persistent moderate to severe pain, usually in the distribution of one or more intercostal nerves. The usual course of pain is limited to the initial 6 to 10 days after surgery, but in a small percentage, it can persist indefinitely. It is a combination of neuropathic (from intercostal nerve injury or neuroma formation) and myofascial pain. Care must be taken not to confuse PTPS with tumor reoccurrence pain. The pain is described as numbness, tingling, burning, itching, or shooting. There is quite often hyperesthesia in the involved dermatome. Treatment involves the use of physical therapy, opioids, antiseizure medications, transcutaneous electrical nerve stimulation, and local anesthetic intercostal nerve blocks. In very severe cases, spinal cord stimulation or spinal analgesics may be indicated.

E. **Postherpetic neuralgia**
   1. **Herpes zoster (HZ)**, resulting from reactivation of varicella zoster (VZ) infection, is characterized by painful, vesicular cutaneous lesions in a dermatomal pattern. Pain may precede visible lesions by 2 to 3 days. HZ is typically self-limited in normal hosts, but in immunocompromised patients it may cause cutaneous dissemination or even potentially fatal systemic and/or CNS infection. Acute HZ pain (acute herpetic neuralgia) typically resolves with healing of cutaneous lesions; however, the risk of persistent postherpetic neuralgia (PHN) increases with age. Even with aggressive therapy, 10% to 30% of individuals older than 60 years presenting with HZ will experience PHN, and up to 50% of persons with PHN may have pain lasting indefinitely.

2. Prevention of postherpetic neuralgia. The incidence and/or duration of PHN is reduced with oral antiviral agents in adults older than 50 years, if therapy is started within 72 hours of onset of rash. Acyclovir (800 mg every 4 hours, five doses daily, for 7 to 10 days) speeds healing of lesions, decreases pain from acute HZ, and may decrease the incidence of PHN. Newer antivirals famciclovir (500 mg every 8 hours for 7 days) or valacyclovir (1,000 mg every 8 hours for 7 days) have been shown to decrease the incidence of PHN with less frequent dosing, which may improve compliance. Addition of systemic corticosteroid to antiviral therapy does not further reduce the risk of PHN, but adding TCA (amitriptyline 25 mg orally at bedtime) may be of benefit. Sympathetic nerve blocks and epidural steroid injections provide excellent pain relief in acute HZ and may reduce PHN. High potency, live attenuated VZ vaccine has been shown to decrease the incidence of HZ and the severity of PHN in adults 60 years of age and older and will likely be used to prevent HZ and PHN in high-risk populations.

3. Treatment of established postherpetic neuralgia is based on the use of systemic analgesics and may include TCAs, anticonvulsants, and/or opioid analgesics. Topical lidocaine 5% patch may be of benefit in PHN associated with cutaneous extra sensitivity (mechanoallodynia).

F. The Opioid toxicity syndrome (OTS) consists of diffuse hyperalgesia, myoclonus, and altered mental status (agitation/delirium or sedation/confusion). Although rare, it is most often seen when patients are on high doses of opioid (often greater than100 mg morphine/hour or equivalent), yet inadequate pain control requires further rapid opioid dose escalation. In such settings, increasing opioid dose may not result in improved pain control, but rather worsened pain (hyperalgesia) and deterioration of mental status. In extreme cases, myoclonus may be nearly continuous and resemble seizure-like activity, but patients are generally conscious and conversant. Dehydration and/or renal insufficiency may increase the risk of opioid toxicity syndrome (OTS). OTS has been most frequently described with systemic morphine, but has been reported with other systemic opioids and with spinal opioid. Opioid-induced facilitation of pain signal transmission (opioid-induced hyperalgesia) appears to be one of the principle factors contributing to OTS.

   Management of OTS requires switching to another opioid (opioid rotation), typically using less than the fully equivalent dose. In extreme cases of OTS, it may be necessary to completely discontinue opioid analgesics temporarily, and rely on nonopioid analgesics (e.g., anticonvulsants or intravenous lidocaine infusion) for pain control. Once OTS symptoms improve, patients may be managed with relatively low doses of another opioid.

G. Cancer pain management in the noncompliant patient. Pain management therapies are less likely to be successful if not used appropriately and consistently. To manage apparent noncompliance, treating health care professionals must identify and manage contributing factors such as: (a) cognitive impairment (due to underlying disease(s), treatments, other factors); (b) psychological/psychiatric disorders (depression/anxiety, personality disorders); (c) substance abuse or dependence; and (d) physical ability to obtain, store, and access prescribed treatments.

   In chronic illness and/or malignancy, patients often develop tolerance (increasing dose requirement) and physical dependence (withdrawal symptoms with abrupt discontinuation) but rarely develop new substance dependence or addiction. In the context of chronic pain in oncology practice, "drug-seeking" behavior likely reflects inadequate pain control, and "substance dependence" or "addiction" is best characterized by impaired control over drug use, compulsive drug use, continued drug use despite harm, and/or drug craving.

   Substance abuse/dependence is rarely diagnosed in patients with terminal disease, but can significantly complicate pain management therapies. It is essential to obtain the patient' cooperation in order to get a thorough substance abuse history and find optimal management strategies. Patients with cancer pain and active substance abuse/dependence will require very close monitoring and multidisciplinary care:

1. Involve psychiatrist, addictionologist especially if substance abuse is recent, ongoing. Encourage participation in a 12-step recovery program (Alcoholics Anonymous, Narcotics Anonymous) if feasible.
2. Analgesics filled by only one prescriber.
3. Use one opioid analgesic, preferably a long-acting formulation, given on a regular schedule. As far as possible, limit access to short-acting or "as-needed" doses of opioid.
4. Optimize use of nonopioid and nonpharmacologic pain therapies.
5. Utilize pill counts and urine toxicology screens, if needed, to help with monitoring of compliance with prescribed therapies and avoidance of other abuse substances.
6. Limit quantity of controlled substances to weekly supply, if compliance is poor. (In extreme cases, it may be necessary for medication to be dispensed daily by home health nurse or even through a substance abuse program.)
7. Utilization of written opioid analgesic guidelines may help patients to understand what is expected regarding appropriate use of analgesic therapies.

Suggested Readings

Cherny NI. The assessment of cancer pain. In: McMahon SB, Koltzenburg M, eds. *Wall and Melzack' textbook of pain*, 5th ed. Philadelphia: Churchill Livingstone, 2006:1099–1125.

Daeninck PJ, Bruera E. Opioid use in cancer pain. Is a more liberal approach enhancing toxicity? *Acta Anaesthesiol Scand* 1999;43:924–938.

Estfan B, LeGrand SB, Walsh D, et al. Opioid rotation in cancer patients: pros and cons. *Oncology* 2005;19:511–516.

Hassenbusch SJ, Cherny NI. Neurosurgical approaches in palliative medicine. In: Doyle D, Hanks G, Cherny NI, et al. eds. *Oxford textbook of palliative medicine*, 3rd ed. Oxford: Oxford University Press, 2004:397–405.

Hassenbusch SJ, Portenoy RK, Cousins M, et al. Polyanalgesic consensus conference 2003: an update on the management of pain by intraspinal drug delivery–report of an expert panel. *J Pain Symptom Manage* 2004;27:540–563.

Lo B, Rubenfeld G. Palliative sedation in dying patients: "we turn to it when everything else hasn't worked". *JAMA* 2005;294:1810–1816.

Mao J. Opioid-induced abnormal pain sensitivity: implications in clinical opioid therapy. *Pain* 2002;100:213–217.

Melzack R, Katz J. Pain assessment in adult patients. In: McMahon SB, Koltzenburg M, eds. *Wall and Melzack' textbook of pain*, 5th ed. Philadelphia: Churchill Livingstone, 2006:291–304.

Murphy KJ, Deramond H. Percutaneous vertebroplasty in benign and malignant disease. *Neuroimaging Clin N Am* 2000;10:535–545.

Opstelten W, van Wijck AJ, Stolker RJ. Interventions to prevent postherpetic neuralgia: cutaneous and percutaneous techniques. *Pain* 2004;107:202–206.

Oxman MN, Levin MJ, Johnson GR, et al. A vaccine to prevent herpes zoster and postherpetic neuralgia in older adults. *N Engl J Med* 2005;352:2271–2284.

Penson RT, Nunn C, Younger J, et al. Trust violated: analgesics for addicts. *Oncologist* 2003;8:199–209.

Quigley C. Opioid switching to improve pain relief and drug tolerability. *Cochrane Database Syst Rev* 2004;(3)CD004847.

Savage SR. Assessment for addiction in pain-treatment settings. *Clin J Pain* 2002;18:S28–S38.

Smith TJ, Staats PS, Deer T, et al. Randomized clinical trial of an implantable drug delivery system compared with comprehensive medical management for refractory cancer pain: impact on pain, drug-related toxicity, and survival. *J Clin Oncol* 2002;20:4040–4049.

Swarm RA, Karanikolas M, Cousins MJ. Anaesthetic techniques for pain control. In: Doyle D, Hanks G, Cherny NI, et al. eds. *Oxford textbook of palliative medicine*, 3rd ed. Oxford: Oxford University Press, 2004:378–396.

Sykes N, Thorns A. The use of opioids and sedatives at the end of life. *Lancet Oncol* 2003;4:312–318.

Wareham D. Postherpetic neuralgia. *Clin Evid* 2005;15:1–9.

World Health Organization. *Cancer pain relief and palliative care: report of a WHO expert committee*. Geneva: World Health Organization, 1990:804.

HOSPICE AND PALLIATIVE CARE

Colleen R. Gilmore

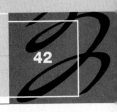

42

"You matter because you are, you matter to the last moment of your life, and we will do all we can not only to help you die peacefully, but to live until you die." Cicely Saunders, M.D.

I. INTRODUCTION. Palliative care and hospice share a philosophy of patient-centeredness, but they differ in terms of the timing of the care and the method of reimbursement. Palliative care is appropriate for patients of any age with any serious medical condition. Hospice is distinctively focused on the end of life. Palliative care and hospice are becoming more prevalent as more people are living with chronic, debilitating, or life-threatening illnesses. With recent advances in oncology, many patients are living longer, even when faced with advanced disease. Patients who have been cured of their cancer may need palliative interventions to help relieve discomfort from transient or permanent side effects from treatments of the disease. This chapter first discusses hospice, which is the older of the two holistic treatment models. It then addresses the more recent emergence and expansion of palliative care, both as a philosophy and as a specialty program.

II. HOSPICE

A. Definition. Hospice care is intensified palliative care that is initiated in the later stages of the patient's illness. A hospice referral is initiated when a patient's disease is no longer responding to active chemotherapy or radiation, the patient has a poor performance status, and/or the patient's quality of life is intolerable. The focus of hospice is on alleviating distress of all types—physiological, psychosocial, and spiritual. The hospice team seeks to help the patient live each day to the fullest and with the best quality as defined by the patient and family. Hospice is a philosophy of care, not a "place to die." Hospice care is most often given in the patient's home. However, hospice patients can be cared for in nursing facilities or in the inpatient hospital setting.

B. History of hospice. The concept of hospice was first developed in the middle of the nineteenth century by a Catholic order, the Sisters of Charity, in Ireland. The sisters found terminally ill people dying in horrible conditions at home, without adequate care from family members. They created clean places where patients could come to die. With the help of national health funds and private philanthropy, the hospice movement spread and flourished in England. By the 1960s, there were 25 hospices in England.

Cicely Saunders, a nurse trained in social work, cared for dying patients in a London hospital. One patient described to her a place he would like to be in during his final days. He left a bequest to the hospital for the establishment of a hospice. Saunders was inspired by the patient and went to medical school. After graduation, she helped open St. Christopher's Hospice in South London in 1967. St. Christopher's was unique for its windows, garden, home-like furnishings, many activities for patients, attention to small details, and for the absence of heroic measures prolonging the dying process. In 1969, St. Christopher's initiated a home care hospice program.

Dr. Saunders presented the concept of hospice care at Yale University in 1974. The first American hospice later opened in New Haven, Connecticut. In 1979, the National Hospice Organization was formed in the United States, and in 1983, the Health Care Finance Administration established the Medicare Hospice Benefit (MHB). In 1987, palliative medicine was first recognized as a specialty in Britain. In

1988, the International Hospice Institute helped form the Academy of Hospice Physicians, now known as the *American Academy of Hospice and Palliative Medicine*.

C. **The hospice team.** The hospice team is an integral part of the hospice philosophy. The team includes a medical director, registered nurses, social workers, chaplains, health aides, volunteers, and other allied health professionals. The patient and his family are the central focus of the team. Members of the hospice team commonly meet at least weekly to discuss the patient and family. All team members provide input from their specialties in an effort to deliver the best interdisciplinary holistic care possible. The team members draw strength and support from one another. Monthly support-group meetings with the spiritual counselor and/or social worker may benefit the team members.

1. **The medical director.** The medical director supervises the medical care of hospice patients; communicates with other attending physicians, fellows, and residents; and provides educational opportunities for medical students who rotate through the hospice program. The medical director does not replace the patient's oncologist, but rather covers for the referring primary physician if he or she is unavailable. The medical director is responsible for overseeing the hospice plan of care. He or she also signs the initial certification along with the primary physician that the patient has 6 months or less to live, which is a requirement of Medicare. Patients who live beyond this certification period are then reassessed by the medical director and recertified quarterly. The hospice medical director is available 24 hours a day, 7 days a week to the hospice staff, and may visit and assess patients when there are complex symptom-management issues. It is imperative that there be a good working relationship between the hospice medical director and the hospital's palliative care physicians and staff to facilitate continuity of care between the inpatient and hospice care settings.

2. **The registered nurse.** When a patient is enrolled to hospice, a primary registered nurse is assigned to care for the patient and family. The hospice nurse has been described as the "eyes and ears" for the physician, because many patients are too weak to be transported to their physician's office. The nurse continually communicates with and assesses the patient through home visits and telephone calls and takes orders from the primary physician or medical director to maintain the patient's comfort. The nurse also provides education and training to the patient's family and caregivers. *Family* is defined broadly as any person who is close to the patient and has made a commitment to care for him or her.

The registered nurse and the family come up with a primary care plan, which sets forth the frequency and types of services needed by the patient. The nurse always does a medication review on admission to make sure the patient and family understand the medication dosages, schedule, and side effects. The nurse assesses the needs for palliative measures and orders needed home medical equipment such as a hospital bed, oxygen, air mattress, wheelchair, and/or bedside commode. A registered nurse is on call 24 hours a day, 7 days a week. If necessary, an on-call nurse will visit the patient at any time of the day or night. The nurse assists the physician in determining whether a patient needs to be admitted as an inpatient for symptom management or respite care in order to relieve the family from the burdens of 24-hour care for a few days. In some situations, the patient will transition from respite care to a nursing facility.

3. **The social worker.** Every hospice patient has a psychosocial assessment by a masters level social worker trained in hospice. Social workers provide support and grief counseling for patients and families, and assess risk for complicated grief reactions. Social workers assess the patient's mental status and provide the patient with the opportunity to do a life review. They encourage the patient and family to share their feelings and discuss their thoughts on death and dying, their fears and regrets, and other things they never had an opportunity to talk about. Social workers help the family with financial and estate planning, advanced directives, and funeral planning. Social workers make referrals to social service agencies, assist patients in nursing home placement, or arrange private-duty nursing care for those who remain at home.

4. **The chaplain.** The hospice chaplain's role is to provide spiritual support and counseling for the patient and family. The chaplain meets with the patient and family and performs a spiritual assessment. Hospice chaplains are ecumenical and nondenominational. Some patients will decline chaplain services because they feel close to and comfortable with their own pastor, rabbi, or spiritual leader. Other patients are estranged from their religion of origin and are open to discussing their spiritual questions and concerns with the chaplain. Many hospice chaplains can perform funerals, weddings, and other religious ceremonies as needed. The chaplain may lead memorial services for patients, their families, and the hospice staff who cared for the patients during the year.

5. **The home health aide.** Home health aides are certified nurses' aides who receive special training through the hospice program. They provide physical care to the patient in the home or residential nursing facility. They assist with bathing, mouth care, turning, and skin care. They teach family members and nursing facility staff about the patient's physical care. They spend a lot of time giving physical touch and comfort to the patient and psychological comfort to the family. Home health aides assist family members in getting the patient up, sometimes with the use of a Hoyer lift. If the patient is not bed-bound, the home health aides assist the patient in getting in and out of the shower or tub. They encourage independence, but as the patient's functioning declines, they gradually provide more physical care. Their companionship is very important to patients and families.

6. **The hospice volunteers.** Hospice volunteers go through an intensive training program. They learn about the phases of dying; confidentiality, safety, and patient and family needs; and the hospice philosophy and team approach. Volunteers who help in the home are included in the patient's plan of care. They may read to or sit with the patient, play music, take a walk with the family, or provide brief respite care. Some hospice volunteers assist in the office by sending out bereavement mailings, compiling patient-education packets, answering phones, typing, cataloguing library books, and giving talks. Hospice volunteers are viewed as a critical part of the hospice team by staff, patients, and families.

7. **Other allied health professionals.** Depending on the patient's needs, other allied health professionals may be included on the hospice team as well. Some hospice patients may benefit from physical therapy, occupational therapy, speech therapy, or nutritional counseling. Others may need psychiatric or psychological services. Some hospices offer complementary therapies to assist with palliative care, and to improve the quality of life. These may include massage therapy, music therapy, healing touch, pet therapy, art therapy, and aroma therapy.

D. **Hospice eligibility criteria.** When is hospice appropriate for a patient? One of a physician's most difficult challenges is to know the right time to initiate a hospice referral. Many patients are referred to hospice very late in their illnesses. Sometimes the patient and family are not ready to discuss hospice until this point. Sometimes the physician is uncomfortable knowing when to raise the issue with the patient or family or when to stop treatment. The patient and family will be more prepared for a hospice referral if the oncologist has maintained an ongoing relationship and open communication with them throughout the course of the illness.

Under Medicare, Medicaid, and most private insurance plans, a patient is eligible for hospice if his physician and the hospice medical director certify that he is terminal and has 6 months or less to live. The patient and caregivers must agree to the philosophy of hospice. That is, they must agree that the focus is on managing symptoms of the disease without the use of life-prolonging measures. The patient needs to have a 24-hour caregiver or be willing to come up with a plan with the hospice team for 24-hour care. The patient could hire 24-hour private-duty nursing care, enter a long-term care facility, arrange for friends or family to take shifts in the patient's own home, or live with a family member. The patient does not have to sign a Do Not Resuscitate (DNR) order to be on hospice. It is the patient's right to choose hospice and still remain full code. The patients may decide after initiating hospice to change their code status.

E. **Funding.** Hospice is covered by a specific MHB. Most private insurance companies and Medicaid offer a similar benefit. When a patient signs for MHB, he or she is electing to have his or her Medicare Part A (hospital benefit) assigned to a Medicare-certified hospice ("Medicare-Certified Agency," or "MCA"). The hospice is then responsible for the patient's plan of care and cannot bill the patient for services. The MCA receives a per diem rate from Medicare that covers all medications for pain and symptom management, durable medical equipment and supplies, nursing care, social services, chaplain visits, and other needed services.

The MHB does not cover private-duty nursing or the cost of room and board at a nursing facility. If the patient is dually eligible for Medicare and Medicaid, the hospice is funded by Medicare and the room and board is covered by Medicaid. If the patient is eligible only for Medicare, the family must pay privately for room and board in a nursing facility.

The MHB provides three levels of care for hospice patients:

1. **Routine home care**—hospice services provided in the patient's home or a nursing facility.

2. **Inpatient respite care**—short-term inpatient admission to promote caregiver well-being. Owing to the physical and psychological stress and strain experienced by the 24-hour care of the family member, respite care is essential. It may be for a few days or the patient may be transferred to a facility from the hospital setting.

3. **Inpatient symptom management**—inpatient admission for more intensive palliative measures. Such admissions would be warranted for severe pain, intractable seizures, uncontrolled bleeding, and intractable nausea/vomiting due to gastrointestinal obstruction. Before admission, the medical director, primary physician, patient, and family discuss the purpose of the hospitalization. The hospice is still responsible for the plan of care and needs to be involved daily and at all levels of decision-making in collaboration with the inpatient staff.

The MHB limits how much active treatment a patient can receive and still be on hospice. The patient's primary physician must discuss with the hospice program on a case-by-case basis the types of services that may be provided to a given patient without disqualifying him or her from hospice. Some measures, such as intravenous hydration, blood transfusions, tube feedings, paracentesis, and thoracentesis may be appropriate for palliation, but must be approved by the hospice medical director first.

F. **Bereavement care.** A very important service for hospice families and caregivers is bereavement care. Bereavement services are provided by hospice programs for at least up to a year after the patient's death. The services are provided by specially trained staff. Depending on the hospice, this service may be provided by the nurse, social worker, chaplain, or specially trained volunteers. Bereavement services include periodic mailings, phone calls, and home visits. Some hospices offer bereavement support groups, and some host annual memorial services. If the family requires additional counseling services, the hospice may choose to provide extended services or refer them to other resources in the community.

III. PALLIATIVE CARE

A. **Definition.** The goal of palliative care is to prevent suffering and support the best quality of life for patients and their families, throughout all phases of illness. Palliative care is a philosophy and an organized structure of care delivery. As a philosophy, palliative care supports the goals of the patient and family, whether for cure, life prolongation, or peace and dignity throughout the course of the illness, the dying process, and death. As a health care–delivery model, palliative care focuses on managing pain and other distressing physical symptoms; coordinating care across settings and disciplines; empowering the patient and family to make decisions; and meeting the psychosocial and spiritual needs of the patient and family according to their values, needs, beliefs, and culture. As with hospice, palliative care is provided by an interdisciplinary team of professionals who have received specialized training and credentialing in the field of palliative care. The team may include physicians; nurses; pharmacists; psychologists; social workers; counselors; chaplains; dieticians;

occupational, speech, and physical therapists; art and music therapists; massage therapists; child-life (pediatric) therapists; trained volunteers; and personal care aides.

Palliative care is appropriate in hospital, nursing home, assisted living, and home care settings. Some intensive care units are establishing specialized palliative teams, because their patients are living longer with serious life-threatening illness, and they need better symptom management and assistance with decision-making. Smaller hospitals and health care settings without a palliative care team can access palliative care resources through tele-medicine or from consultants over the Internet.

Palliative care programs are supported by direct funding from hospitals, philanthropy, fee-for-service, or through grants.

B. **History.** Palliative care developed as an extension of the hospice movement. Health care professionals historically viewed palliative care as the care administered at the end stages of an illness, when curative treatment was no longer feasible. In recent years, palliative care has taken on a broader meaning, to include any measure that is designed to relieve distress at any stage of an illness. One of the driving forces behind the growth of palliative care has been the restrictiveness of the MHB. Many agencies have started up alternative home care programs to offer palliative care to patients who do not meet hospice eligibility criteria. Another driving force has been the dramatic rise in the number of people living with chronic, debilitating, and life-threatening illnesses.

In 2004, five major palliative care organizations in the United States joined together to develop The National Consensus Project for Quality Palliative Care. The purposes of the project were to improve the quality of palliative care programs, reduce the variation among palliative care models, develop greater continuity of care across treatment settings, and encourage collaboration among palliative care programs, hospices, and other health care delivery settings. The end product of the National Consensus Project was a set of Clinical Practice Guidelines designed to promote high-quality and consistent palliative care programming.

C. **Core elements.** The National Consensus Project identified the following "Core Elements" of a palliative care program:

- **Patient population.** Palliative care should be available to patients of all ages who have debilitating, chronic, or life-threatening illnesses, conditions, or injuries.
- **Patient and family centered.** Patient and family uniqueness is respected. The patient defines his or her "family," meaning those significant people who support and care for the patient. The patient and family develop the palliative care plan with support and guidance from the health care team.
- **Timing of palliative care.** Ideally palliative care is initiated at the time of diagnosis of a life-threatening or debilitating condition and continues through a cure, or until death, and into the family's bereavement period.
- **Comprehensive care.** The team performs multidimensional assessments on an ongoing basis, to identify and relieve physical, psychosocial, or spiritual suffering. The team updates the patient and family regarding any changes in the patient's condition, and how they affect future treatments and the goals of the patient and family.
- **Interdisciplinary team.** The palliative care team includes representatives of multiple disciplines. Ideally the team will expand on the basis of the changing needs and goals of the patient and family.
- **Attention to relief of suffering.** The team focuses on preventing or relieving physical, social, psychological, or spiritual distress caused by the illness or its treatments.
- **Communication skills.** It is essential for members of the palliative care team to listen actively to the patient and family, share information appropriately, and communicate effectively with the patient, family, and other health care providers. The team helps the patient and family determine their goals and assists them with making decisions to accomplish those goals.
- **Skill in the care of the dying and the bereaved.** Palliative care specialists understand the signs and symptoms of the dying process and imminent death.

They assess the support needed during different phases of the dying process, and distinguish normal from complicated grief, given the age of the person who is grieving.

■ **Continuity of care across settings.** Palliative care is vitally important in all settings, including hospitals, nursing homes, emergency rooms, primary care providers' offices, the patient's home, assisted living, and some schools and churches. Continuity of support for the patient who is transferring from one setting to another must be assured.

■ **Equitable access.** Palliative care providers should provide equitable access to care for patients regardless of age, diagnosis, race, ethnicity, sexual preference, or ability to pay, and without regard for treatment modality or health care setting.

■ **Quality improvement.** Palliative care services should strive for excellence in quality of care. Palliative care programs should be evaluated regularly and systematically, using both process and outcome measures and validated quality-improvement instruments.

IV. CONCLUSION. Hospice has been providing palliative care and support to patients and the families for many years. The philosophy of patient–family centered care, with an interdisciplinary focus has improved quality of life for many patients and their families. This model has proven to be very cost effective, improved patient and family satisfaction, and has lead to the emergence and growth of palliative care as a specialty service. The palliative care model should be available for patients of all ages and should be initiated at diagnosis of acute, serious, and life-threatening illnesses. Also, patients living with progressive chronic conditions such as advanced heart disease, lung disease, and chronic renal or liver failure would benefit from the palliative care philosophy. The concept of palliation is no longer just for patients who are terminal or actively dying.

Internet Resources

Association for Palliative Medicine (http://www.palliative-medicine.org/)
American Academy of Hospice and Palliative Medicine (http://www.aahpm.org/)
American Board of Hospice and Palliative Medicine (http://www.abhpm.org/)
Caring to the End of Life, a web site for anyone who needs information about palliative care for cancer patients. (http://www.caringtotheend.ca/)
Compassion and Choices (http://compassionandandchoices.org/)
End-of-Life/PalliativeEducationResourceCenter(EPERC) (http://www/eper.mcw.edu/)
Hospice Association of America (HAA) (http://hospice-american.org/)
Hospice and Palliative Nurses Association-Educational products and services for all levels of hospice and palliative care nursing care (http://www.hpna.org/)
International Journal of Palliative Nursing (http://www.ijpn.couk/)
PalliativeCare (http://www.virtualcancercentre.com/asp/documents/what_is_palliative_care .asp?PageType=palliative)
Palliative care (http://www.aromacaring.co.uk/palliative_care.htm)
Palliative Care Drug Information (http://www.palliativedrugs.com/)
The Center to Advanced Palliative Care (CAPC) (http://www.capc.org/)
The National Hospice and Palliative Care Organization (NHPCO) (http://wwwnhpco.org/)

Suggested Readings

Doyle D, Hanks GWC, MacDonald N, eds. *Oxford textbook of palliative medicine.* Oxford: Oxford University Press, 1993.
Health Care Financing Administration. *Medicare hospice benefits.* Baltimore: HCFA, 1999.
Johanson GA. *Physician handbook of symptom relief in terminal care,* 4th ed. Sonoma County Academic Foundation for Excellence in Medicine, 1993.
Kaye P. *Symptom control in hospice and palliative care,* 1st ed. rev. Essex: Hospice Education Institute, 1990.
National Consensus Project for Quality Palliative Care. *Clinical practice guidelines for quality palliative care.* Pittsburgh: National Consensus Project, 2004.
National Hospice Foundation. *The medicare hospice benefits.* Alexandria: National Hospice Foundation, 2000.
Patt RB, ed. *Cancer pain.* Philadelphia: JB Lippincott Co, 1993.

Rossman P. *Hospice: a new approach to humane and dignified care for the dying.* New York: Fawcett Columbine, 1979.

Saunders C, Sykes N, eds. *The management of terminal malignant diseases.* London: Edward Arnold, 1993.

Storey P. *Primer of palliative care.* Gainesville: Academy of Hospice Physicians, 1994.

Twycross R. *Pain relief in advanced cancer.* Edinburgh: Churchill Livingstone, 1994.

Walsh TD, ed. *Symptom control.* London: Blackwell Science, 1989.

Woodruff R. *Palliative medicine.* Melbourne: Asperula Pty, 1996.

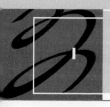

DOSE ADJUSTMENTS OF COMMONLY USED CHEMOTHERAPEUTIC AGENTS IN HEPATIC FAILURE AND RENAL FAILURE

Byron Peters

Renal excretion and biliary excretion represent common routes of elimination of many frequently used chemotherapeutic drugs. If either of these routes of excretion becomes impaired, the risk of decreased clearance of certain chemotherapeutic drugs increases. This decreased clearance can manifest itself as increased toxicity to the patient or may worsen the impaired renal or hepatic function. Therefore, in the presence of diminished renal or hepatic function, recommendations exist to modify dosing of various chemotherapeutic drugs. Although some recommendations are well established, others are not and variations may be found throughout the published literature. The following tables are intended to serve as guidelines for employing dose modifications when renal or hepatic impairment exists in the patient undergoing chemotherapy. Clinical judgment and patient assessment along with recommended dose modifications should dictate the final decision for any dose modification. The reader is cautioned to always refer to the prescribing information for the respective drug before making any treatment or dosing decision.

Dose Adjustments of Commonly Used Chemotherapeutic Agents in Hepatic Failure

Drug	Dose modification (percentage reduction)	Bilirubin (mg/dL)	SGOT (mg/dL)	Alkaline phosphatase
Alemtuzumab	None	—	—	—
Amifostine	None	—	—	—
Arsenic trioxide	None	—	—	—
L-Asparaginase	Use caution	—	—	—
Bevacizumab	None	—	—	—
Bleomycin	None	—	—	—
Bortezomib	Use caution	—	—	—
Busulfan	None	—	—	—
Carboplatin	None	—	—	—
Carmustine	Use caution	—	—	—
Cisplatin	None	—	—	—
Cetuximab	None	—	—	—
Cladribine	None	—	—	—
Cyclophosphamide	25%	3.0–5.0	>180	—
Cyclophosphamide	Hold dose	>5.0	—	—
Cytarabine	Use caution	—	—	—
Dacarbazine	Use caution	—	—	—
Dactinomycin	50%	>3.0	—	—
Daunorubicin	25%	1.2–3.0	60–80	—
Daunorubicin	50%	>3.0	>180	—
Daunorubicin	Hold dose	>5.0	—	—
Docetaxel	Hold dose	>1.5	>60	>2.5 times ULN
Doxorubicin	50%	1.2–3.0	60–80	—
Doxorubicin	75%	3.1–5.0	>180	—
Doxorubicin	Hold dose	>5.0	—	—
Doxorubicin liposomal	50%	1.2–3.0	—	—
Doxorubicin liposomal	75%	3.1–5.0	—	—
Doxorubicin liposomal	Hold dose	>5.0	—	—
Epirubicin	50%	1.2–3.0	2–4 times ULN	—
Epirubicin	75%	>3.0	>4 times ULN	—
Etoposide	50%	1.5–3.0	60–180	—
Etoposide	Hold dose	>3.0	>180	—
Etoposide phosphate	50%	1.5–3.0	60–180	—
Etoposide phosphate	Hold dose	>3.0	>180	—
Fludarabine	None	—	—	—
5-Fluorouracil	Hold dose	>5.0	—	—
Gemcitabine	None	—	—	—

(*continued*)

(continued)

Drug	Dose modification (percentage reduction)	Bilirubin (mg/dL)	SGOT (mg/dL)	Alkaline phosphatase
Idarubicin	25%	1.5–3.0	60–180	—
Idarubicin	50%	3.1–5.0	>180	—
Idarubicin	Hold dose	>5.0	—	—
Ifosfamide	Use caution	—	—	—
Irinotecan	Hold dose	>2.0	>3 times ULN	—
Mechlorethamine	None	—	—	—
Mesna	None	—	—	—
Methotrexate	25%	3.1–5.0	>180	—
Methotrexate	Hold dose	>5.0	—	—
Mitomycin	None	—	—	—
Mitoxantrone	25%	>3.0	—	—
Oxaliplatin	None	—	—	—
Paclitaxel	Hold dose	>5.0	>180 or 1.5 times ULN	—
Pemetrexed	Use caution	—	—	—
Pentostatin	None	—	—	—
Rituximab	None	—	—	—
Streptozocin	Use caution	—	—	—
Topotecan	None	—	—	—
Trastuzumab	None	—	—	—
Vinblastine	50%	>3.0	>180	—
Vincristine	50%	1.5–3.0	60–180	—
Vincristine	Hold dose	>3.0	>180	—
Vinorelbine	50%	2.1–3.0	—	—
Vinorelbine	75%	3.1–5.0	—	—
Vinorelbine	Hold dose	>5.0	—	—

ULN, upper limit of normal.

Dose Adjustments of Commonly Used Chemotherapeutic Agents in Renal Failure

Drug	Dose modification (percentage reduction)	Creatinine clearance (CrCl)
Amifostine	None	—
Arsenic trioxide	Use caution	—
L-Asparaginase	Hold dose	<60 mL/min
Bevacizumab	Hold for severe proteinuria	—
Bleomycin	25%	10–50 mL/min
Bleomycin	50%	<10 mL/min
Bortezomib	None	—
Carboplatin	AUC dose based on CrCl	—
Carmustine	Hold dose	<60 mL/min
Cetuximab	None	—
Cisplatin	50%	30–60 mL/min
Cisplatin	Hold dose	<30 mL/min
Cladribine	Use caution	—
Cyclophosphamide	25%	10–50 mL/min
Cyclophosphamide	50%	<10 mL/min
Cytarabine	Use caution	—
Dacarbazine	Use caution	—
Dactinomycin	None	—
Daunorubicin	50%	S.Cr. >3.0 mg/dL
Docetaxel	None	—
Doxorubicin	25%	<10 mL/min
Doxorubicin liposomal	25%	<10 mL/min
Epirubicin	Use caution	—
Etoposide	25%	10–50 mL/min
Etoposide	50%	<10 mL/min
Etoposide phosphate	25%	10–50 mL/min
Etoposide phosphate	50%	<10 mL/min
Fludarabine	Use caution	—
5-Fluorouracil	None	—
Gemcitabine	Use caution	—
Idarubicin	Use caution	—
Ifosfamide	25–50%	S.Cr. = 2.1–3.0 mg/dL
Ifosfamide	Hold dose	S.Cr. >3.0 mg/dL
Irinotecan	None	—
Mechlorethamine	None	—
Mesna	None	—
Methotrexate	50%	10–50 mL/min
Methotrexate	Hold dose	<10 mL/min
Mitomyciin	25%	<10 mL/min
Mitomyciin	Hold dose	S.Cr. >1.7 mg/dL
Mitoxantrone	None	—
Oxaliplatin	None	—

(continued)

(continued)

Drug	Dose modification (percentage reduction)	Creatinine clearance (CrCl)
Paclitaxel	None	—
Pemetrexed	Dose adjust/hold	<45 mL/min
Pentostatin	Dose adjust	30–60 mL/min
Rituximab	None	—
Streptozocin	Hold dose	<60 mL/min
Topotecan	50%	20–39 mL/min
Topotecan	Hold dose	<20 mL/min
Trastuzumab	None	—
Vinblastine	None	—
Vincristine	None	—
Vinorelbine	None	—

S. Cr., serum creatinine.

Suggested Readings

King PD, Perry MC. Hepatotoxicity of chemotherapy agents. In: Perry MC, ed. *The Chemotherapy Source Book*, 2nd ed. Baltimore: Williams & Wilkins, 1997:709–726.

Noronha V, Mota A, Fogarasi M, et al. Guidelines for chemotherapy and dosing modifications. In: Chu E, DeVita VT, eds. *Physicians' Cancer Chemotherapy Drug Manual 2006.* Sudbury: Jones and Bartlett Publishers, 2006:375–386.

Patterson WP, Reams GP. Renal and electrolyte abnormalities due to chemotherapy. In: Perry MC, ed. *The Chemotherapy Source Book*, 2nd ed. Baltimore: Williams & Wilkins, 1997:727–744.

Thomson Micromedex. *Micromedex® Healthcare Series (Internet database).* Greenwood Village: Thomson Micromedex, 2006. Updated periodically.

Wickersham RM, Novak KK, Schweain SL, eds. *Drug Facts and Comparisons.* St. Louis: Wolters Kluwer Health, 2006.

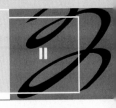

SELECTED CHEMOTHERAPEUTIC REGIMENS

Christine M. Kurtzeborn, Lindsay M. Hladnik, and Kristan M. Augustin

This appendix is a compilation of the common chemotherapeutic regimens reported in the literature and national guidelines for the treatment of patients with cancer. It is not an all-inclusive list, and the regimens are sorted alphabetically by cancer. The chemotherapeutic regimens chosen are not meant to infer superiority or priority over other regimens, but rather to serve as a general reference and starting point for making treatment decisions. No liability will be assumed for use of the appendix, nor for typographic errors. It is highly recommended to refer to the literature and package insert for information pertaining to the patient population participating in the clinical trial, supportive care guidelines (e.g., colony-stimulating factors, antibiotics, etc.), confirmation of dosing, administration rates, scheduling, and duration of therapy. Furthermore, evaluation of the literature and package inserts for dose modification recommendations based on hepatic dysfunction, renal dysfunction, and therapy-related toxicities are encouraged. Alteration in therapy may be necessary as one utilizes good clinical judgement for individualization of therapy according to the patient's response and tolerability.

Regimen	Drug dose	References

AIDS-related malignancies
Kaposi sarcoma

ABV	Doxorubicin 20 mg/m^2 i.v. on day 1 Bleomycin 10 mg/m^2 i.v. on day 1 Vincristine 1 mg i.v. on day 1 Repeat cycle every 14 d	Northfelt DW. *J Clin Oncol* 1998;16: 2445–2451.
BV	Bleomycin 15 IU/m^2 i.v. on day 1 Vincristine 2 mg i.v. on day 1 Repeat cycle every 3 wk	Stewart S. *J Clin Oncol* 1998;16:683–691.
Daunoxome	Liposomal daunorubicin 40 mg/m^2 i.v. on day 1 Repeat cycle every 2 wk	Gill PS. *J Clin Oncol* 1996;14:2353–2364.
Docetaxel	Docetaxel 25 mg/m^2 i.v. on day 1 Repeat cycle weekly × 8	Lim ST. *Cancer* 2004; 103:417–421.
Doxil	Liposomal doxorubicin 20 mg/m^2 i.v. on day 1 Repeat cycle every 3 wk	Northfelt DW. *J Clin Oncol* 1997;15: 653–659. Stewart S. *J Clin Oncol* 1998;16:683–691.
Paclitaxel	Paclitaxel 100 mg/m^2 i.v. over 3 h on day 1 Repeat cycle every 2 wk	Tulpule A. *Cancer* 2002; 95:147–154.
Vinorelbine	Vinorelbine 30 mg/m^2 i.v. on day 1 Repeat cycle every 14 d	Nasti G. *J Clin Oncol* 2000;18:1550–1557.

Non-Hodgkin's lymphoma

CDE	Cyclophosphamide 187.5–200 mg/m^2/d CIVI on days 1–4 Doxorubicin 12.5 mg/m^2/d CIVI on days 1–4 Etoposide 60 mg/m^2/d CIVI on days 1–4 Repeat cycle every 28 d	Spina M. *Cancer* 2001;92:200–206. Sparano JA. *J Clin Oncol* 2004;22: 1491–1500.
CHOP	Cyclophosphamide 750 mg/m^2 i.v. on day 1 Doxorubicin 50 mg/m^2 i.v. on day 1 Vincristine 1.4 mg/m^2 i.v. on day 1 (maximum dose of 2 mg) Prednisone 100 mg p.o. daily on days 1–5 Repeat cycle every 21 d	Vaccher E. *Cancer* 2001;91:155–163. Ratner L. *J Clin Oncol* 2001;19:2171–2178.
CODOX-M/ IVAC	Low-risk patients: CODOX-M only Cyclophosphamide 800 mg/m^2 i.v. on day 1 Cyclophosphamide 200 mg/m^2 i.v. on days 2–5 Doxorubicin 40 mg/m^2 i.v. on day 1	Wang ES. *Cancer* 2003; 98:1196–1205.

(continued)

Regimen	Drug dose	References
	Vincristine 1.5 mg/m^2 i.v. on days 1 and 8 (cycle 1)	
	Vincristine 1.5 mg/m^2 i.v. on days 1, 8, and 15 (cycle 2)	
	Methotrexate 1200 mg/m^2 i.v. over 1 h followed by 240 mg/m^2/h × 23 h with leucovorin	
	Cytarabine 70 mg intrathecal (IT) on days 1 and 3	
	Methotrexate 12 mg IT on day 15	
	High-risk patients:	
	CODOX-M (alternate with IVAC)	
	Cyclophosphamide 800 mg/m^2 i.v. on day 1	
	Cyclophosphamide 200 mg/m^2 i.v. on days 2–5	
	Doxorubicin 40 mg/m^2 i.v. on day 1	
	Vincristine 1.5 mg/m^2 i.v. on days 1 and 8 (cycle 1)	
	Vincristine 1.5 mg/m^2 i.v. on days 1, 8, and 15 (cycle 2)	
	Methotrexate 1200 mg/m^2 i.v. over 1 h followed by 240 mg/m^2/h × 23 h with leucovorin	
	Cytarabine 70 mg IT on days 1 and 3	
	Methotrexate 12 mg IT on day 15	
	IVAC (alternate with CODOX-M)	
	Ifosfamide 1500 mg/m^2 i.v. on days 1–5 (with Mesna)	
	Etoposide 60 mg/m^2 i.v. on days 1–5	
	Cytarabine 2000 mg/m^2 i.v. q12h × 4 on day 1 and 2 g/m^2 i.v. on days 1, 8, and 15 (cycle 2)	
	Methotrexate 12 mg IT on day 5	
Dose-adjusted EPOCH	Etoposide 50 mg/m^2/d CIVI on days 1–4	Little RF. *Blood* 2003; 101:4653–4659.
	Doxorubicin 10 mg/m^2/d CIVI on days 1–4	
	Vincristine 0.4 mg/m^2/d CIVI on days 1–4	
	Cyclophosphamide (cycle 1) 375 mg/m^2 i.v. on day 5 (CD4 + cells ≥100/mm^3) 187 mg/m^2 i.v. on day 5 (CD4 + cells <100 mm^3)	
	Cyclophosphamide (subsequent cycles) Increase by 187 mg/m^2 if nadir ANC >500/μL	

(*continued*)

(continued)

Regimen	Drug dose	References
	Decrease by 187 mg/m^2 if nadir ANC <500/μL or platelets <25000/μL	
	Prednisone 60 mg/m^2/d p.o. daily on days 1–5	
	Repeat cycle every 21 d	
EPOCH	Etoposide 50 mg/m^2/d CIVI on days 1–4	Gutierrez M. *J Clin Oncol* 2000;18: 3633–3642.
	Doxorubicin 10 mg/m^2/d CIVI on days 1–4	
	Vincristine 0.4 mg/m^2/d CIVI on days 1–4	
	Cyclophosphamide 750 mg/m^2 i.v. on day 5	
	Prednisone 60 mg/m^2/d p.o. daily on days 1–5	
	Repeat cycle every 21 d	
Hyper-CVAD	Odd numbered cycles:	Cortes J. *Cancer* 2002; 94:1492–1499.
	Cyclophosphamide 300 mg/m^2 i.v. q12h × 6 starting on day 1	
	Mesna 600 mg/m^2/d CIVI daily × 3 d	
	Vincristine 2 mg i.v. on days 4 and 11	
	Doxorubicin 50 mg/m^2 i.v. on day 4	
	Dexamethasone 40 mg i.v./p.o. on days 1–4 and 11–14	
	Even numbered cycles:	
	Methotrexate 1000 mg/m^2 CIVI on day 1	
	Cytarabine 3000 mg/m^2 i.v. q12h × 4 on days 2 and 3	
	Leucovorin 50 mg i.v. × 1 starting 12 h after the completion of methotrexate, followed by 15 mg i.v. q6h until methotrexate level <0.1 mM	
m-BACOD	Methotrexate 200 mg/m^2 i.v. on day 15	Kaplan LD. *N Engl J Med* 1997;336: 1641–1648.
	Bleomycin 4 U/m^2 i.v. on day 1	
	Doxorubicin 25 mg/m^2 i.v. on day 1	
	Cyclophosphamide 300 mg/m^2 i.v. on day 1	
	Vincristine 1.4 mg/m^2 i.v. on day 1	
	Dexamethasone 3 mg/m^2 p.o. daily on days 1–5	
	Cytarabine 50 mg IT on days 1, 8, 15, and 22	

(continued)

Regimen	Drug dose	References
m-CHOP	Cyclophosphamide 375 mg/m^2 i.v. on day 1 Doxorubicin 25 mg/m^2 i.v. on day 1 Vincristine 1.4 mg/m^2 (maximum dose 2 mg) i.v. on day 1 Prednisone 100 mg p.o. daily on days 1–5	Ratner L. *J Clin Oncol* 2001;19:2171–2178.
Bladder		
Cisplatin/ docetaxel	Cisplatin 75 mg/m^2 i.v. Docetaxel 75 mg/m^2 i.v. Repeat cycle every 3 wk	Dimopoulos MA. *Ann Oncol* 1999;10: 1385–1388.
CMV	Methotrexate 30 mg/m^2 i.v. on days 1 and 8 Vinblastine 4 mg/m^2 i.v. on days 1 and 8 Cisplatin 100 mg/m^2 i.v. on day 2 ($\geq$12 h after methotrexate and vinblastine) Repeat cycle every 21 d	Harker WG. *J Clin Oncol* 1985;3: 1463–1470.
Gemcitabine/ cisplatin	Gemcitabine 1000 mg/m^2 i.v. on days 1, 8, and 15 Cisplatin 70 mg/m^2 i.v. on day 2 Repeat cycle every 28 d	Moore MJ. *J Clin Oncol* 1999;17:2876–2881.
MVAC	Methotrexate 30 mg/m^2 i.v. on days 1, 15, and 22 Vinblastine 3 mg/m^2 i.v. on days 2, 15, and 22 Doxorubicin 15–30[a] mg/m^2 i.v. on day 2 Cisplatin 70 mg/m^2 i.v. on day 2 Repeat cycle every 28 d	Stemberg CN. *Cancer* 1989;64:2448–2458.
Paclitaxel/ carboplatin/ gemcitabine	Paclitaxel 200 mg/m^2 i.v. on day 1 Carboplatin (AUC 5) i.v. on day 1 Gemcitabine 800 mg/m^2 i.v. on days 1 and 8 Repeat cycle every 21 d	Hussain M. *J Clin Oncol* 2001;19: 2527–2533.
Brain		
Carmustine/XRT	Carmustine 80 mg/m^2/d i.v. on days 1–3 Repeat cycle every 8 wk	Green SB. *Cancer Treat Rep* 1983;67: 121–132.
PCV	Lomustine 110 mg/m^2 p.o. on day 1 Procarbazine 60 mg/m^2/d p.o. on days 8–21 Vincristine 1.4 mg/m^2 (maximum dose 2 mg) i.v. on days 8 and 29 Repeat cycle every 6 wk	Glass J. *J Neurosurg* 1992;76:741–745.

(continued)

[a]15 mg if >20 Gy pelvic irradiation in 5 d before.

(continued)

Regimen	Drug dose	References
Temozolomide	Temozolomide 200 mg/m^2/d p.o. daily × 5 d Repeat cycle every 28 d (first cycle, give only 150 mg/m^2/d p.o. daily × 5 d; if no toxicity, then increase dose as above)	Chinot OL. *J Clin Oncol* 2001;19:2449–2455.
Breast		
Abraxane	Abraxane 260 mg/m^2 i.v. on day 1 Repeat cycle every 21 d	Gradishar WJ. *J Clin Oncol* 2005;23: 7794–7803.
AC	Doxorubicin 60 mg/m^2 i.v. on day 1 Cyclophosphamide 600 mg/m^2 i.v. on day 1 Repeat cycle every 21 d	Fisher B. *J Clin Oncol* 1990;8:1483–1496. Fisher B. *J Clin Oncol* 1997;15:1858–1869.
AC→paclitaxel ± trastuzumab	Doxorubicin 60 mg/m^2 i.v. on day 1 Cyclophosphamide 600 mg/m^2 i.v. on day 1 Repeat cycle every 21 d for four cycles Followed by Paclitaxel 175–225 mg/m^2 i.v. on day 1 Repeat cycle every 21 d for four cycles or Paclitaxel 80 mg/m^2 i.v. weekly for 12 wk With ± trastuzumab 4 mg/kg i.v. with first dose of paclitaxel followed by 2 mg/kg i.v. weekly	Henderson IC. *J Clin Oncol* 2003;21: 976–983. Romond EH. *N Engl J Med* 2005;353: 1673–1684.
AC→Paclitaxel	Doxorubicin 60 mg/m^2 i.v. on day 1 Cyclophosphamide 600 mg/m^2 i.v. on day 1 Repeat cycle every 14 d for four cycles Followed by Paclitaxel 175 mg/m^2 i.v. on day 1 Repeat cycle every 14 d for four cycles	Citron ML. *J Clin Oncol* 2003;21:1431–1439. Mamounas EP. *J Clin Oncol* 2005;16: 3686–3696.
AT	Doxorubicin 50 mg/m^2 i.v. on day 1 Docetaxel 75 mg/m^2 i.v. on day 1 Repeat cycle every 21 d	Nabholtz JM. *J Clin Oncol* 2003;21: 968–975. Bontenbal M. *J Clin Oncol* 2005;23: 7081–7088.
AT	Doxorubicin 60 mg/m^2 i.v. on day 1 Paclitaxel 200 mg/m^2 i.v. on day 1 Repeat cycle every 21 d	Biganzoli L. *J Clin Oncol* 2002;20: 3114-3121.

(continued)

Regimen	Drug dose	References
CAF	Cyclophosphamide 100 mg/m^2 p.o. daily on days 1–14 Doxorubicin 30 mg/m^2 i.v. on days 1 and 8 Fluorouracil (5-FU) 500 mg/m^2 i.v. on days 1 and 8 Repeat cycle every 28 d	Bull JM. *Cancer* 1978;41:1649–1657.
Capecitabine	Capecitabine 1250 mg/m^2 p.o. b.i.d. on days 1–14 Repeat cycle every 21 d	Fumoleau P. *Eur J Cancer* 2004;40: 536–542.
Capecitabine/ paclitaxel	Capecitabine 825 mg/m^2 p.o. b.i.d. on days 1–14 Paclitaxel 80 mg/m^2 i.v. on days 1 and 8 Repeat cycle every 21 d	Blum JL. *J Clin Oncol* 2006;24:4384–4390.
Capecitabine/ vinorelbine	Capecitabine 1000 mg/m^2 p.o. b.i.d. on days 1–14 Vinorelbine 25 mg/m^2 i.v. on days 1 and 8 Repeat cycle every 21 d	Welt A. *Ann Oncol* 2005;16:64–69.
CMF	Cyclophosphamide 600 mg/m^2 i.v. on day 1 Methotrexate 40 mg/m^2 i.v. on day 1 5-FU 600 mg/m^2 i.v. on day 1 Repeat cycle every 21 d	Weiss RB. *Am J Med* 1987;83:455–463.
CMF	Cyclophosphamide 100 mg/m^2 p.o. on days 1–14 Methotrexate 40 mg/m^2 i.v. on days 1 and 8 5-FU 600 mg/m^2 i.v. on days 1 and 8 Repeat cycle every 28 d	Bonadonna G. *N Engl J Med* 1976;294: 405–410.
Docetaxel/ bevacizumab	Docetaxel 35 mg/m^2 i.v. on days 1, 8, and 15 Bevacizumab 10 mg/kg i.v. on days 1 and 15 Repeat cycle every 28 d	Ramaswamy B. *Clin Cancer Res* 2006; 12:3124–2129.
Docetaxel/ capecitabine	Docetaxel 75 mg/m^2 i.v. on day 1 Capecitabine 1250 mg/m^2 p.o. b.i.d. on days 1–14 Repeat cycle every 21 d	O'Shaughnessy J. *J Clin Oncol* 2002;20: 2812–2823.
Docetaxel/ trastuzumab	Docetaxel 100 mg/m^2 i.v. on day 1 Repeat cycle every 21 d OR Docetaxel 35 mg/m^2 i.v. weekly Trastuzumab 4 mg/kg i.v. on day 1, followed by 2 mg/kg i.v. weekly	Esteva FJ. *J Clin Oncol* 2002;20:1800–1808. Marty M. *J Clin Oncol* 2005;23:4265–4274.

(continued)

(continued)

Regimen	Drug dose	References
E→CMF	Epirubicin 100 mg/m^2 i.v. on day 1 Repeat cycle every 21 d for four cycles Followed by Cyclophosphamide 750 mg/m^2 i.v. on day 1 or Cyclophosphamide 600 mg/m^2 i.v. on days 1 and 8 Methotrexate 50 mg/m^2 i.v. on day 1 5-FU 600 mg/m^2 i.v. on day 1 Repeat cycle every 21 d for four cycles	Poole CJ. *Proc Am Soc Clin Oncol* 2003;13. Abstract. Rea DW. *J Clin Oncol* 2004;22:595. Abstract.
FAC	5-FU 500 mg/m^2 i.v. on days 1 and 8 or days 1 and 4 Doxorubicin 50 mg/m^2 i.v. on day 1 Cyclophosphamide 500 mg/m^2 i.v. on day 1 Repeat cycle every 21 d	Smalley RV. *Cancer* 1977;40:625–632.
FEC	Cyclophosphamide 75 mg/m^2 p.o. daily on days 1–14 Epirubicin 60 mg/m^2 i.v. on days 1 and 8 5-FU 500 mg/m^2 i.v. on days 1 and 8 Repeat cycle every 28 d	Levine MN. *J Clin Oncol* 1998;16: 2651–2658. Therasse P. *J Clin Oncol* 2003;21: 843–850.
FEC100 ± docetaxel	Cyclophosphamide 500 mg/m^2 i.v. on day 1 Epirubicin 100 mg/m^2 i.v. on day 1 5-FU 500 mg/m^2 i.v. on day 1 Repeat cycle every 21 d Followed by ± Docetaxel 100 mg/m^2 i.v. on day 1 Repeat cycle every 21 d for three cycles	French Adjuvant Study Group. *J Clin Oncol* 2001;19:602–611. Roche H. *San Antonio Breast Cancer Symposium* 2004:27. Abstract.
GT	Paclitaxel 175 mg/m^2 i.v. on day 1 Gemcitabine 1250 mg/m^2 i.v. on days 1 and 8 Repeat cycle every 21 d	Albain KS. *J Clin Oncol* 2004;22:510. Abstract.
Paclitaxel/ trastuzumab	Paclitaxel 175 mg/m^2 i.v. on day 1 Trastuzumab 4 mg/kg i.v. on day 1, followed by 2 mg/kg i.v. weekly Repeat cycle every 21 d	Leyland-Jones B. *J Clin Oncol* 2003;21: 3965–3971. Slamon DJ. *N Engl J Med* 2001;344: 783–792.

(continued)

Regimen	Drug dose	References
TCH/ trastuzumab	Paclitaxel 80 mg/m² i.v. on days 1, 8, and 15 Carboplatin AUC 2 i.v. on days 1, 8, and 15 Repeat cycle every 28 d Trastuzumab 4 mg/kg i.v. on day 1, followed by 2 mg/kg i.v. weekly	Perez EA. *Clin Breast Cancer* 2005;6: 425-432.
TPC	Carboplatin AUC 6 i.v. on day 2 Paclitaxel 175 mg/m² i.v. on day 2 Trastuzumab 4 mg/kg i.v. on day 1, followed by 2 mg/kg i.v. weekly Repeat cycle every 21 d	Robert N. *J Clin Oncol* 2006;24:2786–2792.
Trastuzumab	Trastuzumab 8 mg/kg i.v. on day 1, followed by 6 mg/kg i.v. every 3 wk	Piccart-Gebhart MJ. *N Engl J Med* 2005;353: 1659–1672.
Trastuzumab/ paclitaxel →FEC/ trastuzumab	Paclitaxel 225 mg/m² i.v. on day 1 Trastuzumab 4 mg/kg i.v. × 1 dose with first dose on the day before paclitaxel, followed by 2 mg/kg i.v. weekly for a total of 24 doses Repeat cycle every 21 d for four cycles Followed by 5-FU 500 mg/m² i.v. on days 1 and 4 Epirubicin 75 mg/m² i.v. on day 1 Cyclophosphamide 500 mg/m² i.v. on day 1 Repeat cycle every 21 d for four cycles	Buzdar AU. *J Clin Oncol* 2005;23: 3676–3685.
Vinorelbine	Vinorelbine 25–30 mg/m² i.v. weekly	Fumoleau P. *J Clin Oncol* 1993;11: 1245–1252. Zelek L. *Cancer* 2001;92:2267–2272.
Vinorelbine/ trastuzumab	Trastuzumab 4 mg/kg i.v. on day 1, followed by 2 mg/kg i.v. weekly Vinorelbine 25 mg/m² i.v. weekly (following trastuzumab)	Burstein HJ. *J Clin Oncol* 2001;19: 2722–2730.
Cervical		
Cisplatin/XRT	Cisplatin 40 mg/m² i.v. weekly (maximum dose is 70 mg/wk) Repeat weekly for a maximum of 6 doses XRT: 1.8–2 Gy daily, 5 d per wk for a total of 45 Gy	Keys HM. *N Engl J Med* 1999;340:1154–1161.

(continued)

(continued)

Regimen	Drug dose	References
Cisplatin/5-FU/ XRT	Cisplatin 70 mg/m^2 i.v. on day 1 5-FU 1000 mg/m^2/d CIVI on days 1–4 Repeat cycle every 21 d XRT: 1.7 Gy/day on days 1–5 of each wk for a total of 49.3 Gy (29 fractions)	Peters WA. *J Clin Oncol* 2000;18:1606–1613.
Cisplatin/5-FU/ hydroxyurea/ XRT	Cisplatin 50 mg/m^2 i.v. on days 1 and 29 then 5-FU 4 gm/m^2 CIVI over 96 h beginning on days 1 and 29 Hydroxyurea 2 gm/m^2 p.o. twice weekly 2 h before XRT at weeks 1–6	Rose PG. *N Engl J Med* 1999;340:1144–1153.
Cisplatin/ vinorelbine	Cisplatin 80 mg/m^2 i.v. on day 1 Vinorelbine 25 mg/m^2 i.v. on days 1 and 8 Repeat cycle every 21 d	Pignata S. *J Clin Oncol* 1999;17:756–760. Geggia V. *Oncology* 2002;63:31–37.
Gemcitabine/ cisplatin	Gemcitabine 1250 mg/m^2 i.v. on days 1 and 8 followed by Cisplatin 50 mg/m^2 i.v. on day 1 Repeat cycle every 21 d	Burnett AF. *Gynecol Oncol* 2000;76: 63–66.
Mitomycin-C/ cisplatin	Mitomycin-C 6 mg/m^2 i.v. on day 1 followed by Cisplatin 50 mg/m^2 i.v. on day 1 Repeat every 28 d	Wagenaar HC. *Eur J Cancer* 2001;37: 1624–1628.
Paclitaxel/ carboplatin	Paclitaxel 175 mg/m^2 i.v. on day 1 Carboplatin AUC 5 i.v. on day 1 Repeat cycle every 21 d	Sit AS. *Cancer Invest* 2004;22:368–373.
Paclitaxel/ cisplatin	Paclitaxel 175 mg/m^2 i.v. on day 1 Cisplatin 75 mg/m^2 i.v. on day 1 Repeat cycle every 21 d	Papadimitriou CA. *J Clin Oncol* 1999;17: 761–766.
Paclitaxel/ cisplatin	Paclitaxel 135 mg/m^2 CIVI on day 1 followed by Cisplatin 50–75 mg/m^2 i.v. on day 2 Repeat cycle every 21 d	Moore DH. *J Clin Oncol* 2004;22: 3113–3119. Rose PG. *J Clin Oncol* 1999;17:2676–2680.
Topotecan/ cisplatin	Topotecan 0.75 mg/m^2 i.v. on days 1–3 followed by Cisplatin 50 mg/m^2 i.v. on day 1 Repeat cycle every 21 d	Long HJ. *J Clin Oncol* 2005;23:4626–4633.
Colorectal		
Bevacizumab	Bevacizumab 5 mg/kg i.v. every 2 wk PLUS 5-FU–leucovorin OR IFL OR FOLFOX OR FOLFIRI	Kabbinavar FF. *J Clin Oncol* 2005;23: 3706–3712. Hurwitz HI. *J Clin Oncol* 2005;23: 3502–3508. Giantonio BJ. *ASCO GI Cancers Symposium* 2005;169. Abstract.

(continued)

Regimen	Drug dose	References
Capecitabine	Capecitabine 2500 mg/m^2/d (given as 1250 mg/m^2 b.i.d.) p.o. for 2 wk Repeat cycle every 3 wk	Hoff PM. *J Clin Oncol* 2001;19:2282–2292.
Cetuximab	Cetuximab 400 mg/m^2 first infusion, then 250 mg/m^2 i.v. weekly May be used alone or in combination with irinotecan	Cunningham D. *N Engl J Med* 2004;351: 337–345.
5-FU/leucovorin	Leucovorin 500 mg/m^2 i.v. 5-FU 500 mg/m^2 i.v. given 1 h into leucovorin infusion Weekly for 6 wk followed by 2 wk rest	Petrelli N. *J Clin Oncol* 1989;7:1419–1426.
5-FU/leucovorin	Leucovorin 20 mg/m^2 i.v. on days 1–5 5-FU 425 mg/m^2 i.v. after leucovorin on days 1–5 Repeat cycle at 4 wk, 8 wk, then every 5 wk thereafter	O'Connell MJ. *Cancer* 1989;63:1026–1030.
Irinotecan (every 3 wk)	Irinotecan 300–350 mg/m^2 [b] i.v. over 90 min Repeat cycle every 3 wk	Rougier P. *Lancet* 1998;352:1407– 1412.
Irinotecan/5-FU/ LCV (FOLFIRI)	Irinotecan 180 mg/m^2 i.v. on day 1 Leucovorin 400 mg/m^2 i.v. over 2 h before 5-FU on days 1–2 5-FU 400 mg/m^2 i.v. bolus, then 1200 mg/m^2/d CIVI over 46 h on days 1 and 2 Repeat cycle every 2 wk	Andre T. *Eur J Cancer* 1999;35:1343–1347.
Oxaliplatin/5-FU/ LCV (FOLFOX4)	Oxaliplatin 85 mg/m^2 i.v. on day 1 5-FU 400 mg/m^2 i.v. bolus, followed by 600 mg/m^2 CIVI for 22 h on days 1 and 2 Leucovorin 200 mg/m^2 i.v. (before 5-FU) on days 1 and 2 Repeat cycle every 2 wk	de Gramon A. *J Clin Oncol* 2000;18; 2938–2947.
Oxaliplatin/5-FU/ LCV (FOLFOX6)	Oxaliplatin 100 mg/m^2 i.v. on day 1 5-FU 400 mg/m^2 i.v. bolus, followed by 2400 mg/m^2 CIVI for 46 h Leucovorin 400 mg/m^2 i.v. (before 5-FU) on day 1 Repeat cycle every 2 wk	Tournigand C. *J Clin Oncol* 2004;22: 229–237.

(continued)

[b] For patients older than 69 yr or World Health Organization (WHO) performance status (PS) 2 give 300 mg/m^2 i.v.

(continued)

Regimen	Drug dose	References
Endometrial Cancer		
AP	Doxorubicin 60 mg/m^2 i.v. on day 1 (cycle 1–7 only) Cisplatin 50 mg/m^2 i.v. on day 1 (cycle 8 only) Repeat cycle every 21 d	Randall ME. *J Clin Oncol* 2006;24: 36–44.
AP	Doxorubicin 60 mg/m^2 i.v. on day 1 Cisplatin 60 mg/m^2 i.v. on day 1 Repeat cycle every 28 d	Barrett RJ. *Am J Clin Oncol* 1993;16: 494–496.
Carboplatin/ paclitaxel	Paclitaxel 175 mg/m^2 i.v. on day 1 followed by carboplatin AUC 5–7 i.v. on day 1 Repeat every 28 d	Hoskins PJ. *J Clin Oncol* 2001;19: 4048–4053.
Doxorubicin	Doxorubicin 60 mg/m^2 i.v. on day 1 Repeat cycle every 21 d	Thigpen JT. *J Clin Oncol* 1994;12: 1408–1414.
Paclitaxel	Paclitaxel 175–200 mg/m^2 i.v. on day 1 Repeat cycle every 21 d	Lincoln S. *Gynecol Oncol* 2003;88: 277–281.
Paclitaxel/ cisplatin	Paclitaxel 175 mg/m^2 i.v. on day 1 followed by Cisplatin 75 mg/m^2 i.v. on day 1 Filgrastim 5 μg/kg/d s.c. on day 5 until ANC recovery Repeat cycle every 21 d	Dimopoulos MA. *Gynecol Oncol* 2000;78:52–57.
TAP	Doxorubicin 45 mg/m^2 i.v. on day 1 followed by Cisplatin 50 mg/m^2 i.v. on day 1 Paclitaxel 160 mg/m^2 i.v. on day 2 Filgrastim 5 μg/kg/d s.c. on days 3–12 Repeat cycle every 21 d	Fleming GF. *J Clin Oncol* 2004;22: 2159–2166.
Gastric		
DC	Docetaxel 85 mg/m^2 i.v. on day 1 Cisplatin 75 mg/m^2 i.v. on day 1 Repeat cycle every 21 d	Roth AD. *Ann Oncol* 2000;11:301–306.
DCF	Docetaxel 75 mg/m^2 i.v. on day 1 Cisplatin 75 mg/m^2 i.v. on day 1 5-FU 300 mg/m^2/d CIVI on days 1–14 Repeat cycle every 21 d	Roth AD. *Ann Oncol* 2004;15:759–764.
ECF	Epirubicin 50 mg/m^2 i.v. on day 1 Cisplatin 60 mg/m^2 i.v. on day 1 5-FU 200 mg/m^2/day CIVI on days 1–21 d Repeat cycle every 21 d	Webb A. *J Clin Oncol* 1997;15:261–267. Ross P. *J Clin Oncol* 2002;20:1996–2004. Cunningham D. *N Engl J Med* 2006;355: 11–20.

(continued)

Regimen	Drug dose	References
EOX	Epirubicin 50 mg/m^2 i.v. on day 1 Oxaliplatin 130 mg/m^2 i.v. on day 1 Capecitabine 625 mg/m^2 p.o. b.i.d. Repeat cycle every 21 d	Sumpter K. *Br J Cancer* 2005;92:1976–1983.
FAP	5-FU 300 mg/m^2 i.v. on days 1–5 Doxorubicin 40 mg/m^2 i.v. on day 1 Cisplatin 60 mg/m^2 i.v. on day 1 Repeat cycle every 5 wk	Moertel CG. *J Clin Oncol* 1986;4: 1053–1057.
FLO	Oxaliplatin 85 mg/m^2 i.v. on day 1 5-FU 2600 mg/m^2 CIVI for 24 h on day 1 Leucovorin 500 mg/m^2 i.v. (before 5-FU) on day 1 Repeat cycle every 2 wk	Al-Batran SE. *J Clin Oncol* 2004;22: 658–663.
5-FU	5-FU 500 mg/m^2 i.v. daily on days 1–5 Repeat cycle every 5 wk	Cullinan SA. *J Clin Oncol* 1994;12: 412–416.
5-FU	5-FU 425 mg/m^2 i.v. daily on days 1–5 Leucovorin 20 mg/m^2 i.v. daily on days 1–5 Followed 28 d later with 5-FU 400 mg/m^2 i.v. daily on days 1–4 and 23–25 with XRT Leucovorin 20 mg/m^2 i.v. daily on days 1–4 and 23–25 with XRT Followed 1 mo later and repeated monthly × 2 with 5-FU 425 mg/m^2 i.v. daily on days 1–5 Leucovorin 20 mg/m^2 i.v. daily on days 1–5	MacDonald JS. *N Engl J Med* 2001;345: 725–730.
FOLFOX4	Oxaliplatin 85 mg/m^2 i.v. on day 1 5-FU 400 mg/m^2 i.v. bolus, followed by 600 mg/m^2 CIVI for 22 h on days 1 and 2 Leucovorin 200 mg/m^2 i.v. (before 5-FU) on days 1 and 2 Repeat cycle every 2 wk	De Vita F. *Br J Cancer* 2005;92:1644–1649.
FOLFOX6	Oxaliplatin 100 mg/m^2 i.v. on day 1 5-FU 400 mg/m^2 i.v. bolus, followed by 3000 mg/m^2 CIVI over 46 h on day 1	Louvet C. *J Clin Oncol* 2002;20:4543–4548.

(continued)

(continued)

Regimen	Drug dose	References
	Leucovorin 400 mg/m^2 i.v. (simultaneously with oxaliplatin and before 5-FU) on day 1 Repeat cycle every 2 wk	
FUP	5-FU 1000 mg/m^2/d CIVI on days 1–5 Cisplatin 100 mg/m^2 i.v. on day 2 Repeat cycle every 4 wk	Vanhoefer U. *J Clin Oncol* 2000;18: 2648–2657. Bouche O. *Ann Oncol* 2005;16:1488–1497.
IP	Irinotecan 70 mg/m^2 i.v. on days 1 and 15 Cisplatin 80 mg/m^2 i.v. on day 1 Repeat cycle every 4 wk	Boku N. *J Clin Oncol* 1999;17:319–323.
XELOX	Capecitabine 1000 mg/m^2 p.o. b.i.d. on days 1–14 Oxaliplatin 130 mg/m^2 i.v. on day 1 Repeat cycle every 21 d	Park YH. *Br J Cancer* 2006;94:959–963.
Gestational trophoblastic disease		
EMA-CO	Dactinomycin 0.5 mg/d i.v. on days 1 and 2 Etoposide 100 mg/m^2/d i.v. on days 1 and 2 Methotrexate 100 mg/m^2 i.v. followed by 200 mg/m^2 CIVI over 12 h on day 1 Leucovorin 15 mg i.m./p.o. q12h for 4 doses (starting 24 h after the start of methotrexate) Cyclophosphamide 600 mg/m^2 i.v. on day 8 Vincristine 1 mg/m^2 i.v. on day 8 Repeat cycle every 14 d	Newlands ES. *Br J Obstet Gynecol* 1986;93:63–69.
Methotrexate	Methotrexate 30–50 mg/m^2 i.m. weekly	Homseley HD. *Obstet Gynecol* 1988; 72:413.
Head and neck		
Carboplatin/5-FU	Carboplatin 300–400 mg/m^2 i.v. on day 1 5-FU 600 mg/m^2 i.v. on day 1 Repeat cycle every 21 d	Forastiere AA. *J Clin Oncol* 1992;10: 1245–1251.
Cetuximab	Cetuximab 400 mg/m^2 i.v. over 2 h on day 1, followed by weekly doses of 250 mg/m^2 over 1 h	Bonner JA. *N Engl J Med* 2006;354: 567–578.
Cetuximab/ cisplatin	Cetuximab 400 mg/m^2 i.v. over 2 h on day 1, followed by weekly doses of 250 mg/m^2 over 1 h Cisplatin 100 mg/m^2 i.v. on day 1 (repeat every 4 wk)	Burtness B. *J Clin Oncol* 2005;23:8646–8654.

(continued)

Regimen	Drug dose	References
CF	Cisplatin 75 mg/m^2 i.v. on day 1, immediately followed by 5-FU 1000 mg/m^2/d CIVI for 96 h Repeat cycle every 21 d	Cooper JS. *JAMA* 1999;281:1623–1627.
CF	Cisplatin 100 mg/m^2 i.v. on day 1, immediately followed by 5-FU 1000 mg/m^2/d CIVI for 96 h Repeat cycle every 21 d	Kish JA. *Cancer* 1984;53:1819–1824.
Cisplatin/ docetaxel	Cisplatin 75 mg/m^2 i.v. on day 1 Docetaxel 75 mg/m^2 i.v. on day 1 Repeat cycle every 3 wk	Specht L. *Ann Oncol* 2000;11:845–849.
Cisplatin/XRT	Cisplatin 100 mg/m^2 i.v. on days 1, 22, and 43 Administer concurrently with XRT	Forastiere AA. *N Engl J Med* 2003;349: 2091–2098.
5-FU	5-FU 500 mg/m^2 i.v. daily × 5 Repeat cycle every 5 wk	Ezdinli EZ. *Cancer* 1980;46:2149–2153.
Methotrexate	Methotrexate 40 mg/m^2/wk i.m. Increase dose by 10 mg/m^2 weekly as tolerated (expect tolerable dose of 60 mg/m^2/wk)	Taylor SG. *J Clin Oncol* 1984;2:1006–1011.
Paclitaxel/ carboplatin	Paclitaxel 175 mg/m^2 i.v. on day 1 Carboplatin AUC of 6 i.v. on day 1 Repeat cycle every 21 d	Fountzilas G. *Semin Oncol* 1997;24 (Suppl 2):65–67.
Paclitaxel/ cisplatin	Paclitaxel 175 mg/m^2 i.v. on day 1 Cisplatin 75 mg/m^2 i.v. on day 2 Filgrastim 5 μg/kg/d s.c. on days 4–10 Repeat cycle every 21 d	Hitt R. *Semin Oncol* 1995;22(Suppl 2): 50–54.
TIP	Paclitaxel 175 mg/m^2 i.v. on day 1 Ifosfamide 1000 mg/m^2 i.v. on days 1–3 Mesna 600 mg/m^2/d divided as 400 mg/m^2 i.v. before ifosfamide and 200 mg/m^2 i.v. 4 h after ifosfamide Cisplatin 60 mg/m^2 i.v. on day 1 Repeat cycle every 3–4 wk	Shin DM. *J Clin Oncol* 1998;16:1325–1330.
TPF	Docetaxel 75 mg/m^2 i.v. on day 1 Cisplatin 75–100 mg/m^2 i.v. on day 1 5-FU 1000 mg/m^2 on days 1–4 Repeat cycle every 21 d	Posner M. *J Clin Oncol* 2001;19:1096–1104.
Hepatocellular		
Capecitabine	Capecitabine 1000 mg/m^2 p.o. on days 1–14 Repeat cycle every 21 d	Aguayo A. *Semin Oncol* 2001;28:503–513.

(continued)

(continued)

Regimen	Drug dose	References
Doxorubicin	Doxorubicin 60–75 mg/m^2 i.v. Repeat cycle every 3 wk	Lai CL. *Cancer* 1988;62:479–483.
Intra-arterial cisplatin, doxorubicin, FUDR, and leucovorin	Doxorubicin 30–35 mg/m^2 and Cisplatin 100 mg/m^2 on day 1 by intra-arterial infusion Then floxuridine (FUDR) 60 mg/m^2/d and leucovorin 15 mg/m^2/d by intra-arterial infusion for 4 d Repeat cycle every 5 wk	Patt YZ. *J Clin Oncol* 1994;12:1204–1211.
PIAF	Cisplatin 20 mg/m^2/d i.v. on days 1–4 Doxorubicin 40 mg/m^2 i.v. on day 1 Interferon-α2B 5 MU/m^2 s.c. on days 1–4 5-FU 400 mg/m^2/d i.v. on days 1–4 Repeat cycle every 3 wk	Leung TWT. *Clin Cancer Res* 1999; 5:1676–1681.

Leukemias

Acute lymphocytic leukemia (ALL)

Clofarabine	Clofarabine 52 mg/m^2 i.v. daily on days 1–5 Repeat cycle every 2 to 6 wk	Jeha S. *J Clin Oncol* 2006;24:1917–1923.
Hyper-CVAD ± imatinib	Course I, III, V, and VII: Cyclophosphamide 300 mg/m^2 i.v. q12h × 6 doses on days 1–3 Mesna 600 mg/m^2/d CIVI daily on days 1–3 Vincristine 2 mg i.v. on days 4 and 11 Doxorubicin 50 mg/m^2 i.v. on day 4 Dexamethasone 40 mg i.v./p.o. daily on days 1–4 and 11–14 Filgrastim 10 μg/kg s.c. in divided doses starting on day 5 Course II, IV, VI, and VIII: Methotrexate 200 mg/m^2 i.v. over 2 h followed by 800 mg/m^2 CIVI over 24 h on day 1 with leucovorin rescue Cytarabine 3000 mg/m^2 i.v. q12h × 4 doses on days 2 and 3 Methylprednisolone 50 mg i.v. b.i.d. on days 1–3 Filgrastim 10 μg/kg s.c. in divided doses starting on day 4 ± Imatinib 400 mg p.o. daily on days 1–14 of all intensive chemotherapy courses Refer to the references for IT therapy recommendations	Kantarjian HM. *J Clin Oncol* 2000;18: 547–561. Thomas DA. *Blood* 2004;103:4396–4407.

(continued)

Regimen	Drug dose	References
Larson regimen	Course I (induction <60 years): Cyclophosphamide 1200 mg/m^2 i.v. on day 1 Daunorubicin 45 mg/m^2 i.v. on days 1–3 Vincristine 2 mg i.v. on days 1, 8, 15, and 22 Prednisone 60 mg/m^2/d p.o. on days 1–21 L-Asparaginase 6000 IU/m^2 s.c. on days 5, 8, 11, 15, 18, and 22 Course I (induction ≥60 years): Cyclophosphamide 800 mg/m^2 i.v. on day 1 Daunorubicin 30 mg/m^2 i.v. on days 1–3 Prednisone 60 mg/m^2/d p.o. on days 1–7 Course II (early intensification): Methotrexate 15 mg IT on day 1 Cyclophosphamide 1000 mg/m^2 i.v. on day 1 6-Mercaptopurine 60 mg/m^2/d p.o. on days 1–14 Cytarabine 75 mg/m^2/d s.c. on days 1–4 and 8–11 Vincristine 2 mg i.v. on days 15 and 22 L-Asparaginase 6000 IU/m^2 s.c. on days 15, 18, 22, and 25 Course III (CNS prophylaxis and interim maintenance): IT methotrexate 15 mg IT on days 1, 8, 15, 22, and 29 6-Mercaptopurine 60 mg/m^2/d p.o. on days 1–70 Methotrexate 20 mg/m^2 p.o. on days 36, 43, 50, 57, and 64 Course IV (late intensification): Doxorubicin 30 mg/m^2 i.v. on days 1, 8, and 15 Vincristine 2 mg i.v. on days 1, 8, and 15 Dexamethasone 10 mg/m^2/d p.o. on days 1–14 Cyclophosphamide 1000 mg/m^2 i.v. on day 29	Larson RA. *Blood* 1995;85:2025–2037.

(*continued*)

(continued)

Regimen	Drug dose	References
	6-Thioguanine 60 mg/m^2/d p.o. on days 29–42	
	Cytarabine 75 mg/m^2/d s.c. on days 29–32 and 36–39	
	Course V (maintenance):	
	Vincristine 2 mg i.v. on day 1	
	Prednisone 60 mg/m^2/d p.o. on days 1–5	
	Methotrexate 20 mg/m^2 p.o. on days 1, 8, 15, and 22	
	6-Mercaptopurine 60 mg/m^2/d p.o. on days 1–28	
	Repeat maintenance every 28 d	
Nelarabine	Nelarabine 1500 mg/m^2 i.v. on days 1, 3, and 5	Goekbuget N. *Blood* 2005;106:150. Abstract.
Acute myelogenous leukemia (AML)		
7 + 3	Cytarabine 100 mg/m^2/d CIVI on days 1–7	Rai KR. *Blood* 1981;58:1203–1212.
	Daunorubicin 45 mg/m^2 i.v. on days 1–3 or	Preisler H. *Blood* 1987;69:1441–1449.
	Idarubicin 12 mg/m^2 i.v. on days 1–3 or	Vogler WR. *J Clin Oncol* 1992;10: 1103–1111.
	Mitoxantrone 12 mg/m^2 i.v. on days 1–3	Arlin Z. *Leukemia* 1990;4:177–183.
FLAG ± idarubicin	Fludarabine 30 mg/m^2 i.v. daily on days 1–5	Clavio M. *Haematologica* 1996; 81:513–520.
	Cytarabine 2000 mg/m^2 i.v. daily on days 1–5	Montillo M. *Am J Hematol* 1998;58: 105–109.
	Filgrastim 300 μg s.c. daily starting on day 0	Virchis A. *Br J Haematol* 2004; 124:26–32.
	± Idarubicin 8 mg/m^2 i.v. daily on days 1–3	
Gemtuzumab	Gemtuzumab 9 mg/m^2 i.v. on day 1	Sievers EL. *J Clin Oncol* 2001;19:3244-3251.
	Repeat cycle every 2 wk × 2 doses	
HDAC	Cytarabine 3000 mg/m^2 i.v. over 3 h q12h on days 1, 3, and 5	Mayer RJ. *N Engl J Med* 1994;331:896–903.
MEC	Mitoxantrone 8 mg/m^2 i.v. daily on days 1–5	Greenberg PL. *J Clin Oncol* 2004;22: 1078–1086.
	Etoposide 100 mg/m^2 i.v. daily on days 1–5	
	Cytarabine 1000 mg/m^2 i.v. daily on days 1–5	
Mitoxantrone– etoposide	Mitoxantrone 10 mg/m^2 i.v. daily on days 1–5	Ho AD. *J Clin Oncol* 1988;6:213–217.
	Etoposide 100 mg/m^2 i.v. daily on days 1–5	

(continued)

Regimen	Drug dose	References
Acute promyelocytic leukemia (APL)		
AIDA	All-*trans* retinoic acid (ATRA) 45 mg/m^2/d p.o. in two divided doses	Sanz MA. *Blood* 2004;15:1237–1243.
	Idarubicin 12 mg/m^2 i.v. daily on days 2, 4, 6, and 8	
Arsenic trioxide	Arsenic trioxide 0.15 mg/kg i.v. daily for up to 60 days	Soignet SL. *J Clin Oncol* 2001;19:3852–3860.
ATRA/7+3	ATRA 45 mg/m^2/d p.o. divided into two doses starting on day 1 and continuing until complete response (CR) (maximum of 90 d)	Fenaux P. *Blood* 1999;94:1192–1200.
	Daunorubicin 60 mg/m^2/d i.v. on days 3–5	
	Cytarabine 200 mg/m^2/d CIVI on days 3–10	
Chronic lymphocytic leukemia (CLL)		
Alemtuzumab	Alemtuzumab 30 mg i.v. or s.c. thrice weekly	Keating MJ. *Blood* 2002;99:3554–3561.
	Begin with an initial dose of 3 mg, and increase the dose to 10 mg and then to a final dose of 30 mg as tolerated	Lundin J. *Blood* 2002;100:768–773.
CP	Variation 1: Chlorambucil 30 mg/m^2 p.o. on day 1	Raphael B. *J Clin Oncol* 1991;9:770–776.
	Prednisone 80 mg p.o. daily on days 1–5	Dighiero G. *N Engl J Med* 1992;338: 1506–1514.
	Repeat cycle every 28 d	
	Variation 2: Chlorambucil 0.3 mg/kg p.o. daily on days 1–5	
	Prednisone 40 mg/m^2 p.o. daily on days 1–5	
	Repeat cycle every 28 d	
CVP	Cyclophosphamide 300 mg/m^2 p.o. daily on days 1–5	Raphael B. *J Clin Oncol* 1991;9:770–776.
	Vincristine 1.4 mg/m^2 i.v. on day 1 (maximum dose of 2 mg)	
	Prednisone 100 mg/m^2 p.o. daily on days 1–5	
	Repeat cycle every 21 d	
FC	Fludarabine 30 mg/m^2 i.v. daily on days 1–3	O'Brien S. *J Clin Oncol* 2001;19:1414–1420.
	Cyclophosphamide 250–300 mg/m^2 i.v. daily on days 1–3	Eichhorst BF. *Blood* 2006;107:885–891.
	Repeat cycle every 28–42 d	

(continued)

(continued)

Regimen	Drug dose	References
FCR	See Non-Hodgkin's lymphoma (NHL) for dosing recommendations	
FR	See NHL for dosing recommendations	
PC ± rituximab	Pentostatin 4 mg/m^2 i.v. on day 1 Cyclophosphamide 600 mg/m^2 i.v. on day 1 ± Rituximab 375 mg/m^2 i.v. on day 1 (omit with cycle 1) Repeat cycle every 21 d	Weiss MA. *J Clin Oncol* 2003;21:1278–1284. Lamanna N. *J Clin Oncol* 2006;24: 1575–1581.

Chronic myelogenous leukemia (CML)

Dasatinib	Dasatinib 70 mg p.o. b.i.d.	Hochhaus A. *Blood* 2005;106:41. Abstract. Guihot F. *Blood* 2005; 106:39. Abstract. Talpaz M. *Blood* 2005; 106:40. Abstract.
Imatinib	Imatinib 400 mg p.o. daily (chronic phase) Imatinib 600 mg p.o. daily (accelerated phase or blast crisis)	Kantarjian H. *N Engl J Med* 2002;346: 645–652. Talpaz M. *Blood* 2002;99:1928–1937. Sawyer CL. *Blood* 2002;99:3530–3539.

Hairy cell leukemia

Cladribine	Cladribine 0.1 mg/kg/d CIVI on days 1–7 One cycle only	Saven A. *Blood* 1998;92:1918–1926. Chadha P. *Blood* 2005;106:241–246.
Cladribine	Cladribine 0.12 mg/kg i.v. daily on days 1–5	Robak T. *Eur J Haematol* 1999;62: 49–56.
Pentostatin	Pentostatin 4 mg/m^2 i.v. on day 1 Repeat cycle every 14 d	Grever M. *J Clin Oncol* 1995;13:974–982. Flinn IW. *Blood* 2000; 96:2981–2986.

Myelodysplastic syndrome

Antithymocyte Globulin/ cyclosporine	Antithymocyte globulin 40 mg/kg i.v. daily × 4 d Cyclosporine titrated to maintain level between 200 and 400 mg/dL Methylprednisolone 1 mg/kg i.v. daily × 4 before to each dose of antithymocyte globulin followed by prednisone 60 mg p.o. daily tapered over 1 mo	Yazji S. *Leukemia* 2003;17:2101–2106.

(continued)

Regimen	Drug dose	References
Azacitidine	Azacitidine 75 mg/m^2 s.c. daily × 7 d Repeat cycle every 28 d	Silverman LR. *J Clin Oncol* 2002;20: 2429–2440.
Decitabine	Decitabine 15 mg/m^2 i.v. q8h × 3 d Repeat cycle every 6 wk	Kantarjian H. *Cancer* 2006;106:1794–1803.
Revlimid	Lenalidomide 10 mg p.o. daily	List A. *N Engl J Med* 2005;352:549–557.

Lung cancer

Non–small cell

Regimen	Drug dose	References
Carboplatin/ docetaxel	Docetaxel 75 mg/m^2 i.v. on day 1 Carboplatin AUC 6 i.v. on day 1 Repeat cycle every 3 wk	Fossella F. *J Clin Oncol* 2003;21:3016–3024.
Carboplatin/ gemcitabine	Gemcitabine 1250 mg/m^2 i.v. on days 1 and 8 Carboplatin AUC 5 i.v. on day 1 Repeat cycle every 21 d	Sederholm C. *J Clin Oncol* 2005;23: 8380–8388.
Carboplatin/ paclitaxel	Paclitaxel 225 mg/m^2 i.v. on day 1 Carboplatin AUC 6 i.v. on day 1 Repeat cycle every 3 wk	Kelly K. *J Clin Oncol* 2001;19:3210–3218. Schiller JH. *N Engl J Med* 2002;346: 92–98.
Carboplatin/ paclitaxel	Paclitaxel 200 mg/m^2 i.v. on day 1 Carboplatin AUC 6 i.v. on day 1 Repeat cycle every 3 wk	Greco FA. *Cancer* 2001;92:2142–2147.
Cisplatin/ docetaxel	Docetaxel 75 mg/m^2 i.v. on day 1 Cisplatin 75 mg/m^2 i.v. on day 1 Repeat cycle every 3 wk	Schiller JH. *N Engl J Med* 2002;346: 92–98. Fossella F. *J Clin Oncol* 2003;21:3016–3024.
Cisplatin/ etoposide	Cisplatin 60 mg/m^2 i.v. on day 1 Etoposide 100 mg/m^2 i.v. on days 4, 6, and 8 Repeat cycle every 3–4 wk	Longeval E. *Cancer* 1982;50:2751–2756.
Cisplatin/ gemcitabine	Gemcitabine 1000 mg/m^2 i.v. on days 1, 8, and 15 Cisplatin 100 mg/m^2 i.v. on day 1 Repeat cycle every 4 wk	Sandler AB. *J Clin Oncol* 2000;18: 122–130. Schiller JH. *N Engl J Med* 2002;346: 92–98.
Cisplatin/ paclitaxel	Paclitaxel 175 mg/m^2 i.v. on day 1 Cisplatin 80 mg/m^2 i.v. on day 1 Repeat cycle every 3 wk	Smit EF. *J Clin Oncol* 2003;21:3909–3917.
Cisplatin/ vinorelbine	Vinorelbine 25–30 mg/m^2 i.v. on days 1, 8, 15, and 22 Cisplatin 100 mg/m^2 i.v. on day 1 Repeat cycle every 4 wk	Wozniak AJ. *J Clin Oncol* 1998;16: 2459–2465. Arriagada R. *N Engl J Med* 2004;350: 351–360.

(continued)

(continued)

Regimen	Drug dose	References
Docetaxel	Docetaxel 75 mg/m^2 i.v. on day 1 Repeat cycle every 3 wk	Shepherd FA. *J Clin Oncol* 2000;18: 2095–2103. Fossella FV. *J Clin Oncol* 2000;18: 2354–2362.
Erlotinib	Erlotinib 150 mg p.o. daily	Shepherd FA. *N Engl J Med* 2005;353: 123–132.
Pemetrexed	Pemetrexed 500 mg/m^2 i.v. on day 1 Folic acid 350–1000 μg p.o. daily starting 1 wk before first dose of pemetrexed and continuing until 21 d after the last dose of pemetrexed Vitamin B$_{12}$ 1000 μg i.m. starting 1 wk before the first dose of pemetrexed and repeated every three cycles Dexamethasone 4 mg p.o. b.i.d. on days 0–2 Repeat cycle every 21 d	Hanna N. *J Clin Oncol* 2004;22:1589–1597.
Small cell		
CAV	Cyclophosphamide 1000 mg/m^2 i.v. on day 1 Doxorubicin 45 mg/m^2 i.v. on day 1 Vincristine 2 mg i.v. on day 1 Repeat cycle every 21 d	von Pawel J. *J Clin Oncol* 1999;17: 658–667.
EC	Carboplatin AUC 5–6 i.v. on day 1 Etoposide 100 mg/m^2 i.v. on days 1–3 Repeat cycle every 21–28 d	Okomoto H. *J Clin Oncol* 1999;17: 3540–3545. Skarlos DV. *Ann Oncol* 2001;12:1232–1238.
EP	Etoposide 80 mg/m^2 i.v. on days 1–3 Cisplatin 80 mg/m^2 i.v. on day 1 Repeat cycle every 21 d	Ihde DC. *J Clin Oncol* 1994;12:2022–2034.
Irinotecan/ cisplatin	Irinotecan 60 mg/m^2 i.v. on days 1, 8, and 15 Cisplatin 60 mg/m^2 i.v. on day 1 Repeat cycle every 28 d	Noda K. *N Engl J Med* 2002;346:85–91.
Topotecan	Topotecan 1.5 mg/m^2 i.v. on days 1–5 Repeat cycle every 21 d	von Pawel J. *J Clin Oncol* 1999;17: 658–667.

(continued)

Regimen	Drug dose	References
Lymphoma		
Hodgkin's lymphoma		
ABVD	Doxorubicin 25 mg/m^2 i.v. on days 1 and 15 Bleomycin 10 mg/m^2 i.v. on days 1 and 15 Vinblastine 6 mg/m^2 i.v. on days 1 and 15 Dacarbazine 375 mg/m^2 i.v. on days 1 and 15 Repeat cycle every 28 d	Bonadonna G. *Cancer Treat Rev* 1982;9: 21–35.
BEACOPP (increased dose)	Bleomycin 10 mg/m^2 i.v. on day 8 Etoposide 200 mg/m^2 i.v. on days 1–3 Doxorubicin 35 mg/m^2 i.v. on day 1 Cyclophosphamide 1200 mg/m^2 i.v. on day 1 Vincristine 1.4 mg/m^2 i.v. on day 8 (maximum dose of 2 mg) Procarbazine 100 mg/m^2 p.o. on days 1–7 Prednisone 40 mg/m^2 p.o. on days 1–14 Filgrastim to start on day 8 Repeat cycle every 21 d	Diehl V. *N Engl J Med* 2003;348:2386–2395.
Stanford V	Doxorubicin 25 mg/m^2 i.v. on days 1 and 15 Vinblastine 6 mg/m^2 i.v. on days 1 and 15[c] Mechlorethamine 6 mg/m^2 i.v. on day 1 Vincristine 1.4 mg/m^2 i.v. on days 8 and 22[c] (maximum dose of 2 mg) Bleomycin 5 mg/m^2 i.v. on days 8 and 22 Etoposide 60 mg/m^2 i.v. on days 15 and 16 Prednisone 40 mg/m^2 p.o. every other day Repeat cycle every 28 d	Bartlett NL. *J Clin Oncol* 1995;13: 1080–1088. Horning SJ. *J Clin Oncol* 2002;20: 630–637.
Non-Hodgkin's lymphoma		
Bortezomib	Bortezomib 1.3 mg/m^2 i.v. on days 1, 4, 8, and 11 Repeat cycle every 21 d	Goy A. *J Clin Oncol* 2004;22:6581. Abstract. Goy A. *J Clin Oncol* 2006;24:7512. Abstract.

(continued)

[c] During course III for patients >50 yr, vinblastine reduced to 4 mg/m^2 and vincristine reduced to 1 mg/m^2

(continued)

Regimen	Drug dose	References
CHOP ± rituximab	Cyclophosphamide 750 mg/m^2 i.v. on day 1 Doxorubicin 50 mg/m^2 i.v. on day 1 Vincristine 1.4 mg/m^2 i.v. on day 1 (maximum dose of 2 mg) Prednisone 100 mg p.o. daily on days 1–5 ± Rituximab 375 mg/m^2 i.v. on day 0 Repeat cycle every 21 d	McKelvey EM. *Cancer* 1976;38:1484–1493. Lenz G. *J Clin Oncol* 2005;23:1984–1992. Hiddemann W. *Blood* 2005;106:3725–3732.
CNOP	Cyclophosphamide 750 mg/m^2 i.v. on day 1 Mitoxantrone 10 mg/m^2 i.v. on day 1 Vincristine 1.4 mg/m^2 i.v. on day 1 (maximum dose of 2 mg) Prednisone 50 mg/m^2 p.o. daily on days 1–5 Repeat cycle every 21 d	Pavlovsky S. *Ann Oncol* 1992;3:205–209.
CVP ± rituximab	Cyclophosphamide 750 mg/m^2 i.v. on day 1 Vincristine 1.4 mg/m^2 i.v. on day 1 (maximum dose of 2 mg) Prednisone 40 mg/m^2 p.o. daily on days 1–5 ± Rituximab 375 mg/m^2 i.v. on day 1 Repeat cycle every 21 d	Marcus R. *Blood* 2005;105:1417–1423.
DHAP	Cisplatin 100 mg/m^2 CIVI over 24 h on day 1 Cytarabine 2000 mg/m^2 i.v. q12h × 2 doses on day 2 Dexamethasone 40 mg p.o./i.v. daily on days 1–4 Repeat cycle every 21–28 d	Velasquez WS. *Blood* 1988;71:117–122.
EPOCH	Etoposide 50 mg/m^2/d CIVI on days 1–4 Doxorubicin 10 mg/m^2/d CIVI on days 1–4 Vincristine 0.4 mg/m^2/d CIVI on days 1–4 (dose not capped) Cyclophosphamide 750 mg/m^2 i.v. on day 5 Prednisone 60 mg p.o. daily on days 1–5 Filgrastim daily starting on day 6 Repeat cycle every 21 d	Wilson WH. *J Clin Oncol* 1993;11:1573–1582. Gutierrez M. *J Clin Oncol* 2000;18:3633–3642.
ESHAP	Etoposide 40 mg/m^2 i.v. daily on days 1–4 Methylprednisolone 500 mg i.v. daily on days 1–5	Velasquez WS. *J Clin Oncol* 1994;12:1169–1176.

(continued)

Regimen	Drug dose	References
	Cytarabine 2000 mg/m^2 i.v. on day 5	
	Cisplatin 25 mg/m^2/d CIVI on days 1–4	
	Repeat cycle every 21–28 d	
FC	Fludarabine 20 mg/m^2 i.v. on days 1–5	Flinn IW. *Blood* 2000;96:71–75.
	Cyclophosphamide 600 mg/m^2 i.v. on day 1	
	Filgrastim 5 μg/kg s.c. daily starting on day 8	
	Repeat cycle every 28 d	
FCMR	Rituximab 375 mg/m^2 i.v. on day 1	Forstpointner R. *Blood* 2004;104:3064–3071.
	Fludarabine 25 mg/m^2 i.v. on days 1–3	
	Cyclophosphamide 200 mg/m^2 i.v. on days 1–3	
	Mitoxantrone 8 mg/m^2 i.v. on day 1	
	Repeat cycle every 28 d	
FCR	Fludarabine 25 mg/m^2 i.v. on days 1–3	Keating MJ. *J Clin Oncol* 2005;23: 4079–4088.
	Cyclophosphamide 250 mg/m^2 i.v. on days 1–3	Tam CS. *Cancer* 2006; 106:2412–2420.
	Rituximab 375 mg/m^2 i.v. on day 1 or	
	Rituximab 375 mg/m^2 i.v. on day 1 (cycle 1 only)	
	Rituximab 500 mg/m^2 i.v. on day 1 (cycles 2–6)	
	Repeat cycle every 28 d	
FND	Fludarabine 25 mg/m^2 i.v. on days 1–3	McGlaughlin P. *J Clin Oncol* 1996;14: 1262–1268.
	Mitoxantrone 10 mg/m^2 i.v. on day 1	
	Dexamethasone 20 mg i.v./p.o. daily on days 1–5	
	Repeat cycle every 28 d	
FR	Fludarabine 25 mg/m^2 i.v. daily on days 1–5	Byrd JC. *Blood* 2003;101:6–14.
	Rituximab 50 mg/m^2 i.v. on day 1 (cycle 1 only)	
	Rituximab 325 mg/m^2 i.v. on day 3 (cycle 1 only)	
	Rituximab 375 mg/m^2 i.v. on day 5 (cycle 1 only)	
	Rituximab 375 mg/m^2 i.v. on day 1 (cycles 2–6)	
	Repeat cycle every 28 d	

(continued)

(continued)

Regimen	Drug dose	References
Hyper-CVAD	Course I, III, V, and VII: Cyclophosphamide 300 mg/m^2 i.v. q12h × 6 doses on days 1–3 Mesna 600 mg/m^2/d CIVI daily on days 1–3, Vincristine 2 mg i.v. on days 4 and 11 Doxorubicin 50 mg/m^2 i.v. on day 4 Dexamethasone 40 mg i.v./p.o. daily on days 1–4 and 11–14 Filgrastim 5–10 μg/kg s.c. daily starting on day 5 Course II, IV, VI, and VIII: Methotrexate 200 mg/m^2 i.v. over 2 h followed by methotrexate 800 mg/m^2 CIVI over 22 h on day 1 with leucovorin rescue Cytarabine 3000 mg/m^2 i.v. q12h × 4 doses on days 2 and 3 Filgrastim 5–10 μg/kg s.c. daily starting on day 4 Refer to the references for IT therapy recommendations	Khouri IF. *J Clin Oncol* 1998;16:3803–3809. Thomas DA. *Blood* 2004;104:1624–1630.
Ibritumomab tiuxetan	Rituximab 250 mg/m^2 i.v. on days 1 and 8 Ibritumomab tiuxetan 5 mCi i.v. on day 1 and 0.4 mCi/kg i.v. on day 8 immediately following day 8 rituximab	Witzig TE. *J Clin Oncol* 2002;20:2453–2463. Witzig TE. *J Clin Oncol* 2002;20:3262–3269.
ICE ± rituximab	Ifosfamide 5000 mg/m^2 CIVI over 24 h on day 2 Mesna 5000mg/m^2 CIVI over 24 h on day 2 Carboplatin AUC 5 i.v. on day 2 (maximum dose of 800 mg) Etoposide 100 mg/m^2 i.v. daily on days 1–3 ± Rituximab 375 mg/m^2 i.v. 48 h before start of cycle 1 and on day 1 of each cycle Repeat cycle every 14–15 d	Moskowitz CH. *J Clin Oncol* 1999;17:3776–3785. Kewalramani T. *Blood* 2004;103:3684–3688.
R-EPOCH	Rituximab 375 mg/m^2 i.v. on day 1 Doxorubicin 15 mg/m^2 CIVI on days 2–4 Etoposide 65 mg/m^2 CIVI on days 2–4 Vincristine 0.5 mg CIVI on days 2–4 Cyclophosphamide 750 mg/m^2 i.v. on day 5	Jermann M. *Ann Oncol* 2004;15:511–516.

(continued)

Regimen	Drug dose	References
	Prednisone 60 mg/m^2 daily p.o. on days 1–14	
	Repeat cycle every 21 d	
R–Hyper-CVAD	Course I, III, V, and VII:	Romaguera JE. *J Clin Oncol* 2005;23: 7013–7023.
	Rituximab 375 mg/m^2 i.v. on day 1	
	Cyclophosphamide 300 mg/m^2 i.v. q12h × 6 doses on days 2–4	
	Mesna 600 mg/m^2/d CIVI daily on days 1–3	
	Vincristine 1.4 mg/m^2 (maximum dose of 2 mg) i.v. administered 12 h after the last dose of cyclophosphamide and repeated on day 12	
	Doxorubicin 16.7 mg/m^2/d CIVI on days 5–7	
	Dexamethasone 40 mg i.v./p.o. daily on days 2–5 and 12–15	
	Filgrastim 5 μg/kg s.c. daily starting 24–36 h after the completion of doxorubicin	
	Course II, IV, VI, and VIII:	
	Rituximab 375 mg/m^2 i.v. on day 1	
	Methotrexate 200 mg/m^2 i.v. on day 2 immediately followed by methotrexate 800 mg/m^2 CIVI over 22 h with leucovorin rescue	
	Cytarabine 3000 mg/m^2 i.v. q12h × 4 doses on days 3 and 4	
	Filgrastim 5 μg/kg s.c. daily starting 24–36 h after the completion of chemotherapy	
	Refer to the reference for IT therapy recommendations	
Rituximab	Rituximab 375 mg/m^2 i.v. weekly × 4 doses	Davis TA. *J Clin Oncol* 1999;17:1851–1857.
Tositumomab	Step 1:	Kaminski MS. *J Clin Oncol* 2001;19: 3918–3928.
	Tositumomab 450 mg i.v., followed by tositumomab 35 mg labeled with 5mCi of iodine-131 (^{131}I) on day 1	Kaminski MS. *N Engl J Med* 2005;352: 441–449.
	Step 2:	
	Tositumomab 450 mg i.v., followed by tositumomab 35 mg labeled with an amount of ^{131}I calculated from serial total-body gamma-camera counts 7–14 d after step 1	

(continued)

(continued)

Regimen	Drug dose	References
Melanoma		
Cisplatin/ vinblastine/ dacarbazine/ interferon-α/ interleukin-2	Cisplatin 20 mg/m^2 i.v. daily on days 1–4 Vinblastine 1.6 mg/m^2 i.v. daily on days 1–4 Dacarbazine 800 mg/m^2 i.v. daily on day 1 Interferon-α 9 MU/m^2/d CIVI on days 1–4 Interleukin-2 5 MU/m^2 s.c. daily on days 1–5	Legha SS. *J Clin Oncol* 1998;16:1752–1759. Lewis KD. *J Clin Oncol* 2006;24:3157–3163.
CVD	Cisplatin 20 mg/m^2 i.v. daily on days 2–5 Vinblastine 1.6 mg/m^2 i.v. daily on days 1–5 Dacarbazine 800 mg/m^2 i.v. daily on day 1 Repeat cycle every 21 d	Legha SS. *Cancer* 1989;64:2024–2029.
Dacarbazine	Dacarbazine 250 mg/m^2 i.v. daily on d 1–5 Repeat cycle every 21 d	Middleton MR. *J Clin Oncol* 2000;18: 156–166.
Interferon-α-2B	Interferon-α-2B 20 MU/m^2/d i.v. 5 d per wk for 4 wk, followed by 10 MU/m^2/d s.c. 3 times a wk for 48 wk	Kirkwood JM. *J Clin Oncol* 1996;14:7–17.
Interleukin-2	Interleukin-2 600,000–720,000 IU/kg i.v. every 8 h × 14 consecutive doses over 5 d and after a 6–9 d rest period, repeat an additional 14 doses over 5 d Repeat cycle every 6–12 wk	Atkins MB. *J Clin Oncol* 1999;17:2105–2116.
Temozolomide	Temozolomide 200 mg/m^2 p.o. daily on days 1–5 Repeat cycle every 28 d	Middleton MR. *J Clin Oncol* 2000;18: 156–166.
Temozolomide/ Interferon-α	Temozolomide 200 mg/m^2 p.o. daily on days 1–5 Interferon-α 5 MU/m^2 s.c. 3 times a wk Repeat cycle every 28 d	Kaufmann R. *J Clin Oncol* 2005;23: 9001–9007.
Multiple myeloma		
Dexamethasone	40 mg p.o. daily on days 1–4, 9–12, and 17–20 Repeat cycle every 21 d	Alexanian R. *Ann Intern Med* 1986;105:8–11.
DVD	Pegylated liposomal doxorubicin 40 mg/m^2 i.v. day 1 Vincristine 2 mg i.v. day 1 Dexamethasone 40 mg p.o. daily × 4 Repeat cycle every 28 d	Hussein M. *Cancer* 2002;95:2160–2168. Dimopoulos MA. *Ann Oncol* 2003;14: 1039–1044.

(continued)

Regimen	Drug dose	References
MP	Melphalan 8 mg/m^2 p.o. days 1–4 Prednisone 60 mg/m^2 p.o. days 1–4 Repeat cycle every 28 d	Oken MM. *Cancer* 1997;79:1561–1567.
Revlimid/ dexamethasone	Lenalidomide 25 mg p.o. daily × 21 Dexamethasone 40 mg p.o. daily on days 1–4, 9–12, and 17–20 Repeat cycle every 28 d	Rajkumar SV. *Blood* 2005;106:4050-4053.
Thalidomide/ dexamethasone	Thalidomide initial dose to start at 100–200 mg p.o. every day at bedtime and increase as tolerated Dexamethasone 40 mg p.o. daily on days 1–4, 9–12, and 17–20 Repeat cycle every 28 d	Cavo M. *Blood* 2005;106:35–39. Rajkumar SV. *J Clin Oncol* 2006;24: 431–436.
VAD	Vincristine 0.4 mg/d CIVI days 1–4 Doxorubicin 9 mg/m^2/d CIVI days 1–4 Dexamethasone 40 mg p.o. daily days 1–4, 9–12, 17–20 Repeat cycle every 28–35 d	Barlogie B. *N Engl J Med* 1984;310:1353–1356.
Velcade ± dexamethasone	Bortezomib 1.3 mg/m^2 i.v. on days 1, 4, 8, and 11 ± Dexamethasone 20–40 mg p.o. on days 1, 2, 4, 5, 8, 9, 11, and 12 Repeat cycle every 21 d	Richardson PG. *N Engl J Med* 2003;348: 2609–2617. Jagannath S. *Br J Haematol* 2005;129: 776–783. Richardson PG. *N Engl J Med* 2005;352: 2487–2498.
Ovarian cancer		
Altretamine	Altretamine 260 mg/m^2/d p.o. in 4 divided doses on days 1–14 Repeat cycle every 28 d	Rustin GJ. *J Clin Oncol* 1997;15:172–176.
Carboplatin/ paclitaxel	Carboplatin AUC 5–7.5 i.v. on day 1 Paclitaxel 175 mg/m^2 i.v. on day 1 Repeat cycle every 21 d	Neijt JP. *J Clin Oncol* 2000;18:3084–3092. Ozols RF. *J Clin Oncol* 2003;21:3194–3200. ICON 4. *Lancet* 2003; 361:2099–2106.
Cisplatin/ paclitaxel	Paclitaxel 135 mg/m^2 CIVI over 24 h on day 1 Cisplatin 75 mg/m^2 i.v. on day 2 Repeat cycle every 21 d	McGuire WP. *N Engl J Med* 1996;334:1–6.
Docetaxel	Docetaxel 100 mg/m^2 i.v. on day 1 Repeat cycle every 21 d	Verschraegen CR. *J Clin Oncol* 2000;18: 2733–2739.

(continued)

(continued)

Regimen	Drug dose	References
Docetaxel/ carboplatin	Docetaxel 75 mg/m^2 i.v. on day 1 Carboplatin AUC 5 i.v. on day 1 Repeat cycle every 21 d	Vasey P. *J Natl Cancer Inst* 2004;96: 1682–1691.
Docetaxel/ cisplatin	Docetaxel 75 mg/m^2 i.v. on day 1 followed by Cisplatin 75 mg/m^2 i.v. on day 1 Repeat cycle every 21 d	Vasey PA. *J Clin Oncol* 1999;17:2069–2080.
Etoposide	Etoposide 50 mg/m^2/d p.o. on days 1–21 Repeat cycle every 28 d	Rose PG. *J Clin Oncol* 1998;16:405–410.
Gemcitabine	Gemcitabine 800–1250 mg/m^2 i.v. on days 1, 8, and 15 Repeat cycle every 28 d	Von Minckwitz G. *Ann Oncol* 1999;10: 853–855. Markman M. *Gynecol Oncol* 2003;90: 593–596. Lund B. *J Natl Cancer Inst* 1994;86: 1530–1533.
Gemcitabine/ carboplatin	Gemcitabine 1000 mg/m^2 i.v. on days 1 and 8 Carboplatin AUC 4 on day 1 Repeat cycle every 21 d	Pfisterer J. *J Clin Oncol* 2006;24:4699–4707.
Gemcitabine/ cisplatin	Cisplatin 30 mg/m^2 i.v. on days 1 and 8 Gemcitabine 600–750 mg/m^2 i.v. on days 1 and 8 Repeat cycle every 21 d	Nagourney RA. *Gynecol Oncol* 2003; 88:35–39.
Liposomal doxorubicin	Liposomal doxorubicin 40–50 mg/m^2 i.v. on day 1 Repeat cycle every 21–28 d	Muggia FM. *J Clin Oncol* 1997;15: 987–993.
Topotecan	Topotecan 1.5 mg/m^2/d i.v. on days 1–5 Repeat cycle every 21 d	Brookman MA. *J Clin Oncol* 1998;16: 3345–3352.
Topotecan weekly	Topotecan 4 mg/m^2 i.v. on days 1, 8 and 15 Repeat cycle every 28 d	Levy T. Gynecol Oncol 2004;95:686–690.
Vinorelbine	Vinorelbine 30 mg/m^2 i.v. on days 1 and 8 Repeat cycle every 21 d	Rothenberg ML. *Gynecol Oncol* 2004;95:506–512.
Pancreatic		
5-FU/oxaliplatin	5-FU 2000 mg/m^2 i.v. on days 1, 8, 15, and 22 Folinic acid 200 mg/m^2 i.v. on days 1, 8, 15, and 22 Oxaliplatin 85 mg/m^2 i.v. on days 8 and 22 Repeat cycle every 42 d	Oettle H. *J Clin Oncol* 2005;23:4031. Abstract.

(continued)

Regimen	Drug dose	References
Gemcitabine	Gemcitabine 1000 mg/m^2 i.v. weekly × 7, followed by 1 wk rest, then once weekly × 3 and repeat every 28 d	Burris HA. *J Clin Oncol* 1997;15:2403–2413.
Gemcitabine	Gemcitabine 1000 mg/m^2 i.v. on days 1, 8, and 15 Repeat cycle every 28 d	Neuhaus P. *J Clin Oncol* 2005;23:4013. Abstract.
Gemcitabine/ bevacizumab	Gemcitabine 1000 mg/m^2 i.v. on days 1, 8, and 15[d] Bevacizumab 10 mg/kg i.v. on days 1 and 15 Repeat cycle every 28 d	Kindler HL. *J Clin Oncol* 2005;23: 8033–8040.
Gemcitabine/ capecitabine	Gemcitabine 1000 mg/m^2 i.v. on days 1 and 8 Capecitabine 650 mg/m^2 p.o. b.i.d. on days 1–14 Repeat cycle every 21 d	Hess V. *J Clin Oncol* 2003;21:66–68. Stathopoulos GP. *Ann Oncol* 2004;15: 224–229.
Gemcitabine/ cetuximab	Initial cycle: Cetuximab 400 mg/m^2 (initial dose) i.v. followed by 250 mg/m^2 i.v. weekly × 7 followed by 1 wk rest Gemcitabine 1000 mg/m^2 i.v. weekly × 7 followed by 1 wk rest Additional cycles: Cetuximab 250 mg/m^2 i.v. weekly × 3[e] Gemcitabine 1000 mg/m^2 i.v. weekly × 3 Repeat cycle every 28 d	Xiong HQ. *J Clin Oncol* 2004;22:2610–2616.
Gemcitabine/ cisplatin	Gemcitabine 1000 mg/m^2 i.v. on days 1 and 15 Cisplatin 50 mg/m^2 i.v. on days 1 and 15 Repeat cycle every 28 d	Heinemann V. *J Clin Oncol* 2006;24: 3946–3952.
Gemcitabine/ erlotinib	Gemcitabine 1000 mg/m^2 i.v. weekly × 7, followed by 1 wk rest, then once weekly × 3 Erlotinib 100 mg p.o. daily Repeat 3 wk cycle every 28 d	Moore MJ. *J Clin Oncol* 2005;23:1. Abstract.
Gemcitabine/ oxaliplatin (GemOX)	Gemcitabine 1000 mg/m^2 i.v. over 100 min on day 1 Oxaliplatin 100 mg/m^2 i.v. on day 2 Repeat cycle every 2 wk	Louvet C. *J Clin Oncol* 2005;23:3509–3516. Demols A. *Br J Cancer* 2006;94:481–485.

(continued)

[d]Gemcitabine given before bevacizumab on days 1 and 15
[e]Cetuximab given before gemcitabine

(continued)

Regimen	Drug dose	References
GTX	Capecitabine 750 mg/m^2 p.o. b.i.d. × 14 d Gemcitabine 750 mg/m^2 i.v. on days 4 and 11 Docetaxel 30 mg/m^2 i.v. on days 4 and 11 Repeat cycle every 21 d	Fogelman DR. *Gastrointestinal Cancers Symposium.* 2007:143. Abstract.
Prostate		
Docetaxel	Docetaxel 75 mg/m^2 i.v. Repeat cycle every 21 d	Picus J. *Semin Oncol* 1999;26(5 suppl 7): 14–18.
Docetaxel/ estramustine	Docetaxel 35 mg/m^2 i.v. on day 2 of weeks 1 and 2 Estramustine 420 mg p.o. for the first 4 doses and 280 mg p.o. for the next 5 doses on days 1–3 of weeks 1 and 2 Dexamethasone 4 mg p.o. b.i.d. on days 1–3 of weeks 1 and 2 Repeat cycle every 21 d	Copur MS. *Semin Oncol* 2001;28:16–21.
Docetaxel/ prednisone	Docetaxel 75 mg/m^2 i.v. on day 1 Prednisone 5 mg p.o. daily Repeat cycle every 21 d for up to a total of 10 cycles	Eisenberger MA. *J Clin Oncol* 2004;22:4. Abstract.
Estramustine/ etoposide	Estramustine 15 mg/kg/d p.o. in 4 divided doses × 21 d Etoposide 50 mg/m^2/d p.o. in 2 divided doses × 21 d Repeat cycle every 28 d	Clark PE. *Urology* 2001;57:281–285.
Mitoxantrone/ hydrocortisone	Mitoxantrone 14 mg/m^2 i.v. every 3 wk Hydrocortisone 30 mg every morning and 10 mg every night	Kantoff PW. *J Clin Oncol* 1999;17: 2506–2513.
Mitoxantrone/ prednisone	Mitoxantrone 12 mg/m^2 i.v. on day 1 Prednisone 5 mg p.o. b.i.d. Repeat cycle every 3 wk	Tannock IF. *J Clin Oncol* 1996;14: 1756–1764.
Paclitaxel	Paclitaxel 135–170 mg/m^2 i.v. on day 1 Repeat cycle every 3 wk	Roth BJ. *Cancer* 1993;72:2457–2460.
PE	Paclitaxel 120 mg/m^2 CIVI over 96 h Repeat paclitaxel every 21 d Estramustine 600 mg/m^2/d p.o. in 2–3 divided doses continuously starting 24 h before first paclitaxel Repeat cycle every 21 d	Hudes GR. *J Clin Oncol* 1997;15:3156–3163.

(continued)

Regimen	Drug dose	References
TEC	Estramustine 10 mg/kg/d in divided doses 5 d per wk (start 48 h before chemotherapy) Paclitaxel 60–100 mg/m^2 i.v. weekly Carboplatin AUC 6 i.v. every 4 wk	Kelly WK. *J Clin Oncol* 2001;19:44–53.
Renal cell carcinoma		
Interferon-α-2A/ interleukin-2	Interferon-α-2A 6 MU s.c. thrice weekly Interleukin-2 18 MU/m^2/d CIVI × 5 d every 3 wk for 2 induction cycles and 4 maintenance cycles	Negrier S. *N Engl J Med* 1998;338:1272–1278.
Interferon-α-2B	Interferon-α-2B s.c. thrice weekly Week 1, 5 MU, 5 MU, 10 MU Weeks 2–11, 10 MU 3 times weekly	Medical Research Council Renal Cell College. *Lancet* 1999;353:14–17.
Sorafenib	Sorafenib 400 mg p.o. b.i.d.	Ratain MJ. *J Clin Oncol* 2006;24:2505–2512.
Sunitinib	Sunitinib 50 mg p.o. daily × 4 wk Repeat cycle every 6 wk	Motzer RJ. *JAMA* 2006; 295:2516–2524.
Sarcoma		
Ewing's sarcoma		
CAV alternating with IE	Odd cycles: Cyclophosphamide 1200 mg/m^2 i.v. on day 1 (with Mesna) Doxorubicin 75 mg/m^2 i.v. on day 1 Vincristine 2 mg on day 1 Dactinomycin 1.25 mg/m^2 i.v. on day 1 when cumulative dose of doxorubicin reaches 375 mg/m^2 Even cycles: Ifosfamide 1800 mg/m^2 i.v. on days 1–5 (with Mesna) Etoposide 100 mg/m^2 i.v. on days 1–5	Grier HE. *N Engl J Med* 2003;348:364–701.
HDCAV/IE	Cycles 1, 2, 3, and 6: Cyclophosphamide 2100 mg/m^2 i.v. on days 1 and 2 (with Mesna) Doxorubicin 25 mg/m^2/d CIVI on days 1–3 Vincristine 0.67 mg/m^2/d CIVI on days 1–3 (maximum dose of 2 mg/cycle) Cycles 4, 5, and 7: Ifosfamide 1800 mg/m^2 i.v. on days 1–5 (with Mesna) Etoposide 100 mg/m^2 i.v. on days 1–5	Kolb EA. *J Clin Oncol* 2003;21:3423–3430.

(continued)

(continued)

Regimen	Drug dose	References
VACA	Vincristine 1.5 mg/m²/d i.v. on days 1 and 22 (maximum dose of 2 mg) Doxorubicin 75 mg/m²/d i.v. on day 1 Cyclophosphamide 1400 mg/m²/d i.v. on day 22 (with Mesna) Repeat cycle every 6 wk × 6 THEN Vincristine 1.5 mg/m²/d i.v. on days 1 and 22 (maximum dose of 2 mg) Dactinomycin 0.45 mg/m²/d i.v. on days 1–5 (maximum dose of 0.5 mg) Cyclophosphamide 1400 mg/m²/d i.v. on day 22 (with Mesna) Repeat cycle every 6 wk × 7	Burgert EO. *J Clin Oncol* 1990;8: 1514–1524.
VAIA	Vincristine 1.5 mg/m²/d i.v. on days 1, 8, 15, and 22 Ifosfamide 3000 mg/m²/d i.v. on days 1, 2, 22, 23, 43, and 44 (with Mesna) Doxorubicin 30 mg/m²/d i.v. on days 1, 2, 43, and 44 Dactinomycin 0.5 mg/m²/d i.v. on days 22–24	Paulssen M. *J Clin Oncol* 2001;19: 1818–1829.

Gastrointestinal stromal tumor (GIST)

Imatinib	Imatinib 400 mg p.o. daily	Demetri GD. *N Engl J Med* 2002;347: 472–480.
Sunitinib	Sunitinib 50 mg p.o. daily	Casali PG. *J Clin Oncol* 2006;24:9513. Abstract.

Osteosarcoma

Carboplatin/ ifosfamide	Neoadjuvant therapy: Carboplatin 560 mg/m² i.v. on day 1 Ifosfamide 2650 mg/m² i.v. on days 1–3 (with Mesna) Repeat cycle every 21 d Adjuvant therapy: Carboplatin 560 mg/m² i.v. on day 1 Ifosfamide 2650 mg/m² i.v. on days 1–3 (with Mesna) Doxorubicin 25 mg/m²/d CIVI on days 1–3 Methotrexate 12 gm/m² i.v. with leucovorin rescue × 9	Meyer WH. *J Clin Oncol* 2001;19: 171–182.

(continued)

Regimen	Drug dose	References
	OR Cisplatin 100 mg/m^2 i.v. on day 1 Doxorubicin 25 mg/m^2/d CIVI on days 1–3 Methotrexate 12 gm/m^2 i.v. with leucovorin rescue × 9	
CAV alternating with IE	Odd cycles: Cyclophosphamide 1200 mg/m^2 i.v. on day 1 (with Mesna) Doxorubicin 75 mg/m^2 i.v. on day 1 Vincristine 2 mg on day 1 Dactinomycin 1.25 mg/m^2 i.v. on day 1 when cumulative dose of doxorubicin reaches 375 mg/m^2 Even cycles: Ifosfamide 1800 mg/m^2 i.v. on days 1–5 Etoposide 100 mg/m^2 i.v. on days 1–5	Grier HE. *N Engl J Med* 2003;348:694–701.
Doxorubicin/ cisplatin	Doxorubicin 25 mg/m^2 i.v. on days 1–3 Cisplatin 100 mg/m^2 i.v. on day 1 Repeat cycle every 21 d	Bramwell VHC. *J Clin Oncol* 1992;10: 1579–1591.
Gemcitabine/ docetaxel	Gemcitabine 675 mg/m^2 i.v. on days 1 and 8 Docetaxel 100 mg/m^2 i.v. on day 8 Repeat cycle every 21 d	Leu KM. *J Clin Oncol* 2004;22:1706–1712.
Methotrexate/ doxorubicin/ cisplatin/BCD	Methotrexate 12 gm/m^2 i.v. in weeks 3, 4, 8, 9, 13, 14, 18, 19, 23, 24, 37, and 38 Leucovorin 15 mg/m^2 i.v. q6h × 10 doses in weeks 3, 4, 8, 9, 13, 14, 18, 19, 23, 24, 37, and 38 Doxorubicin 37.5 mg/m^2 i.v. on days 1 and 2 in weeks 5, 10, 25, and 28 Cisplatin 60 mg/m^2 i.v. on days 1 and 2 in weeks 5, 10, 25, and 28 Cyclophosphamide 600 mg/m^2 i.v. in days 1–3 on weeks 15, 31, 34, 39, and 42 Bleomycin 15 mg/m^2 i.v. on days 1–3 in weeks 15, 31, 34, 39, and 42 Dactinomycin 0.6 mg/m^2 i.v. on days 1–3 in weeks 15, 31, 34, 39, and 42 Doxorubicin 30 mg/m^2 i.v. on days 1–3 in week 20	Goorin AM. *J Clin Oncol* 2003;21: 1574–1580.

(continued)

(continued)

Regimen	Drug dose	References
Soft tissue sarcoma		
AD	Doxorubicin 15 mg/m^2/d CIVI daily on days 1–4 Dacarbazine 250 mg/m^2/d CIVI daily on days 1–4 Repeat cycle every 21 d	Antman K. *J Clin Oncol* 1993;11:1276–1285.
AIM	Doxorubicin 50 mg/m^2 i.v. on day 1 Ifosfamide 5000 mg/m^2 CIVI over 24 h on day 1 immediately following doxorubicin Mesna 600 mg/m^2 i.v. before ifosfamide followed by 2500 mg/m^2 CIVI over 24 h on day 1 Mesna 1250 mg/m^2 i.v. over 12 h starting at the end of the ifosfamide infusion Repeat cycle every 21 d	Le Cesne A. *J Clin Oncol* 2000;18: 2676–2684.
Doxil	Doxil 50 mg/m^2 i.v. on day 1 Repeat cycle every 28 d	Judson I. *Eur J Cancer* 2001;37:870–877.
Doxorubicin	Doxorubicin 75 mg/m^2 i.v. on day 1 Repeat cycle every 21 d	Santoro A. *J Clin Oncol* 1995;13:1537–1545.
Gemcitabine/ docetaxel	Gemcitabine 900 mg/m^2 i.v. on days 1 and 8 Docetaxel 100 mg/m^2 i.v. on day 8 Repeat cycle every 21 d	Hensley ML. *J Clin Oncol* 2002;20: 2824–2831.
Gemcitabine/ docetaxel	Gemcitabine 675 mg/m^2 i.v. on days 1 and 8 Docetaxel 100 mg/m^2 i.v. on day 8 Repeat cycle every 21 d	Leu KM. *J Clin Oncol* 2004;22:1706–1712.
MAID	Mesna 2500 mg/m^2/d CIVI daily on days 1–4 Doxorubicin 15 mg/m^2/d CIVI daily on days 1–4 Ifosfamide 2000 mg/m^2/d CIVI daily on days 1–3 Dacarbazine 250 mg/m^2/d CIVI daily on days 1–4 Repeat cycle every 21 d	Antman K. *J Clin Oncol* 1993;11:1276–1285.
Testicular cancer		
BEP	Cisplatin 20 mg/m^2 i.v. on days 1–5 Bleomycin 30 U i.v. on days 2, 9, and 16 Etoposide 100 mg/m^2 i.v. on days 1–5 Repeat cycle every 3 wk × 4	Peckham MJ. *Br J Cancer* 1983;47: 613–619.

(continued)

Regimen	Drug dose	References
EP	Etoposide 100 mg/m^2/d i.v. on days 1–5 Cisplatin 20 mg/m^2/d i.v. on days 1–5 Repeat cycle every 21 d × 2	Motzer RJ. *J Clin Oncol* 1995;13:2700–2704.
TIP	Paclitaxel 250 mg/m^2 i.v. on day 1 Ifosfamide 1500 mg/m^2 i.v. on days 2–5 Cisplatin 25 mg/m^2 i.v. on days 2–5 Mesna 500 mg/m^2 i.v. before and then 4 h and 8 h after each dose of ifosfamide	Kondagunta GV. *J Clin Oncol* 2005;23:6549–55.
VeIP	Vinblastine 0.11 mg/kg i.v. on days 1 and 2 Ifosfamide 1200 mg/m^2 i.v. on days 1–5 Cisplatin 20 mg/m^2 i.v. on days 1–5 Mesna 400 mg/m^2 i.v. before first ifosfamide dose, then 1200 mg/m^2/d on CIVI days 1–5 Repeat cycle every 21 d	Miller K. *J Clin Oncol* 1997;15:1427–1431.
VIP	Etoposide 75 mg/m^2/d i.v. on days 1–5 Ifosfamide 1200 mg/m^2/d i.v. on days 1–5 Cisplatin 20 mg/m^2/d i.v. on days 1–5 Mesna 400 mg/m^2 i.v. before ifosfamide, then 1200 mg/m^2/d CIVI on days 1–5 Repeat cycle every 21 d	Loehrer PJ. *Ann Intern Med* 1988;109:540–546.

AUC, area under the curve; CIVI, continuous intravenous infusion; ANC, absolute neutrophil count; XRT, radiation therapy.